Clinical Neurology

Clinical Neurology

Editor: Thomas Moran

FOSTER ACADEMICS

www.fosteracademics.com

www.fosteracademics.com

FOSTER ACADEMICS

Cataloging-in-Publication Data

Clinical neurology / edited by Thomas Moran.
p. cm.
Includes bibliographical references and index.
ISBN 978-1-63242-534-8
1. Neurology. 2. Nervous system--Diseases. I. Moran, Thomas.
RC346 .C55 2018
616.8--dc23

Foster Academics,
118-35 Queens Blvd., Suite 400,
Forest Hills, NY 11375, USA

ISBN 978-1-63242-534-8 (Hardback)

Printed and bound in China.

Contents

Preface ... IX

Chapter 1 **Ghrelin Modulates the fMRI BOLD Response of Homeostatic and Hedonic Brain Centers Regulating Energy Balance in the Rat** ... 1
Miklós Sárvári, Pál Kocsis, Levente Deli, Dávid Gajári, Szabolcs Dávid, Zsófia Pozsgay, Nikolett Hegedűs, Károly Tihanyi, Zsolt Liposits

Chapter 2 **Hepatic Branch Vagus Nerve Plays a Critical Role in the Recovery of Post-Ischemic Glucose Intolerance and Mediates a Neuroprotective Effect by Hypothalamic Orexin-A** ... 10
Shinichi Harada, Yui Yamazaki, Shuichi Koda, Shogo Tokuyama

Chapter 3 **Temporary Interference over the Posterior Parietal Cortices Disrupts Thermoregulatory Control in Humans** ... 21
Alberto Gallace, Giovanna Soravia, Zaira Cattaneo, G. Lorimer Moseley, Giuseppe Vallar

Chapter 4 **Behavioral and Histopathological Assessment of Adult Ischemic Rat Brains after Intracerebral Transplantation of NSI-566RSC Cell Lines** ... 29
Naoki Tajiri, David M. Quach, Yuji Kaneko, Stephanie Wu, David Lee, Tina Lam, Ken L. Hayama, Thomas G. Hazel, Karl Johe, Michael C. Wu, Cesar V. Borlongan

Chapter 5 **Cortical and Spinal Mechanisms of Task Failure of Sustained Submaximal Fatiguing Contractions** ... 38
Petra S. Williams, Richard L. Hoffman, Brian C. Clark

Chapter 6 **Medulloblastoma in China: Clinicopathologic Analyses of SHH, WNT, and Non-SHH/WNT Molecular Subgroups Reveal Different Therapeutic Responses to Adjuvant Chemotherapy** ... 60
Zhen-Yu Zhang, Jian Xu, Yong Ren, Yu Yao, Kay Ka-Wai Li, Ho-Keung Ng, Ying Mao, Liang-Fu Zhou, Ping Zhong

Chapter 7 **Anatomical Targets Associated with Abrupt versus Gradual Washout of Subthalamic Deep Brain Stimulation Effects on Bradykinesia** ... 68
Scott E. Cooper, Klaus G. Driesslein, Angela M. Noecker, Cameron C. McIntyre, Andre M. Machado, Christopher R. Butson

Chapter 8 **Pressure Pain Thresholds Increase after Preconditioning 1 Hz Repetitive Transcranial Magnetic Stimulation with Transcranial Direct Current Stimulation** ... 78
Tonya M. Moloney, Alice G. Witney

Chapter 9 **Transplantation of Induced Pluripotent Stem Cells Improves Functional Recovery in Huntington's Disease Rat Model** ... 87
Shuhua Mu, Jiachuan Wang, Guangqian Zhou, Wenda Peng, Zhendan He, Zhenfu Zhao, CuiPing Mo, Junle Qu, Jian Zhang

Chapter 10 **Suppression of Motor Cortical Excitability in Anesthetized Rats by Low Frequency Repetitive Transcranial Magnetic Stimulation** 97
Paul A. Muller, Sameer C. Dhamne, Andrew M. Vahabzadeh-Hagh, Alvaro Pascual-Leone, Frances E. Jensen, Alexander Rotenberg

Chapter 11 **Real-Time Dopamine Measurement in Awake Monkeys** 105
Erik W. Schluter, Andrew R. Mitz, Joseph F. Cheer, Bruno B. Averbeck

Chapter 12 **Mechanical Ventilation for Comatose Patients with Inoperative Acute Intracerebral Hemorrhage: Possible Futility of Treatment** 120
Toru Fukuhara, Mizuho Aoi, Yoichiro Namba

Chapter 13 **Increased Hippocampal Excitability in the 3xTgAD Mouse Model for Alzheimer's Disease *In Vivo*** 128
Katherine E. Davis, Sarah Fox, John Gigg

Chapter 14 **Theta-Burst Stimulation of Hippocampal Slices Induces Network-Level Calcium Oscillations and Activates Analogous Gene Transcription to Spatial Learning** 143
Graham K. Sheridan, Emad Moeendarbary, Mark Pickering, John J. O'Connor, Keith J. Murphy

Chapter 15 **Task-Specific and General Cognitive Effects in Chiari Malformation Type I** 157
Philip A. Allen, James R. Houston, Joshua W. Pollock, Christopher Buzzelli, Xuan Li, A. Katherine Harrington, Bryn A. Martin, Francis Loth, Mei-Ching Lien, Jahangir Maleki, Mark G. Luciano

Chapter 16 **Time and Frequency-Dependent Modulation of Local Field Potential Synchronization by Deep Brain Stimulation** 168
Clinton B. McCracken, Zelma H. T. Kiss

Chapter 17 **Deep Brain Stimulation of the Antero-Medial Globus Pallidus Interna for Tourette Syndrome** 181
Perminder S. Sachdev, Adith Mohan, Elisabeth Cannon, John D. Crawford, Paul Silberstein, Raymond Cook, Terrence Coyne, Peter A. Silburn

Chapter 18 **Interdisciplinary Approaches of Transcranial Magnetic Stimulation Applied to a Respiratory Neuronal Circuitry Model** 189
Stéphane Vinit, Emilie Keomani, Thérèse B. Deramaudt, Victoria M. Spruance, Tatiana Bezdudnaya, Michael A. Lane, Marcel Bonay, Michel Petitjean

Chapter 19 **VGF Changes during the Estrous Cycle: A Novel Endocrine Role for TLQP Peptides?** 200
Barbara Noli, Carla Brancia, Filomena D'Amato, Gian-Luca Ferri, Cristina Cocco

Chapter 20 **Short and Long Term Effects of Left and Bilateral Repetitive Transcranial Magnetic Stimulation in Schizophrenia Patients with Auditory Verbal Hallucinations: A Randomized Controlled Trial** **212**
Leonie Bais, Ans Vercammen, Roy Stewart, Frank van Es, Bert Visser, André Aleman, Henderikus Knegtering

Permissions

List of Contributors

Index

Preface

The main aim of this book is to educate learners and enhance their research focus by presenting diverse topics covering this vast field. This is an advanced book which compiles significant studies by distinguished experts in the area of analysis. This book addresses successive solutions to the challenges arising in the area of application, along with it; the book provides scope for future developments.

There are various disorders found in the nervous system. Clinical neurology deals with the treatment and diagnosis of all the diseases related to the nervous system. Some of the tests done in order to diagnose a neurological disorder are MRI, CAT scans and ultrasounds. The aim of this book is to present researches that have transformed this discipline and aided the advancement in treating neurological disorders. For all readers who are interested in neurology, the case studies included in this book will serve as an excellent guide to develop a comprehensive understanding.

It was a great honour to edit this book, though there were challenges, as it involved a lot of communication and networking between me and the editorial team. However, the end result was this all-inclusive book covering diverse themes in the field.

Finally, it is important to acknowledge the efforts of the contributors for their excellent chapters, through which a wide variety of issues have been addressed. I would also like to thank my colleagues for their valuable feedback during the making of this book.

Editor

Ghrelin Modulates the fMRI BOLD Response of Homeostatic and Hedonic Brain Centers Regulating Energy Balance in the Rat

Miklós Sárvári[1]*[❡], Pál Kocsis[2❡], Levente Deli[2], Dávid Gajári[2], Szabolcs Dávid[2], Zsófia Pozsgay[2], Nikolett Hegedűs[2], Károly Tihanyi[2], Zsolt Liposits[1,3]

1 Laboratory of Endocrine Neurobiology, Institute of Experimental Medicine, Hungarian Academy of Sciences, Budapest, Hungary, **2** Preclinical Imaging Center, Gedeon Richter Ltd., Budapest, Hungary, **3** Faculty of Information Technology, Pázmány Péter Catholic University, Budapest, Hungary

Abstract

The orexigenic gut-brain peptide, ghrelin and its G-protein coupled receptor, the growth hormone secretagogue receptor 1a (GHS-R1A) are pivotal regulators of hypothalamic feeding centers and reward processing neuronal circuits of the brain. These systems operate in a cooperative manner and receive a wide array of neuronal hormone/transmitter messages and metabolic signals. Functional magnetic resonance imaging was employed in the current study to map BOLD responses to ghrelin in different brain regions with special reference on homeostatic and hedonic regulatory centers of energy balance. Experimental groups involved male, ovariectomized female and ovariectomized estradiol-replaced rats. Putative modulation of ghrelin signaling by endocannabinoids was also studied. Ghrelin-evoked effects were calculated as mean of the BOLD responses 30 minutes after administration. In the male rat, ghrelin evoked a slowly decreasing BOLD response in all studied regions of interest (ROI) within the limbic system. This effect was antagonized by pretreatment with GHS-R1A antagonist JMV2959. The comparison of ghrelin effects in the presence or absence of JMV2959 in individual ROIs revealed significant changes in the prefrontal cortex, nucleus accumbens of the telencephalon, and also within hypothalamic centers like the lateral hypothalamus, ventromedial nucleus, paraventricular nucleus and suprachiasmatic nucleus. In the female rat, the ghrelin effects were almost identical to those observed in males. Ovariectomy and chronic estradiol replacement had no effect on the BOLD response. Inhibition of the endocannabinoid signaling by rimonabant significantly attenuated the response of the nucleus accumbens and septum. In summary, ghrelin can modulate hypothalamic and mesolimbic structures controlling energy balance in both sexes. The endocannabinoid signaling system contributes to the manifestation of ghrelin's BOLD effect in a region specific manner. In females, the estradiol *milieu* does not influence the BOLD response to ghrelin.

Editor: Marc Claret, Institut d'Investigacions Biomèdiques August Pi i Sunyer, Spain

Funding: This research was supported by the National Science Foundation of Hungary (OTKA K100722) and the National Development Agency of Hungary (NFU-BONUS-HU08/2-2011-0006). The research leading to these results has received funding from the European Community's Seventh Framework Programme (FP7/2007-2013) under grant agreement No. 245009. The funders had no role in study design, data collection and analysis, decision to publish, or preparation of the manuscript.

Competing Interests: PK, LD, DG, SD, ZP, NH and KT are employed by Gedeon Richter Ltd.

* E-mail: sarvari@koki.hu

❡ These authors contributed equally to this work.

Introduction

The hunger signal ghrelin [1] is a potent orexigenic hormone [2] that acts via its G-protein coupled receptor, GHS-R1A [3] within the central nervous system. The expression of GHS-R1A mRNA shows a discrete albeit wide distribution pattern within the neuroaxis [4,5]. The preganglionic neurons of parasympathetic centers in the brainstem, hypothalamic nuclei with longstanding history of contribution to regulation of feeding and energy expenditure, the hippocampal formation and the dopaminergic mesostriatal and mesolimbic systems arising from the rostral mesencephalon are primary targets of direct, receptor-mediated signaling of ghrelin. The binding of radiolabeled ghrelin to identical, GHS-R1A containing loci proves the expression and functional capacity of the receptor protein [6]. In addition to the stomach [7], which provides the major ghrelin supply for the brain, the production of ghrelin in a discrete set of hypothalamic neurons has also been shown [8]. Ghrelin-immunoreactive axons have been detected in rodent [8,9] and *post-mortem* human [10] brains.

Although ghrelin signaling regulates several systems and modulates a wide array of physiological functions in the organism [11,12], a special attention follows its role in the regulation of feeding and energy expenditure [13–16]. Pioneer works have elucidated that ghrelin targets the orexigenic neuropeptide Y/agouti-related protein-synthesizing neuron population in the medial aspect of the arcuate nucleus [1,8,17] that, in turn, relays the orexigenic signal to other hypothalamic feeding centers including the paraventricular nucleus and the lateral hypothalamus [18]. They can respond to the hunger signal and execute effector commands via the endocrine and autonomic systems. These ghrelin-regulated mechanisms ensure the homeostatic control over feeding and energy expenditure [19]. In more recent years, an intriguing concept has emerged about the explicit role of ghrelin in regulation of the reward system [20–24]. Pharmacological targeting of the laterodorsal tegmentum-ventral tegmental area-mesolimbic system axis by GHS-R1A agonists and/or antagonists has shown the involvement of ghrelin in shaping the hedonic component in the control of energy balance [25]. Ghrelin seems to increase the incentive value of rewarding foods [23,26,27], alcohol [28] and abusing drugs [29,30]. It also triggers the cascades of reward seeking behavior [31]. Antagonizing ghrelin signaling centrally offers a challenging approach in the fight against obesity, substance and eating disorders [28,32,33].

A fascinating finding has been that ghrelin modifies the activity of targeted neurons [8,34] and modulates the incoming information of their synaptic afferents. Molecular events downstream from GHS-R1A have not been fully explored yet. A prevailing role has been attributed to PI3K-Akt [35] and AMPK [36] signaling mechanisms at cellular level. Recent studies have revealed that the sirtuin 1/p53 pathway links GHS-R1A activation and AMPK phosphorylation in the hypothalamus [37]. Besides PI3K-Akt and AMPK, additional mechanisms are involved in ghrelin action including the κ-opioid pathway in the hypothalamus [38]. Furthermore, increasing number of evidence indicates that GHS-R1A activation results in changes of endocannabinoid levels in the target cell that, in turn, modify the synaptic input of neuronal afferents via retrograde signaling [39]. Accordingly, CB1 receptors and intact retrograde endocannabinoid signaling mechanisms have been reported essential in the mediation of the orexigenic action of ghrelin in the paraventricular nucleus of the rat [39], and also in the modulation of firing by ghrelin in gonadotropin-releasing hormone (GnRH) neurons of mice [40]. In addition to the cooperation of ghrelin and endocannabinoid signaling systems, the modulatory role of the gonadal hormone 17β-estradiol (E2) has also been raised. Males and females with low E2 levels show a higher response to ghrelin in terms of food intake and body weight gain compared to females with high E2 levels [41], although a recent study has demonstrated no difference in food intake and the signaling pathway downstream to GHS-R1A in response to ghrelin in the two sexes [42].

In the present study, we focused on mapping BOLD responses evoked by ghrelin in the male and female rat brains and on elucidation of the role of endocannabinoid and E2 signaling in the process with special attention to brain centers controlling energy balance.

Materials and Methods

Ethics Statement

All studies were carried out with permission from the Animal Welfare Committee of the Institute of Experimental Medicine, Hungarian Academy of Sciences (Permission Number: A5769-01) and in accordance with the legal requirements of the European Community (Decree 86/609/EEC). In all studies, animal experimentation was conducted in accord with accepted standards of animal care.

Reagents

Rat ghrelin was obtained from Tocris (Bristol, UK). Rimonabant was synthesized by the Synthetic Laboratory of Gedeon Richter Plc (Budapest, Hungary). GHS-R1A antagonist JMV2959 was a kind gift from Aeterna Zentaris GmbH (Frankfurt, Germany).

Animals

Male (n = 20) and female (n = 24) Wistar rats, weighing 240–260 and 170–190 g, respectively, were purchased from Harlan. Rats were housed in light (12:12 light-dark cycle, lights on at 6am) and temperature (21±1°C) controlled environment, with free access to standard food (sniff R/M+H Spezieldiäten GmbH D-59494 Soest) and tap water. The females were surgically ovariectomized (OVX) and half of them were replaced with E2 (OVX+E2) for 10 days as described elsewhere [43]. The average weight of OVX controls (n = 12) and E2 replaced animals (n = 11) was 219.2 g and 207.6 g, respectively. The weight of OVX controls was significantly larger ($p = 0.031$).

MRI Experiments

Functional MRI experiments were performed on a 9.4T ASZ Varian MRI system with a free bore of 210 mm, containing a 120 mm inner size gradient coil (180 µs rise time). For excitation, an actively RF-decoupled 2 channel volume coil system with inner size 72 mm was used and a fix tuned receive-only phase array rat brain coil located directly above the dorsal surface of the animal's head to maximize the signal to noise ratio.

Scout pictures were obtained in planes of coronal and sagittal in order to set the anatomical and functional images. Anatomical scans were acquired using gradient echo multi slice (GEMS) sequence with a field of view, FOV 35×35 mm, slice thickness 1 mm, gap 0.2 mm. Nine slices were received in interleaved order; the scanner's default coronal orientation was slightly changed to get a standard anatomically coronal plane according to the Rat Brain Atlas of Paxinos & Watson [44]. Echo time, TE = 3.83 ms, repetition time, TR = 200 ms, flip angle 45°, averages 3, dummy scans 4, data matrix 192×192, total scan time 2 min.

An interleaved triple-shot gradient-echo echo planar imaging, EPI sequence with compressed segments was used for T2*-weighted MR images. TE = 10 ms, TR = 3000 ms, flip angle 90°, averages 1, dummy scans 4, data matrix 64×64, 1000 repetitions. FOV and slice parameters were the same as in the anatomical setup.

Rats were anaesthetized with isoflurane (5% starting concentration and then 1–1.5% during scanning) administered in compressed air. For intravenous drug administration, a cannula line was inserted and used during the scanning. The anesthetized rat was transferred into the magnet. Body temperature was monitored using a rectal probe and maintained at 37 ± 1°C via a thermostatically controlled air, flowed around the rat. The ventilation was also controlled.

Experiments lasted for 50 min. After 16 min 40 sec (1000 sec) baseline period 20 µg ghrelin was administered i.v. The automated drug administration was performed with an infusion pump controlled by optical signals. GHS-R1 antagonist JMV2959 (6 mg/kg) and rimonabant (3 mg/kg) or were applied i.p. to conscious animals as a pretreatment one hour prior to ghrelin administration. One measurement was performed with each animal. The results of each measurement were stored in the scanner's own file format which were converted to the widely used nifti-format (Neuroimaging Informatics Technology Initiative) using a Matlab script. More detailed technical information about the MRI has been published earlier [45].

Data Analysis

Data analysis was performed as described previously [45]. In brief, displacement was checked and measurements with higher than one voxel movement were excluded. For creating t-maps in the phMRI experiments, paired t-test was performed on each voxel's two time intervals (pre-injection baseline and post-

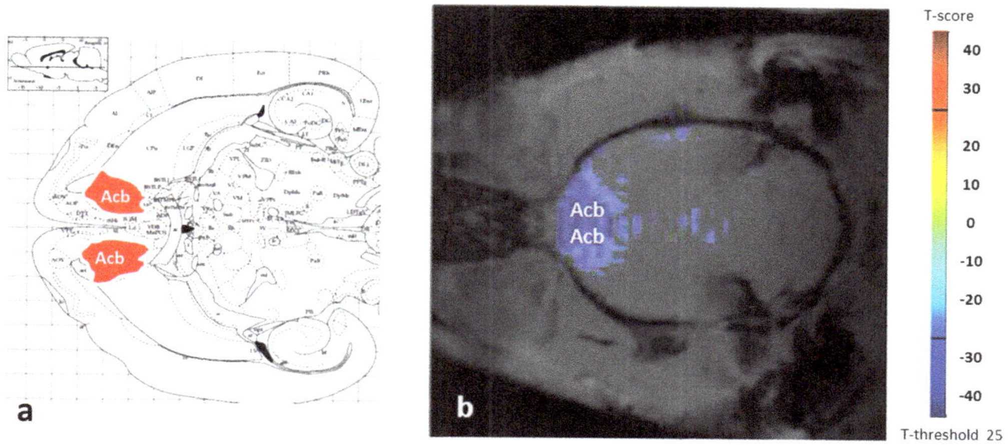

Figure 1. Characteristic fMRI BOLD response to ghrelin in the nucleus accumbens. a. Position of the nucleus accumbens (highlighted in red) is shown in a horizontal scheme of the rat brain [44]. **b.** Ghrelin evoked a negative BOLD response in the nucleus accumbens. Slice thickness is 1 mm.

injection) to evaluate the difference between the baseline signal and post-injection signal. A t-value was ordered to every voxels and voxels over the t value limit were highlighted. Region of interest (ROI) analysis was performed using a Matlab script. ROIs were determined according to the Rat Brain Atlas of Paxinos & Watson [44]. Statistical significance of drug effect was evaluated by multifactorial ANOVA followed by *post-hoc* Fisher test.

List of ROIs and Their Abbreviations

We analyzed the following areas: amygdala (Amyg), arcuate nucleus (ARC), cerebellum (cb), dorsomedial nucleus (DMH), hippocampus (Hipp), lateral hypothalamus (LH), lateral parabrachial nucleus (LPB), laterodorsal tegmental nucleus (LDTg), nucleus accumbens (Acb), nucleus tractus solitarii (Sol), paraventricular nucleus (PVN), parietal associative cortex (PAC), prefrontal cortex (PFC), septum (Sept), striatum (Str), substantia nigra (SN), suprachiasmatic nucleus (SCN), temporal cortex (TC), ventral tegmental area (VTA), ventromedial nucleus (VMH).

Results

BOLD Response to Ghrelin in Homeostatic and Hedonic Brain Centers Regulating Energy Balance in the Male Rat

In the first line of the experiment, the effect of ghrelin (20 µg, i.v.) was tested in either saline or GHS-R1A antagonist JMV2959 (6 mg/kg, i.p.) pretreated male rats. The applied dose of ghrelin corresponds to 25 nM/kg, which induces a marked stimulatory effect in plasma GH levels [46]. ROIs were divided into three groups, each containing well-defined nuclei and anatomical areas as follows: Group I. Reward processing neuronal assembly including the ventral tegmental area, nucleus accumbens, the prefrontal cortex, amygdala, septum and hippocampus. Representative fMRI image showing the nucleus accumbens was presented (Fig. 1). The temporal cortex and associative parietal cortex were included as controls. Group II. Homeostatic feeding centers of the hypothalamus were represented by the arcuate nucleus, ventromedial nucleus, dorsomedial nucleus, paraventricular nucleus, lateral hypothalamus and the circadian rhythm generator suprachiasmatic nucleus. Group III. Brainstem areas regulating hedonic and homeostatic mechanisms of energy balance included the laterodorsal tegmental nucleus, lateral parabrachial nucleus, nucleus tractus solitarii. In addition, we analyzed the main components of the nigrostriatal projection, the substantia nigra and the striatum, and also the 9–10th lobules of cerebellum.

We found a widespread regional response to ghrelin in hedonic and homeostatic centers. The evoked BOLD responses differed from each other in the saline and JMV2959 pretreated groups (Fig. 2). In general, ghrelin decreased the BOLD response in several loci of the neuroaxis, while JMV2959 pretreatment attenuated this effect (Fig. 3). In Group I, the prefrontal cortex (Fig. 2A) and the nucleus accumbens (Fig. 2B) showed the highest response to ghrelin, and also a powerful and significant counteracting effect of JMV2959. Moderate effects of ghrelin were observed in the ventral tegmental area, the hippocampus, septum and the amygdala (Fig. 3). In these loci, the BOLD response was not significant. In Group II, representing the main hypothalamic feeding centers and their modulator systems, ghrelin was also potent in decreasing the BOLD response. Among these structures, the ventromedial nucleus (Fig. 2C), the lateral hypothalamus (Fig. 2D), the paraventricular nucleus (Fig. 2E) and the suprachiasmatic nucleus (Fig. 2F) demonstrated significant BOLD responses. The primary feeding center of the hypothalamus, the arcuate nucleus also displayed a marked response to ghrelin which was attenuated with the antagonist pretreatment (Fig. 3). In Group III, the laterodorsal tegmental nucleus, the lateral parabrachial nucleus, the nucleus tractus solitarii showed weak, non-significant BOLD responses (Fig. 3). A similar activation pattern characterized the additionally examined regions like the striatum, the parietal, temporal cortices and the cerebellar cortex (Fig. 3).

Role of Sex and Estradiol in the Ghrelin-Evoked BOLD Response

In addition to the male, fMRI studies have also been carried out in chronically ovariectomized (OVX) and ovariectomized E2 replaced (OVX+E2) female rats in order to reveal the putative role of sex and the actual E2 *milieu* in the generation of the BOLD response evoked by ghrelin. The examined sets of ROIs were similar to those used in the male rat experiment. Ghrelin resulted in a decrease of the BOLD response in all ROIs both in the OVX ($n = 7$) and OVX+E2 ($n = 7$) groups. The characteristics of the response (slope, duration, maximal effect) were almost identical in

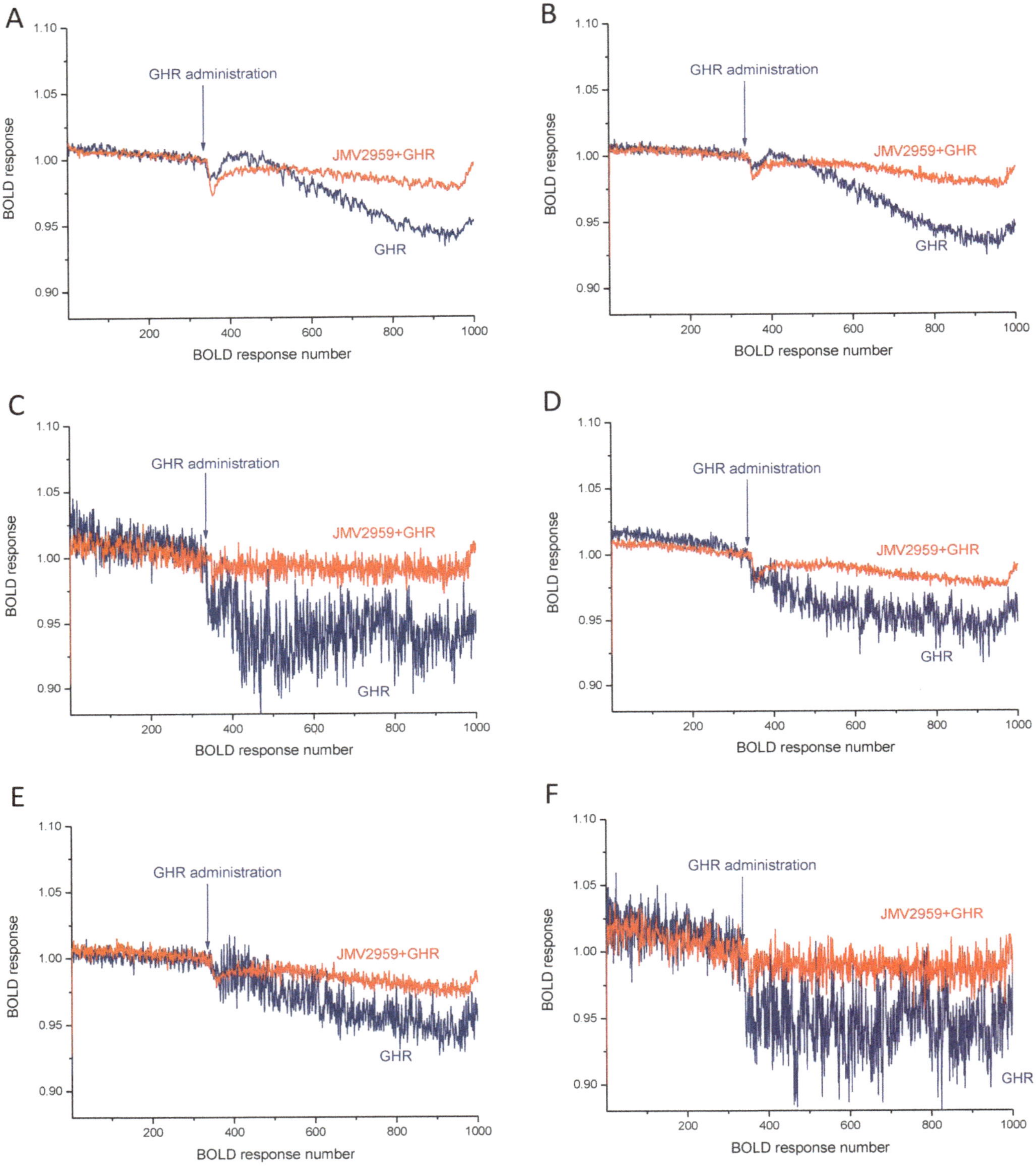

Figure 2. Mean of time response curves of ghrelin's effect on BOLD responses in the prefrontal cortex (A), nucleus accumbens (B), ventromedial nucleus (C), lateral hypothalamus (D), paraventricular nucleus (E) and suprachiasmatic nucleus (F). Blue and red colors indicate pretreatment with saline and GHS-R1A antagonist (JMV2959), respectively. Arrows mark ghrelin (GHR) administration, which started at BOLD response number 333 and lasted to 383 (999–1149 s). For quantifying drug effect, mean of the BOLD responses from 901 to 950 was calculated (2703–2850 s). N = 5–7.

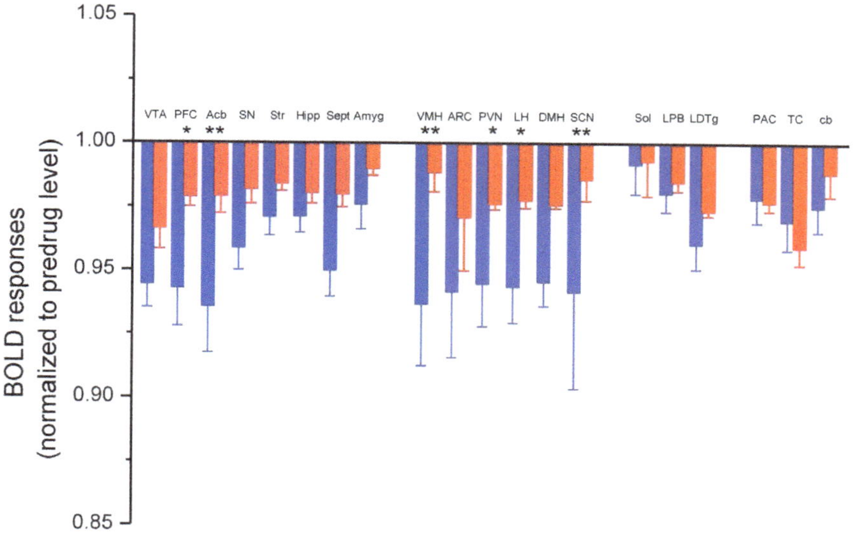

Figure 3. Effect of ghrelin on BOLD responses in reward processing centers, hypothalamic nuclei, brainstem and control areas of the rat brain. The effect of ghrelin after vehicle pretreatment is represented by blue columns and after JMV2959 pretreatment in red columns. Statistically significant differences were found in the prefrontal cortex (PFC), nucleus accumbens (Acb), lateral hypothalamus (LH), paraventricular nucleus (PVN), ventromedial nucleus (VMH) and suprachiasmatic nucleus (SCN). ANOVA and Fisher *post hoc* test *: $p<0.05$; **: $p<0.01$. N = 5–7.

males and females as exemplified in the prefrontal cortex (Fig. 4A), nucleus accumbens (Fig. 4B), ventromedial nucleus (Fig. 4C) and the paraventricular nucleus (Fig. 4D). Seemingly, neither sex nor E2 replacement in OVX females had impact on the ghrelin-evoked BOLD responses in hedonic and homeostatic centers of energy balance.

Effect of Rimonabant on the BOLD Response to Ghrelin

The effect of CB1 receptor antagonist rimonabant (3 mg/kg, i.p.) was tested on the ghrelin response in the third experimental line of the study. The effect of rimonabant was evaluated in various areas by comparing BOLD responses to ghrelin in vehicle (n = 5–7) and rimonabant (n = 7) pretreated animals. Rimonabant highly and significantly attenuated the response to ghrelin in the nucleus accumbens (Fig. 5A) and septum (Fig. 5B). In other ROIs, rimonabant pretreatment did not interfere with the ghrelin-evoked BOLD response in a statistically significant manner (Fig. 6).

Discussion

In this study, we explored the BOLD effects of peripherally administered ghrelin in hedonic and homeostatic centers regulating energy balance in the rat using fMRI. Ghrelin administered to the periphery can act on the brain directly [22,47], or indirectly via vagal afferent [48]. We found a significant BOLD decrease in response to ghrelin in homeostatic feeding centers of the hypothalamus including the ventromedial nucleus, the paraventricular nucleus and the lateral hypothalamic area by comparing the saline and GHS-R1A antagonist pretreated animal groups. Similar significant responses were measured in reward signal processing structures of the telencephalon like the prefrontal cortex, the nucleus accumbens and the septum. These findings are in agreement with recent fMRI studies demonstrating ghrelin-evoked modulation of the brain reinforcement system [49] and key appetite regulatory regions of the hypothalamus [50] in rodents. In addition to the male, we also followed the BOLD response to ghrelin in females, using low (ovariectomized) and high (ovariectomized-E2 replaced) experimental E2 paradigms. The results do not support any sex difference in the ghrelin-evoked BOLD responses or the regulation of the response by the female gonadal hormone, E2. We note that in the male-female comparison we used OVX females with/without E2 replacement and compared them to intact males. For revealing the putative contribution of the endocannabinoid signaling mechanism to the ghrelin-evoked BOLD response, we also examined the effects of ghrelin administration in CB1 receptor blocked male rats and found interaction between the two signaling systems in telencephalic structures. From the results we conclude that i) ghrelin regulates components of the classic mesolimbic reward system, especially the prefrontal cortex, the nucleus accumbens and the septum; ii) ghrelin acts in key hypothalamic feeding centers, the ventromedial nucleus, the paraventricular nucleus and the lateral hypothalamic area; iii) the pattern of BOLD response to ghrelin resembles partly the published expression loci of GHS-R1A mRNA; iv) the effect of ghrelin on BOLD response depends on CB1 signaling in the nucleus accumbens and the septum; and v) ghrelin-evoked BOLD response is independent of sex and the actual E2 *milieu*.

Ghrelin Modulates the BOLD Response of Reward Signal Processing Systems

The ventral tegmental area is a key center in reward processing [51]. It contains the A10 dopaminergic cell group [52] that gives rise to ascending mesocortical and mesolimbic projections that innervate the prefrontal cortex and the nucleus accumbens, respectively [53]. GHS-R1A mRNA has been detected within A10 dopaminergic neurons and cholecystokinin-immunoreactive neurons of the VTA [4]. Ghrelin regulates dopaminergic neurons in the VTA [54]. Via modulation of the mesolimbic dopaminergic system, ghrelin is capable of increasing food intake [14,21,23], modulating hedonic reward value of food, alcohol and addictive chemical substances [22], regulating hyperlocomotion caused by psychostimulant drugs [29,55] and increasing effectiveness of learning and memory [56–58]. Our present findings are in concert with these physiological data by demonstrating that peripheral ghrelin administration causes marked alterations of the BOLD

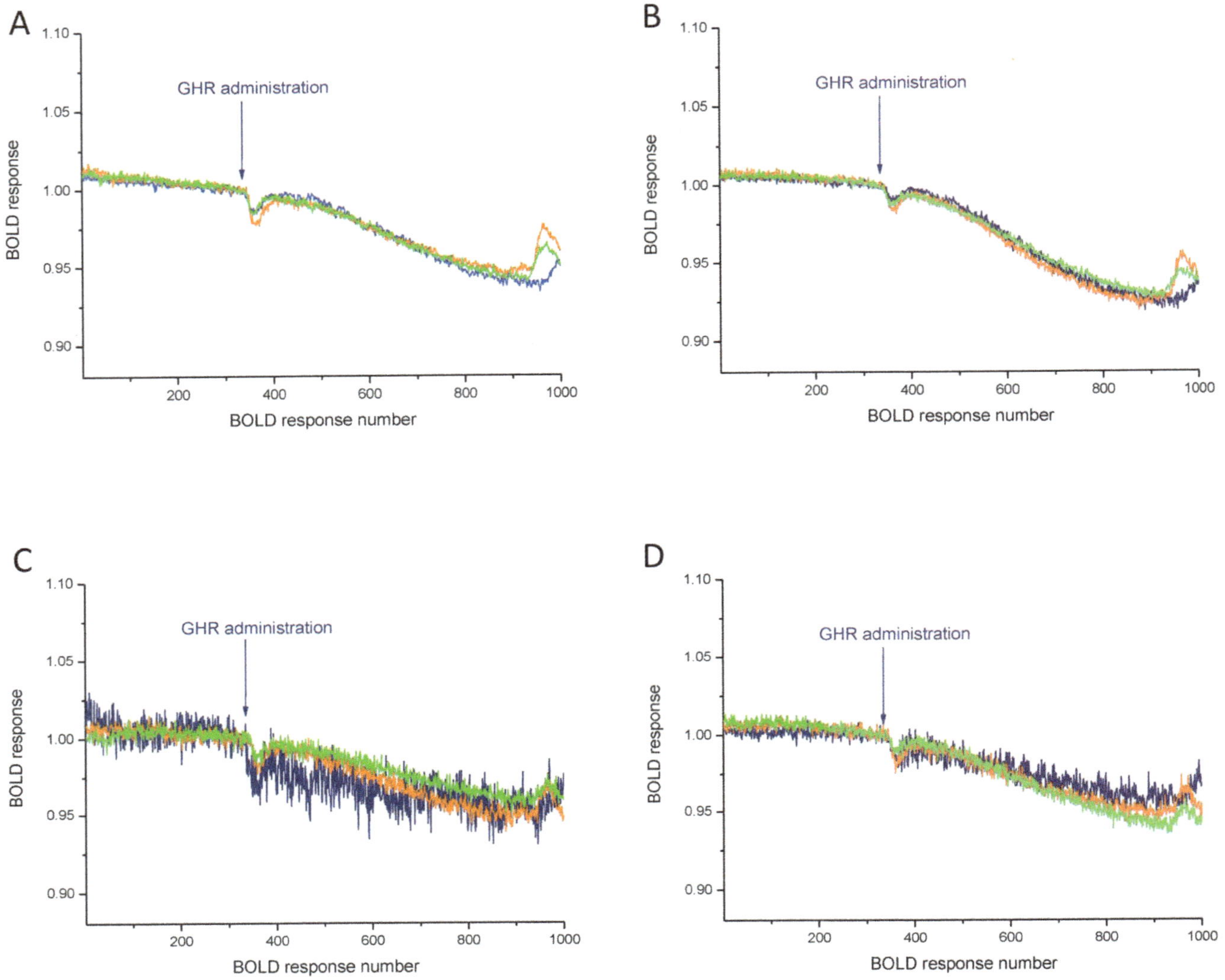

Figure 4. Mean of time response curves of ghrelin's effect on the BOLD responses in the prefrontal cortex (A), nucleus accumbens (B), ventromedial nucleus (C) and paraventricular nucleus (D), in males (blue), ovariectomized females (orange) and ovariectomized females treated with E2 (green). Arrows mark ghrelin administration, which started at BOLD response 333 and lasted to 383 (999–1149 s). For quantifying drug effect mean of the BOLD responses from 901 to 950 was calculated (2703–2850 s). N = 11–14.

response in different structural constituents of the mesolimbic and mesocortical systems. Most notably, it modifies the BOLD response of the nucleus accumbens and prefrontal cortex in a significant manner. The effectiveness of JVM2959 treatment strengthens the view that the manifestation of the ghrelin-evoked BOLD response requires the contribution of GHS-R1A. The facilitative role of GHS-R1A in the regulation of the brain reinforcement system has recently been proposed in the rat based on pharmacological MRI analysis and intracranial self-stimulation [49]. Ghrelin increased the cerebral blood volume (rCBV) in medial and lateral hypothalamic structures and also in mesolimbic reward units, the ventral tegmental area, the nucleus accumbens and septum. The responsiveness of hypothalamic feeding nuclei to ghrelin has also been published in mice using manganase-enhanced MRI [50].

Ghrelin Changes the BOLD Response of Homeostatic Feeding Centers in the Hypothalamus

GHS-R1A is extensively expressed in the rodent hypothalamus [3–5,59,60]. In concert with the distribution pattern of GHS-R1 mRNA expression, we report matching BOLD response from the ventromedial nucleus, the paraventricular nucleus and the lateral hypothalamus. The evoked BOLD effects were attenuated by JMV2959. The arcuate nucleus did also respond to ghrelin, but the effect did not reach statistical significance. The orexigenic effects of ghrelin involve and require AMPK signaling in both the VMH [61] and the PVN [39,62]. In the lateral hypothalamic area, ghrelin evokes Fos immunoreactivity in orexin neurons [63] and also inhibits their electrophysiological activity [9]. Binding of iodinated ghrelin ligand has been reported [6] in all feeding centers of the hypothalamus that showed BOLD response to ghrelin challenge in our study.

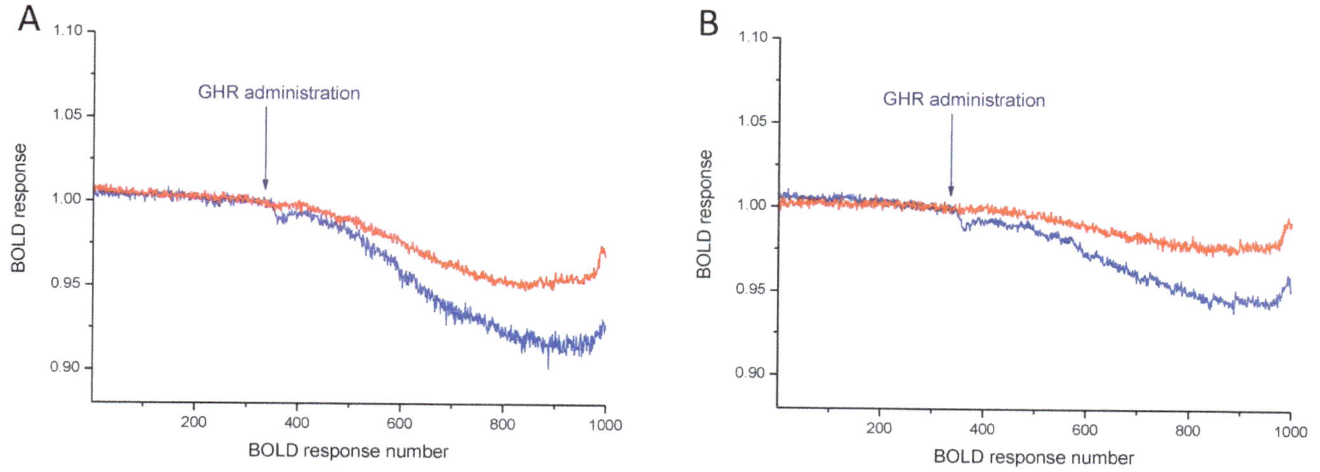

Figure 5. Mean of time response curves of ghrelin's effect on BOLD responses in the nucleus accumbens (A) and septum (B) after vehiculum (blue) or rimonabant pretreatment (red). Arrows mark ghrelin administration, which started at BOLD response 333 and lasted to 383 (999–1149 s). For quantifying drug effect, mean of the BOLD responses from 901 to 950 was calculated (2703–2850 s). N = 5–7.

Pharmacological Blocking of CB1 Signaling Attenuates the Ghrelin-Evoked BOLD Response

Both ghrelin and endocannabinoids regulate energy balance [64,65]. The ghrelin and endocannabinoid signaling mechanisms are interrelated in the hypothalamus. Blocking CB1 receptor by specific antagonists abolishes the orexigenic effect of ghrelin [66]. Ghrelin is also incapable of triggering orexigenic effects in CB1-knockout mice [39]. Activation of GHS-R has been shown to increase the endocannabinoid content of the hypothalamus [39]. Ghrelin inhibits the excitatory inputs to parvocellular paraventricular neurons [39] and gonadotropin-releasing hormone (GnRH) neurons [40] via the cooperation with the endocannabinoid-CB1 system. While the individual regulatory capacity of both the endocannabinoid and ghrelin systems has been confirmed in other parts of the brain as well [67–69], the coupled nature of these signaling mechanisms awaits further studies and clarification. In our fMRI study, the pharmacological inhibition of CB1 by rimonabant abolished the BOLD response to ghrelin in the nucleus accumbens and the septum. This result is in concert with the finding that 2-arachidonoylglycerol signaling through CB1 regulates the activity of forebrain neural circuits that control energy expenditure [70]. The BOLD response of the hippocampus to ghrelin was only partially attenuated by rimonabant. In individual hypothalamic nuclei, the blockade of CB1 receptor did not counteract the BOLD effects of ghrelin. Seemingly, this finding is in conflict with physiological data exploring the coupled nature of ghrelin and endocannabinoid signaling mechanisms. It needs further studies, although, it is also possible that the current resolution power of the used fMRI technology does not allow the

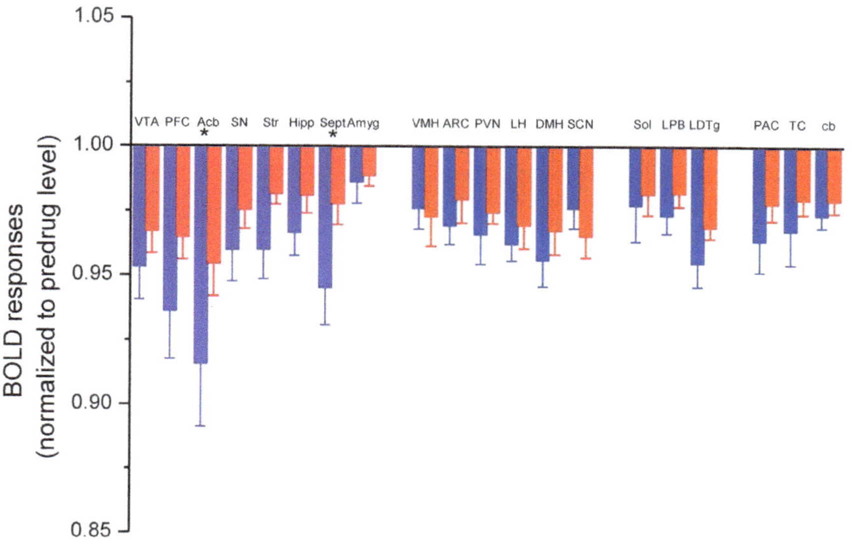

Figure 6. Effect of ghrelin on BOLD responses in reward processing centers, hypothalamic nuclei and brainstem areas. Effect of ghrelin on the BOLD responses was represented by the blue columns after vehicle pretreatment, and red columns after rimonabant pretreatment. Statistically significant differences were found in the nucleus accumbens and septum. ANOVA and Fisher *post hoc* test. *: $p < 0.05$. N = 5–7.

imaging of this particular molecular interaction in small-sized hypothalamic nuclei.

Correlating Human and Rodent fMRI Data about the Central Effects of Ghrelin

The current data and the previously reported fMRI results [49,50] on actions of ghrelin in the CNS are in consensus and suggest that ghrelin exerts the most potent effects on the mesolimbic reward system (VTA, Acb, PFC, Sept) and hypothalamic centers engaged to regulation of feeding and energy expenditure (ARC, VMH, PVN, LH, SCN). Therefore, in rodents, fMRI offers a unique and powerful tool for the exploration of neuronal centers serving the hedonic and homeostatic components of feeding under the challenge of orexigenic and anorexigenic hormones. In humans, ghrelin was reported to modulate the activity of brain regions involved in the control of appetitive behavior [71]. BOLD changes characterized visual information processing centers (occipital gyrus, fusiform gyrus), the insula, as the main gustatory center and limbic structures (substantia nigra, striatum, orbitofrontal cortex, amygdala, caudate and hippocampus) involved in appetite behavior. Fasting levels of ghrelin also correlate with the brain response to pictures of palatable food, with activation of visual, gustatory, limbic reward and hypothalamic centers [72]. A bolus injection of ghrelin in the postprandial period decreases the BOLD response of several brain regions known to control appetite and feeding in humans and it inhibits the response of the CNS to ingested lipid [73]. In the latter study, the response remained essentially unchanged after entering the covariates of body mass index and sex. Our study, also favors the lack of sex specificity of ghrelin action in the rodent brain.

In summary, the present study revealed that ghrelin evokes a marked response in the rodent brain and modulates both the hedonic and homeostatic components of feeding regulating neuronal assemblies. The generated response is not sex specific and the manifestation of ghrelin's effect depends on endocannabinoid signaling in main reward signal processing centers. Furthermore, at the level of CNS, the responses to ghrelin are remarkably similar in humans and rats.

Acknowledgments

We thank Hajni Bekó for her excellent technical support. The authors are indebted to AEterna Zentaris GmbH, Frankfurt, Germany, for the kind donation of JMV2959.

Author Contributions

Conceived and designed the experiments: MS ZL. Performed the experiments: MS PK LD DG. Analyzed the data: PK LD DG SD ZP NH KT. Wrote the paper: ZL MS PK.

References

1. Kojima M, Hosoda H, Date Y, Nakazato M, Matsuo H, et al. (1999) Ghrelin is a growth-hormone-releasing acylated peptide from stomach. Nature 402: 656–660.
2. van der Lely AJ, Tschop M, Heiman ML, Ghigo E (2004) Biological, physiological, pathophysiological, and pharmacological aspects of ghrelin. Endocr Rev 25: 426–457.
3. Howard AD, Feighner SD, Cully DF, Arena JP, Liberator PA, et al. (1996) A receptor in pituitary and hypothalamus that functions in growth hormone release. Science 273: 974–977.
4. Zigman JM, Jones JE, Lee CE, Saper CB, Elmquist JK (2006) Expression of ghrelin receptor mRNA in the rat and the mouse brain. J Comp Neurol 494: 528–548.
5. Mitchell V, Bouret S, Beauvillain JC, Schilling A, Perret M, et al. (2001) Comparative distribution of mRNA encoding the growth hormone secretagogue-receptor (GHS-R) in Microcebus murinus (Primate, lemurian) and rat forebrain and pituitary. J Comp Neurol 429: 469–489.
6. Harrold JA, Dovey T, Cai XJ, Halford JC, Pinkney J (2008) Autoradiographic analysis of ghrelin receptors in the rat hypothalamus. Brain Res 1196: 59–64.
7. Kojima M, Kangawa K (2002) Ghrelin, an orexigenic signaling molecule from the gastrointestinal tract. Curr Opin Pharmacol 2: 665–668.
8. Cowley MA, Smith RG, Diano S, Tschop M, Pronchuk N, et al. (2003) The distribution and mechanism of action of ghrelin in the CNS demonstrates a novel hypothalamic circuit regulating energy homeostasis. Neuron 37: 649–661.
9. Horvath TL, Abizaid A, Dietrich MO, Li Y, Takahashi JS, et al. (2012) Ghrelin-immunopositive hypothalamic neurons tie the circadian clock and visual system to the lateral hypothalamic arousal center. Mol Metab 1: 79–85.
10. Menyhert J, Wittmann G, Hrabovszky E, Szlavik N, Keller E, et al. (2006) Distribution of ghrelin-immunoreactive neuronal networks in the human hypothalamus. Brain Res 1125: 31–36.
11. Kojima M, Kangawa K (2005) Ghrelin: structure and function. Physiol Rev 85: 495–522.
12. Kojima M, Kangawa K (2013) Ghrelin discovery: a decade after. Endocr Dev 25: 1–4.
13. Nakazato M, Murakami N, Date Y, Kojima M, Matsuo H, et al. (2001) A role for ghrelin in the central regulation of feeding. Nature 409: 194–198.
14. Tschop M, Smiley DL, Heiman ML (2000) Ghrelin induces adiposity in rodents. Nature 407: 908–913.
15. Shuto Y, Shibasaki T, Otagiri A, Kuriyama H, Ohata H, et al. (2002) Hypothalamic growth hormone secretagogue receptor regulates growth hormone secretion, feeding, and adiposity. J Clin Invest 109: 1429–1436.
16. Zigman JM, Nakano Y, Coppari R, Balthasar N, Marcus JN, et al. (2005) Mice lacking ghrelin receptors resist the development of diet-induced obesity. J Clin Invest 115: 3564–3572.
17. Willesen MG, Kristensen P, Romer J (1999) Co-localization of growth hormone secretagogue receptor and NPY mRNA in the arcuate nucleus of the rat. Neuroendocrinology 70: 306–316.
18. Zeltser LM, Seeley RJ, Tschop MH (2012) Synaptic plasticity in neuronal circuits regulating energy balance. Nat Neurosci 15: 1336–1342.
19. Castaneda TR, Tong J, Datta R, Culler M, Tschop MH (2010) Ghrelin in the regulation of body weight and metabolism. Front Neuroendocrinol 31: 44–60.
20. Cummings DE, Naleid AM, Figlewicz Lattemann DP (2007) Ghrelin: a link between energy homeostasis and drug abuse? Addict Biol 12: 1–5.
21. Naleid AM, Grace MK, Cummings DE, Levine AS (2005) Ghrelin induces feeding in the mesolimbic reward pathway between the ventral tegmental area and the nucleus accumbens. Peptides 26: 2274–2279.
22. Dickson SL, Egecioglu E, Landgren S, Skibicka KP, Engel JA, et al. (2011) The role of the central ghrelin system in reward from food and chemical drugs. Mol Cell Endocrinol 340: 80–87.
23. Egecioglu E, Jerlhag E, Salome N, Skibicka KP, Haage D, et al. (2010) Ghrelin increases intake of rewarding food in rodents. Addict Biol 15: 304–311.
24. Jerlhag E, Egecioglu E, Dickson SL, Andersson M, Svensson L, et al. (2006) Ghrelin stimulates locomotor activity and accumbal dopamine-overflow via central cholinergic systems in mice: implications for its involvement in brain reward. Addict Biol 11: 45–54.
25. Menzies JR, Skibicka KP, Leng G, Dickson SL (2013) Ghrelin, reward and motivation. Endocr Dev 25: 101–111.
26. Perello M, Sakata I, Birnbaum S, Chuang JC, Osborne-Lawrence S, et al. (2010) Ghrelin increases the rewarding value of high-fat diet in an orexin-dependent manner. Biol Psychiatry 67: 880–886.
27. Skibicka KP, Hansson C, Egecioglu E, Dickson SL (2012) Role of ghrelin in food reward: impact of ghrelin on sucrose self-administration and mesolimbic dopamine and acetylcholine receptor gene expression. Addict Biol 17: 95–107.
28. Jerlhag E, Egecioglu E, Landgren S, Salome N, Heilig M, et al. (2009) Requirement of central ghrelin signaling for alcohol reward. Proc Natl Acad Sci U S A 106: 11318–11323.
29. Jerlhag E, Egecioglu E, Dickson SL, Engel JA (2010) Ghrelin receptor antagonism attenuates cocaine- and amphetamine-induced locomotor stimulation, accumbal dopamine release, and conditioned place preference. Psychopharmacology (Berl) 211: 415–422.
30. Vengeliene V (2013) The role of ghrelin in drug and natural reward. Addict Biol 18: 897–900.
31. Hansson C, Shirazi RH, Naslund J, Vogel H, Neuber C, et al. (2012) Ghrelin influences novelty seeking behavior in rodents and men. PLoS One 7: e50409.
32. Cardona Cano S, Merkestein M, Skibicka KP, Dickson SL, Adan RA (2012) Role of ghrelin in the pathophysiology of eating disorders: implications for pharmacotherapy. CNS Drugs 26: 281–296.
33. Helmling S, Jarosch F, Klussmann S (2006) The promise of ghrelin antagonism in obesity treatment. Drug News Perspect 19: 13–20.
34. Cowley MA (2003) Hypothalamic melanocortin neurons integrate signals of energy state. Eur J Pharmacol 480: 3–11.
35. Kanoski SE, Fortin SM, Ricks KM, Grill HJ (2013) Ghrelin signaling in the ventral hippocampus stimulates learned and motivational aspects of feeding via PI3K-Akt signaling. Biol Psychiatry 73: 915–923.

36. Kola B, Boscaro M, Rutter GA, Grossman AB, Korbonits M (2006) Expanding role of AMPK in endocrinology. Trends Endocrinol Metab 17: 205–215.
37. Velasquez DA, Martinez G, Romero A, Vazquez MJ, Boit KD, et al. (2011) The central Sirtuin 1/p53 pathway is essential for the orexigenic action of ghrelin. Diabetes 60: 1177–1185.
38. Romero-Pico A, Vazquez MJ, Gonzalez-Touceda D, Folgueira C, Skibicka KP, et al. (2013) Hypothalamic kappa-opioid receptor modulates the orexigenic effect of ghrelin. Neuropsychopharmacology 38: 1296–1307.
39. Kola B, Farkas I, Christ-Crain M, Wittmann G, Lolli F, et al. (2008) The orexigenic effect of ghrelin is mediated through central activation of the endogenous cannabinoid system. PLoS One 3: e1797.
40. Farkas I, Vastagh C, Sarvari M, Liposits Z (2013) Ghrelin decreases firing activity of gonadotropin-releasing hormone (GnRH) neurons in an estrous cycle and endocannabinoid signaling dependent manner. PLoS One 8: e78178.
41. Clegg DJ, Brown LM, Zigman JM, Kemp CJ, Strader AD, et al. (2007) Estradiol-dependent decrease in the orexigenic potency of ghrelin in female rats. Diabetes 56: 1051–1058.
42. Lage R, Vazquez MJ, Varela L, Saha AK, Vidal-Puig A, et al. (2010) Ghrelin effects on neuropeptides in the rat hypothalamus depend on fatty acid metabolism actions on BSX but not on gender. FASEB J 24: 2670–2679.
43. Sarvari M, Hrabovszky E, Kallo I, Solymosi N, Toth K, et al. (2011) Estrogens regulate neuroinflammatory genes via estrogen receptors alpha and beta in the frontal cortex of middle-aged female rats. J Neuroinflammation 8: 82.
44. Watson GPaC (1998) The rat brain in stereotaxic coordinates: Academic Press.
45. Kocsis P, Gajari D, Deli L, Gocze KZ, Pozsgay Z, et al. (2013) Effect of tolperisone on the resting brain and on evoked responses, an phMRI BOLD study. Brain Res Bull 99: 34–40.
46. Seoane LM, Tovar S, Baldelli R, Arvat E, Ghigo E, et al. (2000) Ghrelin elicits a marked stimulatory effect on GH secretion in freely-moving rats. Eur J Endocrinol 143: R7–9.
47. Banks WA, Tschop M, Robinson SM, Heiman ML (2002) Extent and direction of ghrelin transport across the blood-brain barrier is determined by its unique primary structure. J Pharmacol Exp Ther 302: 822–827.
48. Date Y, Toshinai K, Koda S, Miyazato M, Shimbara T, et al. (2005) Peripheral interaction of ghrelin with cholecystokinin on feeding regulation. Endocrinology 146: 3518–3525.
49. Wellman PJ, Clifford PS, Rodriguez JA, Hughes S, Di Francesco C, et al. (2012) Brain reinforcement system function is ghrelin dependent: studies in the rat using pharmacological fMRI and intracranial self-stimulation. Addict Biol 17: 908–919.
50. Kuo YT, Parkinson JR, Chaudhri OB, Herlihy AH, So PW, et al. (2007) The temporal sequence of gut peptide CNS interactions tracked in vivo by magnetic resonance imaging. J Neurosci 27: 12341–12348.
51. Tzschentke TM, Schmidt WJ (2000) Functional relationship among medial prefrontal cortex, nucleus accumbens, and ventral tegmental area in locomotion and reward. Crit Rev Neurobiol 14: 131–142.
52. Oades RD, Halliday GM (1987) Ventral tegmental (A10) system: neurobiology. 1. Anatomy and connectivity. Brain Res 434: 117–165.
53. Dahlstroem A, Fuxe K, Olson L, Ungerstedt U (1964) Ascending Systems of Catecholamine Neurons from the Lower Brain Stem. Acta Physiol Scand 62: 485–486.
54. Abizaid A, Liu ZW, Andrews ZB, Shanabrough M, Borok E, et al. (2006) Ghrelin modulates the activity and synaptic input organization of midbrain dopamine neurons while promoting appetite. J Clin Invest 116: 3229–3239.
55. Wellman PJ, Hollas CN, Elliott AE (2008) Systemic ghrelin sensitizes cocaine-induced hyperlocomotion in rats. Regul Pept 146: 33–37.
56. Carlini VP, Monzon ME, Varas MM, Cragnolini AB, Schioth HB, et al. (2002) Ghrelin increases anxiety-like behavior and memory retention in rats. Biochem Biophys Res Commun 299: 739–743.
57. Carlini VP, Ghersi M, Schioth HB, de Barioglio SR (2010) Ghrelin and memory: differential effects on acquisition and retrieval. Peptides 31: 1190–1193.
58. Diano S, Farr SA, Benoit SC, McNay EC, da Silva I, et al. (2006) Ghrelin controls hippocampal spine synapse density and memory performance. Nat Neurosci 9: 381–388.
59. Guan XM, Yu H, Palyha OC, McKee KK, Feighner SD, et al. (1997) Distribution of mRNA encoding the growth hormone secretagogue receptor in brain and peripheral tissues. Brain Res Mol Brain Res 48: 23–29.
60. Bennett PA, Thomas GB, Howard AD, Feighner SD, van der Ploeg LH, et al. (1997) Hypothalamic growth hormone secretagogue-receptor (GHS-R) expression is regulated by growth hormone in the rat. Endocrinology 138: 4552–4557.
61. Lopez M, Lage R, Saha AK, Perez-Tilve D, Vazquez MJ, et al. (2008) Hypothalamic fatty acid metabolism mediates the orexigenic action of ghrelin. Cell Metab 7: 389–399.
62. Kola B, Hubina E, Tucci SA, Kirkham TC, Garcia EA, et al. (2005) Cannabinoids and ghrelin have both central and peripheral metabolic and cardiac effects via AMP-activated protein kinase. J Biol Chem 280: 25196–25201.
63. Olszewski PK, Li D, Grace MK, Billington CJ, Kotz CM, et al. (2003) Neural basis of orexigenic effects of ghrelin acting within lateral hypothalamus. Peptides 24: 597–602.
64. Bermudez-Silva FJ, Cardinal P, Cota D (2012) The role of the endocannabinoid system in the neuroendocrine regulation of energy balance. J Psychopharmacol 26: 114–124.
65. Horvath TL, Diano S, Tschop M (2003) Ghrelin in hypothalamic regulation of energy balance. Current Topics in Medicinal Chemistry 3: 921–927.
66. Tucci SA, Rogers EK, Korbonits M, Kirkham TC (2004) The cannabinoid CB1 receptor antagonist SR141716 blocks the orexigenic effects of intrahypothalamic ghrelin. Br J Pharmacol 143: 520–523.
67. Mechoulam R, Parker LA (2013) The endocannabinoid system and the brain. Annu Rev Psychol 64: 21–47.
68. Katona I, Freund TF (2012) Multiple functions of endocannabinoid signaling in the brain. Annu Rev Neurosci 35: 529–558.
69. Andrews ZB (2011) The extra-hypothalamic actions of ghrelin on neuronal function. Trends Neurosci 34: 31–40.
70. Jung KM, Clapper JR, Fu J, D'Agostino G, Guijarro A, et al. (2012) 2-arachidonoylglycerol signaling in forebrain regulates systemic energy metabolism. Cell Metab 15: 299–310.
71. Malik S, McGlone F, Bedrossian D, Dagher A (2008) Ghrelin modulates brain activity in areas that control appetitive behavior. Cell Metab 7: 400–409.
72. Kroemer NB, Krebs L, Kobiella A, Grimm O, Pilhatsch M, et al. (2013) Fasting levels of ghrelin covary with the brain response to food pictures. Addict Biol 18: 855–862.
73. Jones RB, McKie S, Astbury N, Little TJ, Tivey S, et al. (2012) Functional neuroimaging demonstrates that ghrelin inhibits the central nervous system response to ingested lipid. Gut 61: 1543–1551.

2

Hepatic Branch Vagus Nerve Plays a Critical Role in the Recovery of Post-Ischemic Glucose Intolerance and Mediates a Neuroprotective Effect by Hypothalamic Orexin-A

Shinichi Harada[1], Yui Yamazaki[1], Shuichi Koda[2], Shogo Tokuyama[1]*

1 Department of Clinical Pharmacy, School of Pharmaceutical Sciences, Kobe Gakuin University, Kobe, Japan, **2** Asubio Pharma Co., Ltd., Kobe, Japan

Abstract

Orexin-A (a neuropeptide in the hypothalamus) plays an important role in many physiological functions, including the regulation of glucose metabolism. We have previously found that the development of post-ischemic glucose intolerance is one of the triggers of ischemic neuronal damage, which is suppressed by hypothalamic orexin-A. Other reports have shown that the communication system between brain and peripheral tissues through the autonomic nervous system (sympathetic, parasympathetic and vagus nerve) is important for maintaining glucose and energy metabolism. The aim of this study was to determine the involvement of the hepatic vagus nerve on hypothalamic orexin-A-mediated suppression of post-ischemic glucose intolerance development and ischemic neuronal damage. Male ddY mice were subjected to middle cerebral artery occlusion (MCAO) for 2 h. Intrahypothalamic orexin-A (5 pmol/mouse) administration significantly suppressed the development of post-ischemic glucose intolerance and neuronal damage on day 1 and 3, respectively after MCAO. MCAO-induced decrease of hepatic insulin receptors and increase of hepatic gluconeogenic enzymes on day 1 after was reversed to control levels by orexin-A. This effect was reversed by intramedullary administration of the orexin-1 receptor antagonist, SB334867, or hepatic vagotomy. In the medulla oblongata, orexin-A induced the co-localization of cholin acetyltransferase (cholinergic neuronal marker used for the vagus nerve) with orexin-1 receptor and c-Fos (activated neural cells marker). These results suggest that the hepatic branch vagus nerve projecting from the medulla oblongata plays an important role in the recovery of post-ischemic glucose intolerance and mediates a neuroprotective effect by hypothalamic orexin-A.

Editor: Ken Arai, Massachusetts General Hospital/Harvard Medical School, United States of America

Funding: This study was supported by Grants-in-Aid for Young Scientists (B) (25750366) from the Ministry of Education, Culture, Sports, Science and Technology of Japan. The funders had no role in study design, data collection and analysis, decision to publish, or preparation of the manuscript.

Competing Interests: Dr. Shuichi Koda is an employee of Asubio Pharma Co., Ltd. There are no patents, products in development or marketed products to declare.

* E-mail: stoku@pharm.kobegakuin.ac.jp

Introduction

Stroke is a devastating disease and a leading cause of death and severe disability worldwide [1]. Risk factors associated with stroke include hypertension, dyslipidemia, and obesity [2,3]. Additionally, diabetes mellitus and impaired glucose metabolism (e.g. glucose intolerance) are considered to ones of many important risk factors [4]. Past studies have also suggested that hyperglycemia and/or glucose intolerance following stroke may be associated with greater mortality and reduced functional recovery [5,6]. In a focal cerebral ischemic model, post-ischemic glucose intolerance is one of the triggers of ischemic neuronal damage [7,8,9]. However, the mechanisms remain unclear.

Communication between the brain and peripheral tissues, which occurs via the autonomic nervous system, may be essential for maintaining systemic homeostasis, particularly glucose and energy metabolism [10,11]. In the CNS, the anti-diabetic drug, insulin, suppresses hepatic gluconeogenesis via the hypothalamus and vagus nerve [12,13]. The hepatic branch vagus nerve provides the primary vagal innervation of the rat liver [14]. Therefore, the precise regulation of liver glucose output is necessary to ensure adequate availability of energy sources for the brain.

The orexin family (orexin-A and orexin-B) are hypothalamic neuropeptides [15] possessing many physiological functions, including arousal and energy metabolism such as glucose metabolism, feeding behavior, sleep and wakefulness [16,17]. Importantly, orexin-containing axons are widely distributed in the CNS, particularly in areas involved in autonomic regulation [16,18,19]. Intra-hypothalamic administration of orexin-A enhances insulin-stimulated glucose uptake by activating the sympathetic nervous system [20]. Furthermore, hyperglycemia in diabetic mice is suppressed by intracerebroventricularly (i.c.v.) administration of orexin-A [21]. In our previous reports, intrahypothalamic administration of orexin-A suppressed cerebral ischemic neuronal damage by regulating post-ischemic glucose intolerance, which was achieved by improving impaired hepatic insulin signaling [8]. In other reports, orexin-positive fibers are shown to be distributed throughout the brainstem, including in neurons of the dorsal motor nucleus of the vagus, which is the major source of parasympathetic innervation to peripheral tissues (such as the liver), and neurons in the nucleus of solitary tract

(NTS) [18,19,22]. Hence, we hypothesized that regulation of post-ischemic glucose intolerance in subsequent suppression of developed ischemic neuronal damage showed orexin-A in hypothalamus may be mediated to vagus nerves projected from the medulla oblongata to liver.

In the present study, we examined the influence of hepatic branch vagus nerves projected from the medulla oblongata on the recovery of post-ischemic glucose intolerance, and the neuroprotective effect of intrahypothalamic orexin-A administration.

Materials and Methods

Animals

The present study was conducted in accordance with the Guiding Principles for the Care and Use of Laboratory Animals, adopted by the Japanese Pharmacological Society. All experimental procedures were approved by the ethical committee for animals at Kobe Gakuin University (approval number: A13-25). Experiments were performed on male ddY mice (5 weeks old, 25–30 g) obtained from SLC (Shizuoka, Japan). Animals were housed between 23–24°C on a 12-hr light–dark cycle (lights on 8:00 a.m. to 8:00 p.m.). Food and water were available *ad libitum*.

Drug administration in hypothalamus or medulla oblongata

Intra-hypothalamic administration of 5 pmol/mouse orexin-A (Wako, Osaka, Japan), dissolved in saline, was performed immediately after middle cerebral artery occlusion (MCAO). The selective non-peptide orexin-1 receptor antagonist inhibitor, *N*-(2-methyl-6-benzoxazolyl)-*N'*-1,5-naphthyridin-4-yl urea (SB334867) (Tocris Bioscience, St. Louis, MO, USA), was dissolved in 1% DMSO and administered (intramedullary; 50 or 200 pmol/mouse) 30 min before saline or orexin-A intra-hypothalamic administration. The orexin-A and SB334867 doses and the experimental schedule used here were chosen based on our previous publication [8]. All intra-hypothalamic administrations were performed as previously reported [8,23,24]. The administration volume for orexin-A and SB334867 was 0.2 μL/mouse. Mice were anesthetized with pentobarbital (40 mg/kg) and immobilized on a stereotaxic instrument (SR-5M; NARISHIGE Co., Ltd., Tokyo, Japan). A microsyringe with a 30-gauge stainless-steel needle was used for all experiments. As previously reported [23,24] (but with some modifications), the needle was inserted unilaterally into the hypothalamus (1.3 mm posterior to bregma, 0.5 mm lateral from the midline and 5.7 mm deep) and the medulla oblongata (7.8 mm posterior to bregma, 0.5 mm lateral from the midline and 5.2 mm deep). The injection site of the hypothalamus and medulla oblongata was confirmed with 0.5% trypan blue in saline (0.2 μL/mouse).

Animal model of focal cerebral ischemia

The experimental transient focal ischemia mouse model was induced by performing MCAO, as described previously [25]. Briefly, mice were anesthetized with 2% isoflurane (Abbott Japan, Osaka, Japan) and maintained in an anesthetized state with 1% isoflurane. The common carotid artery (CCA) and external carotid artery were firstly ligated, followed by isolation of the internal carotid artery (ICA). An 8-0 filament (Shirakawa, Fukushima, Japan) coated with a 4-mm thin silicon coat tip (Provil novo Medium; Heraeus Kulzer, Hanau, Germany) was inserted into the left ICA (advanced 9 mm) for 2 h to occlude the left middle cerebral artery (MCA) at its origin through the bifurcation site of CCA. Mice were then anesthetized again, and the occluding filament was gently withdrawn back into the common carotid to allow reperfusion. Sham-operated mice received the same surgery except the filament was not inserted. Body temperature was maintained at 37.0±0.5°C by placing each mouse on a heating pad (FH-100, Unique Medical, Osaka, Japan), which was controlled by a rectal temperature probe (PTE-101, Unique Medical) and a small animal heat controller (ATC-101B, Unique Medical) during surgery and the recovery period. Relative cerebral blood flow (rCBF) was measured by laser Doppler Flowmetry (LDF) (TBF-LN1; Unique Medical) to assess the adequacy of the vascular occlusion and reperfusion, as previously described [25]. MCAO is achieved by a decrease in rCBF to 40% of control values, which is recovered to approximately 100% by reperfusion. In addition, physiological parameters were measured before, during and 30 min after MCAO using a sphygmomanometer (TK-370C; BrainScience Idea, Osaka, Japan) and i-STAT (300F; FUSO Pharmaceutical Industries, Osaka, Japan) [25]. Physiological parameters were within normal physiological ranges in all animals at baseline, during MCAO, and during early reperfusion. We eliminated mice with pricking brain on the silicon coated 8-0 nylon monofilament and unsuccessful infarction on day 3 after MCAO. Thus, the final number of mice was described in each legend. In addition, there are not dead mice by MCAO in present study.

Measurement of fasting blood glucose (FBG) levels

FBG levels were measured, according to previous reports [8,26]. Mice were fasted for 15 h and blood samples (~1.5 μL) were obtained from tail veins. Plasma FBG was measured using the Glucose Pilot (Aventir Biotech, Carlsbad, CA, USA). The increment in FBG was calculated using the following formula: FBG increment = FBG on day 1 after MCAO – FBG before MCAO (pre-MCAO FBG), as previously described [26]. The pre-MCAO FBG level was measured at 48 and 96 h before MCAO.

Measurement of infarct volume

Brains were stained with 2,3,5-triphenyltetrazolium chloride (TTC) (Sigma-Aldrich, St. Louis, MO, USA) to determine infarct volume, as previously demonstrated [8]. Mice were killed on day 3 after reperfusion, and brains were removed, cut (2-mm thick coronal sections) and incubated in saline containing 2% TTC at 37°C for 10 min. Brain slices were then fixed in 4% paraformaldehyde (PFA) at 4°C overnight and scanned. Infarct volumes were measured using the image analysis software, Image J (National Institutes of Health, MD, USA), and Adobe Photoshop Elements 5.0 (Adobe Systems Incorporated, Tokyo, Japan), as previously described [25]. The infarct volume was calculated based on infarct area and intensity (intensity = white intensity of left hemisphere – white intensity of right hemisphere) and according to trapezoid formula.

Neurological examination

Neurological examinations were performed on day 3 after reperfusion using the neurological deficit score (NDS), as previous reported [8,25]. The NDS consists of consciousness (0, normal; 1, restless; 2, lethargic; 3, stuporous; 4, seizures; and 5, death), walking (0, normal; 1, paw; 2, unbalanced walking; 3, circling; 4, unable to stand; and 5, no movement), limb tone (0, normal; 1, spastic; and 2, flaccid), and the pain reflex. The pain reflex was assessed by the tail flick test (pain reflex = latency on day 3 after MCAO – latency before MCAO). NDS points were achieved from the latency difference. A cut-off time of 10 s was used to prevent any injury to the tail. Finally, NDS points assumed total point of consciousness, walking, limb tone and the pain reflex.

Learning and memory tests

A one-trial step-through-type passive avoidance-learning test was performed to examine learning and memory, as described previously [26]. Briefly, the apparatus (Ohara Co., Ltd., Tokyo, Japan) consisted of illuminated and dark compartments (each 4×13×10 cm) adjoining each other through a small gate (3 cm in diameter) with a grid floor, 2.5 mm stainless steel rods set 7 mm apart. In the training trial (2 days after MCAO), mice were placed in the illuminated compartment facing away from the dark compartment. An electric shock (50 V, 3 s in duration) was delivered when mice entered the dark compartment. They were then returned from the dark compartment to the home cage. In the test trial (on day 3 after MCAO and at 24 h after the training trial), mice were placed in the illuminated compartment, and the latency time to enter the dark compartment (maximum of 600 s) was measured.

Locomotor activity

Spontaneous locomotor activity was quantified for 30 min by the open field test, as previously described with some modifications [27,28]. The open field box (30 cm×30 cm×30 cm) consisted of a floor divided into 16 squares (7.5 cm×7.5 cm/square) illuminated by white light. Each mouse was gently placed in the very center of the box and activity was scored as the number of line crossings (i.e. when a mouse removed all four paws from one square and entered another). The open field session was recorded by a camera and the data was analyzed after the session. The open field arena was cleaned with ethanol solution and let dry after testing each mouse.

Western immunoblot analysis

Western immunoblotting was performed, as described previously [23,25,29] but with some modifications. Briefly, the medulla oblongata, liver and skeletal muscle were homogenized in homogenization buffer and diluted with an equal volume of 2× sodium dodecyl sulfate (SDS) sample buffer (0.5 M Tris-HCl [pH 6.8], 10% SDS, 12% β-mercaptoethanol, 20% glycerol, 1% bromophenol blue). Each sample was heated for 3 min at 97°C and protein samples (30 μg) were separated via electrophoresis on 7.5% SDS-polyacrylamide gel and then transferred onto nitrocellulose membranes (BioRad, Hercules, CA, USA) at 15 V for 50 min. Membranes were blocked (60 min at room temperature) in Tris-buffered saline (TBS) (pH 7.6) with 0.1% Tween 20, and either 5% bovine serum albumin (BSA) (Sigma-Aldrich) for insulin receptor (InsR) and tyrosine-phosphorylated (p)-InsR, or 5% skim milk (GE Healthcare, Tokyo, Japan) for orexin-1 receptor, the gluconeogenic regulatory enzymes: phosphoenolpyruvate carboxykinase (PEPCK) and glucose-6-phosphatase (G6Pase), and GAPDH (loading control) (Wako Pure Chemical Industries, Inc., Osaka, Japan). Membranes were incubated with the primary antibodies (in their corresponding blocking solution, overnight at 4°C): rabbit anti-InsR (1:1000, Abcam, Tokyo, Japan), rabbit anti-p-InsR (1:500, Abcam), goat anti-orexin-1 receptor (1:1000, Santa Cruz Biotechnology, Santa Cruz, CA, USA), rabbit anti-PEPCK (1:1000, Santa Cruz Biotechnology) or goat anti-G6Pase (1:500, Santa Cruz Biotechnology), and mouse anti-GAPDH (1:20,000, Chemicon, CA, USA). Blots were then incubated (for 1 h at room temperature) in HRP-conjugated secondary antibodies: anti-rabbit IgG (1:1,000, KPL, Guildford, UK) for InsR, p-InsR and PEPCK, or anti-goat IgG (1:1000, KPL) for orexin-1 receptor and G6Pase, and anti-mouse IgG (1:10,000, KPL) for GAPDH. Immunoreactive bands were visualized with enhanced chemiluminescence western immunoblotting substrate (Pierce; Thermo Scientific, Rockford, IL, USA) followed by a Light-Capture instrument (AE-6981; ATTO, Tokyo, Japan). The signal intensity of immunoreactive bands was analyzed using Cs-Analyzer software (Ver. 3.0) (ATTO) and then normalized to the respective value for GAPDH.

Immunofluorescence

Immunofluorescence was performed, as described previously [30] but with some modifications. Mice were perfused transcardially with 0.1 M phosphate-buffered saline (PBS) (pH 7.4), followed by 4% PFA in 0.1 M PBS, 9 min after intrahypothalamic administration of orexin-A or saline. The brains (which included the medulla oblongata and hypothalamus) were then cut (2-mm thick slices), and slices were incubated and fixed in ice-cold PBS including 4% PFA at 4°C for 3 h, then dehydrated in 10% followed by 20% sucrose for 3 h followed by overnight, respectively at 4°C. Tissues were then embedded and frozen in the Tissue-Tek optimal cutting temperature compound (Sakura Finetek Japan Co., Ltd., Tokyo, Japan) and stored at −80°C until future use. Frozen blocks were cut into 20 μm-thick sections with a cryostat (Leica CM1850; Microsystems GmbH, Wetzlar, Germany), and mounted on a MAS-coated glass slide (Matsunami Glass Ind., Ltd., Osaka, Japan). Sections were post-fixed in 10% formaldehyde at room temperature for 15 min, and subsequently washed with PBS containing 0.1% Tween 20 (PBS-T) 3 times at 5 min intervals. Sections were exposed to 3% BSA in PBS-T for 1 h at room temperature and then incubated (at 4°C for 48 h) with the primary antibodies (in PBS-T with 1% BSA): goat anti-orexin-1 receptor (1:100, Santa Cruz) or mouse anti-cholin acetyltransferase (ChAT; 1:200, Abcam). Sections were incubated (room temperature, 2 h) with the secondary antibody (in 1% BSA): Alexa Fluor 594 goat polyclonal anti-goat (orexin-1 receptor) or -mouse (ChAT) IgG (1:200, Life Technologies Inc., Carlsbad, CA, USA). Sections were then incubated (in PBS-T with 1% BSA, at 4°C for 24 h) with rabbit anti-c-Fos (1:2,000, Santa Cruz) for 24 h or ChAT (1:200) for 48 h. Sections were then washed with PBS-T and incubated (in 1% BSA, at room temperature for 2 h) with the secondary antibody, Alexa Fluor 488 goat polyclonal anti-rabbit (c-Fos) or -mouse (ChAT) IgG (1:200, Life Technologies). After washing, cover-slips were applied to the sections with Fluoromount/Plus (Thermo Shandon Inc., Pittsburgh, PA, USA). Immunoreactive signals were detected with a confocal laser scanning microscope (FV1000, OLYMPUS, Tokyo, Japan).

Selective hepatic branch vagotomy

Hepatic branch vagotomy was performed, as described previously [31,32] but with some modifications. Mice were anesthetized with pentobarbital (65 mg/kg), and the abdominal wall was incised at the midline, the stomach pulled down and the ligaments attaching the liver to the stomach severed. The anterior ligament and the membranous connection of the left lobe of the liver to the diaphragm were cut to provide better visibility of the esophageal-hepatic attachments. The esophageal-hepatic attachment region contains a neurovascular bundle, including the hepatic branch of the vagus nerve. The hepatic branch was selectively transected. Sham vagotomy consisted of the same surgical procedure except for transection of the vagus nerve. MCAO was performed on mice and intrahypothalamic administration of orexin-A or saline was administered on day 7 after surgical recovery.

Statistical analysis

Infarct volume, FBG and quantification of western immunoblots were analyzed via a one-way ANOVA followed by the Scheffe's test and data are presented by the mean ± SEM. The NDS data and one-trial step-through passive avoidance data were analyzed by the Steel-Dwass test with post-hoc nonparametric multiple comparison tests, and data are presented as medians (25th–75th percentile). Significance was reached at values of $p<0.05$ or $p<0.01$.

Results

Effects of hypothalamic administration of orexin-A on FBG levels and ischemic neuronal damage after MCAO

The injection site of orexin-A in the hypothalamus or SB334867, orexin-1 receptor antagonist, in the medulla oblongata was identified using trypan blue (Figure 1A). Orexin-A significantly suppressed the elevation of FBG levels on day 1 after MCAO compared with the saline-treated group (Figure 2B). Furthermore, orexin-A significantly suppressed the development of infarction, increase of NDS score (neurological abnormalities) and decrease of latency by step-through test (memory disturbances) on day 3 after MCAO compared with the saline-treated group (Figure 1C–F). Administration of SB334867 (200 pmol/mouse) in the medulla oblongata significantly inhibited the effects of orexin-A in the medulla oblongata (Figure 1). SB334867 did not affect body weight, blood glucose levels, food intake, drinking volume, and locomoter activity at 3 days or 7 days after administration of saline (vehicle for orexin-A) or 1% DMSO (vehicle for SB334867) (Figure S1). Expression of orexin-1 receptor was not affected by intrahypothalamic administration of orexin-A (Figure S2).

Effects of hypothalamic administration of orexin-A on hepatic and skeletal muscle expression of InsR, p-InsR, PEPCK and G6Pase after MCAO

Compared with the sham group, protein expression of hepatic InsR and p-InsR was significantly decreased on day 1 after MCAO (Figure 2A, B), which was significantly inhibited by orexin-A (Figure 2A, B). Compared with the sham group, expression of hepatic PEPCK and G6Pase protein was significantly increased in the MCAO group (Figure 2C, D), which was significantly decreased by orexin-A (Figure 2C, D). Similarly, in skeletal muscle, MCAO-mediated decrease of InsR and p-InsR levels on day 1 after MCAO was significantly suppressed by orexin-A (Figure 2E, F). The effects of orexin-A were significantly inhibited by administration of SB334867 (200 pmol/mouse) in the medulla oblongata (Figure 2).

Co-localization of c-Fos and orexin-1 receptors after intrahypothalamic administration of orexin-A in the medulla oblongata

c-Fos-positive cells were clearly observed in the medulla oblongata (including the NTS) 90 min after intrahypothalamic administration of orexin-A in this region, and was not seen in the sham group (Figure 3A, D). Orexin-1 receptor positive cells were detected in both saline- and orexin-A-treated groups (Figure 3B, E). Furthermore, orexin-1 receptors were co-localized with c-Fos-positive cells in the NTS of medulla oblongata (Figure 3C, F, and Figure S3).

Co-localization of c-Fos or orexin-1 receptor with ChAT after intrahypothalamic administration of orexin-A in the medulla oblongata

ChAT-positive cells were detected in the medulla oblongata (including the NTS) in both saline- and orexin-A-treated groups (Figure 4). Furthermore, ChAT-positive cells were co-localized with c-Fos and orexin-1 receptors in the NTS of the medulla oblongata (Figure 4, 5, and Figure S4).

Effect of hepatic branch vagotomy on orexin-A-mediated suppression of FBG level and neuronal damage after MCAO

The isolation of the hepatic branch of the vagus nerve is shown in Figure 6A. Hepatic branch vagotomy did not affect non-FBG and FBG levels, body weight, food intake, drinking volume, and the expression of InsR, p-InsR, PEPCK and G6Pase in liver or skeletal muscle (Figure S5, S6). Compared with the saline-treated group, hepatic branch vagotomy inhibited orexin-A-mediated suppression of FBG levels on day 1 after MCAO (Figure 6B). In addition, hepatic branch vagotomy inhibited orexin-A-mediated suppression of infarct development, behavioral abnormality and memory disturbance on day 3 after MCAO (Figure 6C–F).

Effect of hepatic branch vagotomy on orexin-A-mediated effects on InsR, p-InsR, PEPCK and G6Pase after MCAO

On day 1 of MCAO, orexin-A restored MCAO-mediated reduction of hepatic and skeletal muscular protein expression of InsR and p-InsR, and the increase of hepatic PEPCK and G6Pase to control levels. This effect was significantly reversed by hepatic branch vagotomy (Figure 7).

Discussion

In recent years, great attention has been given to the regulation of glucose metabolism by not only the control from individual peripheral tissues, such as the liver, but also by the interaction between the hypothalamus and peripheral tissues [10]. Furthermore, the hypothalamus is the most important brain region for the central regulation of glucose homeostasis, where various hormones and neuropeptides cooperate to produce autonomic outflow to the peripheral tissues, such as liver and skeletal muscle [33,34,35]. Despite this association, its detailed mechanisms still remain unclear.

We recently reported that the regulation of post-ischemic glucose intolerance by intrahypothalamic administration of orexin-A: (1) restored (to sham levels) the decrease of InsR and the increase of gluconeogenic enzymes in the liver, and (2) significantly suppressed cerebral ischemic neuronal damage [8]. In this study, intrahypothalamic administration of orexin-A significantly increased c-Fos-positive cells in the NTS, which contains the nucleus of the vagus nerve [18]. This result is supported by previous reports demonstrating that i.c.v. administration of orexin-A induces c-Fos activation of NTS neurons [36]. Other reports have shown that orexin fibers are distributed throughout the brainstem, including the dorsal motor nucleus of vague neurons (DMN), which is the major source of parasympathetic innervation to the peripheral tissues (such as the liver) and NTS in the CNS [18,19]. In addition, orexin-A directly depolarizes the DMN neurons [37]. The NTS (located in the dorsomedial medulla oblongata) is widely accepted to be crucial for the integration of hepatic control mechanisms [38]. Therefore, in the present study, we hypothesized that hypothalamic orexin-A may regulate liver function, such as glucose metabolism, through parasympathetic nerves projected from the medulla oblongata. Thus, we studied the mechanisms underlying the development of ischemic neuronal damage and the role of post-ischemic glucose intolerance, focusing on communication between the brain and peripheral tissues via parasympathetic nerves.

Our findings reveal that the suppressive effect of hypothalamic orexin-A on the development of post-ischemic glucose intolerance and neuronal damage is mediated by orexin-1 receptor in the medulla oblongata. Furthermore, this receptor mediates hepatic InsR and gluconeogenic enzymes after cerebral ischemic stress.

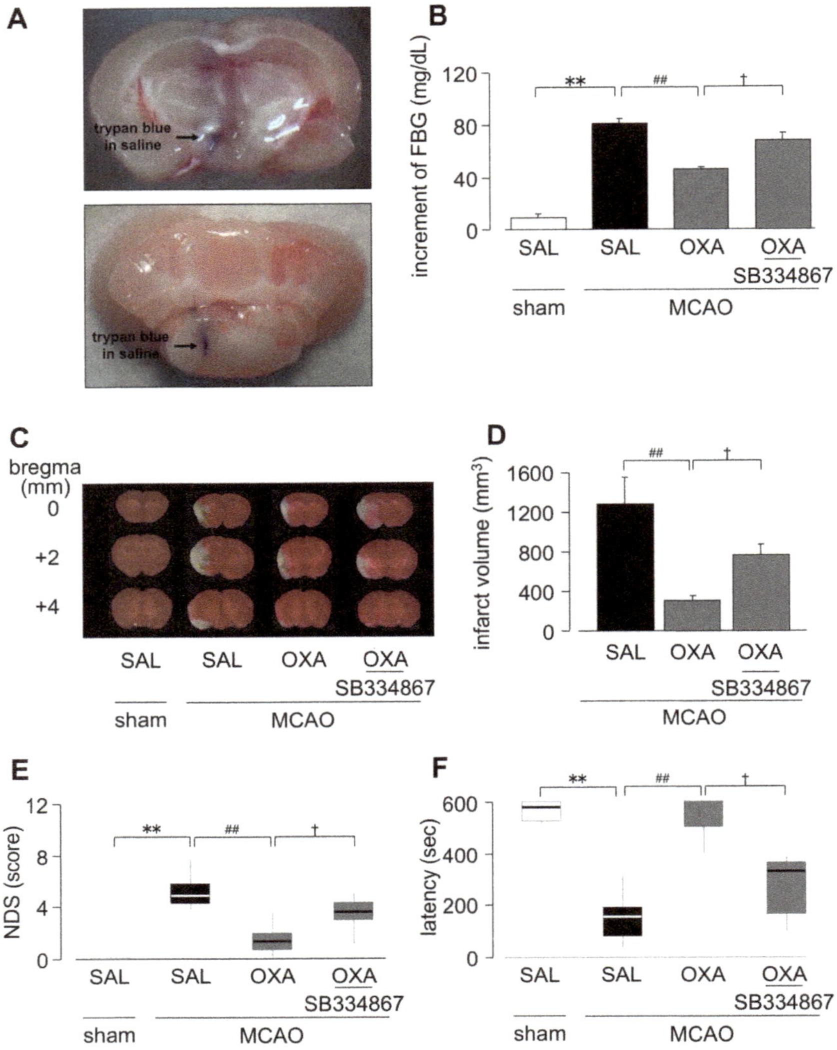

Figure 1. Effects of hypothalamic administration of orexin-A on FBG levels and ischemic neuronal damage after MCAO. Orexin-A (5 pmol/mouse) was intra-hypothalamically administered to mice immediately after MCAO. SB334867 (200 pmol/mouse) was intramedullary administered 30 min before administration of orexin-A. (A) Intra-hypothalamic (upper) or Intra-medullar (lower) administration site (arrow). (B) FBG levels on day 1 after MCAO. (C) Representative photomicrographs of TTC staining on day 3 after MCAO. (D) Quantitative analysis of infarct volume. (B and D) $^{**}P<0.01$, $^{\#\#}P<0.01$, $^{\dagger}P<0.05$. (E) Results of the NDS and (F) the step-through-type passive avoidance learning test on day 3 after MCAO. $^{**}P<0.01$, $^{\#\#}P<0.01$, $^{\dagger}P<0.05$. Sham-treated group: n = 8, MCAO-treated group: n = 6. SAL: saline, OXA: orexin-A.

These results suggest that hypothalamic orexin-A may affect the liver through the medulla oblongata, specifically the parasympathetic nerve (vagus nerve). Orexin-A has been shown to be densely accumulated in the NTS and DMN, which are involved with efferent parasympathetic nerves and thus more effectively the vagus nerve to the liver [36,39]. Moreover, orexin-A activates NTS neurons by modulating a nonselective cationic conductance [40], suggesting that orexin-A may have a functional role in the central parasympathetic nerve control of the NTS. Indeed, hypothalamic orexin-A activated NTS and DMN neurons in the medulla oblongata. Furthermore, these activated neurons were co-localized with orexin-1 receptor and ChAT (cholinergic neuronal marker used for the vagus nerve [41,42]). Therefore, hypothalamic orexin-A-induced effects on liver function (including insulin-induced glucose metabolism) may be mediated by vagus nerves expressing orexin-1 receptor in the NTS of the medulla oblongata. In the hypothalamus, orexin receptors are highly expressed in the LH, the PVN and ARC [43,44]. These areas are involved in origin of sympathetic or parasympathetic (i.e. the vagus nerve) signals to the liver or skeletal muscle [43,44]. In our preliminary study, intrahypothalamic orexin-A activated LHA, ARC and PVN-expressing neurons, which were all co-localized with the orexin-1 receptor (data not shown). These results suggest that orexin neurons projecting from the hypothalamus to the medulla oblongata are involved in hypothalamic orexin-A-mediated effects on liver function. However, whether hypothalamic orexin-A affects liver function through the vagus nerve remains unclear. Therefore, this association is under current investigations using hepatic branch vagotomy mice in our group.

Vagus nerve efferents in the common hepatic branch are important for the suppression of hepatic glucose production when the hypothalamic nutrient sensor is stimulated by nutrient repletion signals, such as insulin or fatty acid oxidation [13,35]. Insulin has been shown over recent years to be a critical

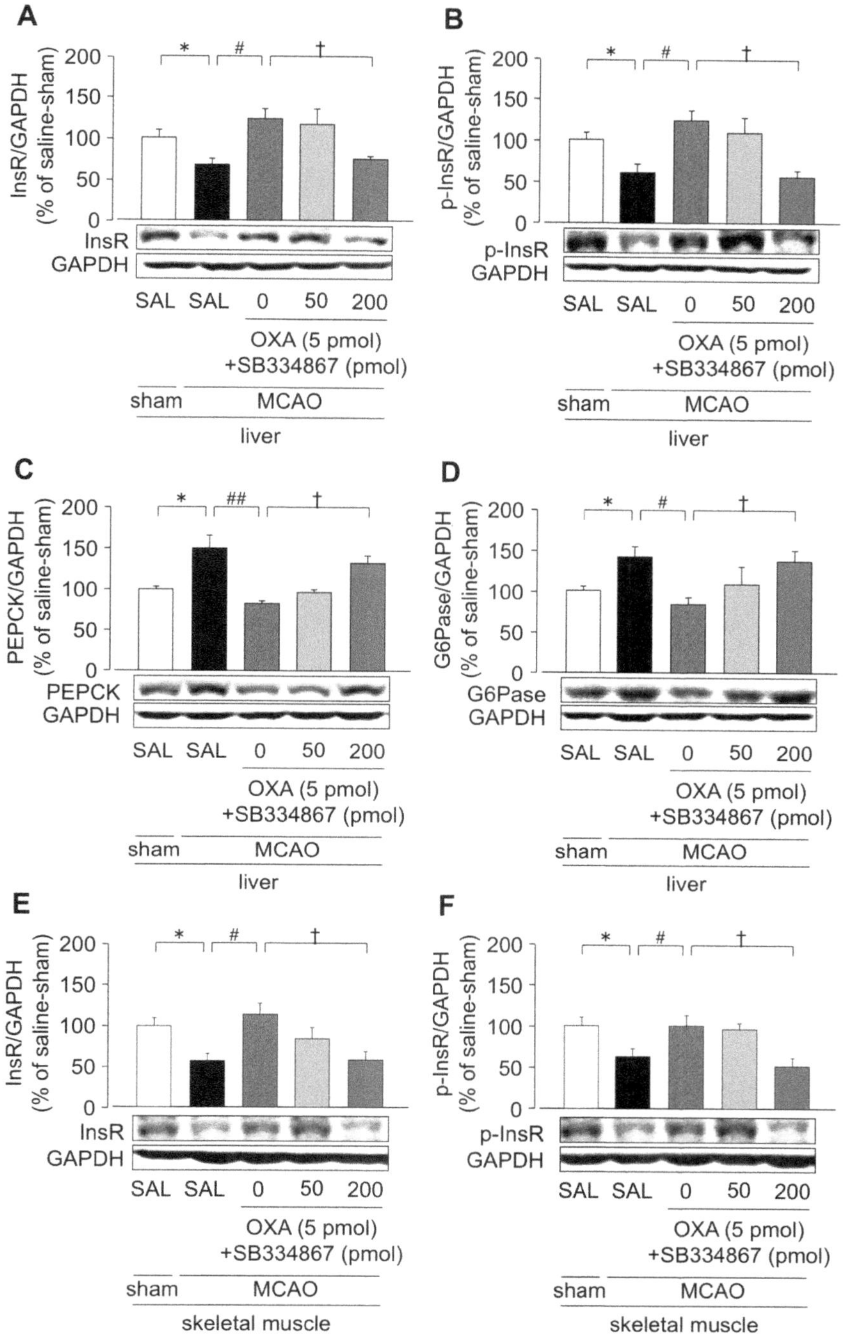

Figure 2. Effects of hypothalamic administration of orexin-A on hepatic and skeletal muscle expression of InsR, p-InsR, PEPCK and G6Pase on day 1 after MCAO. Mice were intrahypothalamically administered with orexin-A immediately after MCAO. SB334867 (50 or 200 pmol/mouse) was intramedullary administered 30 min before orexin-A. Representative western immunoblots and quantification (ratio to GAPDH) as % of sham-SAL of hepatic: InR (A), p-InsR (B), PEPCK (C), G6Pase (D), and skeletal muscular: InsR (E) and p-InsR (F). $^{\#\#}P<0.01$, $^{*}P<0.05$, $^{\#}P<0.05$, $^{\dagger}P<0.05$, Scheffe's test, sham-treated group: n = 6, MCAO-treated group: n = 6. SAL: saline, OXA: orexin-A.

determinant of energy homeostasis and peripheral glucose metabolism [45]. Insulin modifies peripheral glucose metabolism (especially liver glucose synthesis) through insulin receptors localized in the hypothalamus [13,46]. Administration (i.c.v.) of insulin increases insulin sensitivity in peripheral tissues. Furthermore, improved peripheral insulin action is associated with a reduction in hepatic glucose production [13,46,47]. The motor nucleus of the vagus mediates hypothalamic insulin signaling via ATP-sensitive potassium (K_{ATP}) channels, and reaches the liver via the efferent vagus nerve [13]. Furthermore, activation of either insulin signaling or K_{ATP} channels within the hypothalamus is sufficient to decrease blood glucose levels by a substantial inhibition of glucose production, which is largely due to a marked decrease in the hepatic abundance of gluconeogenic enzymes,

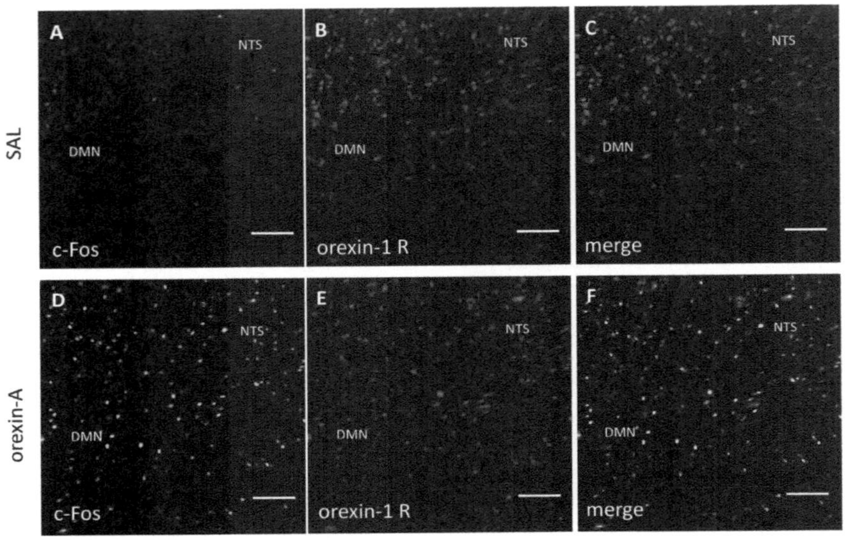

Figure 3. Co-localization of c-Fos and orexin-1 receptors after intrahypothalamic administration of orexin-A in the medulla oblongata. Co-localization (C, F) of c-Fos protein (A, D [green]) and orexin-1 receptor (B, E [red]) after saline or orexin-A was intrahypothalamically administered in the medulla oblongata (including nucleus of solitary tract [NTS]). Scale bar: 100 μm. SAL: saline, orexin-1 R: orexin-1 receptor, DMN: dorsal motor nucleus of the vagus.

such as PEPCK and G6Pase [13,46,47]. Also, effects of central insulin and systemic insulin on hepatic glucose production are suppressed [48]. Therefore, activation of the hypothalamus-medulla oblongata-vagus nerve-liver axis is important for insulin signaling on liver function. Changes in glucose uptake in peripheral tissues after intrahypothalamic (VMH) administration of orexin-A have shown that these orexin-A-affected tissues are mediated by the activation of sympathetic nerve signaling with β2-adrenergic receptors in skeletal muscle [20]. Activation of LH and VMH neurons may regulate InsR substrate activity and glucose production in the liver and skeletal muscle via parasympathetic and sympathetic neurons, respectively [49]. That is, it is through that orexin-A is an important to regulate the glucose metabolism in peripheral organs via the activation of the autonomic nervous system. However, the role of endogenous orexin-A in the central regulation of hepatic glucose homeostasis and the vagus nerve (including the hepatic branch vagus nerve) remains to be clarified. Our findings are the first to show that hypothalamic orexin-A affects the vagus nerve-liver axis, and regulates hepatic insulin regulation. More specifically, hypothalamic orexin-A suppressed post-ischemic glucose intolerance by decreasing hepatic InsR and increasing gluconeogenic enzymes via vagus nerve signaling, and also inhibited neuronal damage. In light with these results, other reports have shown that hypothalamic orexin-A levels are

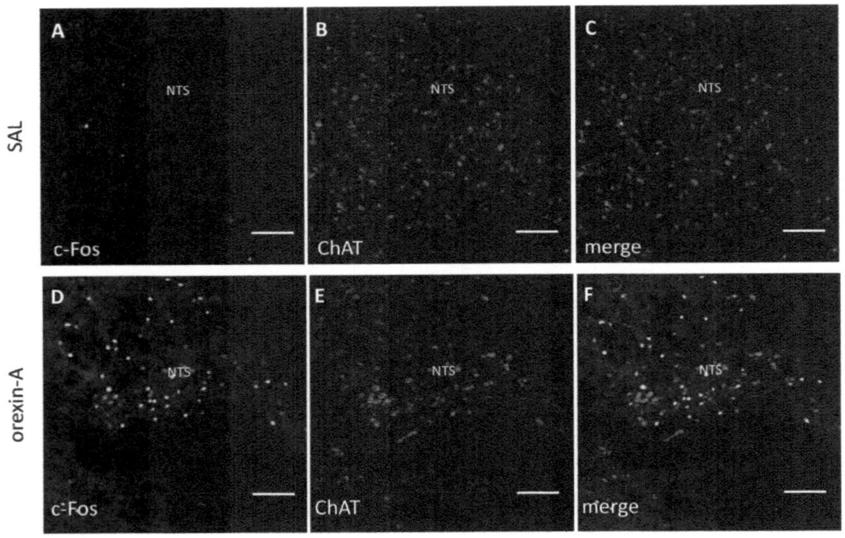

Figure 4. Co-localization of c-Fos and choline acetyltransferase (ChAT) after intrahypothalamic administration of orexin-A in the medulla oblongata. Co-localization (C, F) of c-Fos protein (A, D [green]) and choline acetyltransferase (ChAT) (B, E [red]) after intrahypothalamic administration of saline or orexin-A in the medulla oblongata (including the NTS). Scale bar = 100 μm. SAL: saline.

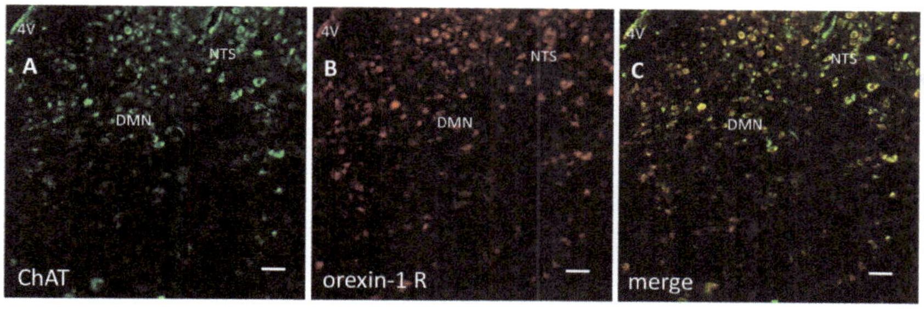

Figure 5. Co-localization of ChAT and orexin-1 receptor in naive mice. Co-localization (C, F) of ChAT (A, D [green]) and orein-1 receptor (B, E [red]) after intrahypothalamic administration of saline or orexin-A in the medulla oblongata (including the NTS). Scale bar = 100 μm. SAL: saline, DMN: dorsal motor nucleus of the vagus, 4V: fourth ventricle.

significantly decreased by cerebral ischemic stress [8]. These results suggest that the development of post-ischemic glucose intolerance may be involved in the reduction of hypothalamic orexin-A-induced activation of orexin neurons projected from the NTS of the medulla oblongata, causing weakness of vagus nerve stimuli and thus, impairing liver function. However, further study is required to fully elucidate the mechanisms of involvement.

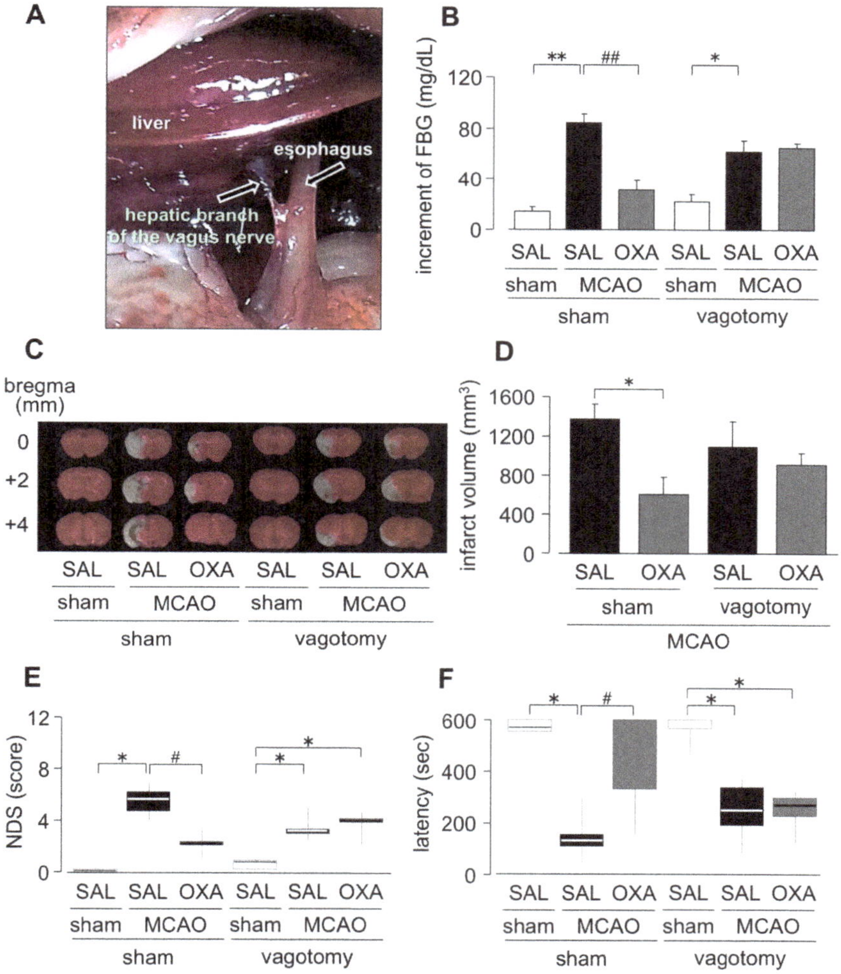

Figure 6. Effect of hepatic branch vagotomy on hypothalamic orexin-A-mediated suppression of FBG levels and neuronal damage on day 1 and 3, respectively after MCAO. Intrahypothalamic administration of orexin-A immediately following MCAO on day 7 after hepatic branch vagotomy. (A) Operative field for selective hepatic nerve of the vagus nerve interruption. (B) FBG levels on day 1 after MCAO. (C) Representative photomicrographs of TTC staining on day 3 after MCAO. (D) Quantitative analysis of the infarct volume. (B and D) $^{**}P<0.01$, $^{\#\#}P<0.01$, $^{*}P<0.05$. (E) Results of the NDS and (F) the step-through-type passive avoidance learning test on day 3 after MCAO. $^{*}P<0.05$, $^{\#}P<0.05$. MCAO/saline-treated group: n = 6, others group: n = 5. SAL: saline, OXA: orexin-A.

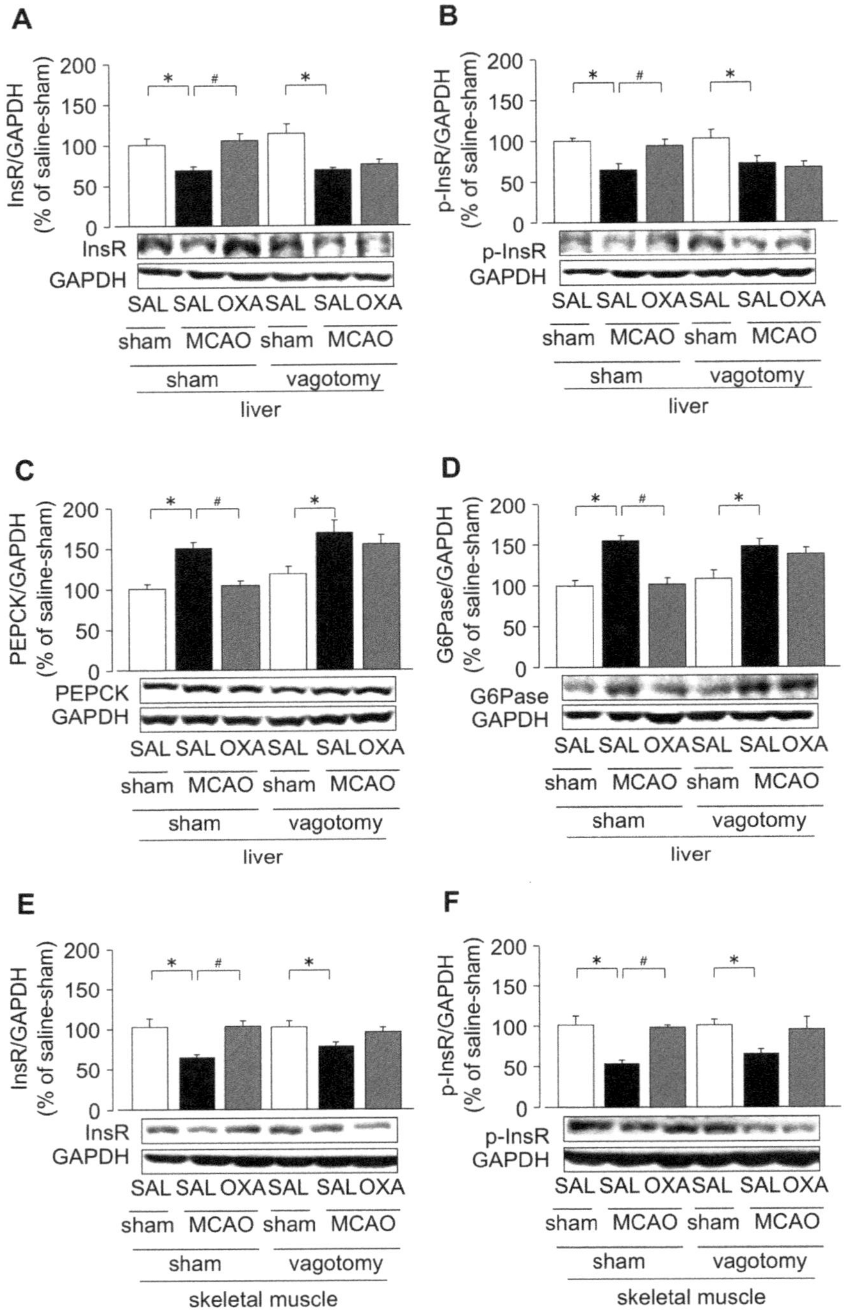

Figure 7. Effect of hepatic branch vagotomy on hypothalamic orexin-A-mediated effects on hepatic and skeletal muscular expression of InsR, p-InsR, PEPCK and G6Pase on day 1 after MCAO. Intrahypothalamic administration of orexin-A immediately following MCAO 7 days after hepatic branch vagotomy. Representative western immunoblots and quantification (ratio to GAPDH) as % of sham-SAL of hepatic: InR (A), p-InsR (B), PEPCK (C), G6Pase (D), and skeletal muscular: InsR (E) and p-InsR (F). $^{*}P<0.05$, $^{\#}P<0.05$. n = 12. SAL: saline, OXA: orexin-A.

Central actions of insulin are reported to induce the activation of signal transducer and activator of transcription (STAT) 3 phosphorylation in the liver [50], suppresses the expression of the transcriptional coactivator of gluconeogenesis, peroxisome proliferator-acivated receptor γ coactivator-1α, and gluconeogenic genes [50,51]. Hypothalamic insulin significantly increases both pAkt/Akt and pSTAT3/STAT3 in the liver [52] and thus, may be involved in vagus nerve stimuli projected to the liver [13]. The α7-nicotinic ACh receptor selective agonist, PNU-282987, enhances STAT3 phosphorylation in the liver and skeletal muscle [53]. Hepatic branch vagus nerve leads to the release of ACh, which then binds to muscarinic and nicotinic acetylcholine receptors [54,55]. Therefore, the regulatory mechanisms of liver function by hypothalamic orexin-A may involve ACh and its receptor, and STAT3. However, this mechanism is still controversial because cholinergic signaling pathways have been reported to not mediate the metabolic effects by the activation of hepatic vagal nerves [56].

However, little is known about the changes in the expression levels of hepatic InsR. Previous reports have shown that polypyrimidine tract-binding protein (PTB) upregulates the expression of insulin and insulin receptor [57,58]. Under conditions activating insulin signaling, PTB promotes the stabilization of mRNAs encoding insulin and insulin receptor, and enhances the translation of insulin receptor mRNA [57]. Furthermore, CCAAT/enhancer-binding proteins (a family of leucine-zipper transcription factors) regulate the transcription of the InsR as part of a larger nuclear protein complex containing transcription factors such as specific protein 1 [59]. Other reports have demonstrated that TNF-α down-regulates insulin signaling by increasing tyrosine phosphatase 1B [60], suggesting that ischemic stress-mediated increases of inflammatory cytokines may affect the transcription or degradation of the InsR.

In previous finding, orexin-1 receptor, a one of orexin-A receptor, immunoreactivity in the cortex that vulnerable brain region to ischemic stress was increased after cerebral ischemia [61] and i.c.v. orexin-A suppressed the development of infarction through increasing the cerebral blood flow [62]. In addition, in others reports, the mechanisms of the neuroprotective effects of orexin-A have been proved to be related with some intracellular signal transduction pathway, such as hypoxia-inducible factor-1α [63]. That is, these reports suggest that indicated the neuroprotective effect of orexin-A was not only involved in the improvement of post-ischemic glucose intolerance, but also other factors (including other neuroprotective mechanisms such as enhances the cerebral blood flow and inhibits ischemic stress-induced increment of HIF-1α).

In conclusion, these findings provide some insight into the therapeutic effectiveness of this endogenous neuropeptide for its communication between brain and peripheral tissues via the autonomic nervous system, specifically the parasympathetic nerve (vagus nerve).

Supporting Information

Figure S1 Changes in body weigh, blood glucose levels, food intake, drinking volume, locomoter activity on day 3 or day 7 after intra-medullar single administration of saline (vehicle of orexin-A) and 1% DMSO (vehicle of SB334867). (A) Body weight on a daily after administration. (B) Blood glucose levels on a daily after administration. (C) Food intake on day 3 or day 7 after administration. (D) Drinking volume on day 3 or day 7 after administration. (E) Locomoter activity on day 3 after administration. (F) Total count of (E). (F) Locomoter activity on day 7 after administration. (H) Total count of (F). n = 3.

Figure S2 Effects of hypothalamic orexin-A on changes in orexin-1 receptor on day 1 after MCAO in medulla oblongata. Mice were intra-hypothalamic administered with orexin-A (5 pmol/mouse) immediately after MCAO. (A) Representative western blots of orexin-1 receptor are shown. (B) Relative levels were analyzed by determining the ratio of orexin-1 receptor/GAPDH on day 1 after MCAO. Results are presented as mean ± S.E.M. n = 4. SAL: saline, OXA: orexin-A.

Figure S3 Immunohistological expression and co-localization of c-Fos and orexin-1 recepter after intrahypothalamic administration of orexin-A in medulla oblongata. (A–F) Photomicrographs illustrating the co-localization (C, F) of c-Fos protein (A, D; green) and orexin-1 receptor (B, E; red) after intra-hypothalamic administration of saline or orexin-A (5 pmol/mouse) in medulla oblongata including nucleus of solitary tract (NTS). Scale bar: 100 µm. SAL: saline, orexin-1 R: orexin-1 receptor, DMN: dorsal motor nucleus of the vagus. The dot square showed Figure 3.

Figure S4 Immunohistological expression and co-localization of c-Fos and choline acetyltransferase after intrahypothalamic administration of orexin-A in medulla oblongata. (A–F) Photomicrographs illustrating the co-localization (C, F) of c-Fos protein (A, D; green) and choline acetyltransferase (ChAT) (B, E; red) after intra-hypothalamic administration of saline or orexin-A (5 pmol/mouse) in medulla oblongata including nucleus of solitary tract (NTS). Scale bar: 100 µm. SAL: saline. The dot square showed Figure 4.

Figure S5 Changes in (A) non-fasting blood glucose levels, (B) fasting blood glucose levels, (C) alteration of body weigh (difference of day 7 – day 0), (D) food intake, (E) drinking volume, (F) locomoter activity on day 7 after hepatic branch vagotomy. n = 3.

Figure S6 Effect of hepatic branch vagotomy on hepatic and/or skeletal muscular InsR, p-InsR, PEPCK and G6Pase expression on day 7. Representative western blots of InR, p-InsR, PEPCK, G6Pase and GAPDH levels are shown. Relative levels were analyzed by determining the ratio of InsR/GAPDH, p-InsR/GAPDH PEPCK/GAPDH and G6Pase/GAPDH on day 1 after MCAO. (A) hepatic InsR, (B) hepetic p-InsR, (C) hepatic PEPCK, (D) hepatic G6Pase, (E) skeletal muscular InsR, (F) skeletal muscular p-InsR. Results are presented as mean ± S.E.M. n = 4. SAL: saline, OXA: orexin-A.

Author Contributions

Conceived and designed the experiments: SH ST. Performed the experiments: SH YY ST. Analyzed the data: SH ST. Contributed reagents/materials/analysis tools: SH SK ST. Wrote the paper: SH ST.

References

1. Go AS, Mozaffarian D, Roger VL, Benjamin EJ, Berry JD, et al. (2013) Heart disease and stroke statistics—2013 update: a report from the American Heart Association. Circulation 127: e6–e245.
2. Kernan WN, Viscoli CM, Inzucchi SE, Brass LM, Bravata DM, et al. (2005) Prevalence of abnormal glucose tolerance following a transient ischemic attack or ischemic stroke. Arch Intern Med 165: 227–233.
3. Saito I (2012) Epidemiological evidence of type 2 diabetes mellitus, metabolic syndrome, and cardiovascular disease in Japan. Circ J 76: 1066–1073.
4. Doi Y, Ninomiya T, Hata J, Fukuhara M, Yonemoto K, et al. (2010) Impact of glucose tolerance status on development of ischemic stroke and coronary heart disease in a general Japanese population: the Hisayama study. Stroke 41: 203–209.
5. Matz K, Keresztes K, Tatschl C, Nowotny M, Dachenhausenm A, et al. (2006) Disorders of glucose metabolism in acute stroke patients: an underrecognized problem. Diabetes Care 29: 792–797.
6. Capes SE, Hunt D, Malmberg K, Pathak P, Gerstein HC (2001) Stress hyperglycemia and prognosis of stroke in nondiabetic and diabetic patients: a systematic overview. Stroke 32: 2426–2432.
7. Yamazaki Y, Harada S, Tokuyama S (2012) Post-ischemic hyperglycemia exacerbates the development of cerebral ischemic neuronal damage through the cerebral sodium-glucose transporter. Brain Res 1489: 113–120.
8. Harada S, Yamazaki Y, Tokuyama S (2013) Orexin-A suppresses postischemic glucose intolerance and neuronal damage through hypothalamic brain-derived neurotrophic factor. J Pharmacol Exp Ther 344: 276–285.

9. Harada S, Fujita-Hamabe W, Tokuyama S (2012) Ischemic stroke and glucose intolerance: a review of the evidence and exploration of novel therapeutic targets. J Pharmacol Sci 118: 1–13.
10. Yamada T, Katagiri H (2007) Avenues of communication between the brain and tissues/organs involved in energy homeostasis. Endocr J 54: 497–505.
11. Imai J, Katagiri H, Yamada T, Ishigaki Y, Suzuki T, et al. (2008) Regulation of pancreatic beta cell mass by neuronal signals from the liver. Science 322: 1250–1254.
12. Bruning JC, Gautam D, Burks DJ, Gillette J, Schubert M, et al. (2000) Role of brain insulin receptor in control of body weight and reproduction. Science 289: 2122–2125.
13. Pocai A, Lam TK, Gutierrez-Juarez R, Obici S, Schwartz GJ, et al. (2005) Hypothalamic K(ATP) channels control hepatic glucose production. Nature 434: 1026–1031.
14. Evans ML, Sherwin RS (2002) Brain glucose metabolism and hypoglycaemia. Diabetes Nutr Metab 15: 294–296; discussion 296.
15. Sakurai T, Amemiya A, Ishii M, Matsuzaki I, Chemelli RM, et al. (1998) Orexins and orexin receptors: a family of hypothalamic neuropeptides and G protein-coupled receptors that regulate feeding behavior. Cell 92: 573–585.
16. de Lecea L, Kilduff TS, Peyron C, Gao X, Foye PE, et al. (1998) The hypocretins: hypothalamus-specific peptides with neuroexcitatory activity. Proc Natl Acad Sci U S A 95: 322–327.
17. Sakurai T (2007) The neural circuit of orexin (hypocretin): maintaining sleep and wakefulness. Nat Rev Neurosci 8: 171–181.
18. Peyron C, Tighe DK, van den Pol AN, de Lecea L, Heller HC, et al. (1998) Neurons containing hypocretin (orexin) project to multiple neuronal systems. J Neurosci 18: 9996–10015.
19. Harrison TA, Chen CT, Dun NJ, Chang JK (1999) Hypothalamic orexin A-immunoreactive neurons project to the rat dorsal medulla. Neurosci Lett 273: 17–20.
20. Shiuchi T, Haque MS, Okamoto S, Inoue T, Kageyama H, et al. (2009) Hypothalamic orexin stimulates feeding-associated glucose utilization in skeletal muscle via sympathetic nervous system. Cell Metab 10: 466–480.
21. Tsuneki H, Sugihara Y, Honda R, Wada T, Sasaoka T, et al. (2002) Reduction of blood glucose level by orexins in fasting normal and streptozotocin-diabetic mice. Eur J Pharmacol 448: 245–252.
22. Davis SF, Williams KW, Xu W, Glatzer NR, Smith BN (2003) Selective enhancement of synaptic inhibition by hypocretin (orexin) in rat vagal motor neurons: implications for autonomic regulation. J Neurosci 23: 3844–3854.
23. Harada S, Fujita-Hamabe W, Tokuyama S (2012) Ameliorating effect of hypothalamic brain-derived neurotrophic factor against impaired glucose metabolism after cerebral ischemic stress in mice. J Pharmacol Sci 118: 109–116.
24. Tsao D, Thomsen HK, Chou J, Stratton J, Hagen M, et al. (2008) TrkB agonists ameliorate obesity and associated metabolic conditions in mice. Endocrinology 149: 1038–1048.
25. Harada S, Hamabe W, Kamiya K, Satake T, Yamamoto J, et al. (2009) Preventive effect of Morinda citrifolia fruit juice on neuronal damage induced by focal ischemia. Biol Pharm Bull 32: 405–409.
26. Harada S, Fujita WH, Shichi K, Tokuyama S (2009) The development of glucose intolerance after focal cerebral ischemia participates in subsequent neuronal damage. Brain Res 1279: 174–181.
27. Dunn AJ, Swiergiel AH (2005) Effects of interleukin-1 and endotoxin in the forced swim and tail suspension tests in mice. Pharmacol Biochem Behav 81: 688–693.
28. Sharma AN, Elased KM, Garrett TL, Lucot JB (2010) Neurobehavioral deficits in db/db diabetic mice. Physiol Behav 101: 381–388.
29. Harada S, Fujita-Hamabe W, Tokuyama S (2011) Effect of orexin-A on post-ischemic glucose intolerance and neuronal damage. J Pharmacol Sci 115: 155–163.
30. Harada S, Nakamoto K, Tokuyama S (2013) The involvement of midbrain astrocyte in the development of morphine tolerance. Life Sci 93: 573–578.
31. Koda S, Date Y, Murakami N, Shimbara T, Hanada T, et al. (2005) The role of the vagal nerve in peripheral PYY3-36-induced feeding reduction in rats. Endocrinology 146: 2369–2375.
32. Bernal-Mizrachi C, Xiaozhong L, Yin L, Knutsen RH, Howard MJ, et al. (2007) An afferent vagal nerve pathway links hepatic PPARalpha activation to glucocorticoid-induced insulin resistance and hypertension. Cell Metab 5: 91–102.
33. Prodi E, Obici S (2006) Minireview: the brain as a molecular target for diabetic therapy. Endocrinology 147: 2664–2669.
34. Marino JS, Xu Y, Hill JW (2011) Central insulin and leptin-mediated autonomic control of glucose homeostasis. Trends Endocrinol Metab 22: 275–285.
35. Mighiu PI, Yue JT, Filippi BM, Abraham MA, Chari M, et al. (2013) Hypothalamic glucagon signaling inhibits hepatic glucose production. Nat Med 19: 766–772.
36. Date Y, Ueta Y, Yamashita H, Yamaguchi H, Matsukura S, et al. (1999) Orexins, orexigenic hypothalamic peptides, interact with autonomic, neuroendocrine and neuroregulatory systems. Proc Natl Acad Sci U S A 96: 748–753.
37. Hwang LL, Chen CT, Dun NJ (2001) Mechanisms of orexin-induced depolarizations in rat dorsal motor nucleus of vagus neurones in vitro. J Physiol 537: 511–520.
38. Lawrence AJ, Jarrott B (1996) Neurochemical modulation of cardiovascular control in the nucleus tractus solitarius. Prog Neurobiol 48: 21–53.
39. Yi CX, Serlie MJ, Ackermans MT, Foppen E, Buijs RM, et al. (2009) A major role for perifornical orexin neurons in the control of glucose metabolism in rats. Diabetes 58: 1998–2005.
40. Yang B, Ferguson AV (2003) Orexin-A depolarizes nucleus tractus solitarius neurons through effects on nonselective cationic and K+ conductances. J Neurophysiol 89: 2167–2175.
41. Tata AM, De Stefano ME, Srubek Tomassy G, Vilaro MT, Levey AI, et al. (2004) Subpopulations of rat dorsal root ganglion neurons express active vesicular acetylcholine transporter. J Neurosci Res 75: 194–202.
42. Bellier JP, Kimura H (2007) Acetylcholine synthesis by choline acetyltransferase of a peripheral type as demonstrated in adult rat dorsal root ganglion. J Neurochem 101: 1607–1618.
43. Marcus JN, Aschkenasi CJ, Lee CE, Chemelli RM, Saper CB, et al. (2001) Differential expression of orexin receptors 1 and 2 in the rat brain. J Comp Neurol 435: 6–25.
44. Trivedi P, Yu H, MacNeil DJ, Van der Ploeg LH, Guan XM (1998) Distribution of orexin receptor mRNA in the rat brain. FEBS Lett 438: 71–75.
45. Kim B, Feldman EL (2012) Insulin resistance in the nervous system. Trends Endocrinol Metab 23: 133–141.
46. Kishore P, Boucai L, Zhang K, Li W, Koppaka S, et al. (2011) Activation of K(ATP) channels suppresses glucose production in humans. J Clin Invest 121: 4916–4920.
47. Obici S, Zhang BB, Karkanias G, Rossetti L (2002) Hypothalamic insulin signaling is required for inhibition of glucose production. Nat Med 8: 1376–1382.
48. Pocai A, Obici S, Schwartz GJ, Rossetti L (2005) A brain-liver circuit regulates glucose homeostasis. Cell Metab 1: 53–61.
49. Shimazu T, Ogasawara S (1975) Effects of hypothalamic stimulation on gluconeogenesis and glycolysis in rat liver. Am J Physiol 228: 1787–1793.
50. Inoue H, Ogawa W, Ozaki M, Haga S, Matsumoto M, et al. (2004) Role of STAT-3 in regulation of hepatic gluconeogenic genes and carbohydrate metabolism in vivo. Nat Med 10: 168–174.
51. Erion DM, Yonemitsu S, Nie Y, Nagai Y, Gillum MP, et al. (2009) SirT1 knockdown in liver decreases basal hepatic glucose production and increases hepatic insulin responsiveness in diabetic rats. Proc Natl Acad Sci U S A 106: 11288–11293.
52. Moore MC, Smith MS, Turney MK, Boysen S, Williams PE (2011) Comparison of insulins detemir and glargine: effects on glucose disposal, hepatic glucose release and the central nervous system. Diabetes Obes Metab 13: 832–840.
53. Xu TY, Guo LL, Wang P, Song J, Le YY, et al. (2012) Chronic exposure to nicotine enhances insulin sensitivity through alpha7 nicotinic acetylcholine receptor-STAT3 pathway. PLoS One 7: e51217.
54. Caulfield MP, Birdsall NJ (1998) International Union of Pharmacology. XVII. Classification of muscarinic acetylcholine receptors. Pharmacol Rev 50: 279–290.
55. Wess J, Eglen RM, Gautam D (2007) Muscarinic acetylcholine receptors: mutant mice provide new insights for drug development. Nat Rev Drug Discov 6: 721–733.
56. Li JH, Gautam D, Han SJ, Guettier JM, Cui Y, et al. (2009) Hepatic muscarinic acetylcholine receptors are not critically involved in maintaining glucose homeostasis in mice. Diabetes 58: 2776–2787.
57. Lee EK, Gorospe M (2010) Minireview: posttranscriptional regulation of the insulin and insulin-like growth factor systems. Endocrinology 151: 1403–1408.
58. Tillmar L, Welsh N (2002) Hypoxia may increase rat insulin mRNA levels by promoting binding of the polypyrimidine tract-binding protein (PTB) to the pyrimidine-rich insulin mRNA 3′-untranslated region. Mol Med 8: 263–272.
59. Foti D, Iuliano R, Chiefari E, Brunetti A (2003) A nucleoprotein complex containing Sp1, C/EBP beta, and HMGI-Y controls human insulin receptor gene transcription. Mol Cell Biol 23: 2720–2732.
60. Nieto-Vazquez I, Fernandez-Veledo S, Kramer DK, Vila-Bedmar R, Garcia-Guerra L, et al. (2008) Insulin resistance associated to obesity: the link TNF-alpha. Arch Physiol Biochem 114: 183–194.
61. Nakamachi T, Endo S, Ohtaki H, Yin L, Kenji D, et al. (2005) Orexin-1 receptor expression after global ischemia in mice. Regul Pept 126: 49–54.
62. Kitamura E, Hamada J, Kanazawa N, Yonekura J, Masuda R, et al. (2010) The effect of orexin-A on the pathological mechanism in the rat focal cerebral ischemia. Neurosci Res 68: 154–157.
63. Yuan LB, Dong HL, Zhang HP, Zhao RN, Gong G, et al. (2011) Neuroprotective effect of orexin-A is mediated by an increase of hypoxia-inducible factor-1 activity in rat. Anesthesiology 114: 340–354.

3

Temporary Interference over the Posterior Parietal Cortices Disrupts Thermoregulatory Control in Humans

Alberto Gallace[1]*, Giovanna Soravia[1], Zaira Cattaneo[1], G. Lorimer Moseley[2,3], Giuseppe Vallar[1,4]

1 Department of Psychology, University of Milano-Bicocca, Milan, Italy, 2 The Sansom Institute for Health Research, University of South Australia, Adelaide, Australia, 3 Neuroscience Research Australia, Sydney, Australia, 4 IRCCS Istituto Auxologico Italiano, Milano, Italy

Abstract

The suggestion has recently been made that certain higher-order cortical areas involved in supporting multisensory representations of the body, and of the space around it, might also play a role in controlling thermoregulatory functions. Here we demonstrate that temporary interference with the function of one of these areas, the posterior parietal cortex, by repetitive transcranial magnetic stimulation, results in a decrease in limb temperature. By contrast, interference with the activity of a sensory-specific area (the primary somatosensory cortex) had no effect on temperature. The results of this experiment suggest that associative multisensory brain areas might exert a top-down modulation over basic physiological control. Such a function might be part of a larger neural circuit responsible for maintaining the integrity of the body at both a homeostatic and a psychological level.

Editor: Nicholas P. Holmes, University of Reading, United Kingdom

Funding: GLM was supported by the National Health & Medical Research Council of Australia ID 571090. G. V. was supported by a Ricerca Corrente Grant from the IRCCS Istituto Auxologico Italiano. A. G. and Z. C. were supported by a Futuro in Ricerca 2012 grant (RBFR12F0BD_003). The funders had no role in study design, data collection and analysis, decision to publish, or preparation of the manuscript.

Competing Interests: The authors have declared that no competing interests exist.

* E-mail: alberto.gallace1@unimib.it

Introduction

A series of studies in the last few years has started to highlight the consequences of higher-order cognitive manipulations on the lower-level mechanisms involved in controlling physiological life-supporting functions [1], [2], see also [3]. In fact, recent findings suggest that psychological illusions regarding the ownership of our body can modulate thermoregulatory [1] and immune [4] system control in neurologically unimpaired participants [5]. For example, eliciting the illusion that a rubber hand is part of a person's body results in a reduction of skin temperature on the hand that is 'replaced' by the artificial one, and in a shift in the perceived temporal order of pairs of tactile stimuli, such that stimuli from the experimental hand are given less weighting (in terms of attentional/processing resources) than stimuli from the other hand [1], [5], [6]. Similarly, researchers have shown in patients with complex regional pain syndrome (CRPS), that changing the position of the affected limb in space can shift from pathological to near-normal the temperature of the affected limb [6], [7], and that this effect depends on the perceived location of the limb, not its true location or alignment [8].

It is important to note that CRPS may occur after stroke involving the posterior parietal cortex [9] and after peripheral limb trauma without stroke. The likelihood of developing CRPS after peripheral trauma is not affected by the severity of the injury, (see [10] for a review). Despite their very different aetiologies, the similarities between post-stroke and post-peripheral trauma CRPS are remarkable, (see [11] for a review). All of these similarities, combined with the recent discovery that cooling of the affected limb in CRPS is positively related to a spatially-defined shift in tactile processing [6], would seem to suggest that the processing of spatial variables occurring in higher-order brain areas, can have an important effect on thermoregulatory control.

In order to account for the rather unexpected findings coming from the study of CRPS patients, as well as for those from bodily illusions in neurologically normal participants, it has recently been suggested that a network of brain areas, named the 'body matrix', might be responsible for maintaining the integrity of the body at both the homeostatic (i.e., thermoregulation) and psychological levels [5]. This neural network might therefore supervise the distribution of cognitive and physiological resources necessary to protect the body surface and the space around it (cf. [12] for the concept of "neuromatrix", a network of brain areas responsible for the subjective experience of pain). Within this network a key role is thought to be played by higher-order (multisensory) areas, such as the posterior parietal cortex (PPC). The PPC is responsible for integrating different (somatotopic and spatial) frames of reference used for the localization of external stimuli and of the position of the body in space, as well as for sustaining a coherent multisensory representation of the body [13]. Following on from these considerations, one might predict that modulation of activity in the PPC may have consequences for homeostatic functions, such as thermoregulatory control.

A number of studies on neurological patients have shown a relationship between brain damage and thermoregulatory control [14–15]. In particular, Naver, Blomstrand, Ekholm, Jensen, Karlsson, and Wallin [16] studied the incidence of symptoms of autonomic dysfunction after the acute phase of stroke. They found that 43% of the patients observed reported a sensation of coldness in the side of the body contralateral to the side of the lesion (contralesional). Moreover, basal skin blood flow and temperature were generally lower in the contralesional side of the patients' bodies. Note, however, that in this study no correlation between the area or size of the lesion and the thermoregulatory dysfunction was reported. Such work was later extended by Riedl, Beckmann, Neundorfer, Handwerker, and Birklein [17] to directly compare autonomic dysfunction in the first few days after stroke to that observed in chronic CRPS, using detailed neurological examination, thermal imaging and evaporation hygrometry. The authors described the two conditions as remarkably similar, leading to the suggestion that autonomic dysfunction have a central origin in the neural system. It is important to note, however, that both studies found no correlation between the area (and side [17]) of the lesion and autonomic control.

As far as a more accurate localization of the brain areas involved in thermoregulatory control is concerned, Ishii, Ohtsuki, Tamaoka, Mizusawa, and Shoji [18] reported two cases of reduced limb temperature following damage to the somatosensory cortex. However, it is worth noting that the presence of subcortical damage and of possible impairment of peripheral nerves in both of these patients undermine any strong conclusion about the causal role of the somatosensory cortex in thermoregulatory control. Satoh, Terada, Onouchi, Takeda, and Kuzuhara [19] also described a patient with somatosensory dysfunction after infarction of the left postcentral gyrus, limited to Brodmann's areas 1 and 2, who showed a decrease in the skin temperature of the right hand. On the basis of this observation, the authors concluded that skin temperature might be controlled somatotopically in the somatosensory cortex, but that further studies were needed in order to clarify the mechanism and the anatomic localization of skin temperature control [19]. To our knowledge, there are no subsequent reports on the possible involvement of the somatosensory cortex on thermoregulatory control in humans (see [20], for the observation of a modulation of body temperature after stimulation of the orbital frontal neocortex in anesthetized rats). In particular, the question of whether or not higher-order cortical areas can modulate the functioning of lower-level physiological mechanisms (as suggested by behavioral evidence; see [5]), still remains unanswered. The present study aimed to clarify this important issue by measuring the effect on body temperature of temporarily interfering with the function of the PPC or S1 using repetitive transcranic magnetic Stimulation (rTMS).

rTMS is a non-invasive technique of brain stimulation that can influence the brain's electrical activity by a pulsed magnetic field. The magnetic field is generated by passing brief current pulses through a coil of wire. An important aspect of rTMS is that the effects of each single pulse can summate with repeated application, leading to effects outlasting a stimulation session [21], [22] and usually to an interference with the stimulated area [22–25].

In order to better explore the neural mechanisms of 'higher order' thermoregulation (i.e., thermoregulatory functions mediated by multisensory associative areas) we used rTMS to interfere with the functioning of PPC or S1. Following on from the body matrix theory [5] highlighted above, our primary hypothesis was that rTMS over PPC (and in particular over the right PPC) would modulate body temperature, but rTMS over S1 would not. Given that the right PPC has been shown to be involved in disorders of body ownership [26], one might expect that the stimulation of this area results in a modulation of body ownership as well as in changes of thermoregulatory control. Finally, considering that previous experiments where bodily illusions were adopted in order to induce changes of thermoregulation have found body-specific effects (e.g., inducing the illusion that the right hand is replaced by a rubber hand results in a reduction of the temperature in the real participant's right hand but not on his/her left hand) one might also expect a body specific modulation of thermoregulatory control following the stimulation of different brain hemispheres.

Methods

Participants

Twenty-four healthy volunteers (12 females) participated in the experiment. Their ages ranged from 20 to 30 years (mean ± S. D. = 24.3±2.5 years). The participants were right-handed, as assessed by a 10-item questionnaire [27], and had no psychiatric, neurological or other relevant medical disorders, as well as no contraindication to TMS [28]. The volunteers gave written informed consent and received course credits in return for their participation. The study reported in this paper was approved by the ethical committee of University of Milano-Bicocca. The experiment was performed in accordance with the ethical standards laid down in the 1991 Declaration of Helsinki.

Materials

Two 17.5 mm×17.5 mm×6 mm 'Thermocron-TC' temperature loggers were used in order to constantly monitor and record the participant's body temperature with an accuracy of 0.07°C (see [29–31]). Readings were then downloaded to a PC by using the proprietary program 'eTemperature'.

The room temperature was measured with a standard mercury thermometer, placed on a desk at approximately 100 cm from the participants. The temperature was recorded three times: 20, 47 and 66 minutes from the beginning of the experimental session. The average temperature measured with this procedure was of 27.5°C (± S.D. of 2.1°C).

The effects of the rTMS stimulation on the participant's perceived ownership of his/her hands were assessed by using two questionnaires (one for each hand) composed of 4 Likert scale questions each (see Appendix S1; cf. [32]).

Procedure

The experiment was performed in a quiet room, with the participants being comfortably seated on a chair in front of a desk. Participants were asked to extend their arms, and rest their hands with their palms down on the desk at a distance of 50 cm from their trunk, and required to reduce to a minimum any body movement for all the duration of the experimental session. The temperature loggers were fixed to the back of the participants' hands with transpiring cotton tape. Temperature values were measured every five seconds for each hand.

The 24 volunteers were randomly assigned to receive rTMS to their left or right hemisphere. Each participant took part in two separate experimental sessions, one for each area stimulated. The two sessions were performed on different days and the order of sessions was counterbalanced across participants. A minimum interval of 24 hours occurred between the first and the second session (mean ± S. D. = 54 h±36.9 h, range 24–216 h).

Each experimental session lasted about 65 minutes, and comprised three phases: 1) baseline pre-TMS phase; 2) rTMS stimulation; and 3) post-rTMS phase (see Figure 1). In the baseline phase, which began after the experimenter had placed the temperature loggers on the participant's hands, the average temperature of the participant's hands was measured for 25 minutes. Hence, rTMS was delivered over PPC or S1 for a period of 20 minutes. Finally, in the last post-rTMS phase the average temperature of the participant's hands was measured again for a period of 20 minutes. At the end of the post-rTMS phase two participants in each group decided to leave the experiment and the remaining participants (N = 10 in each group)

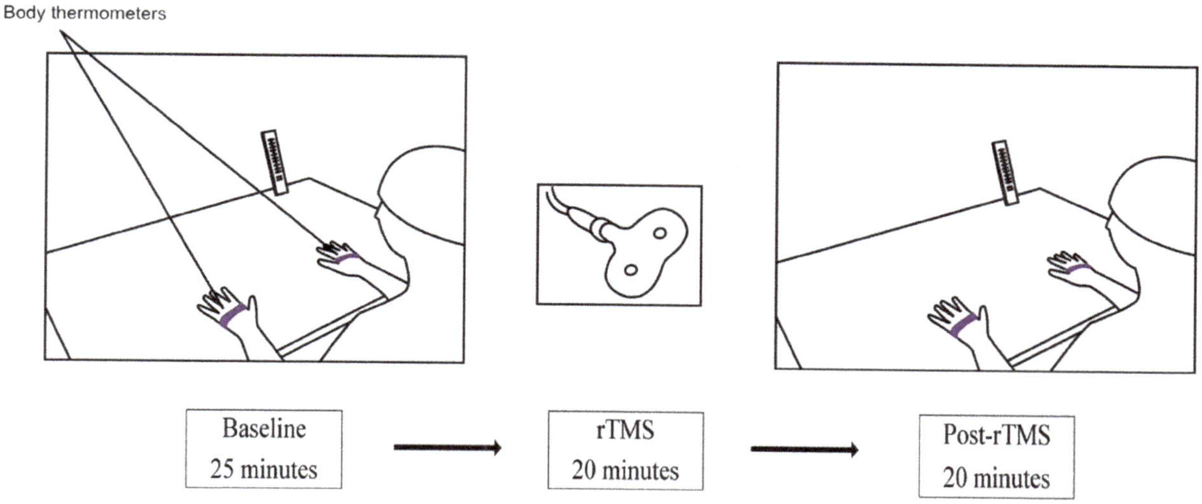

Figure 1. Setup and time course adopted in the present experiment.

were presented with a questionnaire in order to evaluate their sense of ownership regarding their hands (see Appendix S1).

Low-frequency (1 Hz) off-line rTMS was delivered at a fixed intensity of 60% of the maximum stimulator output [33] using a Magstim Super Rapid magnetic stimulator (Magstim, Whitland, UK) and a figure-of-eight coil (70 mm diameter). TMS was applied over the PPC (left or right) and S1 (left or right). The rTMS stimulation sites were individually defined for each participant within the 10–20 electroencephalogram (EEG) coordinate system.

According to previous TMS studies [34], [35], the location of S1 was determined on an individual basis by moving the TMS coil posterior from the scalp location corresponding to the primary motor cortex that was found to produce maximal index finger movements in the contralateral hand. The resting motor threshold value was set to the stimulation level that elicited visible movements of the index finger in five of ten TMS pulses applied to the hand area. The posterior shift was repeated in 5-mm steps until TMS pulses at 120% of the motor threshold produced no visible finger movements and participants reported feeling no muscle twitches in response to the rTMS pulses. For PPC, the area of stimulation corresponded to 1 cm above the position P4 for the right PPC and to 1 cm above the position P3 for the left PPC in the 10:20 EEG system [36], [37]. For both PPC and S1 rTMS, the coil was held tangentially to the scalp, with the handle pointing backwards at an angle of 45° from the midline. For each session, the correct site was marked on the participant's cap and the coil was positioned on that site for the duration of stimulation.

Analysis

The average temperatures measured from both the temperature loggers during the last five minutes of the baseline condition (60 recordings) and the last 19 minutes (228 recordings) of the post-TMS condition were computed. The temperature data recorded during the twenty minutes of rTMS stimulation were not taken into consideration. These data were then submitted to a repeated-measures analysis of variance (ANOVA) with three within-subjects factors (Area: PPC, S1; Time: baseline, pre-rTMS, post-rTMS; Hand: right vs. left), and one between-subjects factor (targeted Hemisphere: right, left). Significant effects were assessed by Newman-Keuls post-hoc multiple comparisons.

The sums of the self-reported ratings of hand ownership from the four questions were also submitted to an ANOVA with two within-subjects factors (Area: PPC, S1; Hand: right, left), and one between-subjects factor (targeted Hemisphere: right, left). Note that, because question 1 referred to ownership, rather than disownership, the participants' responses to question 1 were subtracted from six, in order to make all of the responses homogenous in terms of the ownership effect that was measured (see Table 1, for the means of the responses given by the participants to each item individually).

Results

Figure 2 shows the effects of rTMS (differences between pre and post rTMS values) delivered to the right and left PPC and S1 on temperature of the left and right hand. The temperature in both hands decreased (mean ±SE = : 0.5° Celsius ±0.06° Celsius) after rTMS of the PPC. rTMS to S1 had no effects (mean ± SE: −0.11° Celsius ±0.04° Celsius; see also Figure 3).

The ANOVA showed no significant main effects of Area [$F(1, 22) = 0.21$, $p = .65$, $f^2 = .99$], Time [$F(1, 22) = 1.76$, $p = .20$, $f^2 = .92$], Hand [$F(1, 22) = 0.31$, $p = .58$, $f^2 = .98$], and Hemisphere [$F(1, 22) = 0.03$, $p = .85$, $f^2 = .99$]. Importantly, the Area by Time interaction [$F(1, 22) = 6.27$, $p = .02$, $f^2 = .77$] was significant. Newman-Keuls post-hoc comparisons showed that post rTMS temperature was lower than pre rTMS temperature for PPC stimulation ($p = .04$). No significant differences were reported between pre and post rTMS for S1 stimulation ($p = .52$), nor between S1 and PPC pre rTMS ($p = 0.60$). The Hemisphere by Area [$F(1, 22) = 0.01$, $p = .91$, $f^2 = .99$], Hemisphere by Time [$F(1, 22) = 0.17$, $p = .69$, $f^2 = .99$], Hemisphere by Hand [$F(1, 22) = 1.70$, $p = .21$, $f^2 = .92$], Area by Time by Hemisphere [$F(1, 22) = 0.00$, $p = .96$, $f^2 = .99$], Area by Hand by Hemisphere [$F(1, 22) = 1.82$, $p = .19$, $f^2 = .92$], Area by Time by Hand [$F(1, 22) = 2.59$, $p = .12$, $f^2 = .89$], and Area by Time by Hand by Hemisphere [$F(1, 22) = 0.02$, $p = .90$, $f^2 = .99$] interactions were all not significant.

Figure 4 shows the effects of rTMS delivered to the right and left PPC and S1 on the participants' responses regarding their sense of ownership over the left and right hand. The ANOVA failed to reveal any significant main effect of Area [$F(1,18) = 0.42$, $p = .52$, $f^2 = .97$], Hand $F(1,18) = 1.32$, $p = .26$, $f^2 = .93$] or

Table 1. Mean response to each item of the questionnaire.

LEFT HEMISPHERE																
	PPC								S1							
	Left hand				Right Hand				Left Hand				Right Hand			
	Q. 1	*Q. 2*	*Q. 3*	*Q. 4*	*Q. 1*	*Q. 2*	*Q. 3*	*Q. 4*	*Q. 1*	*Q. 2*	*Q. 3*	*Q. 4*	*Q. 1*	*Q. 2*	*Q. 3*	*Q. 4*
mean response	1.1	1.3	1	1.3	1.1	1	1	1.7	1.1	1.1	1	1.1	1.1	1	1.4	1.7
RIGHT HEMISPHERE																
	PPC								S1							
	Left Hand				Right Hand				Left Hand				Right Hand			
	Q. 1	*Q. 2*	*Q. 3*	*Q. 4*	*Q. 1*	*Q. 2*	*Q. 3*	*Q. 4*	*Q. 1*	*Q. 2*	*Q. 3*	*Q. 4*	*Q. 1*	*Q. 2*	*Q. 3*	*Q. 4*
mean response	1.7	2	1.4	1.8	1.5	1.5	1.3	1.5	1.8	1.9	1.2	1.8	1.1	1	1.3	1.4

Hemisphere [$F(1,18) = 3.52$, $p = .076$, $f^2 = .83$]. The Area by Hand [$F(1,18) = 0.06$, $p = .80$, $f^2 = .99$], Area by Hemisphere [$F(1,18) = 0.42$, $p = .52$, $f^2 = .97$], Hand by Hemisphere [$F(1,18) = 1.72$, $p = .20$, $f^2 = .91$] and Area by Hand by Hemisphere [$F(1,18) = 0.6$, $p = .45$, $f^2 = .96$] interactions were also not significant. That is, no changes in the participants' feelings of ownership regarding their right or left hand were reported after rTMS stimulation of either PPC or S1.

Discussion

We hypothesised that rTMS over PPC would disrupt thermoregulation but rTMS over S1 would not. Our results clearly uphold this hypothesis – temperature of both hands was 0.5 degrees lower after rTMS over PPC, but was not significantly different after rTMS over S1. Our findings provide clear evidence that disruption of higher-order associative brain areas in humans can disrupt homeostatic control.

The results reported here offer additional empirical support for several studies that demonstrate that behavioral manipulations concerning the position of the body in space, as well as the sense of body ownership, can affect thermoregulatory control (see [5] for a review). Moreover, our findings are consistent with a recent model that suggests that a network of brain areas, comprising PPC, the premotor and the insular cortices, might play a crucial role in maintaining the integrity of the body at both the homeostatic (i.e., thermoregulation) and psychological (i.e., in terms of perception and the sense of body ownership) levels [5]. Within this structure, named the 'body matrix', multisensory information regarding the body and the space around it is constantly (and likely automatically) integrated. The results of the experiment reported here fully support this view by showing that a reversible functional interference of PPC, such as that provoked by rTMS, disrupts thermoregulatory control. The results of the present experiment therefore provide the first direct evidence that PPC might exert a top-down modulation of thermoregulatory control. It is, however, relevant to note that previous studies have shown that this brain area is part of a cortical/subcortical network involved in processing information regarding changes of body temperature [38]. That is, the PPC might be involved in both processing incoming signals regarding a variation of core body temperature, as well as in affecting the functioning of those efferent systems responsible for modulating such homeostatic variable.

It is important to highlight that our findings may also be in agreement with a large number of studies suggesting that higher order brain areas involved in integrating multisensory information, and in recalibrating information on the basis of different spatial frames of reference, also play a crucial role in supporting our representation of the body and our sense of body ownership [39–44]. Specifically, the present study extends these findings to suggest that these brain areas, and the PPC in particular, might also exert a top down influence on physiological mechanisms such as thermoregulatory control, related to the protection of the body integrity, a function strictly related to body ownership. This possibility has implications for chronic pain that extend beyond the condition of CRPS. For example, a recent discovery shows a spatially-defined disruption of tactile processing, similar to that observed in CRPS [1], in people with chronic unilateral back pain [45]. One might predict that, if the integration of spatial processing with autonomic control extends to the trunk, then autonomic dysfunction will also be observed in this patients' group. It is, however, worth mentioning that PPC is not a single general multimodal processor, but has distinct functional subregions in the monkey and human (see [46] for a review). Therefore,

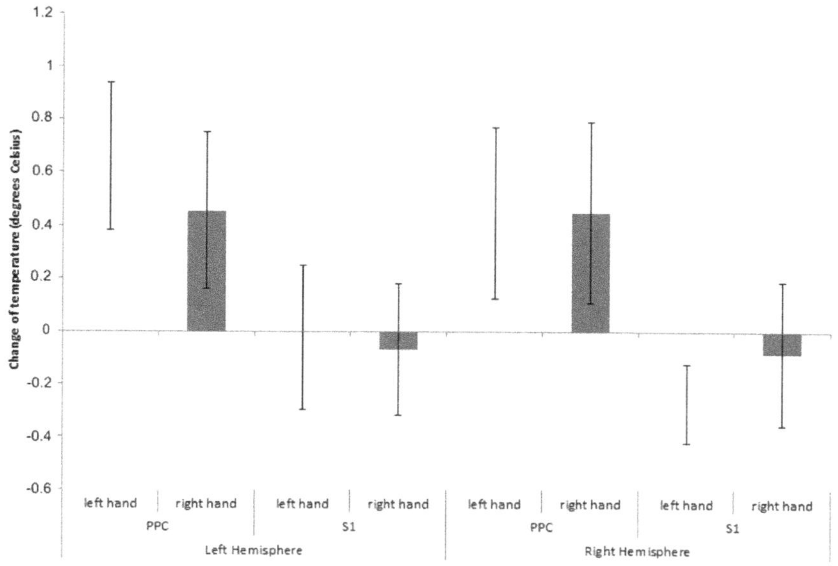

Figure 2. Mean decrease and standard errors of the mean (based on 288 observations per participant) in the temperature of the participants' hands (baseline minus post rTMS) as a function of the stimulated area (PPC = Posterior Parietal Cortex; S1 = Primary Somatosensory Cortex), and of the stimulated brain hemisphere. Temperature is reported using degrees Celsius. Positive values indicate higher temperatures measured in the baseline as compared to the post rTMS condition and viceversa.

further research might also target which specific areas of the PPC are involved in thermoregulatory control.

From a neurological standpoint, lesions of the anterior parietal lobe, including S1, may bring about a contralateral deficit of temperature sensation, together with a deficit of touch, pain, tactile discrimination and stereognosis [47], [48]. Damage to the superior parietal lobule of the PPC affects mainly tactile discrimination and stereognosis [49], and sensorimotor integration [50]. When the inferior parietal lobule of the PPC is damaged, deficits such as tactile agnosia may be found [51]. Although the majority of studies do not report hemispheric asymmetries [52], there is evidence that somatosensory deficits are more frequent after damage to the right hemisphere than to the left [53], which probably reflects a main role of the right hemisphere for somatosensory attention and perception, for both the left contralateral, and the right ipsilateral, sides of the body [54–56]. This hemispheric asymmetry may be related to the fact that awareness of somatosensory events involves their coding in spatial reference frames, an operation for which the right hemisphere is specialized [57–60]. Conversely, more basic processes supported by the body matrix [5], such as thermoregulation, and, as recent evidence suggests - immune regulation [4] - might be more

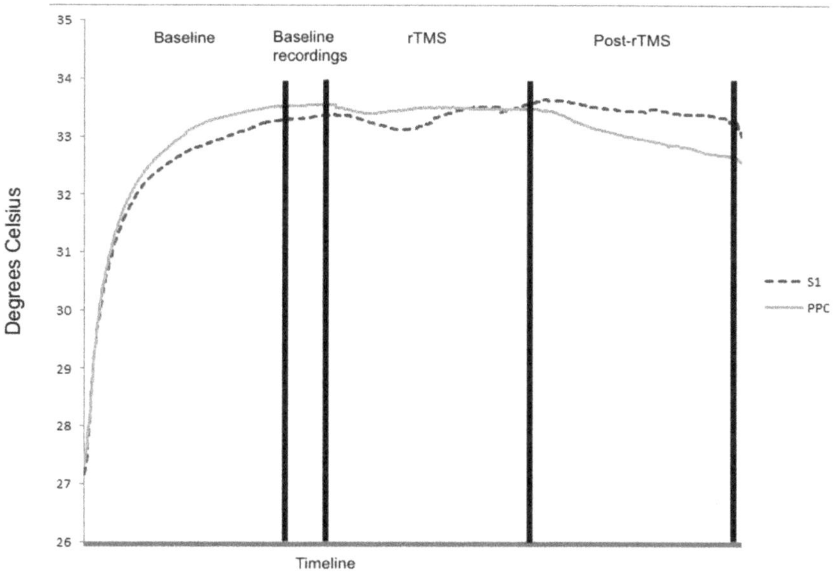

Figure 3. The mean temperatures recorded during all the experiment divided by site of rTMS stimulation.

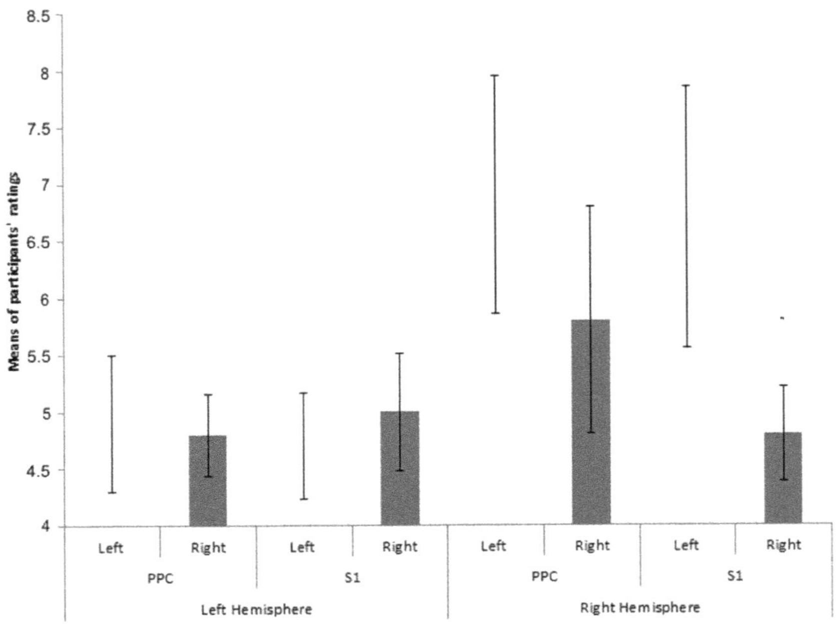

Figure 4. Questionnaire data. Means and standard error of the means of the individual sum of participants' ratings (ranging from 1 to 5) regarding the 4 statements of the questionnaire by stimulated area (PPC = Posterior Parietal Cortex; S1 = Primary Somatosensory Cortex), stimulated brain hemisphere, and participants' hand (left or right). Higher values represent larger sensations of body disownership regarding the specific body part investigated.

symmetrically-distributed across the two cerebral hemispheres. This suggestion would appear to be confirmed by the lack of differences found in the present experiment between rTMS over the right and left PPC on thermoregulatory control.

In the present experiment no differences between the two hands were reported in the decrease of temperature elicited by rTMS over the PPC. By contrast, behavioral experiments have shown body district-specific effects on thermoregulatory control ([1], [5], though see [61], for a lack of body-district specific effects when a full body illusion is elicited). Here one might speculate on whether this lack of more specific effects might be due to the fact that the body matrix likely comprises both motor and perceptual systems [5]. That is, body district-specific effects might be related to the functioning of the motor (i.e., the premotor cortex) rather than to the more perceptual components of the body matrix. Note in fact that one of the ultimate purposes of this cortical network is to protect the body integrity by performing accurate movements. Moreover, there is ample evidence showing that representations posterior to SI, such as those in SII receive inputs from both body sides [62], [63], (cf. [64], for a review on the presence of neurons with bilateral receptive fields also within S1 in animals).

As far as the point of the lack of body specific effects is concerned, it is worth noting here that behavioural experiments where the modulation of thermoregulatory control was confined to a specific body district have adopted the paradigm of the rubber hand illusion [1], [5]. Within such paradigm the participants who are exposed to visuo-tactile synchronous information, start to perceive that a fake hand is part of their own body. One might then argue that, despite of the body specificity of the effect that this illusion exerts on thermoregulatory control, no motor components seems to be involved in generating the phenomenon (in fact the participants keep their arm still). However, one should consider that changes in the perception of where or body is in space, likely involves the access to the body schema, where information regarding the position of the body is continuously updated in order to program accurate movements towards external space. One might therefore speculate that the motor component of the body matrix is activated also under such condition of stimulus presentation. As far as this concept is concerned, it is important to notice that studies on the rubber hand illusion have shown that changes in the perceived position of one's body often occur without any alteration of the participant's sense of body ownership [65].

It should also be considered, that the results reported in the present study might not be due to the fact that interference over PPC disrupts the activity of a network involved in supporting a representation of the body and the sense of body ownership (note in fact that we did not find any changes in body ownership following the stimulation of PPC, see also below). By contrast, they might result from a disruption in the functioning of a network involved in directing attention towards external space. In fact, a number of studies on brain damaged patients, as well as on neurological unimpaired participants, have clearly shown that the PPC is part of a neural circuit involved in the deployment of spatial and selective attention in humans [55], (see also [66], [67] for TMS studies). It is however important to note, that no study has so far directly investigated the role of attentional shifts on thermoregulatory control (though see [8] for the effect of prism adaptation – a procedure that has been shown to modulate spatial attention mechanisms – on thermoregulatory control in patients affected by chronic regional pain syndrome). This topics certainly deserves to be addressed in the near future.

The results from the questionnaire, showed that interference with the functioning of PPC or S1 does not result into an impairment of the participants' sense of body ownership. This result might be taken to suggest that rTMS over PPC might affect in different fashions, physiological and cognitive functions. However, before drawing any conclusion on the basis of this result, one should consider that the participants in our study were not neurologically damaged patients and they certainly knew that the arm in front of them was their own arm. That is, the effect of rTMS might be not as powerful to overcome people's explicit beliefs and expectations regarding their body ownership, but sufficient to alter their (implicitly-controlled) physiological responses. It certainly remains possible that different effects of rTMS might be expected when more robust measuring tools thought to be affected by illusions of body ownership, such as the spatial localization of a person's own body parts, are used instead.

In conclusion, the results of the present experiment show that higher order cortical areas such as PPC might play an important role in sustaining and/or modulating lower level physiological functions such as thermoregulatory control.

Supporting Information

Appendix S1 Ownership of right/left hand questionnaire.

Author Contributions

Conceived and designed the experiments: AG ZC GLM GV. Performed the experiments: GS. Analyzed the data: GS AG. Wrote the paper: AG ZC GS GLM.

References

1. Moseley GL, Olthof N, Venema A, Don S, Wijers M, et al. (2008) Psychologically induced cooling of a specific body part caused by the illusory ownership of an artificial counterpart. Proceedings of the National Academy of Science USA 105: 13169–13173.
2. Tsakiris M, Tajadura-Jiménez AT, Costantini M (2011) Just a heartbeat away from one's body: interoceptive sensitivity predicts malleability of body-representations. Proceedings of the Royal Society Biological Sciences 278: 2470–2476.
3. Kammers MP, Rose K, Haggard P (2011) Feeling numb: Temperature, but not thermal pain, modulates feeling of body ownership. Neuropsychologia 49: 1316–1321.
4. Barnsley N, McAuley J, Mohan R, Dey A, Thomas P, et al. (2011) The rubber hand illusion increases histamine reactivity in the real arm. Current Biology 21: R945–R946.
5. Moseley GL, Gallace A, Spence C (2012) Bodily illusion in health and disease: physiological and clinical perspectives and the concept of a cortical body matrix. Neuroscience & Biobehavioural Reviews 36: 34–46.
6. Moseley GL, Gallace A, Spence C (2009) Space-based, but not arm-based, shift in tactile processing in complex regional pain syndrome and its relationship to cooling of the affected limb. Brain 132: 3142–3151.
7. Moseley GL, Gallace A, Iannetti GD (2012) Spatially defined modulation of skin temperature and hand ownership of both hands in patients with unilateral complex regional pain syndrome. Brain 135: 3676–3686.
8. Moseley GL, Gallace A, di Pietro F, Spence C, Iannetti GD (2013) Limb-specific autonomic dysfunction in complex regional pain syndrome modulated by wearing prism glasses. Pain. doi:pii: S0304-3959(13)00394-1. 10.1016/j.pain.2013.07.026.
9. Petchkrua W, Weiss DJ, Patel RR (2000) Reassessment of the incidence of complex regional pain syndrome type 1 following stroke. Neurorehabilitation and Neural Repair 14: 59–63.
10. Marinus J, Moseley GL, Birklein F, Baron R, Maihöfner C, et al. (2011) Clinical features and pathophysiology of complex regional pain syndrome. Lancet Neurology 10: 637–648.
11. Acerra NE, Souvlis T, Moseley GL (2007) Stroke, complex regional pain syndrome and phantom limb pain: Can Commonalities Direct Future Management? Journal of Rehabilitation Medicine 39: 109–114.
12. Melzack R (1990) Phantom limbs and the concept of a neuromatrix. Trends in Neurosciences 13: 88–92.
13. Ehrsson HH, Holmes NP, Passingham RE (2005) Touching a rubber hand: feeling of body ownership is associated with activity in multisensory brain areas. Journal of Neuroscience 25: 10564–10573.
14. Ellis LB, Weiss S. (1936) Vasomotor disturbance and oedema associated with cerebral hemiplegia. Archives of Neurology & Psychiatry 35: 362–372.
15. Wanklyn P, Isley DW, Greenstein D, Hampton IFG, Roper TA, et al. (1994) The cold hemiplegic arm. Stroke 25: 1765–1770.
16. Naver H, Blomstrand C, Ekholm S, Jensen C, Karlsson T, et al. (1995) Autonomic and thermal sensory symptoms and dysfunction after stroke. Stroke; A journal of cerebral circulation 26: 1379–1385.
17. Riedl B, Beckmann T, Neundorfer B, Handwerker HO, Birklein F (2001) Autonomic failure after stroke–is it indicative for pathophysiology of complex regional pain syndrome? Acta Neurologica Scandinavica 103: 27–34.
18. Ishii K, Ohkoshi N, Tamaoka A, Mizusawa H, Shoji S (1996) Pseudoradicular sensory impairment caused by parietal lesions. Report of two cases. Rinsho Shinkeigaku. Clinical Neurology 36: 951–956.
19. Satoh M, Terada S, Onouchi K, Takeda K, Kuzuhara S (2002) Somatosensory and skin temperature disturbances caused by infarction of the postcentral gyrus: a case report. Journal of Neurology 249: 1404–1408.
20. De Luca B, Monda M, Amaro S, Pellicano MP, Ciuffi LA (1989) Thermogenic changes following frontal neocortex stimulation. Brain Research Bulletin 22: 1003–1007.
21. Robertson EM, Théoret H, Pascual-Leone A (2003) Studies in cognition: The problems solved and created by transcranial magnetic stimulation. Journal of Cognitive Neuroscience 15: 948–960.
22. Hallett M (2007) Transcranial magnetic stimulation: A primer. Neuron, 55: 187–199.
23. Miniussi C, Ruzzoli M, Walsh V (2010) The mechanism of transcranial magnetic stimulation in cognition. Cortex 46: 128–130.
24. Walsh V, Cowey A (2000) Transcranial magnetic stimulation and cognitive neuroscience. Nature Reviews Neuroscience 1: 73–79.
25. Fregni F, Pascual-Leone A (2007) Technology insight: Noninvasive brain stimulation in neurology-perspectives on the therapeutic potential of rTMS and tDCS. Nature Clinical Practice Neurology 3: 383–393.
26. Vallar G, Ronchi R (2009) Somatoparaphrenia: A body delusion. A review of the neuropsychological literature. Experimental Brain Research 192: 533–551.
27. Oldfield RC (1971) The assessment and analysis of handedness: the Edinburgh inventory. Neuropsychologia 9: 97–113.
28. Rossi S, Hallett M, Rossini PM, Pascual-Leone A (2009) Safety, ethical considerations, and application guidelines for the use of transcranial magnetic stimulation in clinical practice and research. Clinical Neurophysiology 120: 2008–2039.
29. Harper Smith AD, Crabtree DR, Bilzon JLJ, Walsh NP (2010) The validity of wireless iButtons and thermistors for human skin temperature measurement. Physiological Measurement 31: 95–114.
30. Hasselberg MJ, McMahon J, Parker K The validity, reliability, and utility of the ibutton for measurement of body temperature circadian rhythms in sleep/wake research. Sleep Medicine In press.
31. van Marken Lichtenbelt WD, Daanen HAM, Wouters L, Fronczek R, Raymann RJEM, et al. (2006) Evaluation of wireless determination of skin temperature using iButtons. Physiology & Behavior 88: 489–497
32. Botvinick M, Cohen J. (1998) Rubber hands "feel" touch that eyes see. Nature 391: 756.
33. Cappelletti M, Barth H, Fregni F, Spelke ES, Pascual-Leone A (2007) rTMS over the intraparietal sulcus disrupts numerosity processing. Experimental Brain Research 179: 631–642.
34. Fiorio M, Haggard P (2005) Viewing the body prepares the brain for touch: effects of tms over somatosensory cortex. European Journal of Neuroscience 22: 773–777.
35. Oliveira FTP, Diedrichsen J, Verstynen T, Duque J, Ivry RB (2010) Transcranial magnetic stimulation of posterior parietal cortex affects decisions of hand choice. Proceedings of the National Academy of Sciences 107: 17751–17756.
36. Herwig U, Satrapi P, Schonfeldt-Lecuona C (2003) Using the international 10–20 EEG system for positioning of transcranial magnetic stimulation. Brain Topography 16: 95–99.
37. Okamoto M, Dan H, Sakamoto K, Takeo K, Shimizu K, et al. (2004) Three-dimensional probabilistic anatomical cranio-cerebral correlation via the international 10–20 system oriented for transcranial functional brain mapping. Neuroimage 21: 99–111.
38. Egan GF, Johnson J, Farrell M, McAllen R, Zamarripa F, et al. (2005) Cortical, thalamic, and hypothalamic responses to cooling and warming the skin in awake humans: a positron-emission tomography study. Proceedings of the National Academy of Sciences 102: 5262–5267.
39. Giummarra MJ, Gibson SJ, Georgiou-Karistianis N, Bradshaw JL (2008) Mechanisms underlying embodiment, disembodiment and loss of embodiment. Neuroscience and Biobehavioural Reviews 32:143–160.
40. Longo MR, Schüür F, Kammers MPM, Tsakiris M, Haggard P (2008) What is embodiment? a psychometric approach. Cognition 107: 978–998.
41. Makin TR, Holmes NP, Ehrsson HH (2008) On the other hand: Dummy hands and peripersonal space. Behavioural Brain Research 191: 1–10.
42. Tsakiris M (2010) My body in the brain: A neurocognitive model of body-ownership. Neuropsychologia 48: 703–712.
43. Tsakiris M, Costantini M, Haggard P (2008) The role of the right temporo-parietal junction in maintaining a coherent sense of one's body. Neuropsychologia 46: 3014–3018.
44. Tsakiris M, Longo MR Haggard P (2010) Having a body versus moving your body: neural signatures of agency and body-ownership. Neuropsychologia 48: 2740–2749.
45. Moseley GL, Gallagher L, Gallace A (2012) Neglect-like tactile dysfunction in chronic back pain. Neurology 79: 327–332.

46. Grefkes C, Fink GR (2005) The functional organization of the intraparietal sulcus in humans and monkeys. Journal of Anatomy 207: 3–17.
47. Bassetti C, Bugousslavsky J, Regli F (1993) Sensory syndromes in parietal stroke. Neurology 43: 1942–1949.
48. Kim JS (2007) Patterns of sensory abnormality in cortical stroke. evidence for a dichotomized sensory system. Neurology 68: 174–180.
49. Freund H-J (2003) Somatosensory and motor disturbances in patients with parietal lobe lesions. Advances in Neurology 93: 179–193.
50. Wolpert DM, Goodbody SJ, Husain M (1998) Maintaining internal representations: The role of the human superior parietal lobe. Nature Neuroscience 1: 529–533.
51. Reed CL, Caselli RJ, Farah MJ (1996) Tactile agnosia. Underlying impairment and implications for normal tactile object recognition. Brain 119: 875–888.
52. Dijkerman HC, de Haan EH (2007) Somatosensory processes subserving perception and action. Behavioral and Brain Sciences 30: 189–201.
53. Sterzi R, Bottini G, Celani MG, Righetti E, Lamassa M, et al. (1993) Hemianopia, hemianaesthesia, and hemiplegia after left and right hemisphere damage: A hemispheric difference. Journal of Neurology Neurosurgery and Psychiatry 56: 308–310.
54. Bottini G, Paulesu E, Gandola M, Loffredo S, Scarpa P, et al. (2005) Left caloric vestibular stimulation ameliorates right hemianesthesia. Neurology 65: 1278–1283.
55. Pardo JV, Fox PT, Raichle ME (1991) Localization of a human system for sustained attention by positron emission tomography. Nature 349: 61–64.
56. Vallar G (2007) A hemispheric asymmetry in somatosensory processing. Behavioral and Brain Sciences 30: 223–224.
57. Gallace A, Spence C (2008) The cognitive and neural correlates of "tactile consciousness": a multisensory perspective. Consciousness and Cognition 17: 370–407.
58. Gallace A, Spence C (2010) The role of the somatosensory cortex in the awareness of tactile information. Psyche 16: 30–67.
59. Kitazawa S (2002) Where conscious sensation takes place. Consciousness and Cognition 11: 475–477.
60. Vallar G (1997) Spatial frames of reference and somatosensory processing: a neuropsychological perspective. In N. . Burgess, K. J. . Jeffery & J. . O'Keefe (Eds.), The Hippocampal and Parietal Foundations of Spatial Cognition (pp. 33–49). Oxford: Oxford University Press.
61. Salomon R, Lim M, Pfeiffer C, Gassert R, Blanke O (2013) Full body illusion is associated with widespread skin temperature reduction. Frontiers in Behavioral Neurosciences 7: 65. doi: 10.3389/fnbeh.2013.00065
62. Blatow M, Nennig E, Durst A, Sartor K, Stippich C (2007) fMRI reflects functional connectivity of human somatosensory cortex. Neuroimage 37: 927–936.
63. Ferretti A, Babiloni C, Gratta CD, Caulo M, Tartaro A, et al.(2003) Functional topography of the secondary somatosensory cortex for nonpainful and painful stimuli: an fMRI study. Neuroimage 20: 1625–1638.
64. Iwamura Y (2000) Bilateral receptive field neurons and callosal connections in the somatosensory cortex. Philosophical Transactions of the Royal Society of London B 355: 267–273.
65. Rohde M, Di Luca M, Ernst MO (2011) The Rubber Hand Illusion: feeling of ownership and proprioceptive drift do not go hand in hand. PloS one 6(6): e21659
66. Blankenburg F, Ruff CC, Bestmann S, Bjoertomt O, Josephs O, et al. (2010) Studying the role of human parietal cortex in visuospatial attention with concurrent TMS-fMRI. Cerebral Cortex 20: 2702–2711.
67. Hung J, Driver J, Walsh V (2005) Visual selection and posterior parietal cortex: effects of repetitive transcranial magnetic stimulation on partial report analyzed by Bundesen's theory of visual attention. Journal of Neuroscience 25: 9602–9612.

4

Behavioral and Histopathological Assessment of Adult Ischemic Rat Brains after Intracerebral Transplantation of NSI-566RSC Cell Lines

Naoki Tajiri[1], David M. Quach[2], Yuji Kaneko[1], Stephanie Wu[2], David Lee[2], Tina Lam[2], Ken L. Hayama[2], Thomas G. Hazel[2], Karl Johe[2], Michael C. Wu[3], Cesar V. Borlongan[1]*

1 Center of Excellence for Aging & Brain Repair, Department of Neurosurgery and Brain Repair, University of South Florida College of Medicine, Tampa, Florida, United States of America, **2** Neuralstem, Inc., Rockville, Maryland, United States of America, **3** Neurodigitech, LLC., San Diego, California, United States of America

Abstract

Stroke is a major cause of death and disability, with very limited treatment option. Cell-based therapies have emerged as potential treatments for stroke. Indeed, studies have shown that transplantation of neural stem cells (NSCs) exerts functional benefits in stroke models. However, graft survival and integration with the host remain pressing concerns with cell-based treatments. The current study set out to investigate those very issues using a human NSC line, NSI-566RSC, in a rat model of ischemic stroke induced by transient occlusion of the middle cerebral artery. Seven days after stroke surgery, those animals that showed significant motor and neurological impairments were randomly assigned to receive NSI-566RSC intracerebral transplants at two sites within the striatum at three different doses: group A (0 cells/μl), group B (5,000 cells/μl), group C (10,000 cells/μl), and group D (20,000 cells/μl). Weekly behavioral tests, starting at seven days and continued up to 8 weeks after transplantation, revealed dose-dependent recovery from both motor and neurological deficits in transplanted stroke animals. Eight weeks after cell transplantation, immunohistochemical investigations via hematoxylin and eosin staining revealed infarct size was similar across all groups. To identify the cell graft, and estimate volume, immunohistochemistry was performed using two human-specific antibodies: one to detect all human nuclei (HuNu), and another to detect human neuron-specific enolase (hNSE). Surviving cell grafts were confirmed in 10/10 animals of group B, 9/10 group C, and 9/10 in group D. hNSE and HuNu staining revealed similar graft volume estimates in transplanted stroke animals. hNSE-immunoreactive fibers were also present within the corpus callosum, coursing in parallel with host tracts, suggesting a propensity to follow established neuroanatomical features. Despite absence of reduction in infarct volume, NSI-566RSC transplantation produced behavioral improvements possibly via robust engraftment and neuronal differentiation, supporting the use of this NSC line for stroke therapy.

Editor: Eva Mezey, National Institutes of Health, United States of America

Funding: CVB received research support from Neuralstem Inc for this study. DMQ, SW, DL, TL, KLH, TGH and KJ are employed by the funder of this study, Neuralstem Inc. CVB is supported by National Institutes of Health, National Institute of Neurological Disorders and Stroke 1R01NS071956-01 and James and Esther King Foundation for Biomedical Research Program. The funder provided support in the form of salaries for authors DMQ, SW, DL, TL, KLH, TGH and KJ, but did not have any additional role in the study design, data collection and analysis, decision to publish, or preparation of the manuscript. The specific roles of these authors are articulated in the 'author contributions' section.

Competing Interests: I have read the journal's policy and have the following conflicts: CVB received research support from Neuralstem Inc for this study. DMQ, SW, DL, TL, KLH, TGH and KJ are employed by the funder of this study, Neuralstem Inc. MCW is employed by Neurodigitech, LLC. CVB is supported by National Institutes of Health, National Institute of Neurological Disorders and Stroke 1R01NS071956-01 and James and Esther King Foundation for Biomedical Research Program.

* E-mail: cborlong@health.usf.edu

Introduction

Stroke is a major unmet clinical need with only one current FDA-approved drug, the tissue plasminogen activator (tPA) [1–5]. The efficacy of tPA is limited to 4.5 hours after stroke onset and benefits only about 3% of ischemic stroke patients [6–8]. The advent of stem cell therapy opens the possibility of regenerating the injured brain and may prove effective in stroke beyond the acute phase of the disease [9–13]. With the increasing diversity of stem cell sources emerging for donor cells in transplantation therapy, many laboratory-to-clinic translational factors must first be considered, dynamics such as the source of the cells, ease of extraction, immunogenicity, capacity for proliferation, and cell yield [14–16]. These concerns may serve as potential limitations respective to the donor cell origin being considered, necessitating the need for a particular stem cell source to be more suitable for a specific disease.

Because stroke is a major cause of death and disability, any treatment that would help stroke patients recover some of the lost motor or cognitive function, would substantially improve their quality of life. Cell-based therapies have emerged as potential methods to treat several neuropathological diseases and injuries, including stroke [1–5,9–13]. Laboratory studies and limited clinical trials have shown that transplantation of neural stem cells (NSCs) in stroke is safe and effective [17–20]. The mechanism of action of stem cell therapy for stroke remains not fully understood,

Table 1. Experimental Treatment Conditions.

Group	Group Size	Test Article	Dose	Survival Time
A	8	Vehicle	0 cells/μL×3 μl/site×3 sites	56+/−4 days
B	8	NSI-566RSC	5,000 cells/μL×3 μl/site×3 sites	56+/−4 days
C	8	NSI-566RSC	10,000 cells/μL×3 μl/site×3 sites	56+/−4 days
D	8	NSI-566RSC	20,000 cells/μL×3 μl/site×3 sites	56+/−4 days

Treatment Summary Table. Table 1 summarizes the 4 treatment groups of randomly assigned stroke animals.

but the two major postulated reparative pathways involve cell replacement and secretion of growth factors [1–5,9–13,21,22]. To date, graft survival and integration with the host remain pressing concerns with cell-based treatment options. The current study set out to investigate those very issues using a human NSC line, NSI-566RSC, in a rat model of ischemic stroke.

Preclinical evidence has demonstrated the safety and efficacy of NSI-566RSC in animal models of the motor neuron disease amyotrophic lateral sclerosis (ALS) [23–26], spinal cord injury [27], and ischemic paraplegia [28]. Larger animal models have also been used to assess safety of NSI-566RSC for CNS transplantation [29,30]. Functional recovery observed in these animal models has been ascribed to neuronal differentiation capacity of NSI-566RSC [25,31], which parallels extensive *in vitro* characterization of these cells similarly demonstrating the cells' ability to display neuronal phenotypic features (i.e., functional motoneurons) [32,33]. The need for immunosuppression in order to augment graft survival and functional effects has been indicated in relevant ALS animal models [30,34]. This translational research portfolio forms the basis for a clinical trial of transplanting NSI-566RSC in ALS patients [35].

Our long-standing interest in stem cell therapy for stroke prompted us to examine the efficacy of NSI-566RSC in an animal model of cerebral ischemia. We report here that intracerebral transplantation of NSI-566RSC at subacute phase of stroke produced behavioral improvements accompanied by graft survival and neuronal differentiation, extending the application of NSI-566RSC for transplantation therapy in ischemic stroke.

Materials and Methods

Subjects

All experiments were conducted in accordance with the National Institute of Health Guide and Use of Laboratory Animals, and were approved by the Institutional Animal Care and Use Committee of the University of South Florida, Morsani College of Medicine. Rats were housed two per cage in a temperature- and humidity-controlled room that was maintained on 12/12 hour-light/dark cycles. They had free access to food and water. All necessary steps were performed to minimize animal pain and stress throughout the study.

Stroke and Transplant Surgery

A total of 32 male Sprague-Dawley rats received middle cerebral artery occlusion (MCAo), a well-established stroke model, as described previously [36–40]. Animals were anesthetized using isoflurane (1.5%–2.5% with oxygen). The scalp skin was shaved and scrubbed with alcohol and chlorhexidine surgical scrub. The animal was fixed in stereotaxic apparatus, then starting slightly behind the eyes, a midline sagittal incision about 2.5 cm long is

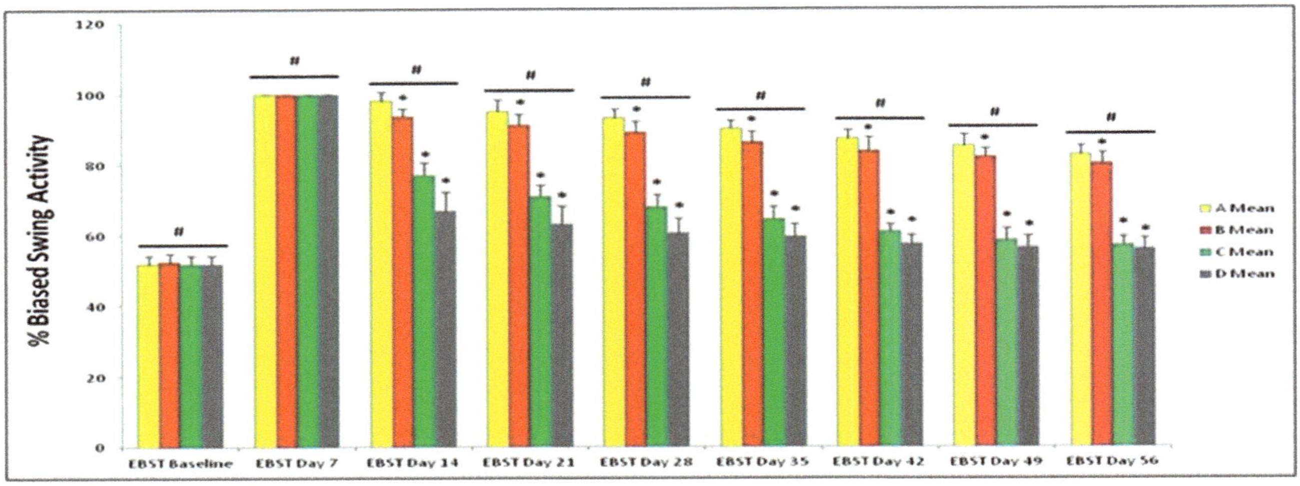

Figure 1. NSI-566RSC cell grafts ameliorate stroke-induced motor deficits. Motor performance was measured by EBST (Figure 1). All animals displayed normal motor behavior at Baseline (i.e., prior to stroke). At day 7 post-stroke, all animals exhibited 100% biased swing behaviors, indicating that all animals received successful stroke. At 14 days post-stroke onwards, dose-dependent and timing-dependent effects of the treatment were recognized, in that the improvement in behavioral performance was in the order of high dose to zero dose as follows: 20,000 cells/μl (D) >10,000 cells/μl (C) >5,000 cells/μl (B)>vehicle infusion only (A). In addition, over time there was a trend of better improvement, with the most significant improvement seen at 56 days post-stroke. *significant <0.05 vs. other treatment groups within time point; #significant <0.05 vs. other time points.

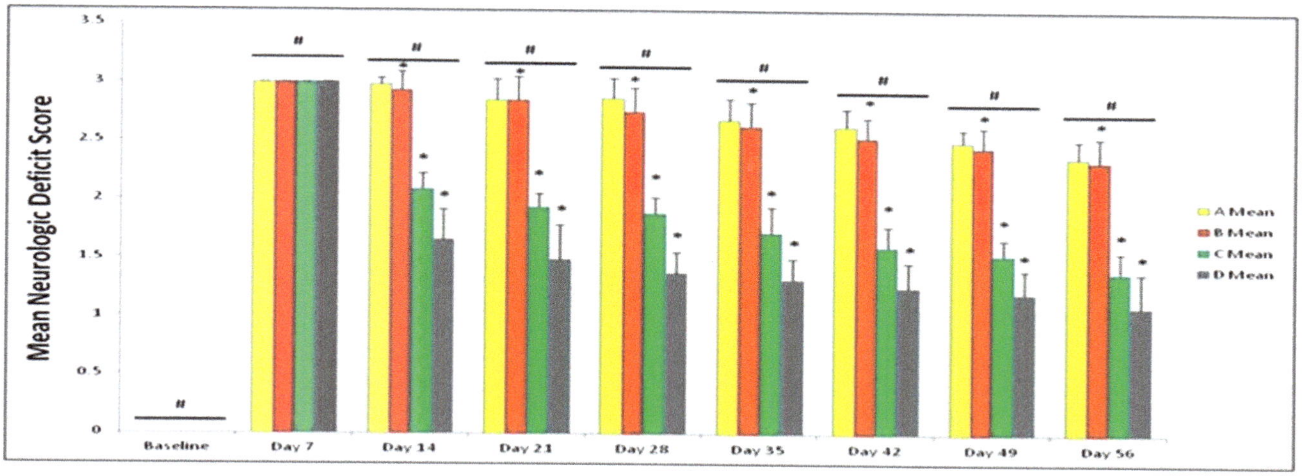

Figure 2. NSI-566RSC cell grafts attenuate stroke-induced neurologic impairments. Neurological function was assessed using a battery of neurological tests (Figure 2). All animals displayed normal neurological function at Baseline (i.e., prior to stroke). At day 7 post-stroke, all animals exhibited significant impairment in neurological function, indicating that all animals received successful stroke. At 14 days post-stroke onwards, dose-dependent and timing-dependent effects of the treatment were recognized, in that the improvement in neurological performance was in the order of high dose to zero dose as follows: 20,000 cells/μl (D) >10,000 cells/μl (C) >5,000 cells/μl (B)>vehicle infusion only (A). In addition, over time there was a trend of better improvement, with the most significant improvement seen at 56 days post-stroke. *significant <0.05 vs. other treatment groups within time point; #significant <0.05 vs. other time points.

made. With the rounded end of a spatula, the skull area was exposed. Using the bregma as reference point (i.e., prior to stroke surgery) laser Doppler recordings were obtained from the following coordinates (AP: +2.0, ML: ±2.0) at pre, during, and post surgery to reveal successful MCAo. The skin on the ventral neck was shaved from the jaw to the manubrium and scrubbed with alcohol and chlorhexidine surgical scrub. A skin incision was made over the right common carotid artery. The external carotid was isolated and ligated as far distally as possible. An incision using a pair of microscissor was made in the stump of the external carotid and a 4-0 nylon filament with a pre-fabricated end was inserted and passed up into the internal carotid artery until resistance was felt (approximately 15–17 mm), which effectively blocked the middle cerebral artery (MCA). The isoflurane was discontinued and the animal placed in a recovery cage over a warming blanket. After 60 minutes, the animal was anesthetized again with isoflurane and the incision opened. The filament causing the occlusion was removed and the stump of the external carotid ligated close to the carotid bifurcation. The skin incision was closed with staples. Finally, the animal was placed in a cage over a warming blanket until full recovery from anesthesia. Forty stroke animals were randomly divided into four Groups A–D (Table 1). They were tested for behavioral and neurological deficits on Day 6 post stroke (baseline), and then treated on Day 7 post stroke. Those animals that showed significant motor and neurological impairments were randomly assigned to receive NSI-566RSC intracerebral transplants at two sites within the striatum at three different doses: group A (0 cells/μl), group B (5,000 cells/μl), group C (10,000 cells/μl), and group D (20,000 cells/μl). The animal was fixed to a stereotaxic apparatus (Kopf Instruments). A 26-gauge Hamilton syringe was then lowered into a small burred skull opening (transplant coordinates were adjusted to 0.5 mm

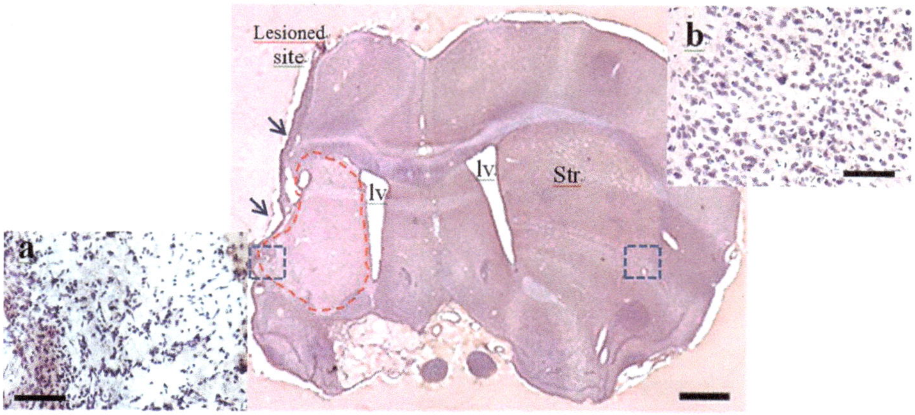

Figure 3. A typical infarct lesion in the striatum and cortex. The tissue damage covers the cortex and infarct striatum (dash area) and areas lateral to infarct core lesion (not shown here). Note the shrinkage and dissolution of the cells in the penumbra (box) compared to the corresponding contralateral side of the brain (Insets a and b). Scale bar = 1.0 mm [lv; lateral ventricles, Str: striatum].

Table 2. Summary of histological assessment of infarct brains transplanted with NSI-566RSC (n = 10 per group)*.

	Stains	Group A-Vehicle	Group B-Low	Group C-Medium	Group D-High	Mean-Total
Freq. of the infarct lesion**	*H&E*	9 (90%)	9 (90%)	9 (90%)	10 (100%)	93%
Freq. of surviving grafts in the striatum	*HuNu*	Not present	10 (100%)	9 (90%)	9 (90%)	93%
	hNSE	Not present	10 (100%)	9 (90%)	8 (80%)	90%
Est. graft size (mm^3)	*HuNu*	Not present	0.85±0.37	0.19±0.05	0.63±0.22	0.56±0.15
	hNSE	Not present	0.99±0.50	0.16±0.04	0.54±0.33	0.58±0.21

Table 2 summarizes the histological assessment of infarct brains that received three different doses of NSI-566RSC cell lines (Group B, C, and D) in comparison with the vehicle (Group A).
*Quantitative analysis did not find statistical difference in graft size across the three dose groups, either by HuNu or by hNSE stain ($p = 0.2002$).
**Freq. of infarct lesion was based on evidence of tissue damage and cellular abnormality such as cell loss, apoptotic bodies in penumbra regions.

anterior and 2.8 mm lateral to bregma and 5.0 mm below the dural surface [41]. Within this single needle pass, 3 deposits of the test articles including 2 into the striatum (5.0 mm and 4.0 mm below the dural surface) and 1 into the cortex (3.0 mm below the dural surface) were made. The target area was the medial striatum and medial cortex which corresponds to the ischemic peri-infarct (or penumbra) area, based on previously established target sites for similar stereotaxic implants [42]. Each deposit consisted of 3 µl volume infused over a period of 3 minutes. All animals received daily immunosuppression (tacrolimus) 1 mg/kg/day IP. All animals were monitored weekly post-grafting for behavioral and neurological outcomes. Animals were euthanized at Day 56 days post-grafting and transcardially perfused with saline and 4% paraformaldehyde.

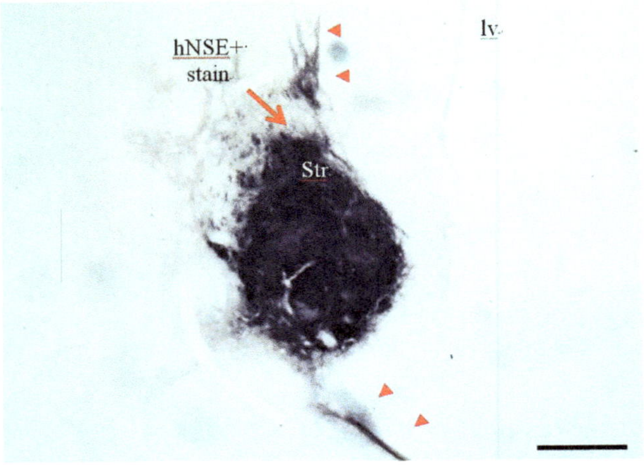

Figure 5. A representative image of hNSE staining in the striatum. Human graft cells were densely confined to the striatum (arrow) with small amounts of hNSE+fibers that extended dorsally and ventrally from the striatum (arrowheads). Scale bar = 0.5 mm [lv; lateral ventricle, Str: striatum].

Behavioral Tests

All investigators testing the animals were blinded to the treatment condition. Animals were subjected to elevated body swing test (EBST) and neurological exam. EBST involved handling the animal by its tail and recording the direction of the swings [36–40]. The test apparatus consisted of a clear Plexiglas box (40×40×35.5 cm). The animal was gently picked up at the base of the tail, and elevated by the tail until the animal's nose was at a height of 2 inches (5 cm) above the surface. The direction of the swing, either left or right, was counted once the animals head moved sideways approximately 10 degrees from the midline position of the body. After a single swing, the animal was placed back in the Plexiglas box and allowed to move freely for 30 seconds prior to retesting. These steps were repeated 20 times for each animal. Intact rats displayed a 50% swing bias, that was, the same number of swings to the left and to the right. A 75% swing bias was used as criterion of successful MCAo. About one hour after the EBST, neurological exam was conducted as previously described [36–40] with minor modifications. Neurologic score for each rat was obtained using 3 tests which included (1) forelimb retraction, which measures the ability of the animal to replace the forelimb after it was displaced laterally by 2 to 3 cm, graded from 0 (immediate replacement) to 3 (replacement after several seconds or no replacement); (2) beam walking ability, graded 0 for a rat that readily traversed a 2.4-cm-wide, 80-cm-long beam to 3 for a rat unable to stay on the beam for 10 seconds; and (3) bilateral forepaw grasp, which measured the ability to hold onto a 2-mm-diameter steel rod, graded 0 for a rat with normal forepaw grasping behavior to 3 for a rat unable to grasp with the forepaws. The scores from all 3 tests were averaged to give a mean neurologic deficit score (maximum possible score, 9 points divided

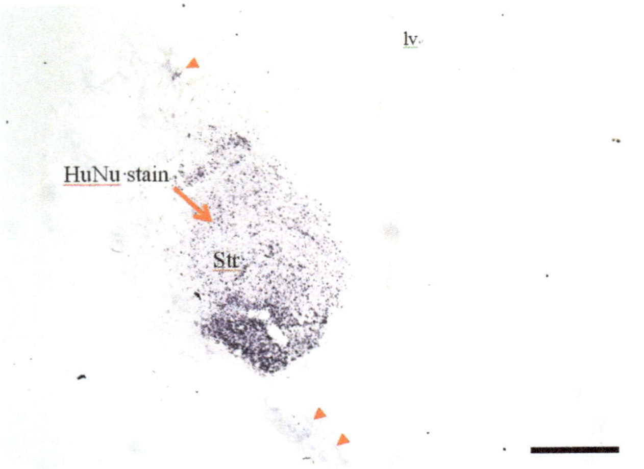

Figure 4. A representative image of HuNu staining in the striatum. HuNu+cells were confined to the striatum of rats receiving the lowest dose of graft cells (Group B). Note that small amounts of HuNu staining extended both dorsally and ventrally from the striatum. Scale bar = 0.5 mm [lv; lateral ventricle, Str: striatum].

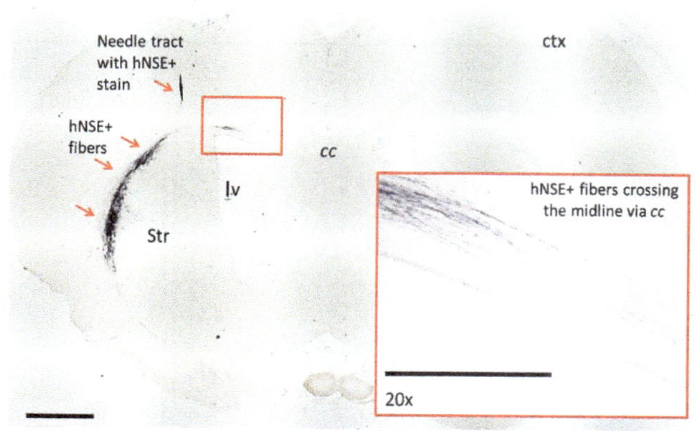

Figure 6. Migration of hNSE+fibers toward the contralateral side of non-infarct region. Needle tract with hNSE+stain was found in the cortex. Additionally, small amounts of hNSE+fibers crossed the *cc contralaterally (inset).* Scale bar = 1.0 mm [lv; lateral ventricle, Str: striatum, ctx: cortex, *cc*: corpus callosum].

by 3 tests = 3). Animals were subjected to both tests at baseline (prior to stroke), then at 7 days after stroke (prior to transplantation) and at weekly intervals over an eight-week period.

Histology

All histological analyses were performed at Neuralstem Inc. (San Diego, CA). Brains were cryoprotected in PBS containing 30% sucrose and later sectioned at 40 μm thickness using a freezing sliding microtome. Every sixth section through the brain was selected for staining.

Immunohistochemistry/Histology

Sections were treated with 3% hydrogen peroxide for 15 minutes, washed 3 times with PBS, and further treated with 0.3% Triton X-100 for 30 minutes followed by wash. Tissue was then blocked in normal horse serum for 90 minutes, and incubated with either mouse anti human nuclei (HuNu; MAB1281; Chemicon International, Temecula, CA; 1:2000) or chicken anti human-specific neuron-specific enolase (hNSE; AB-9698; Chemicon International, Temecula, CA 1:2000) at room temperature overnight. Sections were washed and again blocked with horse serum for 90 minutes, then treated with biotinylated donkey anti-mouse or biotinylated donkey anti-chicken secondary antibody (Jackson ImmunoResearch, West Grove, PA; 1:2000) for 90 minutes. Following wash, sections were incubated with streptavidin conjugated to horseradish peroxidase (Jackson ImmunoResearch, West Grove, PA; 1:5000) for 90 minutes, and then developed with diaminobenzidine containing nickel chloride for 1 minute. The sections were then mounted on gelatin-coated slides, dried, labeled, and cover-slipped. In addition, sections adjacent to sections (1-in-6 series) stained for human stem cells were processed with hematoxylin and eosin (H&E). All slides were examined and scanned using Nikon AZ100 Multizoom microscope (Nikon Instruments, Inc, Japan) for further qualitative and semi-quantitative analyses.

Measurements of Infarct Size

At least 4 coronal sections per brain were processed for H&E. The indirect lesion area, in which the intact area of the ipsilateral hemisphere was subtracted from the area of the contralateral hemisphere, was calculated to reveal cerebral infarction. Scores for infarct lesion were rated accordingly: LOW <30%, MEDIUM 30–60%, HIGH >60%, while scores for volume were rated as follows: Low <1 mm^3, Medium 1–2 mm^3, High >2 mm^3. For calculation of area of infarction in mm2, a separate cohort of animals (n = 8 per group) subjected to the same experimental paradigm were processed for Triphenyltetrazolium chloride (TTC) staining. Anesthetized animals were perfused intracardially with saline. The brain tissue was then removed, immersed in cold saline for 5 minutes, and sliced into 2.0-mm thick sections. The brain slices were incubated in a 2% triphenyltetrazolium chloride (Sigma) dissolved in normal saline for 30 minutes at 37°C and then transferred into a 5% formaldehyde solution for fixation. The area of infarction in each slice was measured using a digital scanner and the Image Tools program (University of Texas Health Sciences Center in San Antonio). The area of infarction in each animal was obtained from largest infarcted brain slice.

Cell Engraftment and Neuronal Phenotype Assessment

The slides were examined at 10X magnification of Nikon AZ100 Multizoom microscope and digitized using a PC-based Image Tools computer program (Nikon, NIS Elements software). Brain sections were blind-coded in assessing cell engraftment index for NSI-566RSC graft survival based on HuNu stained and hNSE stained slides, respectively.

Statistical Analysis

The data were evaluated statistically using either Two-way analysis of variance (ANOVA), or repeated measure of ANOVA and subsequent post hoc compromised t-tests for behavior. These statistical analyses employed a StatView 5.0 software (USA). Statistical significance was preset at $p<0.05$.

Results

NSI-566RSC Cell Grafts Promote Behavioral Recovery in Stroke Animals

Behavioral analyses revealed that all animals included in this study displayed normal behaviors at baseline prior to stroke surgery. At 7 days post-stroke, all animals exhibited the typical stroke-induced behavioral deficits characterized by significantly biased swing activity and impaired neurological performance. However, at 14 days post-stroke (i.e., 7 days post-transplantation onwards), significant recovery of motor (Figure 1) and neurological (Figure 2) functions in stroke animals that received intracerebral transplantation of high doses of 10,000 cells/μl (C) and 20,000 cells/μl (D) of NSI-566RSC compared to vehicle-infused stroke animals (A) or those stroke animals that received the low dose of 5,000 cells/μl (B). ANOVA revealed statistically significant treatment effects (p's<0.01). Post hoc compromised t-tests also revealed dose-dependent treatment effects and post-transplantation timing effects (p's<0.05). There was stable improvement in those stroke transplanted with high doses of cells (Groups C and D) which showed a trend of better improvement over time up to the 56-day study period. Although there was slight improvement in the behavioral performance of vehicle-infused stroke animals and stroke animals that received the low dose of 5,000 cells/μl, the recovery of motor and neurological tests demonstrated by high dose transplanted stroke animals was significantly better throughout the 56-day period compared to vehicle-infused stroke animals or those stroke animals that received the low dose of 5,000 cells/μl (p's<0.05). There were significant dose-dependent differences in the behavioral improvement across treatment groups at post-transplantation periods with the highest dose of 20,000 cells/μl showing the most significant improvement in both motor and

Table 3. Summary of infarct size and graft size.

ID	H&E-infarct	HuNu-Volume	hNSE-Volume
Group A Vehicle	STR+CTX	STR+CTX	STR+CTX
A02	LOW	None	None
A04	LOW	None	None
A13	LOW	None	None
A14	LOW	None	None
A15	HIGH	None	None
A18	LOW	None	None
A19	LOW	None	None
A20	LOW	None	None
A25	LOW	None	None
A26	None	None	None
Group B (5 K cells/μl)			
B01	None	LOW	LOW
B03	LOW	LOW	LOW
B05	HIGH	HIGH	HIGH
B06	MEDIUM	HIGH	LOW
B07	LOW	LOW	LOW
B08	LOW	LOW	LOW
B09	LOW	LOW	LOW
B10	LOW	HIGH	HIGH
B11	LOW	LOW	LOW
B12	LOW	LOW	MEDIUM
Group C (10 K cells/μl)			
C21	LOW	LOW	LOW
C22	LOW	LOW	LOW
C23	LOW	LOW	LOW
C24	MEDIUM	LOW	LOW
C01	LOW	LOW	LOW
C02	LOW	LOW	LOW
C06	MEDIUM	LOW	LOW
C27	LOW	LOW	LOW
C28	LOW	LOW	N/A
C29	None	LOW	LOW
Group D (20 K cells/μl)			
D05	LOW	LOW	LOW
D08	LOW	None	None
D11	HIGH	MEDIUM	HIGH
D16	HIGH	HIGH	LOW
D19	MEDIUM	LOW	LOW
D21	LOW	LOW	LOW
D22	MEDIUM	LOW	LOW
D23	LOW	LOW	LOW
D24	MEDIUM	LOW	LOW
D30	LOW	None	None

Table 3 summarizes the semi-quantitative rating of the infarct size and the size of HuNu (nuclei staining) or hNSE (neuropil staining) positive grafts.
1. Scores for Infarct lesion: LOW <30%, MEDIUM 30–60%, HIGH >60%.
2. Scores for Volume: Low <1 mm^3, Medium 1–2 mm^3, High >2 mm^3.
3. Abbreviations: STR: striatum, CTX: cerebral cortex.

neurological tests (p's<0.05). Similarly, there were significant differences in the behavioral performance among treatment groups at post-transplantation periods with the most significant improvement in both motor and neurological tests seen at day 56 post-transplantation (p's<0.05).

NSI-566RSC Cell Grafts do not Reduce Infarct Size

To confirm infarcts in stroke animals, H&E was used. Infarcts were confirmed in 93% of the animals; infarct size was similar across all groups ($p = 0.2676$) (Figure 3). A summary of infarct frequency for each treatment group is presented for clarity (Table 2). Additionally, we rated the size of the infarct in all animals to get a better approximation of any infarct variability that might have been affected by the grafts, but did not detect any as significant number of outliers across the treatment groups (i.e., only 1 animal each from Groups A–C). Based on these data, infarct size was not reduced by NSI-566RSC cell grafts.

NSI-566RSC Cell Grafts Survive and Display Neuronal Phenotype

To identify the cell graft, and estimate volume, immunohistochemistry was performed using two human-specific antibodies: one to detect all HuNu (Figures 4 & 5), and another to detect hNSE (Figure 6). Tabular summaries of the frequency of surviving grafts and estimated graft size (Table 2 and Table 3) are presented for clarity. Surviving cell grafts were confirmed in 10/10 animals of group A, 9/10 group B, and 9/10 in group C. hNSE and HuNu staining revealed similar graft volume estimates (HuNu volume: $0.56 \pm 0.15\ mm^3$ and hNSE volume: $0.58 \pm 0.21\ mm^3$). hNSE-immunoreactive fibers were also present within the corpus callosum, coursing in parallel with host tracts, suggesting a propensity to follow established neuroanatomical features. Supplementary files are also provided to show individual animal's histology capturing representative images of HuNu and hNSE (Figures S1, S2, S3, S4, S5, S6, S7, S8, and S9).

Discussion

Here, we demonstrated that intracerebral transplantation of NSI-566RSC, a spinal cord-derived NSC line, reduced behavioral deficits associated with ischemic stroke. Significant improvements in both motor and neurological tests were detected in the NSI-566RSC-treated stroke animals. In addition, the results revealed significant dose-dependent differences in the behavioral improvement across treatment groups at post-transplantation periods with the highest NSI-566RSC dose showing the most significant improvement in both motor and neurological tests. Similarly, there were significant differences in the timing of behavioral performance among treatment groups at post-transplantation periods with the most significant improvement in both motor and neurological tests seen at day 56 post-transplantation, indicating that the transplanted stroke animals showed improved recovery over graft maturation period. We observed though that a few transplanted animals did not contain surviving grafts. The reason why some transplanted animals do not have detectable transplanted cells is unknown but it is likely because of graft failure due to immunosuppressant being ineffective to those particular animals.

We used a potent immunosuppressive agent (tacrolimus) to avoid rejection of the human cells, but are aware of the action of this drug in the brain response to ischemia itself or a possible synergic effect with the cell-based therapy proposed in our study. However, in our previous studies, using cyclosporine and tacrolimus [43–45], we came into the conclusion that these immunosuppressant drugs, albeit with neuoroprotective effects, display limited therapeutic window of opportunity, in that the drugs must be administered prior to, during, and/or immediately after the injury. Beyond this very acute time point, such as the present two weeks post-stroke period, we and several others have found that these drugs are not effective. In addition, a vis-à-vis comparison between non-immunosuppressed transplanted stroke animals versus immunosuppressed transplanted stroke animals revealed that immunosuppressed transplanted stroke animals significantly produced functional recovery compared to immunosuppression treatment alone [46]. Moreover, the choice to deliver the cocktail of immunosuppressants in the present study was based on a series of preclinical studies that supported the ongoing clinical trials of the same cells in ALS patients. This cocktail was proven effective in facilitating the graft effects in animal models of ALS, and approved by the FDA for this clinical trial. Accordingly, as we translate these NSCs for stroke clinical application, in keeping with the FDA's requirement and also based on preclinical studies from our group and several others, we maintain the transplant protocol with the immunosuppresion regimen. However, if the transplant procedure was done acutely in stroke, we would be compelled to conduct another vis-à-vis study comparing NSCs with vehicle versus NSCs with immunosuppressants. For the present delayed transplantation regimen, and with the FDA requiring that the same protocol done in ALS be followed in the stroke arena in order to gain entry into the clinic, both scientific and clinical bases support our decision to maintain the NSCs with immunosuppressant regimen.

This study was designed to evaluate the potential therapeutic value of intracerebral dosing of NSI-566RSC in an animal model of adult ischemic stroke. The recovery of motor and neurological tests demonstrated by high dose transplanted stroke animals was significantly better throughout the 56 day study period compared to vehicle-infused stroke animals, or low-dosed transplanted animals. Moreover, there was stable improvement in the high dose animals, and they showed a trend of better improvement over time.

These results demonstrated safety and efficacy of NSI-566RSC in a subacute model of ischemic stroke in rats, indicating a strong proof-of-principle data that NSI-566RSC are potent cell donors for transplantation therapy to treat paralysis in stroke patients. A Phase I trial testing the safety of NSI-566RSC has recently been completed in the treatment of ALS [35]. Our current observations of safety and efficacy of NSI-566RSC in stroke animals mimic similar therapeutic readouts following transplantation of NSI-566RSC in animal models of ALS [23–26], spinal cord injury [27], and ischemic paraplegia [28]. Testing the efficacy of NSI-566RSC in larger stroke animals may be needed, although a safety portfolio already exists in mini-pigs for NSI-566RSC transplantation in CNS [29,30]. That the present transplanted stroke animals exhibited improvement in motor and neurological functions accompanied by NSI-566RSC graft survival and neuronal differentiation also resembled the histopathological outcomes seen in animal models of ALS, spinal cord injury, ischemic paraplegia demonstrating engraftment and neuronal phenotypic persistence in transplanted NSI-566RSC [25,31]. While graft survival and neuronal differentiation have been confirmed, on-going work is investigating the integration of graft into host tissue, determining the neuronal phenotypes of the grafted neurons, and confirming the low proliferation rates of the grafts as suggested from these preliminary histological studies.

Stroke remains a significant unmet clinical need [1–5] with tPA efficacy limited to 4.5 hours after stroke onset and benefits only about 3% of ischemic stroke patients [6–8]. The tPA's narrow therapetuc window has prompted the need for novel treatments, such as stem cell therapy, designed to abrogate stroke beyond the acute phase of the disease [9–13]. Current clinical trials of cell therapy for stroke have pursued adult stem cells (.e.g., bone marrow and placenta) and NSCs, based on ample laboratory evidence demonstrating safety and efficacy of these cells [4,5,42,47–49]. Optimization of clinical outcomes has been a key translational research effort for cell therapy for stroke [10,13,50–52]. With myriad stem cell sources in transplantation therapy, many laboratory-to-clinic translational factors have been recognized including well-defined donor stem cells, cell isolation and propagation, immunogenicity, capacity for proliferation, and cell yield [14–16]. Although NSC transplantation has been shown effective in stroke models [19,53,54], the mechanism of action remains elusive, in particular graft survival and integration with the host have yet to be fully understood in the stroke brain. Here, we provide evidence of a regenerative pathway involving robust NSI-566RSC engraftment and neuronal differentiation that accompanied behavioral improvements despite absence of cerebral infarct reduction. Axonal growth with long fibers from NSC grafts extended to the corpus callosum and traversed with host tracts, indicating graft-host integration recapitulating endogenous neuroanatomical landmarks. In addition, while on-going clinical trials of cell therapy have targeted the acute and chronic phase of stroke, the present study suggests the sub-acute phase as an equally effective therapeutic window for NSI-566RSC transplantation in ischemic stroke.

Supporting Information

Figure S1 HuNu staining in vehicle-infused group. No detectable HuNu staining is observed.

Figure S2 HuNu staining in low dose-transplanted group. HuNu staining is detected in all transplanted stroke brain.

Figure S3 HuNu staining in medium dose-transplanted group. HuNu staining is detected in all transplanted stroke brain except for one brain (C29).

Figure S4 HuNu staining in high dose-transplanted group. HuNu staining is detected in all transplanted stroke brain except for one brain (D30).

Figure S5 hNSE staining in vehicle-infused group. No detectable hNSE staining is observed.

Figure S6 hNSE staining in low dose-transplanted group. hNSE staining is detected in all transplanted stroke brain.

Figure S7 hNSE staining in medium dose-transplanted group. hNSE staining is detected in all transplanted stroke brain except for one brain (C29).

Figure S8 hNSE staining in high dose-transplanted group. hNSE staining is detected in all transplanted stroke brain except for two brains (D08 and D30).

Figure S9 Area of infarction. TTC staining reveals area of infarction (mm^2) in the laragest infarcted slice. *$p<0.05$ versus A or B.

Author Contributions

Conceived and designed the experiments: KJ CVB. Performed the experiments: NT DMQ YK SW DL TL KLH TGH KJ MCW CVB. Analyzed the data: NT KJ MCW CVB. Contributed reagents/materials/analysis tools: KJ MCW CVB. Wrote the paper: NT KJ CVB.

References

1. Tajiri N, Dailey T, Metcalf C, Mosley YI, Lau T, et al. (2013) In vivo animal stroke models: a rationale for rodent and non-human primate models. Transl Stroke Res 4: 308–321.
2. Kaneko Y, Pabon MM, Dailey T, Weinbren NL, Rizzi J, et al. (2013) The battle of the sexes for stroke therapy: female- versus male-derived stem cells. CNS Neurol Disord Drug Targets 12: 405–412.
3. Kaneko Y, Tajiri N, Shinozuka K, Glover LE, Weinbren NL, et al. (2012) Cell therapy for stroke: emphasis on optimizing safety and efficacy profile of endothelial progenitor cells. Curr Pharm Des 18: 3731–3734.
4. Borlongan CV, Glover LE, Tajiri N, Kaneko Y, Freeman TB (2011) The great migration of bone marrow-derived stem cells toward the ischemic brain: therapeutic implications for stroke and other neurological disorders. Prog Neurobiol 95: 213–228.
5. Borlongan CV (2011) Bone marrow stem cell mobilization in stroke: a 'bonehead' may be good after all! Leukemia 25: 1674–1686.
6. Tan Tanny SP, Busija L, Liew D, Teo S, Davis SM, et al. (2013) Cost-effectiveness of thrombolysis within 4.5 hours of acute ischemic stroke: experience from Australian stroke center. Stroke 44: 2269–2274.
7. Saver JL, Fonarow GC, Smith EE, Reeves MJ, Grau-Sepulveda MV, et al. (2013) Time to treatment with intravenous tissue plasminogen activator and outcome from acute ischemic stroke. JAMA 309: 2480–2488.
8. Fisher M, Albers GW (2013) Advanced imaging to extend the therapeutic time window of acute ischemic stroke. Ann Neurol 73: 4–9.
9. Chopp M, Steinberg GK, Kondziolka D, Lu M, Bliss TM, et al. (2009) Who's in favor of translational cell therapy for stroke: STEPS forward please? Cell Transplant 18: 691–693.
10. Stem Cell Therapies as an Emerging Paradigm in Stroke P (2009) Stem Cell Therapies as an Emerging Paradigm in Stroke (STEPS): bridging basic and clinical science for cellular and neurogenic factor therapy in treating stroke. Stroke 40: 510–515.
11. Hess DC, Borlongan CV (2008) Cell-based therapy in ischemic stroke. Expert Rev Neurother 8: 1193–1201.
12. Hess DC, Borlongan CV (2008) Stem cells and neurological diseases. Cell Prolif 41 Suppl 1: 94–114.
13. Borlongan CV, Chopp M, Steinberg GK, Bliss TM, Li Y, et al. (2008) Potential of stem/progenitor cells in treating stroke: the missing steps in translating cell therapy from laboratory to clinic. Regen Med 3: 249–250.
14. Sanberg PR, Eve DJ, Metcalf C, Borlongan CV (2012) Advantages and challenges of alternative sources of adult-derived stem cells for brain repair in stroke. Prog Brain Res 201: 99–117.
15. Sanberg PR, Eve DJ, Cruz LE, Borlongan CV (2012) Neurological disorders and the potential role for stem cells as a therapy. Br Med Bull 101: 163–181.
16. Rodrigues MC, Voltarelli J, Sanberg PR, Allickson JG, Kuzmin-Nichols N, et al. (2012) Recent progress in cell therapy for basal ganglia disorders with emphasis on menstrual blood transplantation in stroke. Neurosci Biobehav Rev 36: 177–190.
17. Borlongan CV, Tajima Y, Trojanowski JQ, Lee VM, Sanberg PR (1998) Transplantation of cryopreserved human embryonal carcinoma-derived neurons (NT2N cells) promotes functional recovery in ischemic rats. Exp Neurol 149: 310–321.
18. Nelson PT, Kondziolka D, Wechsler L, Goldstein S, Gebel J, et al. (2002) Clonal human (hNT) neuron grafts for stroke therapy: neuropathology in a patient 27 months after implantation. Am J Pathol 160: 1201–1206.
19. Stroemer P, Patel S, Hope A, Oliveira C, Pollock K, et al. (2009) The neural stem cell line CTX0E03 promotes behavioral recovery and endogenous neurogenesis after experimental stroke in a dose-dependent fashion. Neurorehabil Neural Repair 23: 895–909.
20. Sinden JD, Vishnubhatla I, Muir KW (2012) Prospects for stem cell-derived therapy in stroke. Prog Brain Res 201: 119–167.
21. Teng YD, Benn SC, Kalkanis SN, Shefner JM, Onario RC, et al. (2012) Multimodal actions of neural stem cells in a mouse model of ALS: a meta-analysis. Sci Transl Med 4: 165ra164.
22. Teng YD, Yu D, Ropper AE, Li J, Kabatas S, et al. (2011) Functional multipotency of stem cells: a conceptual review of neurotrophic factor-based

evidence and its role in translational research. Curr Neuropharmacol 9: 574–585.
23. Xu L, Shen P, Hazel T, Johe K, Koliatsos VE (2011) Dual transplantation of human neural stem cells into cervical and lumbar cord ameliorates motor neuron disease in SOD1 transgenic rats. Neurosci Lett 494: 222–226.
24. Xu L, Yan J, Chen D, Welsh AM, Hazel T, et al. (2006) Human neural stem cell grafts ameliorate motor neuron disease in SOD-1 transgenic rats. Transplantation 82: 865–875.
25. Xu L, Ryugo DK, Pongstaporn T, Johe K, Koliatsos VE (2009) Human neural stem cell grafts in the spinal cord of SOD1 transgenic rats: differentiation and structural integration into the segmental motor circuitry. J Comp Neurol 514: 297–309.
26. Hefferan MP, Galik J, Kakinohana O, Sekerkova G, Santucci C, et al. (2012) Human neural stem cell replacement therapy for amyotrophic lateral sclerosis by spinal transplantation. PLoS One 7: e42614.
27. van Gorp S, Leerink M, Kakinohana O, Platoshyn O, Santucci C, et al. (2013) Amelioration of motor/sensory dysfunction and spasticity in a rat model of acute lumbar spinal cord injury by human neural stem cell transplantation. Stem Cell Res Ther 4: 57.
28. Cizkova D, Kakinohana O, Kucharova K, Marsala S, Johe K, et al. (2007) Functional recovery in rats with ischemic paraplegia after spinal grafting of human spinal stem cells. Neuroscience 147: 546–560.
29. Raore B, Federici T, Taub J, Wu MC, Riley J, et al. (2011) Cervical multilevel intraspinal stem cell therapy: assessment of surgical risks in Gottingen minipigs. Spine (Phila Pa 1976) 36: E164–171.
30. Usvald D, Vodicka P, Hlucilova J, Prochazka R, Motlik J, et al. (2010) Analysis of dosing regimen and reproducibility of intraspinal grafting of human spinal stem cells in immunosuppressed minipigs. Cell Transplant 19: 1103–1122.
31. Yan J, Xu L, Welsh AM, Hatfield G, Hazel T, et al. (2007) Extensive neuronal differentiation of human neural stem cell grafts in adult rat spinal cord. PLoS Med 4: e39.
32. Lunn JS, Pacut C, Backus C, Hong Y, Johe K, et al. (2010) The pleotrophic effects of insulin-like growth factor-I on human spinal cord neural progenitor cells. Stem Cells Dev 19: 1983–1993.
33. Guo X, Johe K, Molnar P, Davis H, Hickman J (2010) Characterization of a human fetal spinal cord stem cell line, NSI-566RSC, and its induction to functional motoneurons. J Tissue Eng Regen Med 4: 181–193.
34. Yan J, Xu L, Welsh AM, Chen D, Hazel T, et al. (2006) Combined immunosuppressive agents or CD4 antibodies prolong survival of human neural stem cell grafts and improve disease outcomes in amyotrophic lateral sclerosis transgenic mice. Stem Cells 24: 1976–1985.
35. Glass JD, Boulis NM, Johe K, Rutkove SB, Federici T, et al. (2012) Lumbar intraspinal injection of neural stem cells in patients with amyotrophic lateral sclerosis: results of a phase I trial in 12 patients. Stem Cells 30: 1144–1151.
36. Garbuzova-Davis S, Rodrigues MC, Hernandez-Ontiveros DG, Tajiri N, Frisina-Deyo A, et al. (2013) Blood-brain barrier alterations provide evidence of subacute diaschisis in an ischemic stroke rat model. PLoS One 8: e63553.
37. Tajiri N, Acosta S, Glover LE, Bickford PC, Jacotte Simancas A, et al. (2012) Intravenous grafts of amniotic fluid-derived stem cells induce endogenous cell proliferation and attenuate behavioral deficits in ischemic stroke rats. PLoS One 7: e43779.
38. Borlongan CV, Kaneko Y, Maki M, Yu SJ, Ali M, et al. (2010) Menstrual blood cells display stem cell-like phenotypic markers and exert neuroprotection following transplantation in experimental stroke. Stem Cells Dev 19: 439–452.
39. Matsukawa N, Yasuhara T, Hara K, Xu L, Maki M, et al. (2009) Therapeutic targets and limits of minocycline neuroprotection in experimental ischemic stroke. BMC Neurosci 10: 126.
40. Borlongan CV, Hayashi T, Oeltgen PR, Su TP, Wang Y (2009) Hibernation-like state induced by an opioid peptide protects against experimental stroke. BMC Biol 7: 31.
41. Paxinos G, Watson C (2007) The Rat Brain in Stereotaxic Coordinates: Hard Cover Edition: Academic press.
42. Yasuhara T, Matsukawa N, Hara K, Maki M, Ali MM, et al. (2009) Notch-induced rat and human bone marrow stromal cell grafts reduce ischemic cell loss and ameliorate behavioral deficits in chronic stroke animals. Stem Cells Dev 18: 1501–1514.
43. Dailey T, Eve DJ, Tajiri N, Lau T, Mosley YI, van Loveren H, Sanberg PR, Kaneko Y, Borlongan CV. (2013) Different sources of stem cells for transplantation therapy in stroke. In: *Cell-Based Therapies in Stroke*. Jolkkonen J, Walczak P (eds). Springer. 29–46.
44. Borlongan CV, Yu G, Matsukawa N, Xu L, Hess DC, et al. (2005) Acute functional effects of cyclosporine-A and methylprednisolone treatment in adult rats exposed to transient ischemic stroke. Life Sci 76: 1503–1512.
45. Osman MM, Lulic D, Glover L, Stahl CE, Lau T, et al. (2011) Cyclosporine-A as a neuroprotective agent against stroke: its translation from laboratory research to clinical application. Neuropeptides 45: 359–368.
46. Borlongan CV, Tajima Y, Trojanowski JQ, Lee VM, Sanberg PR (1998) Transplantation of cryopreserved human embryonal carcinoma-derived neurons (NT2N cells) promotes functional recovery in ischemic rats. Exp Neurol 149: 310–321.
47. Mays RW, Borlongan CV, Yasuhara T, Hara K, Maki M, et al. (2010) Development of an allogeneic adherent stem cell therapy for treatment of ischemic stroke. J Exp Stroke Transl Med 3: 34–46.
48. Chen J, Shehadah A, Pal A, Zacharek A, Cui X, et al. (2013) Neuroprotective effect of human placenta-derived cell treatment of stroke in rats. Cell Transplant 22: 871–879.
49. Yang B, Xi X, Aronowski J, Savitz SI (2012) Ischemic stroke may activate bone marrow mononuclear cells to enhance recovery after stroke. Stem Cells Dev 21: 3332–3340.
50. Borlongan CV (2009) Cell therapy for stroke: remaining issues to address before embarking on clinical trials. Stroke 40: S146–148.
51. Savitz SI (2013) Cell therapies: careful translation from animals to patients. Stroke 44: S107–109.
52. Sinden JD, Muir KW (2012) Stem cells in stroke treatment: the promise and the challenges. Int J Stroke 7: 426–434.
53. Pollock K, Stroemer P, Patel S, Stevanato L, Hope A, et al. (2006) A conditionally immortal clonal stem cell line from human cortical neuroepithelium for the treatment of ischemic stroke. Exp Neurol 199: 143–155.
54. Guzman R, De Los Angeles A, Cheshier S, Choi R, Hoang S, et al. (2008) Intracarotid injection of fluorescence activated cell-sorted CD49d-positive neural stem cells improves targeted cell delivery and behavior after stroke in a mouse stroke model. Stroke 39: 1300–1306.

5

Cortical and Spinal Mechanisms of Task Failure of Sustained Submaximal Fatiguing Contractions

Petra S. Williams[1,2]*, Richard L. Hoffman[1], Brian C. Clark[1,3,4]

1 Ohio Musculoskeletal & Neurological Institute (OMNI), Ohio University, Athens, Ohio, United States of America, **2** Department of Physical Therapy and Athletic Training, Northern Arizona University, Flagstaff, Arizona, United States of America, **3** Department of Biomedical Sciences, Ohio University, Athens, Ohio, United States of America, **4** Department of Geriatric Medicine and Gerontology, Ohio University, Athens, Ohio, United States of America

Abstract

In this and the subsequent companion paper, results are presented that collectively seek to delineate the contribution that supraspinal circuits have in determining the time to task failure (TTF) of sustained submaximal contractions. The purpose of this study was to compare adjustments in supraspinal and spinal excitability taken concurrently throughout the performance of two different fatigue tasks with identical mechanical demands but different TTF (i.e., force-matching and position-matching tasks). On separate visits, ten healthy volunteers performed the force-matching or position-matching task at 15% of maximum strength with the elbow flexors to task failure. Single-pulse transcranial magnetic stimulation (TMS), paired-pulse TMS, paired cortico-cervicomedullary stimulation, and brachial plexus electrical stimulation were delivered in a 6-stimuli sequence at baseline and every 2–3 minutes throughout fatigue-task performance. Contrary to expectations, the force-matching task TTF was 42% shorter (17.5±7.9 min) than the position-matching task (26.9±15.11 min; $p<0.01$); however, both tasks caused the same amount of muscle fatigue ($p=0.59$). There were no task-specific differences for the total amount or rate of change in the neurophysiologic outcome variables over time ($p>0.05$). Therefore, failure occurred after a similar mean decline in motorneuron excitability developed ($p<0.02$, ES = 0.35–0.52) coupled with a similar mean increase in measures of corticospinal excitability ($p<0.03$, ES = 0.30–0.41). Additionally, the amount of intracortical inhibition decreased ($p<0.03$, ES = 0.32) and the amount of intracortical facilitation ($p>0.10$) and an index of upstream excitation of the motor cortex remained constant ($p>0.40$). Together, these results suggest that as fatigue develops prior to task failure, the increase in corticospinal excitability observed in relationship to the decrease in spinal excitability results from a combination of decreasing intracortical inhibition with constant levels of intracortical facilitation and upstream excitability that together eventually fail to provide the input to the motor cortex necessary for descending drive to overcome the spinal cord resistance, thereby contributing to task failure.

Editor: François Hug, The University of Queensland, Australia

Funding: This work was supported in part by grant R15HD065552 from the National Institutes of Health's Eunice Kennedy Shriver National Institute of Child Health and Human Development to B. C. Clark. Additionally, internal support for this work was provided by a grant from the Research and Scholarly Affairs Committee at the Ohio University Heritage College of Medicine. The funders had no role in study design, data collection and analysis, decision to publish, or preparation of the manuscript.

Competing Interests: B. C. Clark has received consulting fees from Regeneron Pharmaceuticals, Inc., and Abbott Laboratories. No other conflicts were reported. Dr. B. C. Clark's participation as a consultant for Regeneron Pharmaceuticals, Inc.

* E-mail: petra.williams@nau.edu

Introduction

For healthy individuals performing sustained contractions, fatigue is an expected and normal physiologic reaction that inevitably leads to task failure [1,2]. Muscle fatigue is defined as the gradual decline in maximum muscle force capacity relative to pre-fatigue values and can be viewed as the development of activity dependent weakness that resolves with rest [1,3,4]. During sustained submaximal contractions, muscle fatigue will be present *prior* to task failure; however, task performance will continue for a period of time without appreciable disruption [1,3,5–7]. As task duration increases, muscle fatigue will progress to a degree such that it interferes with the capacity to sustain the precise amount of submaximal force output required (e.g. force output fluctuates around the target force) impeding accuracy of performance and eventually prohibiting effective task performance. Task failure becomes the point in time when the force output required for successful task performance can no longer be sustained as demanded by the activity [5].

It is well accepted that there is not one single cause of fatigue; instead, the physiologic mechanisms behind the decline in force output that prohibits indefinite task performance are specific to the task demands (i.e., contraction intensity, duration, mode, muscle group, joint angle, limb posture, and stabilization) that collectively stress different regions of the neuromuscular pathway responsible for the contraction in order to sustain the required force output [1,3,4,7–12]. In general, it has been shown that the nervous system's failure to maintain sufficient activation of the muscle is a significant contributor to task failure in sustained submaximal contractions as compared to maximal contractions [1,5,6,8,13,14]. Additionally, under otherwise identical mechanical demands during sustained submaximal contractions, neurophysiologic measures have also been found to differ with load compliance (e.g. exert a constant force against a rigid restraint or hold an equivalent inertial weight) which requires individuals to attend to distinct performance feedback variables, to either force output (*force-matching task*) or joint angle position (*position-matching task*) [5,7,12,15,16]. Typically, submaximal contractions performed with the elbow flexors at an intensity up to 30% of maximum force result in the same amount of muscle fatigue at task failure; however, the time to task failure (TTF) is nearly twice as long for the force-matching task compared to the position-matching task [12,15,16].

The excitatory drive to the muscle by the motorneurons during sustained submaximal contractions can be modulated by supraspinal inputs from descending pathways, spinal inputs from interneurons and peripheral afferents, and also by intrinsic changes of the motorneuron itself [1,7,17–19]. Evoked potentials elicited by transcranial magnetic stimulation (TMS) of the motor cortex and electrical stimulation of the spinal tracts or the peripheral nerve during task performance provide evidence about the state of nervous system excitability and have been suggested to be an indirect assessment of the amount of nervous system activation [20,21]. It is important to recognize that this experimental strategy does not directly assess the amount of activation provided to the motor pool from the motor cortex or spinal afferents rather it examines the responsivity of the nervous system to external stimulation at the time of stimulation from which interpretations about the segmental state of activity are made [21]. Inferences about the state of activation in a region relative to another are more plausible when cortical, spinal and peripheral measures are evoked concurrently, in real-time and also during different states of activation (i.e., fatigued vs. non-fatigued, resting vs. active) [22–24].

The amplitude of a motor evoked potential (MEP) evoked by a single suprathreshold TMS pulse to the motor cortex provides a composite index of excitability of the entire voluntary motor pathway, as the size of the response depends upon both cortical and spinal excitability [1,25,26]. During sustained submaximal contractions, much like the voluntary electromyographic (EMG) signal, MEP amplitude has been shown to increase as task duration increases [1,22,27,28]. This increase in responsivity to the external stimulus has been attributed to enhanced voluntary drive both to and from the motor cortex and to increased descending drive to recruit motorneurons in order to sustain neural output and thus muscle activation [21–23,28,29]. These findings are consistent with evidence from single motor unit studies that report progressive recruitment of new, unfatigued motor units to sustain force output that underlies the increase in voluntary EMG amplitude throughout task performance [17,30,31].

When evoked during a voluntary contraction, the MEP is followed by an electrical silent period (SP), observed as a transient cessation of ongoing EMG activity consistent with an interruption in volitional drive to the cortex and withdrawal of descending input to the spinal motorpool [32]. In non-fatiguing contractions, the SP duration has been attributed to an initial short period of spinal refractoriness that recovers (~50msec) combined with a longer period of cortical inhibition (up to ~200 msec) [29,32]. During fatiguing contractions, the SP duration also increases, and this increase has been assumed to be due to the same mechanism of enhanced cortical inhibition reported for a longer SP with non-fatiguing contractions [1,15,33,34]. This interpretation of increased SP duration with fatiguing contractions has posed a conundrum in that despite an increase in cortical excitability as measured by the increased in MEP amplitudes, there also appears to be a concurrent increase in cortical inhibition [1,15,35]. This raises the question as to the segmental contribution of intracortical circuits within the motor cortex, and also of "upstream" inputs to the motor cortex, to task failure during sustained submaximal contractions [1,15,22,34,36]. In other words, during task performance does active cortical inhibition develop or is there insufficient intracortical facilitation and "upstream input" that limits the capacity of supraspinal structures to sustain sufficient excitatory drive to the motorneuron pool and thus contribute to task failure?

Paired-pulse TMS protocols, including short-interval intracortical inhibition (SICI) and intracortical facilitation (ICF), provide a strategy to more directly evaluate the excitability of intracortical interneuron networks within the motor cortex [20,37–39]. The effect of a subthreshold conditioning pulse that activates the cortical interneurons on the MEP amplitude of a subsequent suprathreshold test pulse is compared relative to a single MEP. When separated by interstimulus intervals (ISI) of 2–5msec, the evoked MEP amplitude decreases and the SICI ratio of the test MEP to the single MEP is less than 1.0 reflecting intracortical inhibition [38,40]. An ISI of 12–25msec increases the test MEP amplitude and generally, the ratio is greater than 1.0, which is interpreted as representing ICF [20,37]. These two measures of intracortical excitability have rarely been used to monitor the ongoing adjustments in intracortical excitability related to fatigue [41–43] and, to date, have not been employed to examine intracortical networks during the performance of submaximal contractions sustained to task failure.

Electrical stimulation to the spinal cord tracts at the cervicomedullary junction transynaptically activates the motor neuron pool and elicits a cervicomedullary evoked potential (CMEP) regarded as a segmental index of spinal alpha-motorneuron excitability [44,45]. The CMEP response latency suggests that the CMEP reflects a monosynaptic relationship between the corticospinal tract and the motorneuron without influence from presynaptic inhibition of the corticospinal tract [45,46]. Collision experiments have demonstrated that MEPs and CMEPs are transmitted in the same axons of the corticospinal tract; therefore, it is practical to compare the two responses to differentiate cortical relative to spinal motorneuron adaptations as fatigue develops [44–46]. A technique introduced by McNeil et al., where MEPs and CMEPs are evoked during the SP (i.e., stimulating during the period of electrical silence after a single suprathreshold TMS pulse) provides a strategy to assess the excitability of the corticospinal system and the motorneurons independent of upstream voluntary drive to the cortex and descending drive during a fatiguing contraction [22,23,47].

In the non-fatigued state, the amplitudes of a MEP or a CMEP evoked in the SP are less than those evoked in the presence of voluntary activation such that a ratio of the SP evoked response to the single control pulse is typically <1.0 [22,47]. In addition, the MEP ratio is also less than the CMEP ratio suggesting the added presence of intracortical inhibition in the non-fatigued state [22,47]. The ratio of the MEP evoked in the SP to the single MEP is referred to as long-interval intracortical inhibition (LICI) and is thought to be influenced by cortical inhibition mechanisms similar to those influencing the SP duration in the non-fatigued state [1,24]. The cortically evoked MEP amplitude depends upon composite cortical and spinal excitability–whether or not it is evoked in the SP–and recent work by McNeil et al., suggests that the term long-interval inhibition (LII) may be a more accurate label for this ratio as opposed to LICI [22,23,47,48].

During the performance of sustained submaximal contractions where subjects were asked to maintain a consistent level of voluntary EMG activity (as opposed to force output), the amplitudes of the CMEP evoked in the SP and the MEP evoked in the SP declined in parallel to each other and to values well-below pre-fatigue measures [23]. McNeil and colleagues concluded that because the values for the cortical and spinal measures declined in parallel, as opposed to seeing a greater decline in the cortically evoked MEPs, the motor cortex is not actively inhibited during sustained submaximal contractions. Instead, they propose that the motorneurons become progressively resistant to stimulation as the task progresses which suggests that changes in LII as well as in SP duration are more likely due to decreased motorneuron excitability rather than to increased cortical inhibition when measured in the fatigued state [22,23,47–49].

Studies examining the functional significance of neurophysiologic adjustments to the difference in TTF between the force-matching and the position-matching tasks have provided valuable insight into the spinal mechanisms that limit the duration of sustained submaximal contractions. The shorter TTF for the position-matching task has been associated with a greater reduction in H-reflex amplitude (a global index of spinal excitability) [27,50] and no decline in 1a pre-synaptic inhibition measured by the conditioned H-reflex (an indirect index of pre-synaptic inhibition) when compared to the force-matching task (where 1a pre-synaptic inhibition declines) [17]. To date, only one study has investigated the differences in supraspinal excitability between the two tasks using single pulse TMS [27]. Non-significant differences were observed in the rates of increase in MEP amplitude and EMG amplitude; however, at task failure the longer duration force-matching task had greater MEP and EMG amplitude and a longer SP duration while the shorter duration position-matching task had greater rate and amount of reduction in H-reflex amplitude. Together these results suggest insufficient motor unit recruitment contributed to early position-matching task failure [7,15,27]. While inconclusive regarding supraspinal mechanisms the results from this study, when combined with prior reports from single motor unit studies about recruitment threshold and discharge rates, have been interpreted to suggest that the shorter TTF for the position-matching is associated with decreased facilitation of the motorneuron pool from peripheral afferents due to sustained or even increased pre-synaptic inhibition of the Ia afferent by descending inputs in order to manage force fluctuations as opposed to intrinsic changes to the motorneuron itself [5,15].

The neurophysiologic studies reviewed here have provided convincing evidence to support the conclusion that early task failure is associated with a faster rate of motor unit recruitment by descending inputs in order to compensate for a rapid decline in spinal excitability [12,17,22,23,27,29,31]; nevertheless, these findings do not rule out the potential that supraspinal mechanisms influencing descending drive also contribute to task failure as despite the compensation, task failure remains inevitable. Studies that have employed single pulse TMS suggest that there is a simultaneous increase in both cortical excitability (i.e., increase MEP amplitude) and inhibition (i.e., increase SP duration) [1,15,22,33–36]. Therefore, the purpose of this study was to delineate supraspinal adjustments, including intracortical facilatory and inhibitory circuits and voluntary drive "upstream" of the motor cortex, relative to concurrent spinal adjustments in excitability to determine the functional significance on the difference in TTF for the force-matching and position-matching tasks. We used a combination of single-pulse TMS, paired-pulse TMS and paired cortico-cervicomedullary stimulation as alone these measures do not directly quantify the amount of neural activation; however, if interpreted relative to the others greater inference to the state of nervous system activity is possible [20,21,51]. We hypothesized that the shorter TTF for the position-matching task would be associated with a greater rate of reduction in alpha-motorneuron excitability and a greater rate of increase in the measures cortical excitability, without an associated increase in measures of intra-cortical inhibition.

Methods

Subjects

Ten healthy, right-handed individuals volunteered to participate in this study (5 men, 5 women; 24.5±3.10 yrs, 174.5±12.5 cm, 75.73±20.92 kg). Prior to participation, each subject attended an orientation session where they completed a series of questionnaires to confirm they were free from any known contraindications to either stimulation (magnetic or electrical) or exercise due to a neurologic disorder, cardiovascular disease, or musculoskeletal injury in the upper extremities. Subjects identified themselves as highly active (n = 2, 1 male, 1 female,) moderately active (n = 5, 3 male, 2 female), or low active (n = 3, 1 male, 2 female) based on the Lipid Research Clinics Physical Activity Questionnaire [52], but denied participating in resistance training in the prior 3-months. Handedness was evaluated using the Edinburgh Handedness Inventory (mean score: 74±19%) with scores greater than 40% indicating right hand dominance [53]. During the orientation, subjects were familiarized to the neurophysiologic testing methods and the experimental procedures, but they remained naïve to the prior research on differences in TTF for the two tasks.

Ethics Statement

The Institutional Review Board at Ohio University approved the study protocol, and all study participants provided written informed consent.

General Overview of the Experiment and Testing Sessions

Subjects participated in two experimental sessions separated by 5–8 days (mean days separating sessions: 6.5±1.1 days) conducted at the same time of day for each subject. Subjects were randomly assigned to a counterbalanced order of fatigue-task conditions (Force-matching task visit 1:2 men and 3 women; Position-matching task visit 1:3 men and 2 women). During each testing session, subjects performed one of two sustained submaximal fatiguing contraction tasks with the elbow flexors of the non-dominant arm at an intensity equal to 15% of maximal voluntary contraction (MVC) until volitional task failure. The two fatigue tasks followed an identical protocol and had identical mechanical demands, including identical net muscle force, joint angle, limb posture and stabilization, but differed in load compliance (i.e., force-matching vs. position-matching task). The difference in load compliance required the subjects to attend to distinct performance feedback variables during each task; either the force output from the elbow flexors (*force-matching task*) or the joint angle position of the elbow joint (*position-matching task*). During the force-matching task, subjects were asked to sustain a consistent 15% MVC force output for as long and as accurately as possible as they pulled against a force transducer tethered to the chair whose length, when taut, prevented the elbow from flexing more than 90°. For the position-matching task, subjects supported a free-hanging, untethered weight equivalent to 15% MVC force and focused on maintaining the elbow joint position at 90° as long and as precisely as possible until task failure. Subjects received task-specific visual feedback about either the force output or joint position throughout task performance. Muscle activation patterns of the biceps brachii and brachioradialis muscles were examined during the respective tasks by quantifying the amplitude of the interference electromyogram signals. Adjustments in cortical, spinal, and muscle excitability during task performance were assessed prior to and during the fatigue tasks. Here, a sequence of 6 electrical and magnetic stimuli were delivered to the motor cortex (TMS), the cervicomedullary junction, and the brachial plexus at regular intervals. The performance outcomes were TTF, and muscle fatigue quantified as the reduction in MVC force immediately following the fatigue task. Eight neurophysiologic outcome measures were quantified from the evoked responses: 1) MEP amplitude, 2) SP duration, 3) MEP amplitude elicited during the corticospinal SP (MEP in SP), 4) paired-pulse MEP ratio of long interval inhibition (LII), 5) paired-pulse MEP ratio of SICI, 6) paired-pulse MEP ratio of ICF, 7) CMEP's elicited during the SP (CMEP in SP; as an index of motorneuron excitability independent from descending drive), and 8) M_{max} (used as an index of muscle excitability and to permit normalization of all of the neurophysiologic amplitude evoked potential measures). To permit analysis of changes in the neurophysiologic outcome variables between fatigue-tasks and relative to each other during the fatigue-tasks, the outcome variables were normalized and expressed as a percentage of the baseline pre-fatigue value.

The experimental protocol for both testing sessions was identical and consisted of three phases (**Figure 1**). Subjects were positioned in a custom-made chair, fit with a wrist orthosis, and prepped for EMG recordings. Phase 1 started by testing the elbow flexor MVC to measure pre-fatigue strength and determine the 15% MVC target force to be sustained during the fatigue tasks. Subjects then performed several 15% MVC short-duration (3–5 sec) force-matching contractions during which the stimulation intensities for TMS, cervicomedullary, and peripheral nerve stimulation were determined. The values for the target force and the stimulus intensities identified in test session 1 were confirmed during test session 2, and used for both test sessions. During phase 2, a total of 3 pre-fatigue baseline values for each neurophysiologic outcome variable were obtained. At the conclusion of the baseline testing, subjects were given a break before starting the fatigue task. For phase 3, subjects performed either the force-matching or the position-matching fatigue task to task failure. One-minute into the fatigue task, subjects were asked their rating of perceived exertion (RPE) using the Modified Borg 0–10 scale [54], which was immediately followed by a 60-sec sequence of 6 total magnetic and electrical stimulation pulses (1 every 10-secs). The RPE/stimulation measures were repeated every 2-min up to 7 minutes (i.e., 1, 3, 5, and 7-mins), after which they were taken every 3-min (e.g. 10, 13, 16-min, etc.) until task failure. Subjects were not informed of the timing of stimulation or their contraction times. A final RPE was taken at task failure. Five seconds after task failure, subjects performed one last MVC. Subjects were only told their TTF after completing both test sessions.

Experimental Setup and Mechanical Recordings

To provide consistent mechanical demands between the two tasks, the upper limb position, proximal segment stabilization, and joint torque (force×moment arm) were identical. Subjects were seated in an upright adjustable chair with the left arm positioned next to the body in 10–15° of humeral abduction which placed the olecranon process of the elbow joint on the small padded rest used to support the weight of the upper arm. This shoulder joint alignment has been shown to minimize stress on the rotator cuff muscles during fatigue-task performance [55]. The elbow rest did not restrict motions of the humerus or the forearm. With the torso resting against the back of the chair and the shoulder joint aligned with 0° flexion/extension, the humerus was vertical and the forearm parallel to the ground to position the elbow joint at 90°. The forearm was in neutral rotation with the thumb pointed towards the ceiling. The shoulder joint was oriented in neutral rotation so that when the elbow flexed, the thumb aimed towards the acromion process of the shoulder, not the subject's chin. To obviate the use of the hand and wrist muscles during testing as well as to provide a secure attachment for the loads, the forearm and hand were immobilized in a pre-fabricated Wrist-Hand-Thumb-Orthosis (Model 100, Orthomerica, Newport Beach, CA). This composite arm posture has been found to provide a consistently significant difference in TTF between the force-matching and position-matching tasks with the elbow flexors for loads below 45% MVC for both men and women between ages 18 and 45 years [16,17,56,57]. A 14-inch computer monitor that provided visual feedback about task performance was placed 1-meter in front of the subject and the height aligned at eye level to ensure that subjects would not alter their sitting posture (and therefore their arm position) in order to view the screen [58]. It is important to note that external supports (i.e. straps) were not used to restrict motions at the shoulder or the torso in order to equalize the demand placed on synergists, proximal joints, and postural stabilizers between the two fatigue-tasks. A schematic illustration of the experimental setup is shown in **Figure 2**.

The loads were attached on the ulnar side of the wrist to the bend of a "U" shaped bolt that was secured around the orthosis just proximal to the wrist joint. This permitted the load to slide unrestricted in the frontal plane thus uncoupling forearm pronation and supination motions from elbow joint flexion angle. For the MVC tests and the 15% MVC force-matching task, the orthosis was tethered to an anchor point on the chair base. The length of the tether was set so that when it was pulled taut by the vertically directed force of the contracting elbow flexors, the elbow joint was flexed to 90° with the forearm parallel to the ground. Unlike in other studies where the orthosis was clamped into place, restricting forearm motion in all planes [16,17,31,57,59,60], the tether only prevented further elbow flexion beyond 90°; no other motions in the arm were restricted. During the position-matching task, the total weight suspended from the orthosis was equivalent to 15%MVC. To ensure consistent torque demands between tasks, the moment arm length for the force was the measured distance between the "U" bolt and the posterior elbow on the padded rest and the forearm parallel to the ground with the humerus vertical creating a 90° angle at the elbow joint. Elbow flexor force (N) was measured with an isometric force transducer (TSD121C, 0–100kg range, Biopac Systems Inc., Goleta, CA) placed in series between the orthosis and either the anchor point of the tether or the suspended weight. The force transducer signal was differentially scaled (i.e. calibrated) to measure the MVC (Range 125.7–491.5N) and the 15% MVC target force (Range 13.3–76.2N) to enhance signal resolution at the submaximal force level. The force signal was sampled at 2.5 kHz and smoothed at 200 samples/sec (MP 150, BioPac Systems, Inc. Goletta, CA) then displayed on the computer screen to provide visual feedback to the subject. Elbow joint position (degrees) in the sagittal plane (flexion/extension) was measured with an electrogoniometer (TSD130B Twin-Axis Goniometer 150, (−)90°− (+)90° range, BioPac Systems, Goleta, CA) secured to the skin over the lateral side of the humerus and forearm using double-sided surgical tape. The position signal was sampled at 2.5kHz and displayed as visual feedback.

Strength Testing of the Elbow Flexors

Elbow flexor strength was defined as the maximal MVC value for the elbow flexors and was assessed at the start of each session and again just after task failure. To establish baseline MVC, subjects performed a minimum of three maximum isometric contractions by pulling against the tethered force transducer. Subjects were instructed to gradually increase their elbow flexion

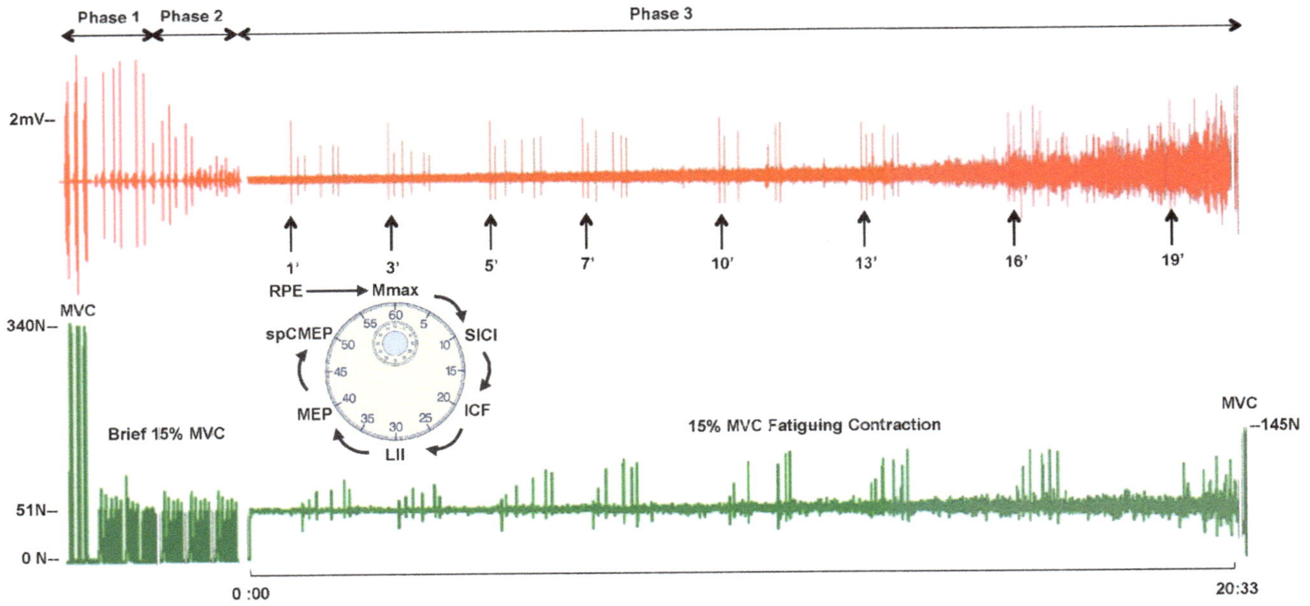

Figure 1. Experimental protocol. *(Top)* The three phases of the testing protocol. Phase 1 involved strength testing and stimulus intensity determination for evoked signals; in Phase 2 pre-fatigue baseline measures for evoked signals were taken 3 times; and in Phase 3 subjects performed the sustained, submaximal fatigue task during which the stimulus protocol was delivered at predetermined intervals. At task failure subjects performed a final MVC. *(Middle)* Representative trace of the biceps electromyogram (EMG) and time points when this subject received the stimulus protocol (see clock insert for sequence delivered over 60 seconds). *(Bottom)* Representative trace of the recorded force signal during the force-matching task. This subject's time to task failure was 20:30 minutes. *ICF: intracortical facilitation; LII: long interval inhibition; MEP: motor evoked potential; Mmax: maximum compound muscle action potential; MVC: maximum voluntary contraction; N: newtons; RPE: rating of perceived exertion; SICI: short interval intracortical inhibition; spCMEP: cervicomedullary evoked potential elicited in the silent period.*

force to maximum over 3-secs and then to hold that maximum force for 3-sec before relaxing. Standard verbal encouragement was provided [1] throughout the contraction and subjects were given visual feedback of their force output on the computer monitor. There was a 1–2 minute rest between each contraction. Subjects performed additional contractions if the MVC trials were not within 5% of each other or if subjects produced more force with each successive trial. One final MVC was performed ~5-secs after fatigue task failure (5-secs was required to reconnect the tether to the force transducer after the position-matching task). Baseline MVC for each session was defined as the greatest force output from that session and was used to compare to the final MVC performed after task failure. The highest force output during test session 1 was used as the reference level for the 15% MVC target force that was used in both test sessions. Baseline MVC did not differ between test sessions for the entire subject set (n = 10 Test session 1 MVC: 276.39±101.67 N, Test session 1 MVC: 272.0±102.85 N; $p = 0.40$) or for women (n = 5 Test session 1 MVC: 187.05±33.0 N, Test session 2 MVC: 183.90±36.07 N; $p = 0.56$) or for men (n = 5 Test session 1 MVC: 365.72±47.09 N, Test session 2 MVC: 360.39±54.44 N; $p = 0.42$).

Force-Matching and Position-Matching Fatigue Tasks

During the fatigue-tasks, subjects were asked to sustain a submaximal fatiguing contraction with the elbow flexors equivalent to 15% of their MVC until task failure under two different conditions. Subjects focused their attention on either maintaining a consistent 15% MVC force output during the force-matching task or preventing their elbow joint angle from moving away from 90°-flexion during the position-matching task. Task-specific visual feedback of force output or joint position was displayed as a horizontal line that spanned the width of the computer screen. To optimize real-time performance feedback, a 100-ms time window was used to display the signal permitting the horizontal line to fluctuate above and below the target line with increases and decreases in force output or joint angle. For both fatigue-tasks, subjects were instructed, and reminded throughout task performance, to keep the signal line representing their force output or the elbow joint position as close to the target line for as long as possible. Limb position, including elbow contact on the padded rest, and postural alignment were monitored by close visual inspection and corrective verbal feedback regarding compensations was provided by the same investigator (PSW) for all test sessions. Task failure during the force-matching fatigue-task occurred when subjects could no longer sustain their force output within ±5% of the target force (i.e. 15% MVC±1.50% MVC) or when subjects could not perform the task without compensations for ≥5 seconds. For the position-matching task, task failure occurred when subjects could not keep the elbow joint flexed within ±10° of the 90° target position (i.e. between 80° and 100°) or if, as with the force-matching task, the subjects could not correct their compensations for ≥5 seconds. Typical compensations included forearm supination, shoulder extension, shoulder adduction with external rotation or shoulder abduction with internal rotation. For both tasks, the visual feedback failure criteria spanned a 10-cm bandwidth around the target line on the computer screen, such that the resolution for the visual gain during the force-matching task was 0.5% MVC/cm and 2°/cm during the position-matching task [31,59,61].

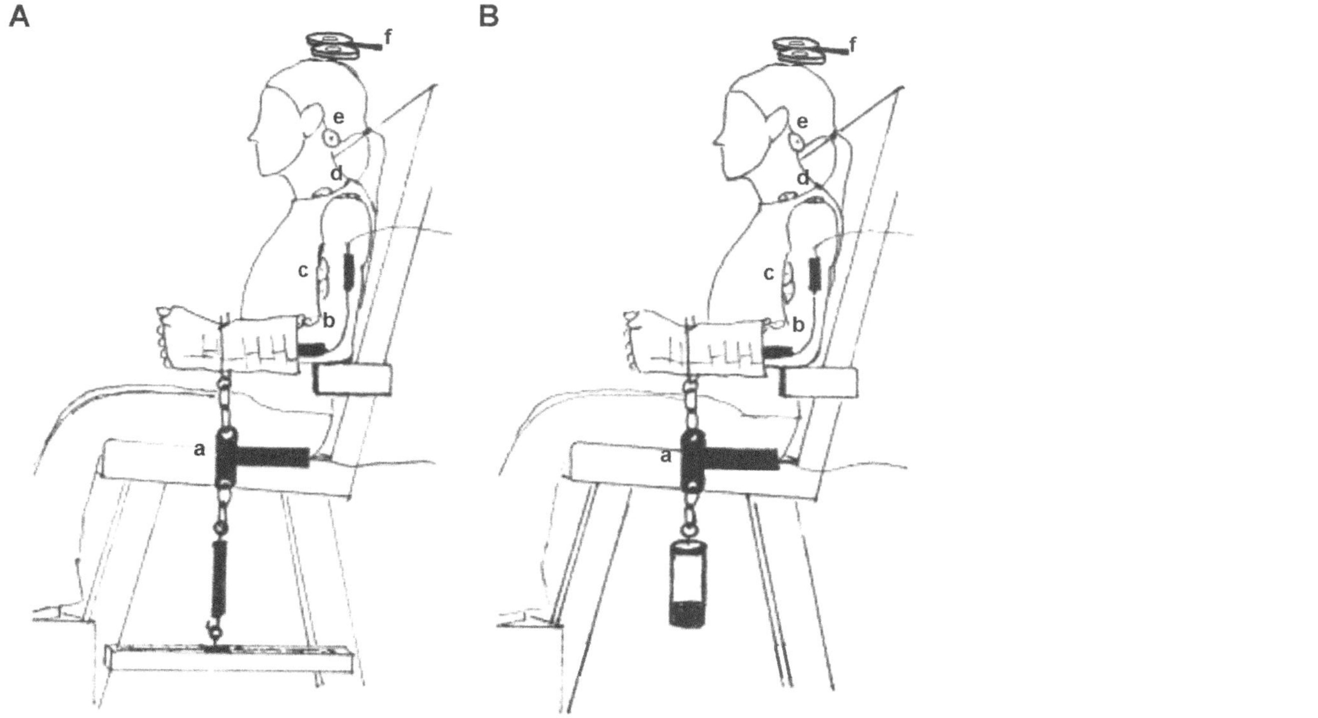

Figure 2. Experimental setup and subject positioning for the force-matching task (A) and the position-matching task (B). Special care was taken to ensure that the mechanical demands of each task were identical, and no external restraints were used to restrict motions of the torso, shoulder, elbow, or forearm in either test session. A. During the force-matching task the orthosis was anchored to the chair base via an adjustable length tether that became taut with the elbow flexed to 90°. The force transducer (a), placed in series between the anchor and the orthosis, measured the amount of force exerted by the elbow flexors through the tether against the anchor. The force output (15% MVC) was displayed on a computer monitor to provide visual feedback. The elbow joint angle was determined and confirmed by an electrogoniometer (b), electromyographic signals were recorded from the biceps brachii and brachioradialis muscles (c), electrical stimulation was delivered at Erb's point (d) and the cervicomedullary junction (e), and transcranial magnetic stimulation was delivered to the motor cortex (f). B. During the position-matching fatigue-task the magnitude of the suspended weight was equivalent to 15% MVC confirmed by the force transducer (a), and the elbow joint angle, measured via an electrogoniometer, was displayed on a computer monitor to provide visual feedback (b). An identical electromyographic (c), electrical stimulation (d and e), and transcranial magnetic stimulation (f) setup as described for the force-matching task was also implemented for the position-matching task.

Electrical Recordings

Voluntary and evoked EMG signals were recorded from the biceps brachii and the brachioradilais muscles using bipolar surface electrodes (Ag-AgCl, 8-mm diameter, interelectrode distance 25-mm, Trace 1, Nikomed, Huntingdon Valley, PA) located longitudinally over the muscle bellies on shaved, abraded and cleaned skin. The reference electrode was placed on the medial epidcondyle. EMG signals were amplified (1,000x), band-pass filtered (10–500 Hz), and sampled at 2,500 Hz (MP150, BioPac Systems Inc., Goleta, CA).

Brachial Plexus Stimulation

Electrical stimulation (single pulses, 100-µsec pulse width) to the brachial plexus at Erb's point in the supraclavicular fossa were delivered using a constant current stimulator (Digitimer D7SAH, Digitimer Ltd., Hertfordshire, UK) to evoke a M_{max} in the biceps and brachioradialis muscles both before and during the fatiguing contractions. The anodal electrode (Ag-AgCl, 8 mm) was placed on the acromion and the cathodal electrode (Ag-AgCl, 8mm) at the optimal stimulating point in the supraclavicular fossa. The intensity of the electrical stimulus was gradually increased until the evoked M-wave amplitude in the biceps plateaued. A supramaximal stimulus intensity (100–400 mA) equivalent to 120% of the plateau value was used to evoke the M_{max} response during the 15% MVC baseline and fatiguing contractions. The amplitude of the biceps M_{max} under resting conditions was used as the reference value for the target size of an unconditioned MEP and unconditioned CMEP (i.e.~50%M_{max}, see below) and the mean value did not change significantly between visits (Test session 1:9.57±2.78 mV, Test session 2:9.13±3.97 mV; $p = 0.72$).

Transcranial Magnetic Stimulation

Single and paired monophasic magnetic pulses were delivered over the right motor cortex region for the left upper extremity using a hand-held 70-mm figure-of-8 focal coil connected to a BiStim[2] stimulator (Jali Medical Inc. Woburn, MA) attached to two Magstim 200[2] stimulators (The Magstim Co Ltd, Whitland, UK). For cortical paired-pulse protocols one stimulator delivered the conditioning stimulus (CS) and the other the test stimulus (TS). To induce a current field that flowed perpendicular to the central sulcus, from posterior-lateral to anterior-medial direction in the brain, the coil was positioned tangential to the lateral surface of the head and angled 45° from the sagittal plane so that the stimulator handle was pointed in a posterior-lateral direction [62]. With the coil in this location and current flow in this direction, studies evaluating MEP latency, single motor unit behavior, and epidural recordings within the spinal cord have shown that the TMS pulse primarily activates the axons of both excitatory and inhibitory interneurons that then synapse on the corticospinal tract neurons, rather than activating the corticospinal system directly [37,63]. Therefore, unlike peripheral nerve or cervicomedullary electrical stimulation, which elicits a single synchronous activation of motorneurons, the TMS pulse evokes a descending volley of action potentials in the corticospinal neurons that are temporally summated by the motorneuron pool [64].

The optimal spatial location on the head where the TMS pulse consistently evoked the largest MEP peak-to-peak amplitude in the contralateral biceps muscle at rest (i.e. the motor hotspot) was found by moving the coil in 1-cm steps over the anatomical location of the upper extremity region of the motor cortex while delivering slightly suprathreshold stimuli. Once found, this position was marked with a sticker to ensure consistent coil placement during all TMS protocols for that day. Active motor threshold (AMT) was defined as the minimum stimulator intensity (reported as % of Stimulator Output: % SO) that evoked an MEP with a peak-to-peak amplitude ≥ twice the amplitude of the background interference EMG associated with the 15% MVC force task in at least 50% of the trials [65]. To determine AMT, subjects performed short-duration 15% MVC force-matching contractions (3 to 5-secs) during which a single pulse was delivered. The subject maintained the force output to the target force line after the TMS pulse until instructed to relax. The maximum EMG baseline peak-to-peak amplitude was quantified across the 500 milliseconds prior to the stimulus artifact and averaged across 4 trials. To confirm AMT, the stimulator intensity was varied by 3% of SO and 4 more trials conducted with the process repeating until AMT was determined. AMT values were consistent between test sessions (Test session 1 AMT: 50±9% SO; Test session 2 AMT: 46±8% SO, $p=0.17$).

The CS intensity used for the first stimulus pulse in the paired-pulse protocols for SICI and ICF was set as 70% of AMT for each session (Test session 1 CS: 35±6% SO, Test session 2 CS: 33±6% SO, $p=0.17$) [39,66]. The stimulator intensity was then increased to establish the suprathreshold TS intensity, which was used for single pulse MEP (i.e. unconditioned MEP), the TS (i.e. second stimulus pulse) in SICI and ICF, and for both the CS and TS in the LII paired-pulse protocol. The TS was defined as the stimulus intensity that, when delivered alone during a 15%MVC contraction, was sufficient to evoke an unconditioned MEP amplitude ~50% of the resting M_{max} amplitude and with a SP duration greater than 75-msec in the biceps. The value for the TS was consistent between sessions (Test session 1 TS: 75±14% SO, Test session 2 TS: 72±11% SO, $p=0.21$) and was equivalent to 150±24% of AMT during test session 1 and 157±30% of AMT during test session 2 ($p=0.22$). The interstimulus intervals (ISI) between the CS and TS were 3-msec to assess SICI and 15-msec for ICF. Both LII and paired cortico-cervicomedullary stimulation had a 75-msec ISI. The SP duration was consistent between sessions at baseline (Visit 1:133±20msec, Visit 2:129±20 msec, $p=0.46$) and therefore, sufficiently long enough for the 75-msec ISI used for the LII and paired cortico-cervicomedullary stimulation paired pulse protocols (see below).

Paired Cortico-Cervicomedullary Stimulation

Direct stimulation of the descending spinal tracts is considered to be the best available method to assess motorneuron excitability because the corticospinal/motorneuron synapse is not modified by Ia presynpatic inhibition, unlike both the H-reflex and the F-wave [46]. Stimulation at the cervicomedullary junction is preferable because there is less of a chance of activating the spinal nerve roots and the bend in the corticospinal tract, as it crosses to the contralateral side of the body in the medullary pyramids, facilitates current activation of the spinal cord tract axons [45]. Recent work comparing the change in MEP and CMEP amplitudes during sustained submaximal fatiguing contractions have found that both the MEP and CMEP amplitudes continue to increase relative to their baseline values and follow a similar pattern of response, but the CMEP amplitude compared to the MEP amplitude (both normalized to M_{max}) is lower [67]. McNeil et al., using a paired pulse cortico-cervicomedually electrical stimulation protocol where a conditioned CMEP is evoked during the SP after a suprathreshold TMS pulse during an active contraction, found that the conditioned CMEP amplitude progressively declined to below pre-fatigue values during fatiguing maximal contractions and sustained submaximal contractions [22,23,47]. They concluded that the motor cortex is not actively inhibited during sustained submaximal contractions but instead that the motorneurons become progressively resistant to stimulation. When evoked during the fatiguing contraction, the CMEP represents the excitability of the spinal motor circuits in the presence of supraspinal drive [22,23,47]. If, however, the CMEP is evoked during the SP (analogous to a conditioned MEP in LII), the conditioned CMEP offers a more direct view of the motorneuron responsiveness during fatigue independent of descending inputs [22,29,47,48].

For this experiment, electrical stimulation (single pulse, 100-μsec pulse duration) of the descending spinal tracts at the cervicomedullary junction was delivered using the same constant current stimulator previously described. The electrical current was passed between two self-adhesive surface electrodes (Ag-AgCl, 8 mm) that were affixed to the skin just medial to the mastoid processes on the soft-tissue adjacent to the inferior occiput with the anode on the left side of the spinal column [45]. The stimulus intensity (200–500 mA) was set to evoke, during brief 15% MVC force-matching contractions, an unconditioned CMEP (i.e. CMEP delivered alone) with a peak-to-peak amplitude ~50% M_{max}, and equivalent to the MEP amplitude evoked in response to the TS. The mean amplitude for the unconditioned CMEP did not differ between sessions (Test session 1 CMEP: 3.73±1.72 mV; Test session 2 CMEP: 4.57±3.34 mV; $p=0.41$). As the stimulus intensity increased, the CMEP latency was monitored to be sure it did not "jump" (i.e. sudden 1–2 msec decrease in the latency) indicating that the cervical spinal nerve roots were activated by the stimulus masking the spinal cord tract activation [68]. The paired cortico-cervicomedullary electrical stimulation protocol is analogous to LII, except that the spinal cord stimulation replaces the second TMS pulse [22,23]. One of the TMS stimulators delivered the first pulse (suprathreshold TS intensity) to the motor cortex to evoke an unconditioned MEP followed by a SP and simultaneously triggered the electrical stimulator to stimulate the cervicomedullary junction after a 75-msec ISI to evoke the CMEP during the SP.

Data Analysis

For each fatigue-task, the TTF was measured from the recorded torque output signal starting from when the torque signal reached the target force and ending when the failure criteria were met. The amplitude of the voluntary EMG signal was quantified by calculating the root mean squared (RMS) EMG from the biceps and brachioradialis over a 0.5-sec epoch surrounding peak force during the pre-fatigue MVC, prior to the stimulation sequence for the pre-fatigue baseline measures, and prior to the start of each stimulation series during the fatiguing contractions. These data were normalized to the pre-fatigue MVC values for each respective muscle.

The outcome measures for all of the evoked signals were analyzed off-line using the AcqKnowledge software package version 4.2.0 (Biopac Systems Inc. Goleta, CA). Peak-to-peak amplitude, rather than response area, was used to be consistent with recommendations for analyzing TMS protocols [69,70]. Before further analysis, to control for individual and non-experimental influences on the interpretation of the evoked responses as well as for changes in the muscle fiber excitability associated with fatigue, all evoked responses were normalized to the corresponding M_{max} amplitude recorded at each time point [27,71–73]. Ratios representing SICI, ICF, and LII were calculated by dividing the corresponding conditioned MEP amplitude by the single-pulse unconditioned MEP amplitude evoked during the same fatigue-stimulus protocol time point. The pre-fatigue values for each dependent variable represent the average of the three baseline measures normalized to the average pre-fatigue M_{max}; therefore, the pre-fatigue ratio values for SICI, ICF, and LII were calculated from these averages.

In order to assess changes in alpha-motorneuron, corticospinal and intracortical excitability between fatigue-tasks and also relative to each other, all of the evoked outcome variables were calculated as the ratio of the fatigue value divided by the baseline pre-fatigue value, expressed as a percentage [22,23]. To examine the effect of volitional drive on corticospinal excitability as measured by MEP amplitude during the fatigue-tasks, the 1) normalized MEP evoked in the SP (MEP in SP%pre-fatigue) when volitional drive has been temporarily suspended and the 2) normalized unconditioned MEP (MEP%pre-fatigue) evoked during ongoing volitional output were compared. To examine changes in corticospinal and motorneuron excitability during the SP without volitional drive 3) normalized CMEP evoked in the SP (CMEP in SP%pre-fatigue) was compared with the MEP in SP%pre-fatigue. To compare changes in intracortical inhibition and facilitation the normalized ratios for 4) SICI (SICI%pre-fatigue) and 5) ICF (ICF%pre-fatigue), were examined. To assess changes in the composite measures of corticospinal inhibiton, normalized ratios for 6) LII (LII%pre-fatigue) and 7) SP duration (SP%pre-fatigue) were also compared. **Figure 3** outlines the neurophysiologic outcome variables.

To examine the time-course of changes in the neurophysiologic measures during the fatigue-tasks, the data were compared over time in 20% intervals of the TTF calculated for each individual's TTF (Pre-fatigue, 20%, 40%, 60%, 80% and 100% of TTF). The absolute times relative to the TTF were found for each individual and the responses measures for the stimuli delivered closest to that time, or the average of two stimuli delivered within an equal time frame on either side of the time point, were used. The last stimulus protocol was delivered within 0.73±0.48 minutes of the TTF and represents the final measure and is thus considered to represent 100% of TTF even if the subject continued to contract for a short period of time after the stimulation protocol was finished.

Statistical Analysis

SPSS version 20 for Mac (SPSS Inc, Chicago, IL) was used for the statistical analyses. Data are reported as mean±SD in the text with effect size (ES = partial η^2) and means±SE in the figures. An α of 0.05 was required for statistical significance. A paired *t*-test was used to compare the TTF between the two respective tasks and task-specific baseline values for the neurophysiologic outcomes from each muscle. Two-way repeated measures ANOVA (RM ANOVA) was used to compare changes in MVC with TASK (2:Force, Position) and TIME (2:pre-fatigue, task failure) as repeated factors. A mixed model ANOVA with TASK (2: POSITION, FORCE) as a repeated factor and GENDER (2: women, men) was used to compare the TTF between women and men. The effect of target force was analyzed by an ANCOVA (TASK, GENDER WITH TARGET FORCE COVARIED). Simple linear regression was then used to examine relationships between TTF and target force.

Analysis of the serial measures of muscle activation (i.e., RMS EMG) during the fatigue-task protocols was conducted using a three-way RM ANOVA with MUSCLE (Biceps, Brachioradialis), TASK and TIME (6:Pre-Fatigue, 20,40, 60, 80, Task-Failure) as factors. A significant interaction of MUSCLE × TIME was found for the brachioradialis; thus, the analyses of the eight neurophysiologic outcome variables were conducted separately for the biceps and the brachioradialis. A two-way RM ANOVA with TASK and TIME (6:Pre-Fatigue, 20,40, 60, 80, Task-Failure) as factors was used to explore for task-specific differences in RPE as well as the eight neurophysiologic outcome variables normalized to pre-fatigue baseline. An interaction for TASK × TIME was used to examine for differences in rate of change for the outcomes. To compare pairs of outcome variables a three-way RM ANOVA with TASK, TIME, and STIMULUS was used (e.g. STIMULUS 2 levels: MEP in SP%pre-fatigue and CMEP in SP%prefatigue). When a significant main effect and/or interaction terms were observed a follow-up post-hoc Sidak test was used to control for alpha inflation.

Sample size for the present study was based on previous data comparing the time to task failure for the force and position matching tasks, and was powered (power = 0.80) to detect significant differences in the time to task failure between the tasks at a P<0.05 [17]. However, with relatively small sample sizes, as in the present study, rather large differences may not reach statistical significance and result in Type II error. Therefore, effect sizes (here, referring to partial eta^2, which represents the proportion of total variation attributable to the factor, partialling out other factors from the total non-error variation) are reported as an additional statistical parameter to aid in interpretation of the findings.

Results

Performance Outcomes

Time to task failure and decline in MVC (Figures 4 and 5). The mean TTF for the position-matching task was 1.5 times longer than the mean TTF for the force-matching task (26.9±15.11 min vs. 17.5±7.9 min, $p<0.01$, ES = 0.60). The decline in MVC following the fatigue tasks did not differ between the two task conditions (Position-matching MVC %-Decline: 30.09±18%, Force-Matching MVC %-Decline: 30.07±15%; MVC TASK × TIME: $p = 0.59$). Individual values for TTF for the respective tasks are illustrated in Figure 5A. Interestingly, women exhibited a greater magnitude of difference in TTF ($TTFDiff_{P-F}$) between the two fatigue-tasks (TASK × GENDER: $p<0.01$); however, when the absolute 15% MVC target-force was statistically covaried, the effect of GENDER on $TTFDiff_{P-F}$ was no longer significant (TASK × GENDER: $p = 0.81$; it should be noted that TASK MAIN EFFECT persisted in the covariate analysis, $p<0.01$). There was an inverse relationship between the absolute value for the 15% MVC Target force and the $TTFDiff_{P-F}$ ($r = -0.85$, $p<0.01$). The absolute value for the target force predicted a significant amount of the between-subject variability in TFF for the position-matching task ($r^2 = 0.81$, $p<0.01$) and the force-matching task ($r^2 = 0.72$, $p<0.01$), as well as for the $TTFDiff_{P-F}$ ($r^2 = 0.73$, $p<0.01$). Thus, stronger subjects with a higher absolute target force were more likely to have similar TTF between the two tasks, whereas weaker subjects with a lower absolute target force had a greater difference

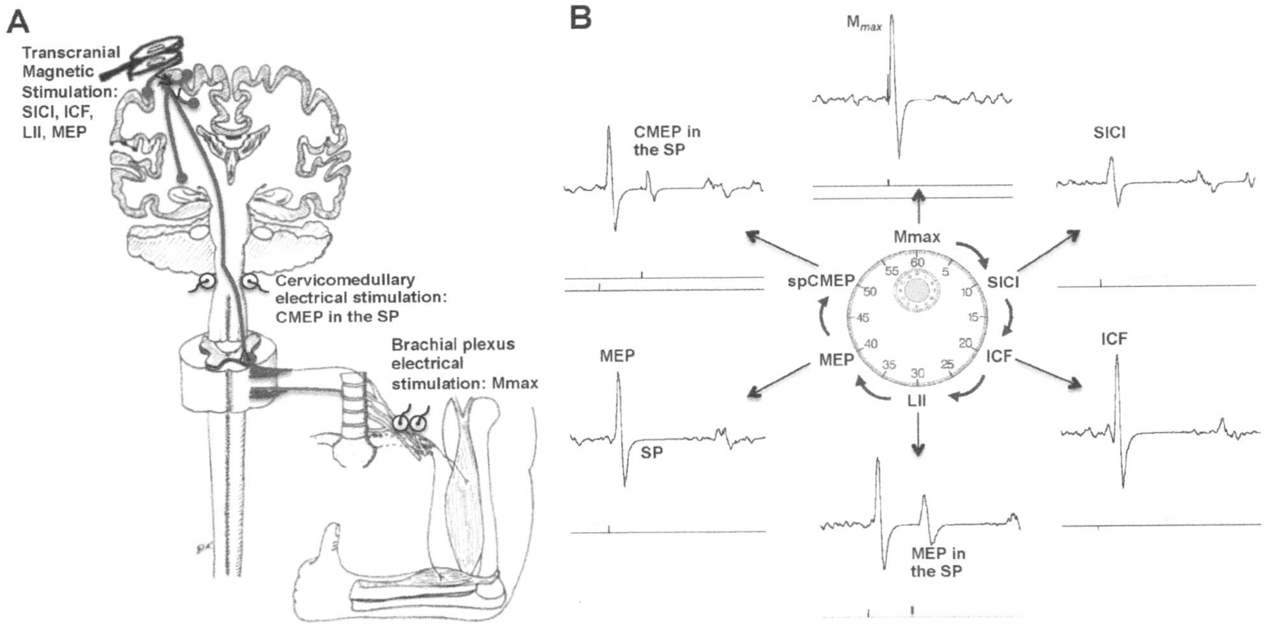

C

Peripheral pathway:
1. Muscle excitability→ Mmax amplitude*

Corticospinal pathway:
2. Corticospinal excitability→ MEP amplitude
3. Corticospinal inhibition→ SP duration

Intracortical circuits:
4. Intracortical inhibition→ SICI ratio
5. Intracortical facilitation→ ICF ratio

Fatigue state of corticospinal pathway and spinal motorneurons (volitional drive suspended):
6. Corticospinal excitability in the silent period→ MEP amplitude elicited in SP
7. Motorneuron excitability in the silent period→ CMEP amplitude elicited in SP

Upstream input effect on corticospinal pathway:
8. MEP amplitude (2) compared to MEP amplitude elicited in SP (6)→ LII ratio

Figure 3. Stimulation sites (A), example evoked potentials (B), and neurophysiologic outcome variables quantified from electromyographic recordings (C). A. Single and paired pulse stimuli were delivered to the motor cortex, the spinal cord at the cervicomedullary junction and the peripheral nerve at the brachial plexus. B. Sample electromyographic recordings of evoked potentials from a single subject elicited by the six stimuli in the protocol sequence. C. Eight neurophysiologic outcome variables were quantified from the evoked potentials. As the SP reflects a temporary cessation of voluntary drive, stimuli delivered during the SP were used to examine the fatigue state of the corticospinal pathway and spinal motorneurons. For intracortical circuits, the amplitude of a conditioned MEP elicited by paired pulse TMS is compared to the amplitude of the single pulse MEP in a ratio. The effect of upstream drive to the motor cortex was examined by comparing the amplitude of the MEP elicited in the SP to the amplitude of the single pulse MEP. This was also quantified as the ratio of long interval inhibition (LII ratio). *All cortical and cervicomedullary evoked potentials were normalized to M_{max}.

in TTF between tasks with a significantly longer TTF for the position-matching task.

Rating of perceived exertion. RPE increased throughout both fatigue tasks from 0 to equivalent mean values of 9.5±0.26 during the force-matching task and 9.7±0.21 for the position-matching task (Time $p<0.01$, ES = 0.96). The RPE values between pre-fatigue and 80% of TTF were significantly greater than the previous interval (post hoc pairwise comparison $p<0.01$) and then plateaued between 80% and 100% TTF ($p = 0.72$).

Neurophysiologic Outcomes

Pre-fatigue baseline measures of muscle activation and the eight neurophysiologic outcome variables for the biceps and brachioradialis are presented in **Table 1**. Prior to the fatigue tasks, the SP duration was significantly longer in the position-matching task than the force-matching task for both muscles ($p<0.001$). There were no significant differences in the pre-fatigue measures, in either the biceps or the brachioradialis, for muscle activation ($p>0.10$), the amplitudes for M_{max} ($p>0.10$), unconditioned MEP ($p>0.05$), conditioned MEP elicited in the silent period (MEP in SP: $p>0.10$), and conditioned CMEP elicited in the SP (CMEP in SP: $p>0.10$) nor were there significant baseline differences in the calculated ratios for SICI ($p>0.10$), ICF ($p>0.05$), and LII ($p>0.10$).

Muscle activation (Figure 6). There were no differences in the amounts of muscle activation throughout the performance of the two fatigue tasks to task failure (Task × Muscle × Time: $p = 0.21$, ES = 0.16); however, the rate of muscle activation was greater for the brachioradialis (Muscle × Time: p = 0.03 ES = 0.31). Although the amount of muscle activation in the brachioradialis was greater during the force matching task, the difference was not statistically significant (Muscle × Task: $p = 0.19$, ES = .0.18; Muscle: $p = 0.08$, ES = 0.31). At task failure the Biceps EMG had increased to 25.95±10.88%MVC and 28.12±17.21%MVC and the Brachioradialis EMG increased to 39.30±18.31%MVC and 27.59±13.23%MVC for the force-matching and position-matching tasks respectively (Time: p = 0.00 ES = 0.78; Sidak post hoc test p<0.05 between all TTF intervals except 80%TTF vs.100%TTF).

M_{max}. During the fatigue-tasks, the M_{max} amplitude did not change throughout either fatigue-task (Biceps Time: $p = 0.38$ ES = 0.10; Brachioradialis Time: $p = 0.74$ ES = 0.03) nor

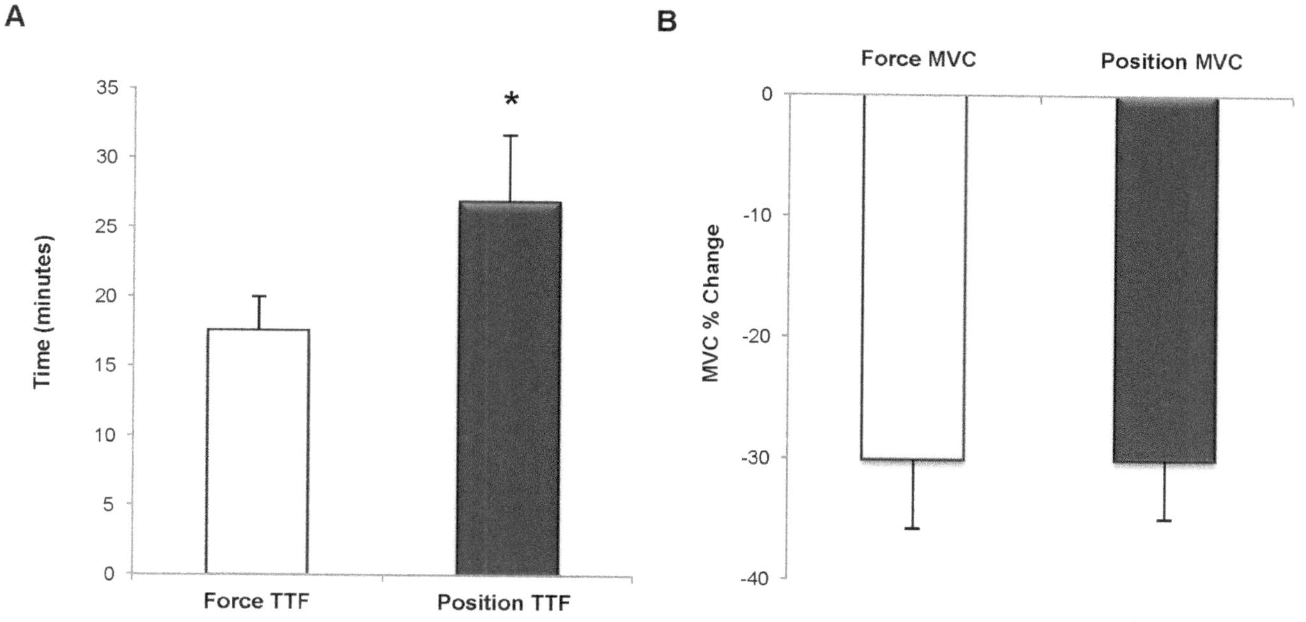

Figure 4. Time to task failure (A) and percent change in elbow flexor maximum voluntary contraction force (B). A. The time to task failure (TTF) for the position-matching task was longer than the TTF for the force-matching task ($p<0.01$, ES = .60). B. There was no difference between the two fatigue-tasks in the amount of muscle fatigue as measured by the percent decline in maximum voluntary contraction (MVC) force at task-failure ($p = 0.59$).

differ significantly between fatigue-tasks (Task: Biceps $p = 0.68$ ES = 0.02; Brachioradialis $p = 0.07$ ES = 0.33).

MEP amplitude (Figure 7A). The amplitude of the unconditioned MEP gradually increased in the biceps to 157.60±85.33%pre-fatigue baseline and to 147.60±79.57%pre-fatigue baseline (Time: $p = 0.03$, ES = 0.33) and in the brachioradialis to 226.13±153.49%pre-fatigue baseline and to 223.80±125.95%pre-fatigue baseline (Time: $p = 0.01$, ES 0.41) by task failure for the force-matching and position-matching tasks respectively. There were no significant post hoc pair-wise

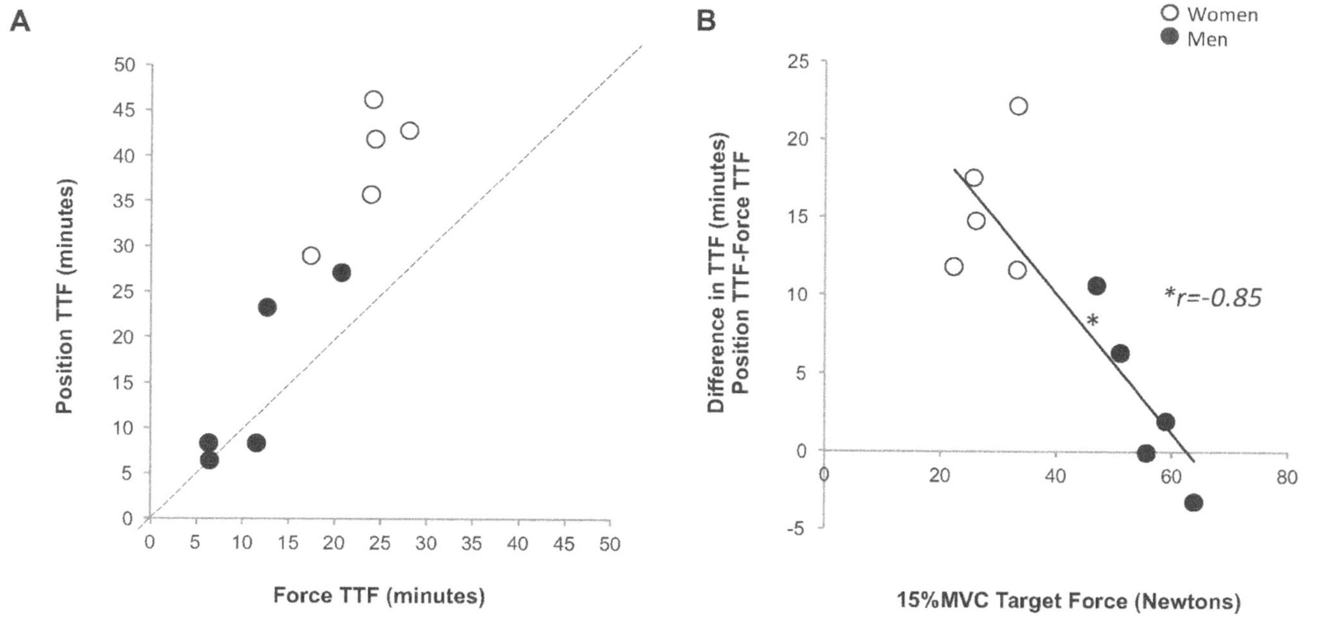

Figure 5. Individual time to task failure (A) and time to task failure difference with target force (B). (*Open circles*) Women (*Filled circles*) Men A. When compared to the force-matching task, 80% of the subjects had a greater time to task failure (TTF) during the position-matching task. The dashed line represents an equivalent TTF for both fatigue-tasks. B. There was inverse relationship between the magnitude of the difference in TTF (position-matching TTF − force-matching TTF) of the two fatigue-tasks and the absolute value of the target force (*$r = -0.85$, $p<0.01$).

Table 1. Pre-fatigue baseline values for the neurophysiologic outcome variables.

BICEPS				BRACHIORADIALIS			
Force	*Position*	*p*	ES	*Force*	*Position*	*p*	ES
RMS EMG %pre-fatigue MVC							
13.07±6.43	11.27±6.83	0.39	0.08	13.24±5.01	10.22±3.36	0.06	0.33
M_{max} mV							
6.69±3.60	9.74±4.78	0.11	0.26	7.50±.4.65	8.20±3.73	0.67	0.02
MEP %M_{max}							
69.49±28.65	51.93±15.83	0.08	0.31	49.63±25.99	44.98±24.68	0.27	0.13
SP duration msec							
127.97±19.69*	146.47±22.19*	**0.00**	0.74	127.97±26.48*	150.20±27.48*	**0.00**	**0.67**
MEP in SP %M_{max}							
44.58±21.52	30.03±18.88	0.10	0.28	31.82±17.95	25.00±19.38	0.16	0.21
CMEP in SP %M_{max}							
46.84±29.98	33.92±26.99	0.19	0.18	36.43±21.52	26.29±23.06	0.19	0.19
SICI ratio							
0.75±0.27	0.69±0.27	0.55	0.04	0.87±0.29	0.78±0.32	0.16	0.20
ICF ratio							
1.04±0.18	1.07±0.17	0.61	0.03	1.30±0.39	1.01±0.11	0.07	0.33
LII ratio							
0.73±0.48	0.60±0.41	0.14	0.23	0.77±0.46	0.55±0.34	0.12	0.25

Data are mean values (±SD) of the three pre-fatigue baseline measures taken during short duration 3–5sec 15%MVC task-specific contractions. Asterisks (*) signify a task-specific difference between baseline values (*p* values <0.05 are indicated by bold text). *ES: Effect size partial eta^2; ICF: intracortical facilitation; LII: long interval inhibition; MEP: motor evoked potential; Mmax: maximum compound muscle action potential; MVC: maximum voluntary contraction; RMS EMG: root mean squared electromyographic amplitude; SICI: short interval intracortical inhibition; SP: silent period; spCMEP: cervicomedullary evoked potential elicited in the silent period.*

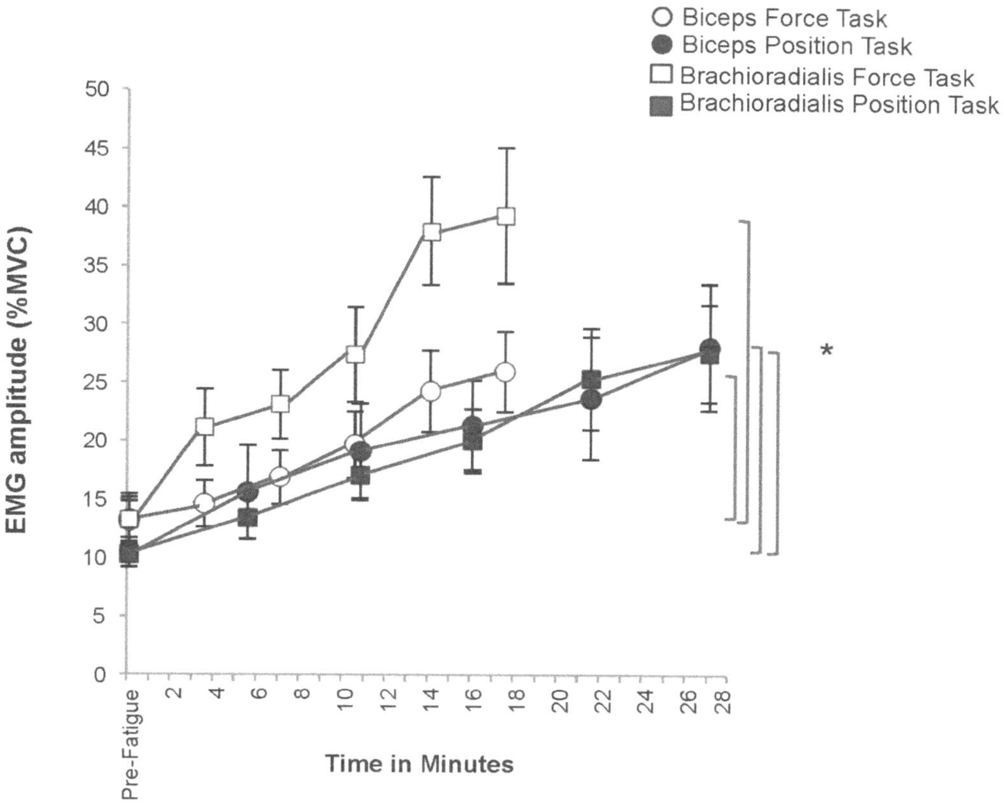

Figure 6. Muscle activation of the biceps and brachioradialis during the force-matching and position-matching tasks. The EMG amplitude (% of pre-fatigue MVC) increased in both muscles throughout both fatigue tasks (*$p = 0.00$) but did not differ between tasks or muscles. The rate of muscle activation was greater for the brachioradialis during fatigue task performance ($p = 0.03$). Each data point represents the mean EMG (% of pre-fatigue MVC) at 20% intervals of the TTF relative to each individual's TTF during each task. **The respective TTF interval was significantly greater than all previous intervals except 80% vs. 100%TTF.

comparisons for TIME ($p>0.05$). No task-specific differences were found for the amount of increase in MEP amplitude (TASK: Biceps $p = .91$ ES = 0; Brachioradialis $p = 0.38$ ES = 0.09) or for the rate of change in MEP amplitude (TASK × TIME: Biceps $p = 0.82$ ES = 0.03; Brachioradialis $p = 0.56$ ES = 0.07).

Silent period duration (Figure 7B). At task failure, the SP duration had increased in the biceps to 112.97±6.68%pre-fatigue baseline and to 109.11±3.53%pre-fatigue baseline (TIME: $p<0.01$, ES = 0.37) and in the brachioradialis to 115.25±6.36%pre-fatigue baseline and to 107.97±3.17%pre-fatigue baseline (TIME: $p = 0.02$, ES = 0.36) for the force-matching and position-matching tasks respectively. There were no significant post hoc pair-wise comparisons for TIME ($p>0.05$). There were no task-specific differences for the amount of change (TASK: Biceps $p = 0.24$ ES = 0.15; Brachioradialis $p = 0.07$ ES = 0.34) or for rate of change in SP duration (TASK × TIME: Biceps $p = 0.33$ ES = 0.12; Brachioradialis $p = 0.13$ ES = 0.18).

MEP elicited during the silent period (Figure 8A). During both fatiguing contractions, the amplitude of the MEP in SP gradually increased in the biceps to 197.22±41.60%pre-fatigue baseline and to 164.74±35.57%pre-fatigue baseline (TIME: $p = 0.01$, ES = 0.30) and in the brachioradialis to 175.77±30.39%pre-fatigue baseline and to 193.41±36.66%pre-fatigue baseline (TIME: $p = 0.01$, ES 0.38) for the force-matching and position-matching tasks respectively. There were no significant post hoc pair-wise comparisons for TIME ($p>0.05$). No task-specific differences were found for either the amount of change (TASK: Biceps $p = .83$ ES = 0.01; Brachioradialis $p = 0.86$ ES = 0) or the rate of change in MEP in SP amplitude (TASK × TIME: Biceps $p = 0.53$ ES = 0.08; Brachioradialis $p = 0.78$ ES = 0.03).

CMEP elicited in the silent period (Figure 8B). The amplitude of the CMEP in SP gradually decreased in the biceps to 74.41±18.40%pre-fatigue baseline and to 58.93±11.01%pre-fatigue baseline (TIME: $p = 0.02$, ES = 0.35) and in the brachioradialis to 35.42±8.72%pre-fatigue baseline and to 55.89±13.19%pre-fatigue baseline (TIME: $p<0.00$, ES = 0.52) for the force-matching and position-matching tasks respectively at task failure. Significant pairwise comparisons for TIME were found in the brachioradialis between pre-fatigue and the 40%TTF and 100%TTF intervals. There were no significant post hoc pair-wise comparisons for TIME in the biceps ($p>0.05$). There were no task-specific differences in the overall amount of change (TASK: Biceps $p = 0.36$ ES = 0.09; Brachioradialis $p = 0.40$ ES = 0.08) or in the rate of change for CMEP in SP amplitude (TASK × TIME: Biceps $p = 0.61$ ES = 0.06; Brachioradialis $p = 0.52$ ES = 0.07).

Short-Interval intracortical inhibition ratio (Figure 9A). In both fatiguing contractions, the SICI ratio increased to 146.63±22.81%pre-fatigue baseline in the force-matching task and to 191.72±41.40%pre-fatigue baseline for the position-matching task (TIME: $p = 0.02$, ES = 0.35) indicating decreasing intracortical inhibition in the biceps. There were no significant post hoc pair-wise comparisons for Time ($p>0.05$). The

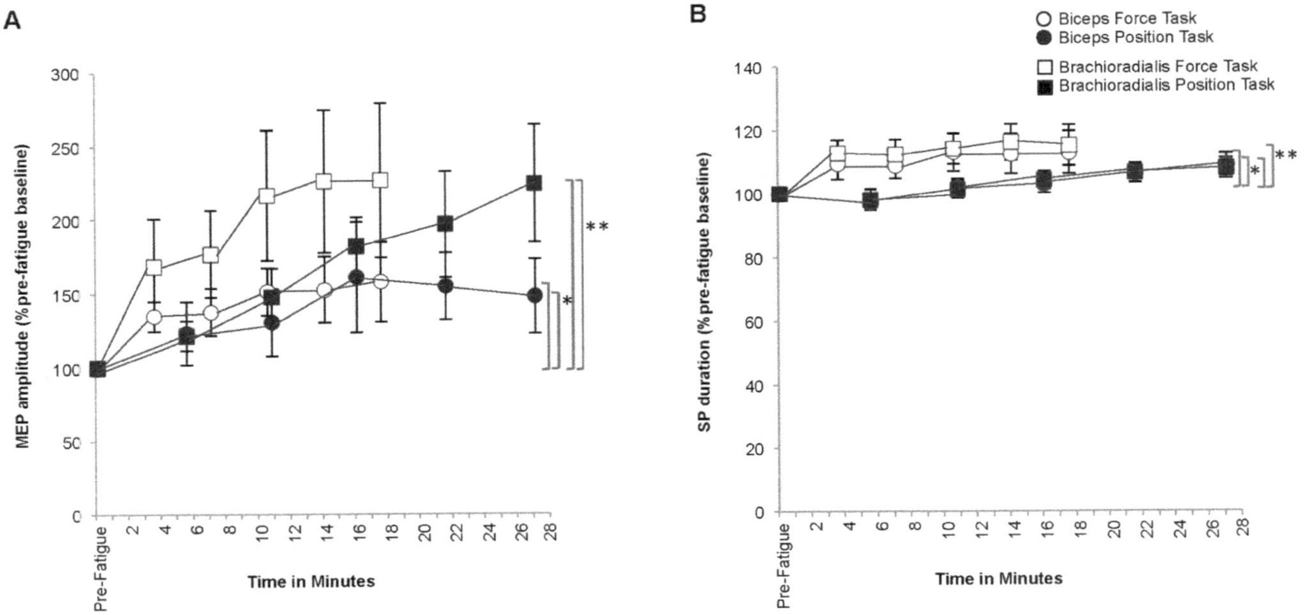

Figure 7. Motor evoked potential amplitude (A) and silent period duration during the force-matching and position-matching tasks (B). A. The motor evoked potential (MEP) amplitude (%pre-fatigue baseline) increased during both fatigue-tasks in the biceps (*$p = 0.03$) and the brachioradialis (**$p = 0.01$). B. Silent period (SP) duration (%pre-fatigue baseline) increased throughout both fatigue tasks in the biceps (*$p < 0.01$) and the brachioradialis (**$p < 0.01$).

changes in the SICI ratio for the brachioradialis, while greater than baseline, were not statistically significant (force-matching: 113.61±16.01%pre-fatigue baseline, position-matching: 120.23±13.02%pre-fatigue baseline; TIME: $p = 0.12$ ES = 0.17). There were no task-specific differences in the amount of change (TASK: Biceps $p = .52$ ES = 0.05; Brachioradialis $p = 0.26$ ES = 0.14) or the rate of change in SICI ratio (TASK ×

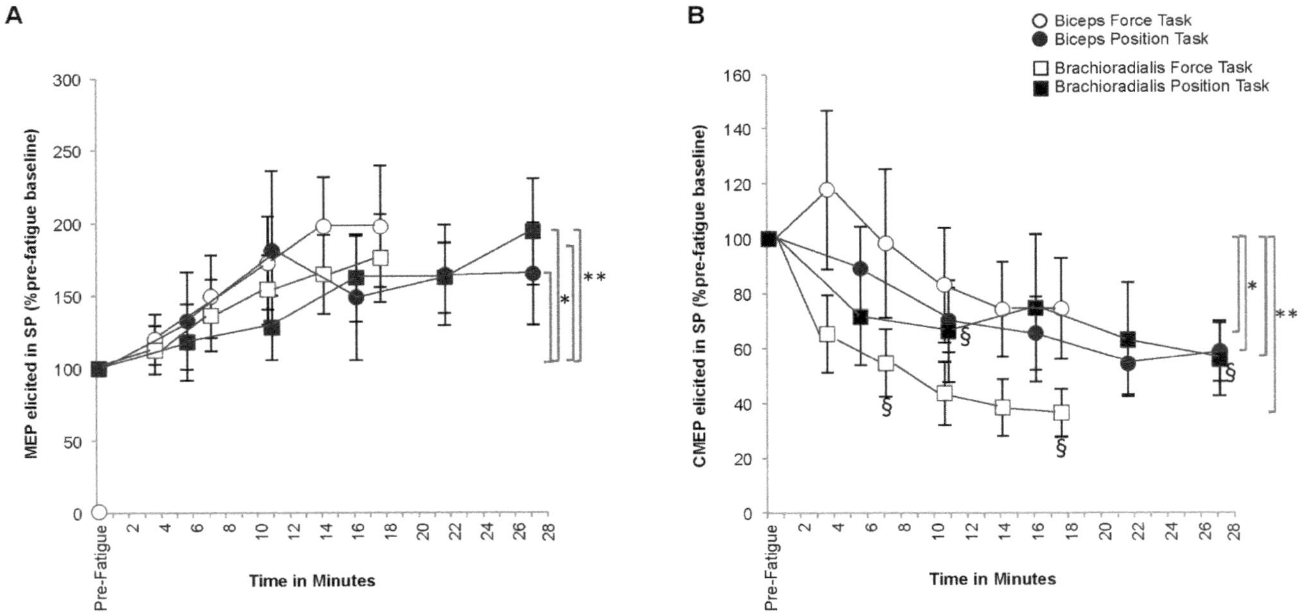

Figure 8. Cortically-evoked response elicited in the silent period (A) and cervicomedullary-evoked response elicited in the silent period (B). A. The amplitude (% of pre-fatigue baseline) of the motor evoked potential elicited in the silent period (MEP elicited in SP) increased progressively to task failure during both fatigue-tasks in the biceps (*$p = 0.01$) and the brachioradialis (**$p = 0.01$). B. The amplitude (%pre-fatigue baseline) of the cervicomedullary-evoked potential elicited in the SP (CMEP elicited in SP) progressively decreased throughout the fatiguing contractions to task failure in the biceps (*$p = 0.02$) and the brachioradialis (**$p < 0.001$).

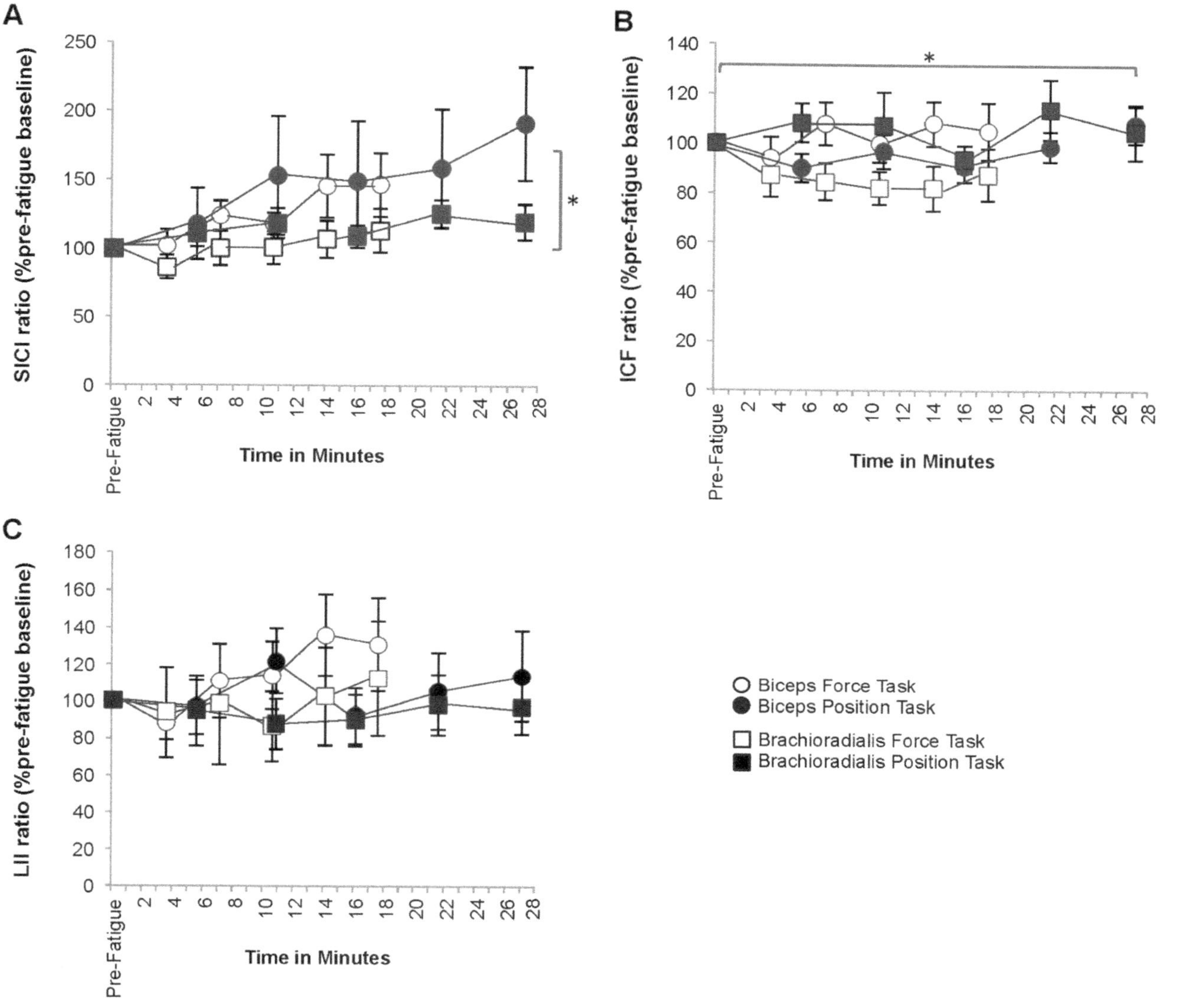

Figure 9. Short interval intracortical inhibition ratio (A), intracortical facilitation ratio (B) and long-interval inhibition ratio (C). A. The value for the ratio (%pre-fatigue baseline) of short interval intracortical inhibition (SICI ratio) progressively increased throughout the fatigue-tasks in the biceps (* $p = 0.03$), which is consistent with *decreasing* intracortical inhibition and did not change in the brachioradialis ($p > 0.10$). B. The value for the intracortical facilitation (ICF) ratio (%pre-fatigue baseline) did not change during fatigue-task performance in either muscle ($p > 0.10$) and, in the brachioradialis, remained greater than baseline during the position-matching task and less than baseline in the force-matching task (* $p = 0.20$). C. The value for long interval inhibition (LII) ratio (%pre-fatigue baseline) did not differ between the fatigue-tasks nor change during fatigue-task performance ($p > 0.50$).

TIME: Biceps $p = 0.58$ ES = 0.06; Brachioradialis $p = 0.52$ ES = 0.07).

Intracortical facilitation ratio (Figure 9B). The ICF ratio did not significantly change in either muscle during either fatiguing contraction (TIME: Biceps $p = 0.10$ ES = 0.18; Brachioradialis $p = 0.69$ ES = 0.04). There was a task-specific difference in the overall value for the ICF ratio in the brachioradialis with the mean value throughout the force-matching task (87.11±16.44%pre-fatigue baseline) significantly lower than during the position-matching task (104.69±12.65%pre-fatigue baseline; TASK: $p = 0.02$, ES = 0.47), but not for the biceps (TASK: $p = 0.40$, ES = 0.08). There was no difference in the rate of change in ICF ratio (TASK × TIME: Biceps $p = 0.72$ ES = 0.06; Brachioradialis $p = 0.21$ ES = 0.15).

Long interval inhibition ratio (Figure 9C). There were no changes in the LII ratio throughout the fatiguing contractions (TIME: Biceps $p = 0.41$ ES = 0.09, Brachioradialis $p = 0.91$ ES = 0.03) nor were there any task-specific differences in the overall value for the LII ratio (TASK: Biceps $p = 0.55$ ES = 0.04, Brachioradialis $p = 0.82$ ES = 0.01) in either muscle.

MEP vs. MEP elicited in the silent period (Figure 10A). Measures of corticospinal excitability with (MEP) and without volitional drive (MEP in SP) progressively increased in both muscles throughout both fatigue tasks to task failure (TIME: Biceps MEP: 152.62±20.71%pre-fatigue baseline, MEP in SP:181.03±29.52%pre-fatigue baseline $p = 0.00$, ES 0.41; Brachioradialis MEP: 224.89±41.98%pre-fatigue baseline, MEP in SP 184.14±28.05%pre-fatigue baseline $p = 0.01$, ES = 0.46). There were no significant differences between tasks and stimuli in

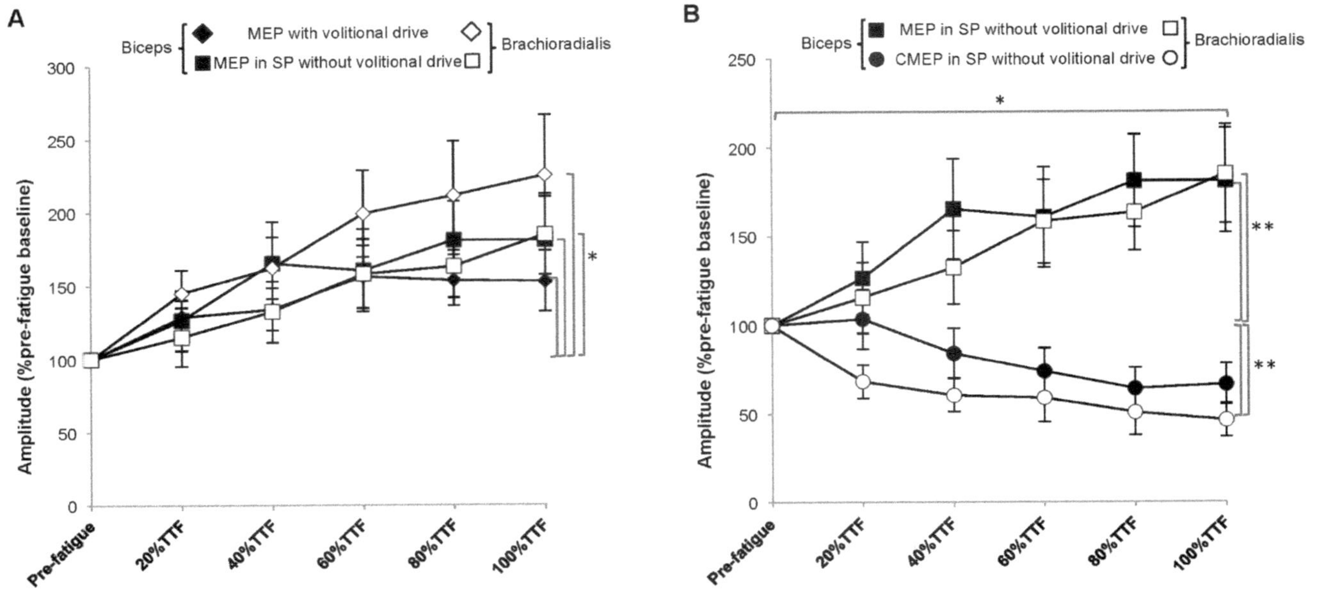

Figure 10. Comparisons of corticospinal excitability with and without volitional drive (A) and corticospinal and spinal excitability without volitional drive (B). A. The amount of corticospinal excitability (%pre-fatigue baseline) both with volitional drive (MEP) and without volitional drive (MEP in SP) increased throughout fatigue task performance in both muscles (*p<0.01). There were no differences found between tasks; therefore, values were pooled across tasks for clarity. B. The amount of corticospinal excitability (%pre-fatigue baseline) without volitional drive (MEP in SP) progressively increased and was greater throughout task performance in both muscles (*$p<0.001$) relative to the amount of spinal excitability (%pre-fatigue baseline) without volitional drive (CMEP in SP) which progressively decreased throughout fatigue-task performance in both muscles (**$p=0.00$). There were no differences found for task therefore, values were pooled across tasks for clarity.

either muscle (Stimulus × Task × Time: Biceps $p=0.23$ ES = 0.14; Brachioradialis $p=0.67$ ES = 0.04).

MEP elicited in the silent period vs. CMEP elicited in the silent period (Figure 10B). Measures of the fatigue state of corticospinal excitability (MEP in SP), were significantly greater throughout fatigue task performance relative to the fatigue state measures of spinal excitability (CMEP in SP) (Stimulus × Time: Biceps $p=0.00$, ES 0.42; Brachioradialis $p=0.00$, ES = 0.61), but there were no differences between tasks (Stimulus × Task × Time: Biceps $p=0.34$ ES = 0.12, Brachioradialis $p=0.87$ ES = 0.04). The mean MEP elicited in SP was significantly greater than the mean CMEP elicited in the SP during fatigue task performance (Stimulus: Biceps MEP in SP152.32±19.32%pre-fatigue baseline, CMEP in SP 82.12±10.11%pre-fatigue baseline, $p=0.17$, ES = 0.49; Brachioradialis MEP in SP 142.30±17.05%pre-fatigue baseline, CMEP in SP 64.05±8.42%pre-fatigue baseline, $p=0.00$, ES = 0.77).

SICI ratio vs. ICF ratio (Figure 11A). In the biceps, the mean value for SICI increased to 169.20±25.5% of pre-fatigue baseline during the fatigue-tasks while the ICF ratio did not change (106.4±7.72%pre-fatigue baseline) indicating a reduction in short interval intracortical inhibition during the fatigue tasks with sustained intracortical facilitation (Stimulus × Time: $p=0.01$, ES = 0.46). There were no significant differences found for the brachioradialis ($p>0.05$).

LII ratio vs. SP duration (Figure 11B and Figure 12). Initial analyses comparing the LII ratio with the SP duration did not reveal any significant effects ($p>0{,}05$); therefore, the LII ratio was further analyzed individually. During the fatiguing contractions, the mean value for the normalized LII ratio in the biceps was 113.3±10.9%pre-fatigue baseline and 105.0±11.4% and in the brachioradialis 99.0±20.8%pre-fatigue baseline and 94.5±10.7%pre-fatique baseline during the force-matching task and position-matching tasks respectively which suggests no increase in corticospinal inhibition during the fatigue tasks (Task × Time: Biceps $p=0.62$ ES = 0.06, Brachioradialis $p=0.78$ ES = 0.34).

To explore the relationship between SP duration and measures of corticospinal and motorneuron excitability in the SP, a final 3-way RM-ANOVA (Task (2), Time (6), Stimulus (3)) comparing the normalized values for SP duration, CMEP evoked during the SP, and MEP evoked during the SP was completed (**Figure 12**) in the biceps and the brachioradialis. This analysis revealed that during the fatiguing contractions, in the biceps as the SP duration increased to 111.0±3.4%pre-fatigue, the MEP in SP increased to 181.0±29.5%pre-fatigue while the CMEP in SP amplitude decreased to 66.7±11.6% of pre-fatigue values (Stimulus × Time: $p=0.00$, ES 0.36). Similar results were found in the brachioradialis (SP duration: 111.6%±3.8%pre-fatigue baseline, MEP in SP: 184.6±27.7%pre-fatigue baseline, CMEP in SP: 46.2±9.3%pre-fatigue baseline; Stimulus × Time: $p=0.00$, ES 0.50). Significant pairwise comparisons for Stimulus were found between the CMEP elicited in the SP with the MEP elicited in the SP and the SP duration in both muscles greater overall ($p<0.05$).

Discussion

The purpose of this study was to compare the task specific differences in the adjustments in cortical and spinal excitability that developed during the performance of the force-matching and position-matching tasks with the elbow flexors in order to further delineate the contribution of supraspinal mechanisms to task failure during sustained submaximal contractions. There were five main findings from this experiment. First, contrary to expectations, the duration of the position-matching task with the elbow flexors was 45% longer than the force-matching task when

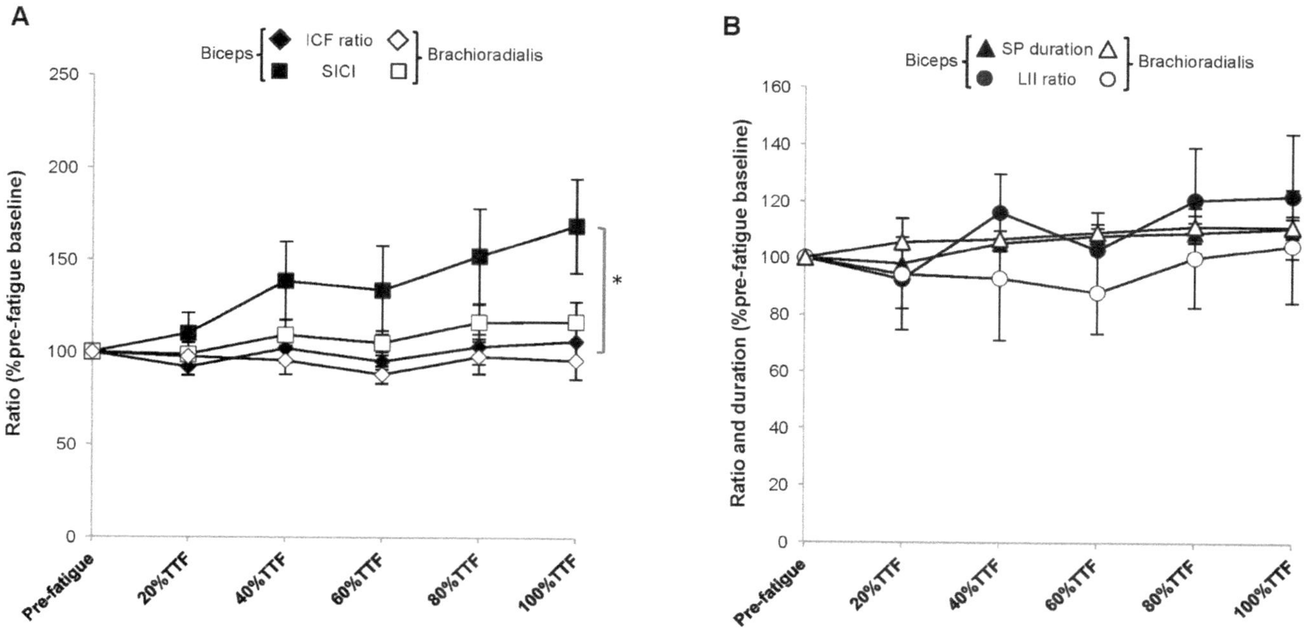

Figure 11. Comparisons between intracortical inhibition and facilitation (A) and long interval inhibition with silent period duration (B). A. In the biceps, the amount of short interval intracortical inhibition (SICI ratio %pre-fatigue baseline) increased during fatigue task performance indicating a *reduction* in inhibition while the amount of intracortical facilitation (ICF ratio %pre-fatigue baseline) remained unchanged (*$p = 0.01$); however, there were no differences found in the brachioradialis for either variable ($p > 0.05$). Values were pooled across tasks for clarity as there were no differences found by task. B. Comparison of the ratio for long interval inhibition (LII as %pre-fatigue baseline) and the duration of the silent period (SP duration as %pre-fatigue baseline) did not demonstrate significance when compared by task, time and stimulation protocol suggesting no change in composite corticospinal inhibition. Values were pooled across tasks for clarity.

performed under identical mechanical demands without proximal stabilization or restraint of the forearm. Second, there were no significant task-specific differences found for the total amount of change and the rate of change for the eight neurophysiologic outcome variables in the biceps muscle. Third, the amount of corticospinal excitability (i.e., MEP and MEP elicited in the SP) increased throughout fatigue task performance while the amount of spinal excitability (i.e., CMEP elicited in the SP) decreased. Fourth, the amount of intracortical inhibition within the motor cortex decreased or was sustained (i.e., SICI ratio) during fatigue task performance. Both ICF within the motor cortex (i.e., ICF ratio) and upstream excitation of the motor cortex (i.e. MEP vs. MEP elicited in the SP, LII ratio) remained constant. Lastly, the increase in the duration of the SP followed the progressive decrease in spinal excitability throughout fatigue-task performance but deviated from the progressive increase in corticospinal excitability. Below, these key results will be discussed further.

Task-specific Differences in Performance

Consistent with the paradigm identified in prior studies with the elbow flexors comparing the task duration of two sustained submaximal contractions that differ by load compliance, both tasks resulted in the same amount of muscle fatigue, amount of muscle activation, and change in RPE despite significant differences in contraction times [15,59]. Contrary to our initial hypothesis, the duration of the position-matching task was found to be nearly 42% longer than the duration of the force-matching task. Therefore, the shorter TTF for the force-matching task observed here is in disagreement with the majority of the current literature comparing the task duration between the force-matching and position-matching tasks [11,16,17,27,50,57,59,74–78].

Prior studies examining sustained submaximal contractions (i.e. ≤30%MVC) of the elbow flexors with the upper extremity positioned next to the body, the elbow flexed to 90° and the forearm in neutral as in this study have consistently found the position-matching task TTF to be on average 40% *shorter* than the force-matching task TTF [16,17,27,57,59]. The most common results reported for studies comparing the TTF for the two tasks performed by extremity muscles (i.e. ankle dorsiflexors, knee extensors, wrist extensors, first dorsal interossei) [11,50,74–76,78] and for the elbow flexors in a different arm posture [57,77,79] are for a 21–53% increase in TTF for the force-matching task depending upon contraction intensity and muscle tested. However, while most common, the paradigm is far from ubiquitous and has several caveats. The magnitude of difference in TTF for the force-matching task over the position-matching task has been found to depend upon: 1) the intensity of the submaximal contraction [15,16,75]; 2) the posture of the limb and the body [57,77]; and 3) the amount of proximal stabilization and limb support provided during task performance [11,76,80]. The effect of these conditions is to reduce and even eliminate the difference in TTF between the two tasks due to the total amount of muscle activation required by not only the primary movers but also synergists, accessory muscles and postural stabilizers [16,57,74]. Thus, while this is not the first study to find results about task duration that differ from the most common result, this is the first extremity muscle study to report the direct opposite result: the TTF for the position-matching task with the elbow flexors was 42% longer than the force-matching task. Recently, one study evaluating the trunk extensors has also reported similar results [79]. Two aspects of the experimental setup used in this study may have contributed to the reversal in

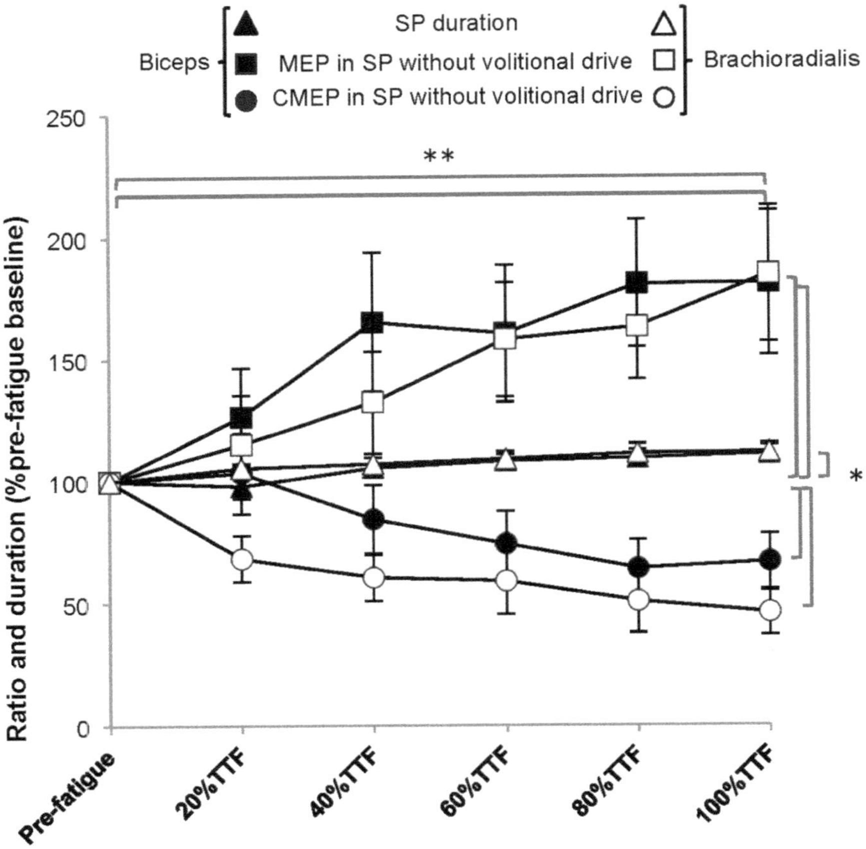

Figure 12. Comparisons between silent period duration with corticospinal and spinal excitability measured during the silent period. The duration of the silent period (SP duration %pre-fatigue baseline) progressively increased during fatigue task performance to task failure as the amount of corticospinal excitability (%pre-fatigue baseline) measured during the silent period (MEP in SP without volitional drive) progressively increased and the amount of spinal excitability (%pre-fatigue baseline) measured in the silent period (CMEP in SP without volitional drive) progressively decreased in both muscles (*$p = 0.00$). The value for the MEP elicited in the SP as well as the SP duration remained above baseline and were significantly greater than the mean value for the CMEP elicited in the SP which was below baseline for both muscles (**$p<0.05$).

task duration result: 1) subject stabilization and 2) sensitivity of the visual feedback.

Prior to discussing the factors that could explain the unexpected TTF, to ensure the validity of the experimental strategy and therefore its usefulness for addressing the stated hypotheses about neural mechanisms of task failure in sustained submaximal contractions, it is worth highlighting the performance results that were consistent with prior force-matching/position-matching studies. First, despite the differences in TTF, the amount of muscle fatigue, as measured by the decline in MVC force at task failure, was similar for the two tasks (i.e. 30±15% and 30±18%) and comparable to the results reported from prior studies of the elbow flexors using a 15% MVC [17,59]. Second, at task failure, the amount of perceived effort reported by subjects, using the RPE scale, increased to the same value for both tasks. Therefore, consistent with the paradigm, at task failure both tasks ended with the same amount of physical and perceptual fatigue/exertion despite having a 42% difference in task duration [12,15,16,59]. Third, consistent with the intensity/duration characteristics of sustained submaximal contractions (i.e. lower intensity contractions have a longer duration), the absolute target force the individual subjects exerted with the elbow flexors was a significant contributor to the TTF for both the force-matching and the position-matching tasks [18,55] and eliminated the gender differences found for TTF [81]. Additionally, the magnitude of the absolute target force explained 73% of the variability in the difference in TTF between the two tasks. The stronger subjects who sustained a higher absolute target force were more likely to have similar TTF for both tasks, whereas weaker subjects with a lower absolute target force had a greater difference in TTF between tasks with a significantly longer position-matching TTF. The difference in TTF has been attributed to faster and/or greater recruitment of the motor pool during the shorter task [17,31]. Therefore, for the stronger subjects with a higher magnitude absolute target force, most likely a greater proportion of the motor pool was recruited at the start of both fatigue tasks in order to produce the force output needed for task performance leaving fewer unrecruited motor units available to be recruited as the contraction duration progressed thus eliminating the difference in TTF.

Task Specific Differences in Measures of Supraspinal and Spinal Excitability

There were no differences found between the force-matching and the position-matching tasks for either the mean total amount of change or the rate of change for the eight neurophysiologic measures of segmental excitability in the biceps. Additionally, there were no significant task-specific differences in the total amount of change in muscle activation for both muscles. Although the brachioradialis had a greater rate of activation during fatigue task performance, this difference was not task specific. The only significant task-specific difference was found in the brachioradialis muscle for the ICF ratio where the mean value was greater than baseline for the position-matching task and less than baseline throughout the force-matching task; however, this value did not change with fatigue. Thus, it is unlikely that this one difference could explain the difference we found in the TTF between the force-matching and position-matching tasks because the value for ICF did not change as fatigue developed and remained constant to task failure. Instead, this finding may suggest a task-specific difference in intracortical control mechanisms of the brachioradialis necessary for performance but unrelated to fatigue [20,37]. Together these results suggest that the net amount and rate of change in segmental excitability, as measured by the eight variables, that developed with fatigue did not differ between the two tasks.

The only prior study comparing cortical and spinal excitability measures between the two tasks found equivalent changes in corticospinal excitability, as measured by MEP amplitude, and a task specific difference in spinal excitability, measured with the H-reflex, such that the shorter duration position-matching task had both a greater and faster decline in spinal excitability [27]. The shorter duration of the position-matching task was ascribed to a decline in neural activation of the muscle secondary to a decrease in peripheral sensory afferent drive to the motor pool from the muscle spindle Ia afferent fiber due to the effect that inertial load compliance has on the sensitivity of the stretch reflex–this as opposed to a reduction in descending motor drive or adaptations intrinsic to the motorneuron that modulate firing rates [5,15,17,27,74]. This disfacilitation is suggested to be mediated by presynaptic inhibition of the Ia afferent fiber by descending inputs thereby permitting more sensory feedback to be delivered to supraspinal centers which can then be used to adjust the drive to the motor pool via long loop reflex control [17,27]. Evidence to support this hypothesis include the task-specific differences in H-reflex amplitude [27] and decline in Ia presynaptic inhibition (i.e., less inhibition) during the longer duration force-matching task [17]. The purpose of the increased presynaptic inhibition in the position-matching task is suggested to permit greater cortical influence over the motor pool to minimize force fluctuations [15,82].

Prior studies using the force-matching/position-matching task paradigm to investigate neural mechanisms associated with task failure have suggested that there are fundamental differences in central neural control strategies that are driven by the task demands, specifically the compliance or stiffness of the load [5,7,11,12,15,16,57,59,74]. This same rationale of a different neural control strategy may explain the shorter duration found in this study for the force-matching task and, in addition to differences in load compliance, could be driven by two specific elements of the experimental setup used in this study: 1) the absence of stabilization and limb constraint during task performance and 2) the sensitivity of the visual feedback.

It is well understood that less stabilization requires that more muscles are used to perform the task and if more muscles perform the task, then there is an overall greater level of central neural drive [5,16,57,83]. Greater stabilization has been associated with less muscle activation of prime movers and accessory muscles as well as a longer TTF for the force-matching task [16,57,74,77]. It should be noted, that to date, co-activation ratios between the agonist prime movers (e.g., biceps) and antagonists (e.g., triceps) have been found to be the same between the two tasks and therefore do not to contribute to the differences in TTF [27,67,74,75]. In this study, every effort was made to ensure equivalent mechanical demands during task performance. Therefore, external supports (e.g., straps) were not used to restrict motions at the shoulder or the torso in order to equalize the demand placed on synergists, proximal joints, and postural stabilizers between the two fatigue-tasks. Additionally, in both tasks the arm was free to move in all degrees of freedom with the tether used in force-matching task only limiting the amount of elbow flexion. This is different the typical setup used for the force-matching task where the orthosis is clamped to a frame that effectively holds the forearm in the target position and prevents motion [11,16,17,27,50,57,59,74,75,77,78]. Accordingly, the shorter task duration found in this study for the force-matching task could be related to the overall amount of muscle activity needed within the upper extremity and torso to perform the task.

Two studies using lower limb muscles have compared the TTF across three conditions: the typical free-motion position matching task, a more restrained position-matching task, and the typical setup for the force-matching task [11,76]. When a greater amount of restraint was provided to the limb during the position-matching task, the difference in TTF between the force-matching and position-matching tasks was reduced by half [11,76]. This suggests that with more restraint there were less degrees of freedom to control during the position-matching task as well as less compensatory movements to prevent at other joints. One additional "benefit" of restraint and stabilization from external supports during task performance is that it is easier for synergist muscles from both proximal and distal joints to assist in isometric task performance. Indeed, the intention of effective stabilization during isometric task performance is to minimize joint motion that could occur at other joints; however, just because the joint motions are restricted does not mean that these other muscles are not producing force. For example, greater activation was recorded in the rectus femoris muscle during the force-matching task performed by the dorsiflexors. It was suggested that the hip flexion action of the rectus femoris could assist in task performance as both the foot and leg were restrained [74].

In this study, because the subjects were unrestrained, they were closely monitored and were specifically instructed that no other joint or body motions were permitted that would put tension through the tether connecting the wrist to the force transducer (e.g. no lateral trunk lean, no shoulder shrugging), they could only bend the elbow aiming the thumb towards the ceiling. Because subjects were not stabilized and the limb was not restrained in either fatigue task, the demands placed upon postural stabilizers and accessory muscles, in order to maintain postural alignment and to prevent limb motions in the transverse and frontal planes of motion, were most likely equivalent in this study. Thus, the difference in TTF may be more related to the degree control needed to manage these multiple degrees of freedom within the body. In other words, in addition to the quantity of muscles that needed to be activated for task performance, the two tasks may have required different intracortical control strategies perhaps reflected by differences in the excitability of intracortical circuits to achieve the correct task performance. This type of control would need to be constant throughout task performance, and thus would be independent from the amount and/or rate of change measures of segmental excitability.

The second potential source for the longer duration position-matching task may be due a difference in the sensitivity of or resolution of the visual feedback to detect fluctuations in output. From a motor control perspective, both of these tasks can be considered to be analogous to a sustained visuomotor tracking task because the only way the subject knows that the force output is correct is through constant visual feedback [84–86]. From prior studies, the shorter duration task is considered to be the more difficult task by subjects during task performance even though the mechanical demands, torque output, and amount of muscle fatigue at task failure are equivalent between the two tasks [12,15]. Indeed in this study, subjects anecdotally reported that the force-matching task was "harder" specifically because it was more challenging to keep the feedback line steady. For both tasks, the verbal instructions given to the participant were to "keep the line as close to the target line for as long as you possibly can without using compensations at other joints." A prior study comparing the effect of visual feedback signal gain during the position-matching task found an increase in TTF for a wider bandwidth of performance [87]. This suggests that had the boundary been wider, performance could have lasted longer. Perhaps it is not just the boundary but also the sensitivity to fluctuations in output that occur within that boundary that matters [85]. The on-screen bandwidth set as the criteria for defining task failure was the same for the two tasks such that the decline in performance output resulted in a similar drop in the net elbow flexor torque for each task. However, the sensitivity of the force transducer to detect fluctuations in force output within that bandwidth and thus project those fluctuations on screen as visual feedback to the subject may have been greater than the sensitivity of the electrogoniometer for detecting the effect of those force fluctuations had on joint angle position. Therefore, during the position-matching task, slight fluctuations in motor output may not be as visually obvious to the participant as compared to the force-matching task and therefore would not merit the need for corrective action by the subject in response to the visual feedback order to maintain their feedback line close to the target line. This suggests that the two tasks may have differed not only in load compliance but also in the demand for feedback-driven corrections in motor output requiring greater cortical control. Together these results, in combination with prior studies about the differences in proximal stabilization and the effect of visual feedback on force control, suggests that there is something more than/other than load compliance that make the TTF for these two tasks differ.

Supraspinal Contributions to Task Failure

Although there were no task-specific differences found for the changes in excitability in the biceps and for only one variable in the brachioradialis, the data from this experiment adds to the growing understanding of the neurologic mechanisms involved in the decline in force output that limits the duration of a sustained submaximal contraction by investigating the contribution of supraspinal adjustments stemming from changes in intracortical and corticospinal excitability relative to concurrent changes in spinal excitability. At task failure for both the force-matching and position-matching tasks, a similar amount of decline in motorneuron excitability developed as measured by the amplitude of the CMEP elicited in the SP. Additionally, the amount of increase in corticospinal excitability, as measured by the single pulse MEP, was also similar at task failure for both tasks. Therefore, consistent with prior research, both fatigue-tasks ended secondary to a decline in motorneuron excitability coupled with a failure of supraspinal input to successfully sustain motorneuron activity [22,23,27]. That task failure occurred for both the force-matching and position-matching tasks after a similar mean decline in motorneuron excitability coupled with a similar mean increase in corticospinal excitability suggests that, in general, the motor cortex is able to compensate for changes in spinal excitability until a particular amount of change develops. At that point, unless more drive is provided from the motor cortex or to the motor cortex, failure occurs. These findings are consistent with the general mechanism for task failure proposed from single motor unit studies, namely task duration is determined by the rate of recruitment of the motor pool by descending drive to compensate for the declining force output from active motor units [12,17,22,23].

The next question to answer then is *why is the motor cortex eventually unable to sustain activation of the motor pool?* To address this question, two competing hypotheses/questions posed in the literature [1,15,29] were addressed by the data in this experiment: 1) Is there evidence to support that the cortex itself becomes inhibited, analogous to the spinal cord, which would then decrease the amount of descending drive? 2) Is there evidence to suggest that there is a lack of excitatory drive provided from upstream sources to the motor cortex that would be needed to sustain descending drive?

During the performance of both fatigue-tasks, the duration of the SP increased, which would suggest an increase in intracortical inhibition; however, the direct measures of intracortical excitability do not support this interpretation. First, the amount of intracortical inhibition, as indexed by the value of the SICI ratio, progressively decreased throughout fatigue-task performance to between 147–192% for both tasks in the biceps and to 114–121% in the brachioradialis (although not statistically significant $p = 0.12$). In general, SICI is considered to be mediated locally within the motor cortex such that changes in SICI are interpreted to reflect selective focusing of cortical excitability and corticospinal outputs involved in task performance in the muscle used for voluntary contractions [66,88]. In addition, prior studies that have used SICI to assess the intracortical changes that develop during fatigue associated with sustained or intermittent MVCs found significant decreases in intracortical inhibition localized to the muscle participating in the task [41–43]. Second, the amount of ICF, indexed by the ICF ratio, while greater in the brachioradialis throughout the duration of the force-matching task, the amount of intracortical facilitation did not change during either fatigue-task indicating that there was neither an increase nor decrease in the amount of facilitation within the motor cortex. The ICF ratio, like the SICI ratio, is thought to reflect changes in local motor cortex excitability [20,37]. One prior study investigating fatigue associated with the performance of intermittent MVCs reported the same result as found in this experiment [42]. Because of the way that that SICI and ICF are evoked through the paired-pulse protocol that investigates the effect of a subthreshold stimulus, that selectively activates the intracortical neurons, on the amplitude of the MEP evoked by the second stimulus, the values for SICI and ICF reflect the excitability of the intracortical circuitry within the motor cortex that synapse upon the corticospinal projections to the motor pool [39,40,63,89]. Therefore, when the normalized values for SICI and ICF were compared to each other, there was a significantly lower amount of intracortical inhibition at task failure for the biceps and no significant change in inhibition in the brachioradialis; however, the amount of intracortical facilitation did not increase as fatigue progressed.

The amount of change that occurred in corticospinal excitability assessed in the presence of voluntary drive, as indexed by the single unconditioned MEP, did not significantly differ from the amount of change in corticospinal excitability measured during the SP when volitional drive was temporarily suspended during both fatigue tasks. Both values increased in both muscles to between 150% and 225% of baseline. If the motor cortex were becoming progressively inhibited as the traditional interpretation of the increased duration of the SP implies, then the amount of change in excitability for the MEP elicited in the SP should not have increased as much as the single MEP evoked in the presence of volitional drive. Additionally, the magnitude of change for the single, unconditioned MEP was not significantly greater than the magnitude of change for the MEP elicited in the SP, which suggests that upstream input to the motor cortex remained consistent relative to the level of ongoing output from the motor cortex as fatigue developed. Further support for this result comes from the lack of change in the value for the LII ratio throughout task performance. This value is the ratio of the two MEP values: the value for the MEP elicited in the SP independent from volitional drive to the value for the MEP evoked in the presence of volitional drive. Therefore, the LII ratio could be considered to represent the effect of volitional drive on corticospinal excitability. Taken together, when compared to the amount of change in the amplitude of the CMEP elicited in the SP (**Figure 10**), these results indicate that increases in corticospinal excitability are not accompanied by active increases in inhibition within the motor cortex. Instead these results indicate that the increase in intracortical excitability that drives the amount of descending drive needed to overcome spinal cord resistance is mediated by decreasing intracortical inhibition that exceeds the amount of change in intracortical facilitation and excitation delivered to the motor cortex from upstream drive. Therefore, the supraspinal mechanisms that limit task duration are most likely mediated by inadequate upstream excitatory drive to the motor cortex, as opposed to increased intracortical inhibition, as the increased SP duration would imply. Upstream drive can be influenced by the level of motivation as reflected by the RPE [1,9]. It can also be affected by sensory afferents from the periphery to the cortex including both Ia proprioceptive afferents as discussed in the previous section about task differences as well as inputs from the group III and IV metaboreceptors [1,5,12]. Recent evidence suggests that the group III and IV afferents have a greater effect on cortical excitability compared to spinal excitability [90]. Finally, when the normalized values for the changes in LII ratio were compared to the normalized SP duration, there was no interaction. Instead, when the normalized SP was compared to the normalized values for the cortical and spinal measures evoked during the SP the results suggest that as the duration of the SP increase, the amount of spinal excitability decreases while the amount of cortical excitability independent from ongoing volitional drive increases. Therefore, these results also support the conclusion that the change in SP duration that occurs during fatiguing contractions is most likely mediated by the progressive decline in spinal excitability and not to an increase in intracortical inhibition as with non-fatiguing contractions.

Limitations

Although there were no task-specific differences for the total amount of change in spinal and supraspinal excitability that developed over time during fatigue task performance, it should be noted that the effect sizes for some of the pre-fatigue baseline values as well as for two fatigue-task values from the brachioradialis suggest that a main effect for task, independent of contraction duration, may be present. The sample size for this study was calculated from data from previously published studies comparing the time to task failure for the force and position matching tasks and was powered (power = 0.80) to detect significant differences in the time to task failure between the tasks at a $p<0.05$ [17]. Thus, this study was likely underpowered to detect differences under baseline conditions between the two tasks and further work is required to more fully investigate this issue.

Conclusion

The concurrent use of single pulse, paired-pulse TMS and paired cortio-cervicomedullary stimulation used in this experiment during the performance of the two fatigue tasks (i.e., force-matching and position-matching) provided a unique opportunity to both localize and compare adjustments in segmental excitability in the nervous system to determine the functional significance of the changes to task duration. Although task-specific differences in the neurophysiologic variables were not found in this study, these results do add to a growing body of work that supports the efficacy of the two-task approach to explore the neural mechanisms of task failure. That the opposite task was found to have the shorter TTF (i.e. force-matching <position-matching) in comparison to most reports, supports the conclusion of a task specific difference in central neural command in motor unit recruitment [5,17,87]; however, the source of the task specificity may be due to factors other than load compliance such as the amount of stabilization provided to the body and limb and the corrective demand driven by the sensitivity of the visual feedback within the same range of gain [85,86].

The collective neurophysiologic results across both tasks suggest that, as fatigue develops prior to task failure, the increase in corticospinal excitability observed in relationship to the progressive decline in spinal excitability is the product of decreasing values of intracortical inhibition combined with unchanged values of intracortical facilitation and "upstream" excitability of the motor cortex. Therefore, despite an increase in SP duration, there was no evidence of enhanced intracortical inhibition; instead, these results suggest that the capacity of supraspinal inputs to continue to override spinal resistance is limited by a lack of increase in intracortical facilitation and "upstream" drive to the motor cortex. These results also support the conclusion that during fatiguing submaximal contractions, the increase in SP duration is most likely due to spinal mechanisms reducing motorneuron excitability and therefore, would be best viewed as a measure of composite corticospinal inhibition and not intracortical inhibition as with non-fatiguing contractions [22,47].

In our subsequent companion paper we present an experiment designed to explore the results presented here that insufficient facilitation and upstream drive to the motor contributes to task failure. Specifically, we address the question of whether anodal transcranial direct current stimulation (tDCS), a non-invasive focal neurostimulation using weak direct electrical currents known to transiently increase cortical excitability, delivered to the motor cortex during the performance of a sustained submaximal contraction increases TTF when compared to a sham tDCS condition.

Author Contributions

Conceived and designed the experiments: PW BC. Performed the experiments: PW RH. Analyzed the data: PW. Contributed reagents/materials/analysis tools: BC. Wrote the paper: PW BC.

References

1. Gandevia SC (2001) Spinal and Supraspinal Factors in Human Muscle Fatigue. Physiol Rev 81: 1725–1789.
2. Kluger BM, Krupp LB, Enoka RM (2013) Fatigue and fatigability in neurologic illnesses: Proposal for a unified taxonomy. Neurology 80: 409–416.

3. Bigland-Ritchie B, Woods JJ (1984) Changes in muscle contractile properties and neural control during human muscular fatigue. Muscle Nerve 7: 691–699.
4. Enoka RM, Stuart DG (1992) Neurobiology of muscle fatigue. J Appl Physiol 72: 1631–1648.
5. Barry BK, Enoka RM (2007) The neurobiology of muscle fatigue: 15 years later. Integr Comp Biol 47: 465–473.
6. Bigland-Ritchie B, Cafarelli E, Vollestad NK (1986) Fatigue of submaximal static contractions. Acta Physiol Scand Suppl 556: 137–148.
7. Enoka RM, Duchateau J (2008) Muscle fatigue: what, why and how it influences muscle function. J Physiol 586: 11–23.
8. Bigland-Ritchie B (1981) EMG and fatigue of human voluntary and stimulated contractions. In: Porter R, Whelan J, editors. Human Muscle Fatigue: Physiologic Mechanisms London: Pitman Medical. 130–156.
9. Enoka RM (2012) Muscle fatigue - from motor units to clinical symptoms. J Biomech 45: 427–433.
10. Hunter SK, Critchlow A, Shin IS, Enoka RM (2004) Fatigability of the elbow flexor muscles for a sustained submaximal contraction is similar in men and women matched for strength. J Appl Physiol 96: 195–202.
11. Yoon T, Hawe R, Hunter SK (2009) Variation in limb support influences the time to task failure for a postural contraction. J Mot Behav 41: 393–395.
12. Maluf KS, Enoka RM (2005) Task failure during fatiguing contractions performed by humans. J Appl Physiol 99: 389–396.
13. Bigland-Ritchie B (1981) EMG/force relations and fatigue of human voluntary contractions. Exerc Sport Sci Rev 9: 75–117.
14. Place N, Bruton JD, Westerblad H (2009) Mechanisms of fatigue induced by isometric contractions in exercising humans and in mouse isolated single muscle fibres. Clin Exp Pharmacol Physiol 36: 334–339.
15. Enoka RM, Baudry S, Rudroff T, Farina D, Klass M, et al. (2011) Unraveling the neurophysiology of muscle fatigue. J Electromyogr Kinesiol 21: 208–219.
16. Rudroff T, Justice JN, Holmes JR, Matthews SD, Enoka RM (2011) Muscle activity and time to task failure differ with load compliance and target force for elbow flexor muscles. J Appl Physiol 110: 125–136.
17. Baudry S, Rudroff T, Pierpoint LA, Enoka RM (2009) Load type influences motor unit recruitment in biceps brachii during a sustained contraction. J Neurophysiol 102: 1725–1735.
18. Duchateau J, Balestra C, Carpentier A, Hainaut K (2002) Reflex regulation during sustained and intermittent submaximal contractions in humans. J Physiol 541: 959–967.
19. Nordstrom MA, Gorman RB, Laouris Y, Spielmann JM, Stuart DG (2007) Does motoneuron adaptation contribute to muscle fatigue? Muscle Nerve 35: 135–158.
20. Reis J, Swayne OB, Vandermeeren Y, Camus M, Dimyan MA, et al. (2008) Contribution of transcranial magnetic stimulation to the understanding of cortical mechanisms involved in motor control. J Physiol 586: 325–351.
21. Rothwell JC (2008) TMS measures and voluntary motor function. In: Wassermann EM, Epstein CM, Ziemann U, Walsh V, Paus T et al., editors. The Oxford Handbook of Transcranial Stimulation. New York: Oxford University Press. 171–184.
22. McNeil CJ, Martin PG, Gandevia SC, Taylor JL (2009) The response to paired motor cortical stimuli is abolished at a spinal level during human muscle fatigue. J Physiol 587: 5601–5612.
23. McNeil CJ, Giesebrecht S, Gandevia SC, Taylor JL (2011) Behaviour of the motoneurone pool in a fatiguing submaximal contraction. J Physiol 589: 3533–3544.
24. Reis J, Robertson EM, Krakauer JW, Rothwell J, Marshall L, et al. (2008) Consensus: Can transcranial direct current stimulation and transcranial magnetic stimulation enhance motor learning and memory formation? Brain Stimul 1: 363–369.
25. Goss DA, Hoffman RL, Clark BC (2012) Utilizing transcrancial magnetic stimulation to study the human neuromuscular system. Journal of Visualized Experiments: JoVE 20.
26. Kobayahsi M, Pascual-Leone A (2003) Transcranial magnetic stimulation in neurology. Lancet Neurology 2: 145–156.
27. Klass M, Levenez M, Enoka RM, Duchateau J (2008) Spinal mechanisms contribute to differences in the time to failure of submaximal fatiguing contractions performed with different loads. J Neurophysiol 99: 1096–1104.
28. Sidhu SK, Cresswell AG, Carroll TJ (2012) Motor cortex excitability does not increase during sustained cycling exercise to volitional exhaustion. J Appl Physiol 113: 401–409.
29. Rothwell JC (2009) The fatigued spinal cord. J Physiol 587: 5517–5518.
30. Adam A, De Luca CJ (2003) Recruitment order of motor units in human vastus lateralis muscle is maintained during fatiguing contractions. J Neurophysiol 90: 2919–2927.
31. Mottram CJ, Jakobi JM, Semmler JG, Enoka RM (2005) Motor-unit activity differs with load type during a fatiguing contraction. J Neurophysiol 93: 1381–1392.
32. Chen R, Lozano AM, Ashby P (1999) Mechanism of the slient period following transcranial magnetic stimulation. Exp Brain Res 128: 539–542.
33. Taylor JL, Butler JE, Allen GM, Gandevia SC (1996) Changes in motor cortical excitability during human muscle fatigue. J Physiol 490 (Pt 2): 519–528.
34. Taylor JL, Gandevia SC (2008) A comparison of central aspects of fatigue in submaximal and maximal voluntary contractions. J Appl Physiol 104: 542–550.
35. Sacco P, Thickbroom GW, Byrnes ML, Mastaglia FL (2000) Changes in corticomotor excitability after fatiguing muscle contractions. Muscle and Nerve 23: 1840–1846.
36. Taylor JL, Todd G, Gandevia SC (2006) Evidence for a supraspinal contribution to human muscle fatigue. Clin Exp Pharmacol Physiol 33: 400–405.
37. Di Lazzaro V, Pilato F, Oliviero A, Dileone M, Saturno E, et al. (2006) Origin of facilitation of motor-evoked potentials after paired magnetic stimulation: direct recording of epidural activity in conscious humans. J Neurophysiol 96: 1765–1771.
38. Nakamura HK, Kawaguchi Y, Tsuji H (1997) Intracortical facilitation and inhibition after transcranial magnetic stimulation in conscious humans. Journal of Physiology 498.3: 817–823.
39. Rothwell JC, Day BL, Thompson PD, Kujirai T (2009) Short latency intracortical inhibition: one of the most popular tools in human motor neurophysiology. J Physiol 587: 11–12.
40. Kujirai T, Caramia MD, Rothwell JC, Day BL, Thompson PD et al. (1993) Corticocortical inhibition in human motor cortex. Journal of Physiology 471: 501–519.
41. Benwell NM, Sacco P, Hammond GR, Byrnes ML, Mastaglia FL, et al. (2006) Short-interval cortical inhibition and corticomotor excitability with fatiguing hand exercise: a central adaptation to fatigue? Exp Brain Res 170: 191–198.
42. Maruyama A, Matsunaga K, Tanaka N, Rothwell JC (2006) Muscle fatigue decreases short-interval intracortical inhibition after exhaustive intermittent tasks. Clin Neurophysiol 117: 864–870.
43. Vucic S, Cheah BC, Kiernan MC (2011) Dissecting the mechanisms underlying short-interval intracortical inhibition using exercise. Cereb Cortex 21: 1639–1644.
44. Taylor JL, Gandevia SC (2004) Noninvasive stimulation of the human corticospinal tract. J Appl Physiol 96: 1496–1503.
45. Ugawa Y, Rothwell JC, Day BL, Thompson PD, Marsden CD (1991) Percutaneous Electrical Stimulation of Corticospinal Pathways at the Level of the Pyramidal Decussation in Humans. Ann Neurol 29: 418–427.
46. Martin PG, Hudson AL, Gandevia SC, Taylor JL (2009) Reproducible measurement of human motoneuron excitability with magnetic stimulation of the corticospinal tract. J Neurophysiol 102: 606–613.
47. McNeil CJ, Martin PG, Gandevia SC, Taylor JL (2011) A novel way to test human motoneurone behaviour during muscle fatigue. Physiology News: 29–31.
48. McNeil CJ, Giesebrecht S, Khan SI, Gandevia SC, Taylor JL (2011) The reduction in human motoneurone responsiveness during muscle fatigue is not prevented by increased muscle spindle discharge. J Physiol 589: 3731–3738.
49. Gandevia SC (2008) Voluntary muscle strength and endurance: 'The mechanism of voluntary muscle fatigue' by Charles Reid. Experimental Physiology 93.9: 1030–1033.
50. Baudry S, Maerz AH, Gould JR, Enoka RM (2011) Task- and time-dependent modulation of Ia presynaptic inhibition during fatiguing contractions performed by humans. J Neurophysiol 106: 265–273.
51. Petersen NC, Butler JE, Taylor JL, Gandevia SC (2010) Probing the corticospinal link between the motor cortex and motoneurones: some neglected aspects of human motor cortical function. Acta Physiol (Oxf) 198: 403–416.
52. Ainsworth BE, Jacobs DR, Leon AS (1993) Validity and reliability of self-reported physical activity status: the Lipid Research Clinics questionnaire. Med Sci Sports Exerc 25: 92–98.
53. Oldfied R (1971) The assessment and anlaysis of handedness: the Edinburgh Inventory. Neuropsychologia 9: 97–113.
54. Borg GA (1982) Pyschophysical basis of perceived exertion. Med Sci Sports Exerc 14: 377–381.
55. Rudroff T, Christou EA, Poston B, Bojsen-Moller J, Enoka RM (2007) Time to failure of a sustained contraction is predicted by target torque and initial electromyographic bursts in elbow flexor muscles. Muscle Nerve 35: 657–666.
56. Hunter SK, Lepers R, MacGillis CJ, Enoka RM (2003) Activation among the elbow flexor muscles differs when maintaining arm position during a fatiguing contraction. J Appl Physiol 94: 2439–2447.
57. Rudroff T, Barry BK, Stone AL, Barry CJ, Enoka RM (2007) Accessory muscle activity contributes to the variation in time to task failure for different arm postures and loads. J Appl Physiol 102: 1000–1006.
58. Harrison DD, Harrison SO, Croft AC, Harrison DE, Troyanovich SJ (1999) Sitting biomechanics part I: Review of the literature. Journal of Manipulative and Physiological Therapeutics 22: 594–609.
59. Hunter SK, Ryan DL, Ortega JD, Enoka RM (2002) Task differences with the same load torque alter the endurance time of submaximal fatiguing contractions in humans. J Neurophysiol 88: 3087–3096.
60. Hunter SK, Enoka RM (2003) Changes in muscle activation can prolong the endurance time of a submaximal isometric contraction in humans. J Appl Physiol 94: 108–118.
61. Mottram CJ, Christou EA, Meyer FG, Enoka RM (2005) Frequency modulation of motor unit discharge has task-dependent effects on fluctuations in motor output. J Neurophysiol 94: 2878–2887.
62. Zijdewind I, Butler JE, Gandevia SC, Taylor JL (2006) The origin of activity in the biceps brachii muscle during voluntary contractions of the contralateral elbow flexor muscles. Exp Brain Res 175: 526–535.
63. Di Lazzaro V, Oliviero A, Profice P, Saturno E, Pilato F, et al. (1998) Comparison of descending volleys evoked by transcranial magnetic and electric stimulation in conscious humans. Electroencephalogr Clin Neurophysiol 109: 397–401.

64. Rothwell JC (2012) Overview of neurophysiology of movement control. Clin Neurol Neurosurg 114: 432–435.
65. Damron LA, Dearth DJ, Hoffman RL, Clark BC (2008) Quantification of the corticospinal silent period evoked via transcranial magnetic stimulation. J Neurosci Methods 173: 121–128.
66. Ortu E, Deriu F, Suppa A, Tolu E, Rothwell JC (2008) Effects of volitional contraction on intracortical inhibition and facilitation in the human motor cortex. J Physiol 586: 5147–5159.
67. Levenez M, Garland SJ, Klass M, Duchateau J (2008) Cortical and spinal modulation of antagonist coactivation during a submaximal fatiguing contraction in humans. J Neurophysiol 99: 554–563.
68. Taylor JL (2006) Stimulation at the cervicomedullary junction in human subjects. J Electromyogr Kinesiol 16: 215–223.
69. Rossini PM, Barker AT, Berardelli A, Caramina MD, Caruso G, et al. (1994) Non-invasive electrical and magnetic stimulation of the brain, spinal cord and roots: basic principles and procedures for routine clinical application. Report of an IFCN committee. Electroencephalogr Clin Neurophysiol 91: 79–92.
70. Groppa S, Oliviero A, Eisen A, Quartone A, Cohen LG, et al. (2012) A practical guide to diagnostic transcranial magnetic stimulation: Report of an IFCN committee. Clin Neurophysiol 123: 858–882.
71. Dearth DJ, Umbel J, Hoffman RL, Russ DW, Wilson TE, et al. (2010) Men and women exhibit a similar time to task failure for a sustained, submaximal elbow extensor contraction. Eur J Appl Physiol 108: 1089–1098.
72. Farina D, Merletti R, Enoka RM (2004) The extraction of neural strategies from the surface EMG. J Appl Physiol 96: 1486–1495.
73. Keenan KG, Farina D, Merletti R, Enoka RM (2006) Amplitude cancellation reduces the size of motor unit potentials averaged from the surface EMG. J Appl Physiol 100: 1928–1937.
74. Hunter SK, Yoon T, Farinella J, Griffith EE, Ng AV (2008) Time to task failure and muscle activation vary with load type for a submaximal fatiguing contraction with the lower leg. J Appl Physiol 105: 463–472.
75. Maluf KS, Shinohara M, Stephenson JL, Enoka RM (2005) Muscle activation and time to task failure differ with load type and contraction intensity for a human hand muscle. Exp Brain Res 167: 165–177.
76. Poortvliet PC, Tucker KJ, Hodges PW (2013) Changes in constraint of proximal segments effects time to task failure and activity of proximal muscles in knee position-control tasks. Clin Neurophysiol 124: 732–739.
77. Rudroff T, Poston B, Shin IS, Bojsen-Moller J, Enoka RM (2005) Net excitation of the motor unit pool varies with load type during fatiguing contractions. Muscle Nerve 31: 78–87.
78. Rudroff T, Justice JN, Matthews S, Zuo R, Enoka RM (2010) Muscle activity differs with load compliance during fatiguing contractions with the knee extensor muscles. Exp Brain Res 203: 307–316.
79. Thomas JS, Ross AJ, Russ DW, Clark BC (2011) Time to task failure of trunk extensor muscles differs with load type. J Mot Behav 43: 27–29.
80. Bojsen-Moller J, Schwartz S, Magnusson SP (2011) Limited difference in time to failure between sustained force and position control contractions with the knee extensors. Scand J Med Sci Sports 21: e48–55.
81. Hunter SK, Enoka RM (2001) Sex differences in the fatiguability of arm muscles depends on absolute force during isometric contractions. J Appl Physiol 91: 2686–2694.
82. Shemmell J, Krutky MA, Perreault EJ (2010) Stretch sensitive reflexes as an adaptive mechanism for maintaining limb stability. Clin Neurophysiol 121: 1680–1689.
83. Le Bozec S, Bouisset S (2004) Do bimanual isometric push efforts in humans stop as a consequence of postural muscle exhaustion? Neurosci Lett 356: 61–65.
84. Lauber B, Leukel C, Gollhofer A, Taube W (2012) Time to task failure and motor cortical activity depend on the type of feedback in visuomotor tasks. PLoS One 7: e32433.
85. Lee Hong S, Newell KM (2008) Visual information gain and the regulation of constant force levels. Exp Brain Res 189: 61–69.
86. Lee Hong S, Brown AJ, Newell KM (2008) Compensatory properties of visual information in the control of isometric force. Perception & Psychophysics 70: 306–313.
87. Mottram CJ, Hunter SK, Rochette L, Anderson MK, Enoka RM (2006) Time to task failure varies with the gain of the feedback signal for women, but not for men. Exp Brain Res 174: 575–587.
88. Ridding MC, Taylor JL, Rothwell JC (1995) The effect of voluntary contraction on cortico-cortical inhibition in human motor cortex. Journal of Physiology 487.2: 541–548.
89. Chen R (2004) Interactions between inhibitory and excitatory circuits in the human motor cortex. Exp Brain Res 154: 1–10.
90. Martin PG, Weerakkody N, Gandevia SC, Taylor JL (2008) Group III and IV muscle afferents differentially affect the motor cortex and motoneurones in humans. J Physiol 586: 1277–1289.

Medulloblastoma in China: Clinicopathologic Analyses of SHH, WNT, and Non-SHH/WNT Molecular Subgroups Reveal Different Therapeutic Responses to Adjuvant Chemotherapy

Zhen-Yu Zhang[1]⁹, Jian Xu[1]⁹, Yong Ren[2], Yu Yao[1]*, Kay Ka-Wai Li[3], Ho-Keung Ng[3], Ying Mao[1], Liang-Fu Zhou[1], Ping Zhong[1]*

1 Department of Neurosurgery, Huashan Hospital, Fudan University, Shanghai, China, **2** Department of Pathology, Wuhan General Hospital of Guangzhou Command, People's Liberation Army, Wuhan, China, **3** Department of Anatomical and Cellular Pathology, Prince of Wales Hospital, The Chinese University of Hong Kong, Hong Kong, China

Abstract

Medulloblastoma (MB) is one of the most common primary central nervous system tumors in children. Data is lacking of a large cohort of medulloblastoma patients in China. Also, our knowledge on the sensitivity of different molecular subgroups of MB to adjuvant radiation therapy (RT) or chemotherapy (CHT) is still limited. The authors performed a retrospective study of 173 medulloblastoma patients treated at two institutions from 2002 to 2011. Formalin-fixed paraffin embedded (FFPE) tissues were available in all the cases and sections were stained to classify histological and molecular subgroups. Univariate and multivariate analyses were used to investigate prognostic factors. Of 173 patients, there were 118 children and 55 adults, 112 males and 61 females. Estimated 5-year overall survival (OS) rates for all patients, children and adults were 52%, 48% and 63%, respectively. After multivariate analysis, postoperative primary radiation therapy (RT) and chemotherapy (CHT) were revealed as favorable prognostic factors influencing OS and EFS. Postoperative primary chemotherapy (CHT) was found significantly improving the survival of children ($p<0.001$) while it was not a significant prognostic factor for adult patients. Moreover, patients in WNT subtype had better OS ($p=0.028$) than others (SHH and Non-SHH/WNT subtypes) given postoperative adjuvant therapies. Postoperative primary RT was found to be a strong prognostic factor influencing the survival in all histological and molecular subgroups ($p<0.001$). Postoperative primary CHT was found significantly to influence the survival of classic medulloblastoma (CMB) (OS $p<0.001$, EFS $p<0.001$), SHH subgroup (OS $p=0.020$, EFS $p=0.049$) and WNT subgroup (OS $p=0.003$, EFS $p=0.016$) but not in desmoplastic/nodular medulloblastoma (DMB) (OS $p=0.361$, EFS $p=0.834$) and Non-SHH/WNT subgroup (OS $p=0.127$, EFS $p=0.055$). Our study showed postoperative primary CHT significantly influence the survival of CMB, SHH subgroup and WNT subgroup but not in DMB and Non-SHH/WNT subgroup of MB.

Editor: Javier S Castresana, University of Navarra, Spain

Funding: This study was supported by Shanghai Talents Development Funds (No. 2011063 to YY). The funders had no role in study design, data collection and analysis, decision to publish, or preparation of the manuscript.

Competing Interests: The authors have declared that no competing interests exist.

* E-mail: yu_yao04@126.com (YY); zhp2288991@126.com (PZ)

⁹ These authors contributed equally to this work.

Introduction

Medulloblastoma is one of the most common primary central nervous system tumors in children, with an estimated incidence of 0.5/100,000 children [1,2]. In contrast, medulloblastoma represents a rare tumor in adults and comprises less than 1% of adult primary brain neoplasms [3]. Current managements of medulloblastoma are mainly based on the results of several prospective studies initiated in North America and Europe [4]. For children, surgical resection followed by craniospinal irradiation (CSI) and chemotherapy (CHT) is the typical treatment modality [4–7]. Although there lack prospective clinical trials confirming the benefit of CHT in treating adult patients, there is a trend towards a combined treatment strategies including CHT for adults[8].

Recent progress on medulloblastoma gene expression profiling demonstrated the disease is heterogeneous and consists of different molecular subgroups: SHH, WNT and Non-SHH/WNT medulloblastoma [9–12]. These molecular subgroups have been demonstrated to differ in demographic, genetic and clinical aspects. Of note, patients with WNT medulloblastoma survived significantly longer than patients with other subgroups of medulloblastoma, and there is a consensus that patients in this subgroup may be over treated with the possibilities of reducing current therapies such as RT and CHT [11]. Nevertheless, how to reduce adjuvant therapies in WNT medulloblastoma remains unclear. For instance, is it safe to remove CHT from current treatment modality for WNT medulloblastoma? Since our knowledge on the sensitivity of different molecular subgroups to adjuvant RT or CHT is still limited, it may be difficult to answer this question.

In the past decades, clinical and pathological prognostic factors for patients with medulloblastoma have been discussed by numerous reports. However, there are few reports on large cohorts of medulloblastoma patients in China and relevant data are very limited [13]. We performed a retrospective study of medulloblastoma to investigate underlying prognostic factors, and focused on the sensitivity of different molecular subgroups of medulloblastoma to current adjuvant therapies.

Patients and Methods

Ethics Statement

This study was approved by the Ethics Committee of Huashan Hospital, Fudan University and Southwest Hospital, Third Military Medical University. Since this is a retrospective study, written informed consent was not given by patients for their clinical records to be used in this study. However, clinical records of all patients in this study were anonymized and de-identified prior to analysis. Ethics Committee of Huashan Hospital, Fudan University and Southwest Hospital, Third Military Medical University had waived the need for written informed consent from the patients.

Patients and clinical data

A total of 173 medulloblastoma patients pathologically diagnosed in Huashan Hospital (Shanghai, China) and Southwest Hospital (Chongqing, China) between January 2002 and October 2011 were included in this study. Clinical data were collected from medical charts and follow-up data were collected by telephone interviews or clinic follow-ups. These data included age, sex, neurological symptoms, symptom duration, neuroimaging findings, extent of resection, CSF shunting, postoperative primary radiation therapy (RT), postoperative primary CHT and patients' clinical outcomes.

Classifications of histological and molecular subgroups

Formalin-fixed paraffin embedded (FFPE) tissues from primary tumor resection were available in all the cases. Haematoxylin & eosin (H&E) stained sections of tumors were reviewed and classified according to the 2007 WHO classification of tumors of central nervous system [14]. One histological subtype is medulloblastoma with extensive nodularity (MBEN), which is closely related to desmoplastic/nodular medulloblastoma (DMB) [14]. There were only 4 specimens classified as MBEN in our series and we added the 4 cases into DMB. Thus, there were 3 histological subtypes in our study: classic medulloblastoma (CMB), DMB and large-cell/anaplastic medulloblastoma (AMB). Immunohistochemistry for molecular subgroups of medulloblastoma was undertaken and evaluated according to the protocol illustrated by Ellison et al with modifications [9]. SHH subgroups, WNT subgroups and non-SHH/WNT subgroups were categorized by different immunoreactivities to two antibodies: β-catenin (BD #610154; 1:800; antigen retrieval, citrate buffer 20 min Bond), GAB1 (Abcam #ab27439; 1:50; antigen retrieval, citrate buffer 20 min Bond) (**Table S1**).

Statistical analysis

Overall survival(OS)was measured from the date of diagnosis to the date of death or last follow-up. Event-free survival(EFS)was measured from the date of diagnosis to the date of disease recurrence, death, or last follow-up. Survival curves were constructed using Kaplan-Meier methods. Differences in OS and EFS between subgroups of patients were analyzed using log-rank test (univariate analysis). Suitable prognostic factors for multivariate analysis were selected based on the p-value (<0.10) in univariate analysis. These factors were subsequently put into Cox proportional hazards regression model to identify independent prognostic factors (multivariate analysis). Statistical significance was defined as p-value being less than 0.05. Data statistics were performed using software IBM SPSS Statistics 19 (IBM Corp., Armonk, NY, USA).

Results

Patients' characteristics

There were 118 children ($3 \le \text{age} < 16$ years) and 55 adults ($\text{age} \ge 16$ years) with a children to adults ratio of 2.1:1. The median age at diagnosis was 12 years (range, 3–45 years). A male preponderance was observed in our cohort: 112 (65%) were male and 61 (35%) were female with a male to female ratio of 1.8:1. The most common symptoms were headache (69%) and nausea/vomiting (55%), which were associated with increased intracranial pressure. Cerebellar dysfunctional symptoms such as ataxia (40%) and diplopia (6%) were also common. Duration of symptoms varied from 0.5 day to 1.5 years and median duration of symptoms was 1.1 month. Except for those patients with missing information (26 cases), 63 (43%) patients had tumor infiltrating brainstem or IV ventricle floor. Radiological examinations revealed hydrocephalus in 111 patients (70%), with missing data in 15 cases (**Table 1**).

Treatment characteristics

All patients underwent tumor resection: 114 patients (69%) had gross total resection, 36 patients (31%) had subtotal resection and the extent of resection in 7 cases could not be evaluated based on our data. Perioperative CSF shunting was performed in 53 patients (34%) with missing data in 17 patients. In the entire cohort, 139 patients (80%) received postoperative primary RT and 98 patients (57%) received postoperative primary CHT (**Table 1**). There were 94 patients (54%) who underwent postoperative primary RT followed by sequential CHT, 47 patients (27%) who received only postoperative primary RT, 7 patients (4%) who received only postoperative primary CHT and 25 (15%) patients who underwent neither postoperative primary RT nor CHT.

Survival analysis for prognostic factors

The median follow-up time for all patients was 38.0 months with a range of 0.1 to 118.9 months. Estimated 5-year overall survival rates for all patients, children and adults were 52%, 48% and 63%, respectively. Estimated 5-year event-free survival rates for all patients, children and adults were 45%, 42% and 52%, respectively (**Figure S1**). Univariate analysis of prognostic factors for the entire cohort revealed that absence of brainstem or IV ventricle floor involvement by the tumor, gross total resection of the tumor, reception of postoperative primary RT and CHT were favorable factors significantly influencing OS and EFS (**Table 1**). The p-values of other two parameters (age and CSF shunting) were less than 0.10. Therefore, the 6 clinical parameters (age, CSF Shunting, involvement of brain stem or IV ventricle floor, extent of resection, RT and CHT) were put into multivariate analysis, in which postoperative primary RT and CHT were identified as independent prognostic factors significantly impacting OS and EFS (**Table 2**). The influence of postoperative primary adjuvant therapies to the survival of children and adults with medulloblastoma was further studied by univariate analysis (**Table S2**). Postoperative RT was a favorable prognostic factor for both children and adults ($p<0.001$). Postoperative primary CHT

Table 1. Univariate analysis of prognostic factors for OS and EFS in medulloblastoma patients (n = 173).

Factors	No. of cases	5-year OS(%)	p-value	5-year EFS(%)	p-value
Sex					
Male	112	49.8	0.216	43.2	0.384
Female	61	55.5		48.6	
Age					
Children	118	47.6	0.090	41.9	**0.047**
Adult	55	62.7		51.7	
Location					
Midline	152	50.2	0.219	43.7	0.228
Lateral	21	65.3		54.9	
Involvement[a]					
Yes	63	43.3	**0.002**	35.2	**0.001**
No	84	63.8		55.2	
Unknown	26				
Tumor Size					
<3 cm	110	56.8	0.314	47.7	0.444
≥3 cm	37	44.2		41.8	
Unknown	26				
Extent of resection					
Gross total	114	60.9	**0.002**	53.9	**<0.001**
Subtotal	52	42.7		33.0	
Unknown	7				
CSF Shunting					
Yes	53	45.8	0.074	41.1	0.055
No	103	56.0		47.5	
Unknown	17				
RT[b]					
Yes	139	58.4	**<0.001**	49.3	**<0.001**
No	34	8.0		8.0	
CHT[c]					
Yes	98	62.1	**<0.001**	51.2	**0.001**
No	75	38.9		38.9	
Institution					
A	153	53.3	0.184	46.9	0.238
B	20	40.0		40.0	

[a]involving brain stem or IV ventricle floor by the tumor.
[b]indicating postoperative primary radiation therapy.
[c]indicating postoperative primary chemotherapy.
Institution A = Huashan Hospital.
Institution B = Southwest Hospital.

significantly improved the survival of children (OS p = 0.001, EFS p = 0.003) while it was not a significant prognostic factor for adult patients.

Survival analysis for histological and molecular subgroups

There were 119 CMB, 45 DMB and 9 AMB according to WHO classification. Univariate analysis for OS and EFS between the three histological groups did not find significant differences (**Table 3**). Immunohistochemical staining classified 173 cases into three molecular subgroups (**Figure 1**): SHH subgroup (40 cases), WNT subgroup (37 cases) and Non-SHH/WNT subgroup (96 cases). Univariate analysis for OS and EFS between the three molecular groups did not find significant differences initially. However, after excluding 25 cases who did not receive any postoperative primary adjuvant therapies (RT or CHT), it was found that patients of WNT subgroup had significantly better OS than patients of other subgroups (SHH subgroup and Non-SHH/WNT subgroup) (**Table 3, Figure S2**).

We further studied the influence of postoperative primary adjuvant therapies to the survival of different histological and molecular subgroups of medulloblastoma by univariate analysis. Due to the limited number (9 cases) of AMB, it was not included in the analysis. Postoperative primary RT was found to be a strong

Table 2. Multivariate analysis of prognostic factors for OS and EFS in patients with medulloblastoma (n = 173).

Factors	OS		EFS	
	OR(95%CI)	p-value	OR(95%CI)	p-value
Age (Children vs. Adults)	0.69(0.38–1.26)	0.229	0.73(0.42–1.25)	0.251
CSF Shunting(Yes vs. No)	0.71(0.42–1.20)	0.202	0.73(0.45–1.20)	0.201
Involvement[a] (Yes vs. No)	0.60(0.29–1.22)	0.157	0.70(0.36–1.40)	0.306
Complete resection (Yes vs. No)	1.23(0.58–2.58)	0.590	1.56(0.78–3.10)	0.208
RT[b] (Yes vs. No)	8.18(4.52–14.80)	**<0.001**	6.74(3.83–11.87)	**<0.001**
CHT[c] (Yes vs. No)	1.75(1.04–2.96)	**0.036**	1.63(1.00–2.65)	**0.050**

OR: odds ratio, CI: confidence interval.
[a]involving brain stem or IV ventricle floor by the tumor.
[b]indicating postoperative primary radiation therapy.
[c]indicating postoperative primary chemotherapy.

prognostic factor influencing the survival in all histological and molecular subgroups. Postoperative primary CHT was found significantly influence the survival of CMB, SHH subgroup and WNT subgroup but not in DMB and Non-SHH/WNT subgroup (**Table S3, Figure 2**).

Discussion

The utility of several prognostic factors, either clinical or pathological, for predicting the clinical outcomes of medulloblastoma patients have been controversially discussed for a long time. Moreover, the sensitivity of different molecular subgroups of MB to current adjuvant therapies is poorly understood. In this study, we analyzed clinical outcomes and prognostic factors in 173 medulloblastoma patients treated at two institutions in China from 2002 to 2011.

There are no infants (age<3 years) in our series. Infants with medulloblastoma usually have a worse outcome compared to older children and adults, mainly due to absence of postoperative RT [15–17], so the survivals of our series may be higher than those of the entire group of patients in China. Authors of prospective clinical trials and retrospective studies on medulloblastoma patients mostly considered children (age≥3 years) and adults as different groups of subjects and focused on either one of the two groups. Meanwhile, several reports, including large population-based study, did not find significant difference in survivals between children and adults [8,17,18]. The role of sex in predicting the outcomes of medulloblastoma patients is also controversial. There are a few series showing female patients having better prognosis both in children and adults [19–21], while others did not find sex influencing treatment outcomes significantly [22]. Our data revealed no independent prognostic significance according to age groups (<16 years vs. ≥16years) and sex in medulloblastoma patients.

The role of two clinical parameters—involvement of brainstem or IV ventricle floor by the tumor at diagnosis and extent of tumor resection, on medulloblastoma patients' outcomes has been contraversial and numerous clinical studies yielded different results [23–34]. In the present study, absence of brainstem or IV ventricle floor involvement by the tumor and complete tumor resection significantly correlated with better OS and EFS in our series in the univariate analysis. Nonetheless, these two prognostic factors both lost significance in the multivariate analysis. Possible explanations for this may be that the two factors were intertwined with each

Table 3. Univariate analysis of histological and molecular subgroups for OS and EFS in medulloblastoma patients (n = 173).

Factors	No. of cases	5-year OS(%)	p-value	5-year EFS(%)	p-value
Histological subgroups					
CMB	119	51.7	0.187	46.7	0.643
DMB	45	61.0		45.7	
AMB	9	18.5		18.5	
Molecular subgroups					
SHH	40	50.4	0.182	40.9	0.277
WNT	37	69.2		59.2	
Non-SHH/WNT	96	45.9		41.0	
Molecular subgroups[a]					
WNT	30	83.3	**0.028**	78.6	0.081
Other	118	54.9		44.6	

CMB = Classic medulloblastoma, DMB = Desmoplastic/nodular medulloblastoma, AMB = Large-cell/anaplastic medulloblastoma, SHH = SHH pathway medulloblastoma, WNT = WNT pathway medulloblastoma, Non-SHH/WNT = Non-SHH/WNT pathway medulloblastoma.
[a]those patients who did not receive any adjuvant therapies after primary resection were excluded.

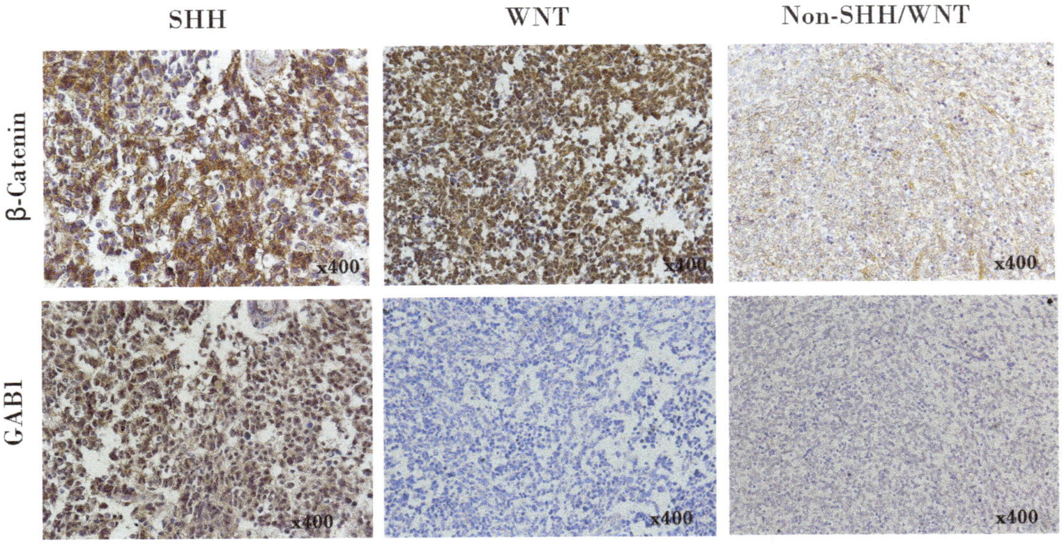

Figure 1. Molecular classification of medulloblastoma by immunohistochemical staining. 173 cases were classified into SHH subgroup (β-Catenin cytoplasmic-positive, GAB1 cytoplasmic-positive), WNT subgroup (β-Catenin nuclear+cytoplasmic-positive, GAB1-negative) and Non-SHH/WNT subgroup (β-Catenin cytoplasmic-positive, GAB1-negative). Representative photomicrographs of each subgroup are shown.

other, or that the sample size was not enough to reveal significance. Although the true prognostic value of brainstem or IV ventricle floor involvement and extent of resection are still undetermined, it appears advisable to attain the greatest extent of resection as long as serious surgical complications are avoided.

The use of postoperative RT has provided the greatest improvement in control of tumors and was an integral component of curative treatments of medulloblastoma patients for many years. The commonly used RT dose is 54 Gy to the posterior fossa, and a standard dose around 35 Gy for lesion-free craniospinal target [22,29,35]. Notably, there were 34 patients who did not receive postoperative primary RT in our cohort due to various reasons (e.g. refusal or incompliance). The clinical outcomes for these patients were dismal: only 8.0% of the patients survived at the time of 5 years, and most of them had tumor recurrence within the first year after primary resection.

Chemotherapy has been a very important part of treatment for medulloblastoma in the past several years. For children with medulloblastoma, several studies have showed a benefit for the use of CHT in either average-risk or high-risk children with medulloblastoma [7,22,34]. Due to the rarity of adult medulloblastoma, there was only one prospective study on treatments of this group until now [36]. The study concluded CHT was helpful in reducing the risk of recurrence and death in high-risk adult patients. However, the role of CHT in average-risk adults with medulloblastoma is still unconfirmed. Our study demonstrated the prognostic significance of CHT for better OS and EFS in children but not in adults. The true value of CHT in adults with medulloblastoma requires further prospective clinical trials.

In recent years, the discovery of WNT subtype in medullolastoma and its relatively favorable outcomes with current therapies have raised the possibility of reducing intensity of adjuvant therapies [6,9–12]. Since our cohort does not include infant patients and WNT subtype was uncommon in this group of patients by previous study [10], the proportion of WNT subtype in our series (21%) is high than other studies which included infants (~15%) [9,10]. Initially, patients of WNT subtype did not have a significantly better survival than patients of other molecular subtypes in our series. However, after 25 patients missing primary adjuvant therapies were excluded, a significant survival benefit had been found in patients of WNT subtype than patients with other subtypes. This finding is consistent with previous studies, suggesting the sensitivity of WNT subtype of medulloblastoma to adjuvant therapies and a possibility of reduction in adjuvant therapies. Another important result is that postoperative CHT was found significantly influence the survival of CMB, SHH subgroup and WNT subgroup of MB. Current trend in treating WNT subgroup of MB is to decrease the intensity of therapy [11]. Our finding suggested that WNT subgroup was sensitive to CHT and it would be risky to remove or defer CHT after primary tumor resection in this subgroup. We also found that postoperative primary CHT did not significantly influence the survival of patients with DMB and Non-SHH/WNT medulloblastoma. Rieken et al analyzed 20 patients with DMB and found the addition of postoperative adjuvant CHT did not bring significant survival benefit, like ours [37]. We postulate that the limited sample size of patients with DMB may be the reason and studies of more patients are needed to confirm the role of CHT in DMB. For Non-SHH/WNT medulloblastoma, more recent studies have reclassified this subgroup into Group 3 and Group 4 [10–12]. Patients of Group 4 medulloblastoma had an intermediate prognosis as patients of SHH medulloblastoma do, while patients of Group 3 medulloblastoma had the worst outcome [10,11]. Our data revealed no significant difference between the survivals of patients who received adjuvant CHT and who did not in Non-SHH/WNT subgroup, and this insensitivity to current CHT of the subgroup may be one of the reasons explaining the dismal outcome of Group 3 medulloblastoma. However, further detailed studies are necessary to explore the role of CHT in Non-SHH/WNT medulloblastoma.

One of the limitations of this study is the unavailability of detailed information of postoperative RT and CHT, since detailed protocols of RT and CHT were acquired only in a minority of our cohort. Radiation area/dose and type of chemotherapy are

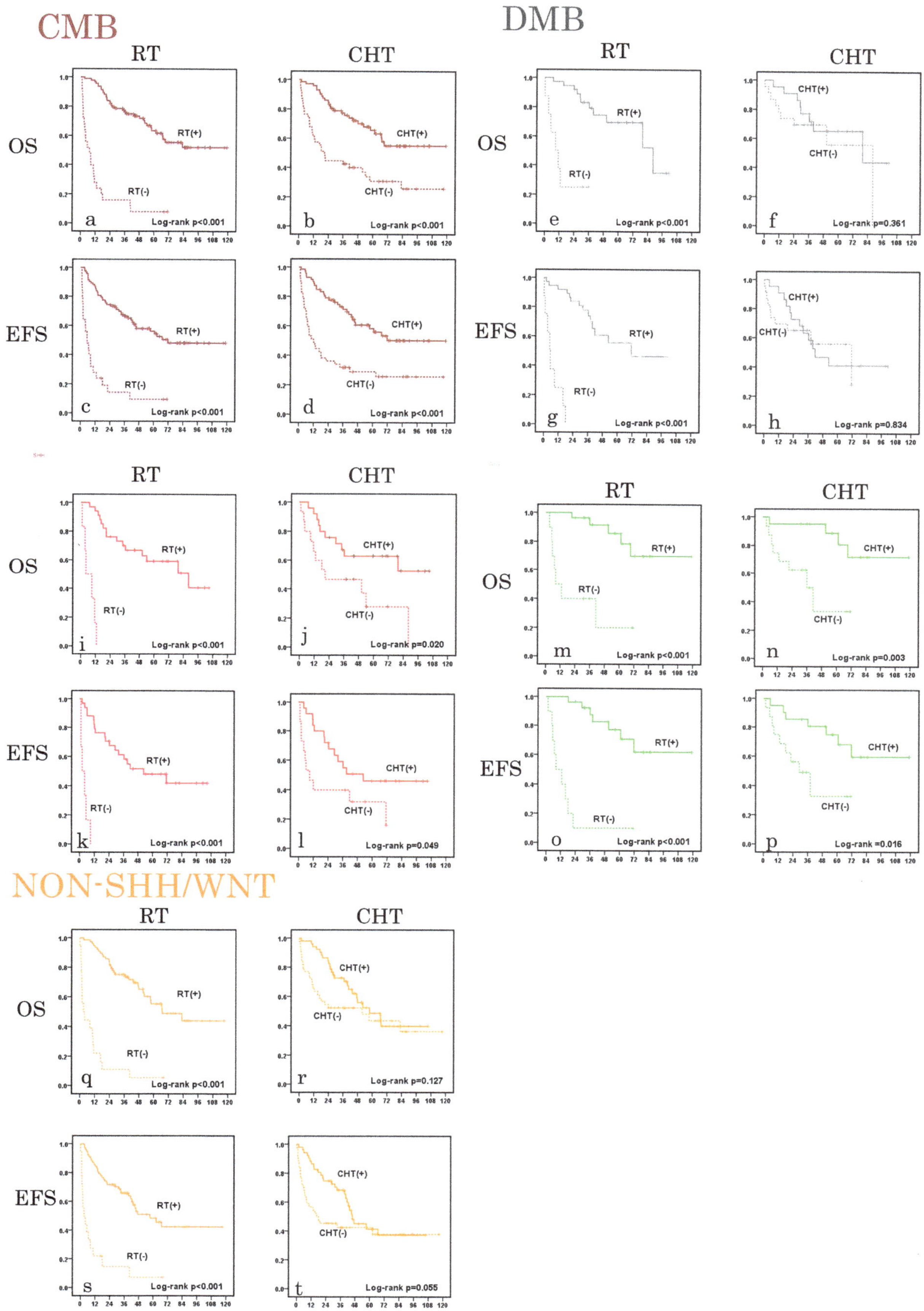
CMB
DMB
NON-SHH/WNT
RT
CHT
OS
EFS
a Log-rank p<0.001
b Log-rank p<0.001
c Log-rank p<0.001
d Log-rank p<0.001
e Log-rank p<0.001
f Log-rank p=0.361
g Log-rank p<0.001
h Log-rank p=0.834
i Log-rank p<0.001
j Log-rank p=0.020
k Log-rank p<0.001
l Log-rank p=0.049
m Log-rank p<0.001
n Log-rank p=0.003
o Log-rank p<0.001
p Log-rank =0.016
q Log-rank p<0.001
r Log-rank p=0.127
s Log-rank p<0.001
t Log-rank p=0.055
RT(+)
RT(-)
CHT(+)
CHT(-)

Figure 2. Univariate analysis of overall survival (OS) and event-free survival (EFS) of histological and molecular subgroups of medulloblastoma. a–d: OS and EFS analysis in classic medulloblastoma (CMB, dark red) according to postoperative radiation therapy (RT) and chemotherapy (CHT). e–h: OS and EFS analysis in desmoplastic/nodular medulloblastoma (DMB, grey) according to postoperative RT and CHT. i–l: OS and EFS analysis in SHH medulloblastoma (red) according to postoperative RT and CHT. m–p: OS and EFS analysis in WNT medulloblastoma (green) according to postoperative RT and CHT. q–t: OS and EFS analysis in Non-SHH/WNT medulloblastoma (yellow) according to postoperative RT and CHT. Numbers on the Y axis indicate probability of survival in medulloblastoma patients. Numbers of the X axis indicate the follow-up time (months).

considered as prognostic factors significantly affecting clinical outcome of MB patients [1,4,18,24]. The findings of current study would be strengthened if details of RT and CHT were complete in all the cases and be demonstrated comparable across subgroups of MB. Future studies with more detailed data are needed to further confirm the findings.

In conclusion, we have reported a large series of medulloblastoma patients in China. Our data demonstrated that the administration of adjuvant CHT to children could significantly improve the survival of this group. Moreover, postoperative primary CHT was found significantly influence the survival of CMB, SHH subgroup and WNT subgroup but not in DMB and Non-SHH/WNT subgroup. The role of postoperative CHT in DMB and Non-SHH/WNT medulloblastoma needs further study.

Supporting Information

Figure S1 Survival curves of medulloblastoma patients. a: Overall survival of 173 medulloblastoma patients. **b**: Event-free survival of 173 medulloblastoma patients. **c**: Overall survival of 118 children with medulloblastoma. **d**: Event-free survival of 118 children with medulloblastoma. **e**: Overall survival of 55 adults with medulloblastoma. **d**: Event-free survival of 55 adults with medulloblastoma. Numbers on the Y axis indicate probability of survival in medulloblastoma patients. Numbers of the X axis indicate the follow-up time (months).

Figure S2 Survival analysis between WNT subgroup (green) and other molecular subgroups (SHH and Non-SHH/WNT subgroups, blue). a: OS analysis revealed WNT subgroup had significantly better survival than other groups; **b**: EFS analysis revealed WNT subgroup had a trend to significantly better survival than other groups.

Table S1 Immunoreactivity patterns of SHH, WNT, and non-SHH/WNT molecular subgroups*.

Table S2 Univariate analysis of postoperative adjuvant therapies for OS and EFS in children and adults with medulloblastoma (n = 173).

Table S3 Univariate analysis of postoperative adjuvant therapies for OS and EFS in patients with different histological and molecular subgroups of medulloblastoma (n = 173).

Author Contributions

Conceived and designed the experiments: YY PZ. Performed the experiments: ZYZ JX YR. Analyzed the data: ZYZ JX. Contributed reagents/materials/analysis tools: YR KK-WL H-KN. Wrote the paper: ZYZ JX YY. Provided clinical samples: YM LFZ PZ. Revised for important intellectual content: H-KN KK-WL.

References

1. Packer RJ, Cogen P, Vezina G, Rorke LB (1999) Medulloblastoma: clinical and biologic aspects. Neuro Oncol 1: 232–250.
2. Sarkar C, Pramanik P, Karak AK, Mukhopadhyay P, Sharma MC, et al. (2002) Are childhood and adult medulloblastomas different? A comparative study of clinicopathological features, proliferation index and apoptotic index. J Neurooncol 59: 49–61.
3. Wrensch M, Minn Y, Chew T, Bondy M, Berger MS (2002) Epidemiology of primary brain tumors: current concepts and review of the literature. Neuro Oncol 4: 278–299.
4. Packer RJ, Vezina G (2008) Management of and prognosis with medulloblastoma: therapy at a crossroads. Arch Neurol 65: 1419–1424.
5. Packer RJ, Sutton LN, Goldwein JW, Perilongo G, Bunin G, et al. (1991) Improved survival with the use of adjuvant chemotherapy in the treatment of medulloblastoma. J Neurosurg 74: 433–440.
6. Gajjar A, Chintagumpala M, Ashley D, Kellie S, Kun LE, et al. (2006) Risk-adapted craniospinal radiotherapy followed by high-dose chemotherapy and stem-cell rescue in children with newly diagnosed medulloblastoma (St Jude Medulloblastoma-96): long-term results from a prospective, multicentre trial. Lancet Oncol 7: 813–820.
7. von Hoff K, Hinkes B, Gerber NU, Deinlein F, Mittler U, et al. (2009) Long-term outcome and clinical prognostic factors in children with medulloblastoma treated in the prospective randomised multicentre trial HIT'91. Eur J Cancer 45: 1209–1217.
8. Rieken S, Mohr A, Habermehl D, Welzel T, Lindel K, et al. (2011) Outcome and prognostic factors of radiation therapy for medulloblastoma. Int J Radiat Oncol Biol Phys 81: e7–e13.
9. Ellison DW, Dalton J, Kocak M, Nicholson SL, Fraga C, et al. (2011) Medulloblastoma: clinicopathological correlates of SHH, WNT, and non-SHH/WNT molecular subgroups. Acta Neuropathol 121: 381–396.
10. Kool M, Korshunov A, Remke M, Jones DT, Schlanstein M, et al. (2012) Molecular subgroups of medulloblastoma: an international meta-analysis of transcriptome, genetic aberrations, and clinical data of WNT, SHH, Group 3, and Group 4 medulloblastomas. Acta Neuropathol 123: 473–484.
11. Taylor MD, Northcott PA, Korshunov A, Remke M, Cho YJ, et al. (2012) Molecular subgroups of medulloblastoma: the current consensus. Acta Neuropathol 123: 465–472.
12. Northcott PA, Korshunov A, Witt H, Hielscher T, Eberhart CG, et al. (2011) Medulloblastoma comprises four distinct molecular variants. J Clin Oncol 29: 1408–1414.
13. Liu Y, Zhu Y, Gao L, Xu G, Yi J, et al. (2005) Radiation treatment for medulloblastoma: a review of 64 cases at a single institute. Jpn J Clin Oncol 35: 111–115.
14. Louis DN, Ohgaki H, Wiestler OD, Cavenee WK, Burger PC, et al. (2007) The 2007 WHO classification of tumours of the central nervous system. Acta Neuropathol 114: 97–109.
15. Sun LM, Yeh SA, Wang CJ, Huang EY, Chen HC, et al. (2002) Postoperative radiation therapy for medulloblastoma—high recurrence rate in the subfrontal region. J Neurooncol 58: 77–85.
16. Johnston DL, Keene D, Bartels U, Carret AS, Crooks B, et al. (2009) Medulloblastoma in children under the age of three years: a retrospective Canadian review. J Neurooncol 94: 51–56.
17. Curran EK, Le GM, Sainani KL, Propp JM, Fisher PG (2009) Do children and adults differ in survival from medulloblastoma? A study from the SEER registry. J Neurooncol 95: 81–85.
18. Roldan G, Brasher P, Vecil G, Senger D, Rewcastle B, et al. (2008) Population-based study of medulloblastoma: outcomes in Alberta from 1975 to 1996. Can J Neurol Sci 35: 210–215.
19. Weil MD, Lamborn K, Edwards MS, Wara WM (1998) Influence of a child's sex on medulloblastoma outcome. JAMA 279: 1474–1476.
20. Wolff JE, Huettermann U, Ritter J, Straeter R, Palm D, et al. (1998) Medulloblastoma: experience of a single institution. Klin Padiatr 210: 234–238.
21. Riffaud L, Saikali S, Leray E, Hamlat A, Haegelen C, et al. (2009) Survival and prognostic factors in a series of adults with medulloblastomas. J Neurosurg 111: 478–487.
22. Paulino AC (2002) Current multimodality management of medulloblastoma. Curr Probl Cancer 26: 317–356.

23. Menon G, Krishnakumar K, Nair S (2008) Adult medulloblastoma: clinical profile and treatment results of 18 patients. J Clin Neurosci 15: 122–126.
24. Padovani L, Sunyach MP, Perol D, Mercier C, Alapetite C, et al. (2007) Common strategy for adult and pediatric medulloblastoma: a multicenter series of 253 adults. Int J Radiat Oncol Biol Phys 68: 433–440.
25. Chan AW, Tarbell NJ, Black PM, Louis DN, Frosch MP, et al. (2000) Adult medulloblastoma: prognostic factors and patterns of relapse. Neurosurgery 47: 623–631, 631–632.
26. Malheiros SM, Franco CM, Stavale JN, Santos AJ, Borges LR, et al. (2002) Medulloblastoma in adults: a series from Brazil. J Neurooncol 60: 247–253.
27. Carrie C, Lasset C, Alapetite C, Haie-Meder C, Hoffstetter S, et al. (1994) Multivariate analysis of prognostic factors in adult patients with medulloblastoma. Retrospective study of 156 patients. Cancer 74: 2352–2360.
28. Choux M, Lena G, Hassoun J (1983) Prognosis and long-term follow-up in patients with medulloblastoma. Clin Neurosurg 30: 246–277.
29. Herrlinger U, Steinbrecher A, Rieger J, Hau P, Kortmann RD, et al. (2005) Adult medulloblastoma: prognostic factors and response to therapy at diagnosis and at relapse. J Neurol 252: 291–299.
30. Albright AL, Wisoff JH, Zeltzer PM, Boyett JM, Rorke LB, et al. (1996) Effects of medulloblastoma resections on outcome in children: a report from the Children's Cancer Group. Neurosurgery 38: 265–271.
31. Del CJ, Bolek TW, McCollough WM, Maria BL, Kedar A, et al. (1998) Medulloblastoma: time-dose relationship based on a 30-year review. Int J Radiat Oncol Biol Phys 42: 147–154.
32. Zeltzer PM, Boyett JM, Finlay JL, Albright AL, Rorke LB, et al. (1999) Metastasis stage, adjuvant treatment, and residual tumor are prognostic factors for medulloblastoma in children: conclusions from the Children's Cancer Group 921 randomized phase III study. J Clin Oncol 17: 832–845.
33. Frost PJ, Laperriere NJ, Wong CS, Milosevic MF, Simpson WJ, et al. (1995) Medulloblastoma in adults. Int J Radiat Oncol Biol Phys 32: 951–957.
34. Packer RJ, Sutton LN, Elterman R, Lange B, Goldwein J, et al. (1994) Outcome for children with medulloblastoma treated with radiation and cisplatin, CCNU, and vincristine chemotherapy. J Neurosurg 81: 690–698.
35. Whelan HT, Krouwer HG, Schmidt MH, Reichert KW, Kovnar EH (1998) Current therapy and new perspectives in the treatment of medulloblastoma. Pediatr Neurol 18: 103–115.
36. Brandes AA, Franceschi E, Tosoni A, Blatt V, Ermani M (2007) Long-term results of a prospective study on the treatment of medulloblastoma in adults. Cancer 110: 2035–2041.
37. Rieken S, Gaiser T, Mohr A, Welzel T, Witt O, et al. (2010) Outcome and prognostic factors of desmoplastic medulloblastoma treated within a multidisciplinary treatment concept. BMC Cancer 10: 450.

7

Anatomical Targets Associated with Abrupt versus Gradual Washout of Subthalamic Deep Brain Stimulation Effects on Bradykinesia

Scott E. Cooper[1]*, Klaus G. Driesslein[2], Angela M. Noecker[3], Cameron C. McIntyre[3], Andre M. Machado[1], Christopher R. Butson[2]

1 Cleveland Clinic, Center for Neurological Restoration, Cleveland, Ohio, United States of America, **2** Medical College of Wisconsin, Departments of Neurology & Neurosurgery, Biotechnology and Bioengineering Center, Milwaukee, Wisconsin, United States of America, **3** Case Western Reserve University, Department of Biomedical Engineering, Cleveland, Ohio, United States of America

Abstract

The subthalamic nucleus (STN) is a common anatomical target for deep brain stimulation (DBS) for the treatment of Parkinson's disease. However, the effects of stimulation may spread beyond the STN. Ongoing research aims to identify nearby anatomical structures where DBS-induced effects could be associated with therapeutic improvement or side effects. We previously found that DBS lead location determines the rate – abrupt vs. gradual – with which therapeutic effect washes out after stimulation is stopped. Those results suggested that electrical current spreads from the electrodes to two spatially distinct stimulation targets associated with different washout rates. In order to identify these targets we used computational models to predict the volumes of tissue activated during DBS in 14 Parkinson's patients from that study. We then coregistered each patient with a stereotaxic atlas and generated a probabilistic stimulation atlas to obtain a 3-dimensional representation of regions where stimulation was associated with abrupt vs. gradual washout. We found that the therapeutic effect which washed out gradually was associated with stimulation of the zona incerta and fields of Forel, whereas abruptly-disappearing therapeutic effect was associated with stimulation of STN itself. This supports the idea that multiple DBS targets exist and that current spread from one electrode may activate more than one of them in a given patient, producing a combination of effects which vary according to electrode location and stimulation settings.

Editor: Guglielmo Foffani, Hospital Nacional de Parapléjicos, Spain

Funding: Supported by K23NS052523 from www.nimh.nih.gov. The funders had no role in study design, data collection and analysis, decision to publish, or preparation of the manuscript.

Competing Interests: The authors have declared that no competing interests exist.

* Email: coopers2@ccf.org

Introduction

The subthalamic nucleus (STN) is a common anatomical target for deep brain stimulation (DBS) for the treatment of Parkinson's disease [1], and is being assessed for treatment of other disorders [2–4]. Over the past decade studies on subthalamic deep brain stimulation have looked for anatomical targets that optimize clinical outcomes [5–11]. However, the problem of relating electrode location to clinical results poses several challenges. First, although the location of the stimulating electrode contact within the brain can be determined from post-operative imaging, clinical effects derive not from that single point but from a surrounding *volume* of tissue activated (VTA) by the spread of electrical current, and this volume must be estimated. Second, the electrode is surrounded by multiple anatomical structures, each of which may be associated with different stimulation effects. Thus, the actual effects observed will be a mixture, reflecting overlap between VTA and different anatomical structures. Since many structures cannot be imaged *in vivo*, individual patient data must be coregistered with a detailed neuroanatomical atlas to identify these possible structures. Third, any data-based attempt at relating VTAs to clinical effects must employ some form of averaging whereby VTAs of multiple patients are combined to estimate a probability distribution function for clinical effects conditional on stimulation location.

We previously described two spatially distinct and therapeutically effective stimulation sites in the vicinity of the STN, distinguishable by the rate at which therapeutic effects on bradykinesia "wash out" after stimulation is turned off [12]. There was a statistically significant relationship between the location of active electrode contacts and the proportion of fast vs. slow washout. We found that when electrodes were located laterally most of the DBS effect disappeared abruptly, after which a small amount of residual effect washed out in a slow, gradual fashion. When electrodes were located medially, very little of the effect disappeared abruptly and most of it washed out slowly. This suggested that electrical current was spreading from the electrodes to two spatially distinct stimulation targets, with one or the other target activated preferentially according to electrode position. However, because of the difficulties enumerated above, we could not determine what neuroanatomical structures were actually responsible for the fast- and slow-washout effects. To address this, in the present paper, we use previously published approaches to identify these potentially different targets. We begin by estimating

VTAs using patient-specific computational models [13]. Next, we coregister the VTAs with a detailed anatomical atlas [14]. Finally we combine VTAs from multiple patients to generate a probabilistic stimulation atlas (PSA) of bradykinesia washout effects [16,17]. This approach illustrates how stimulation targets can be elucidated by combining outcomes from multiple patients.

Methods

Design and conduct of the study was approved by, and written informed consent obtained per the Cleveland Clinic Institutional Review Board.

Patients

14 Parkinson's patients in [12] had sufficient perioperative clinical data available to reconstruct electrode locations for VTA computations; four subjects were excluded due to: 1) operated at another institution 2) "frameless" stereotaxic system used (incompatible with Cicerone software 3) incomplete surgical records and 4) incomplete radiological records. All had a diagnosis of PD by a movement disorders neurologist, clear levodopa response, and were non-demented. All had a minimum of 5 years disease duration and were at least 5 months post-implantation on the tested (dominant) side (range: 5–74 months). All had completed the initial postoperative period of DBS adjustments, and the median time since last adjustment was 14 months. Details of patient characteristics and stimulator settings appear in Table 1. Average values were (mean ± standard deviation): Age 61.8±5.9 years; Disease duration 14.5±5.2 years; Unified Parkinson's Disease Rating Scale (UPDRS) OFF med/OFF stim motor score 30.9±11.3; preoperative total daily levodopa equivalent 1096±553.9 mg; percent reduction in daily levodopa equivalent from pre- to post-operatively (at time of testing) 46±34%; time since surgery 26.5±26.3 months.

Experimental Procedure

Experimental procedure was described in [12]; we summarize here briefly as follows: Bradykinesia measurements were made at 2-minute intervals, and each measurement lasted 20 seconds. During each measurement, patients rapidly tapped the tips of the thumb and index finger together (UPDRS item 3.4 [17]). An angular velocity transducer (model G-1, NeuroKinetics, Edmonton, Alberta, Canada) was taped to the proximal index finger. As a measure of bradykinesia, we used total power in the angular velocity signal in the 1–10 Hz band (lower power = greater bradykinesia).

Patients came to the lab in the OFF-medication state, medications withheld for an average of 12 hours (range 10–16 hours). At the start of each experiment, DBS was ON at clinically optimized settings established prior to and independently of this study. Details of stimulator settings are provided in Table 2. Average values were (mean ± standard deviation): frequency 147.5±24.9 Hz; Pulse width 75±15.6 µsec, Amplitude 3.2±0.51 volts. 6 patients were stimulated in monopolar mode, 7 patients bipolar, and one had two negative and one positive contact.

For twenty minutes, bradykinesia was measured every two minutes. Then the stimulator contralateral to the dominant hand was turned off, and measurements continued every two minutes for a further 50 minutes. At the conclusion of this time, the stimulator was turned back on, and measurements were again made every two minutes for a further 20 minutes.

The following procedure was used for turning off/on the stimulator: Patients were told beforehand that their stimulator settings would be changed at some point during the experiment, but the exact nature and timing of the change was obscured from them by having the experimenter press ineffective buttons on the programmer device at random while the patient performed a distractor task (visual choice reaction time task) for 4 minutes. Half-way through this procedure, the real, effective button was pressed which turned the stimulator off/on.

Curves were then fit to the bradykinesia versus time data using Nelder-Mead iterative minimization of summed, squared error [18]. An example is shown in Figure 1. The abrupt loss of stimulation effect appears as a discontinuity between the curve during the initial stimulation-on baseline interval, vs. during the stimulation-off interval. The further, gradual decrease from that time to the eventual plateau represents the slow washout of residual therapeutic effect. Of the total change in bradykinesia, from baseline to plateau, the percent which occurred abruptly was measured by the "%STEP" parameter.

The curve fit to the stimulation-off interval was a first-order exponential function of time. We found that the curve fit to the stimulation-on interval could be either first-order exponential, first-order linear, or zeroth-order linear function of time without affecting the relationship between electrode location and the %STEP parameter. In the present paper, for the baseline interval, we use the zeroth-order linear function (i.e. a simple mean of baseline values).

Patient-Specific VTA Models

We generated patient-specific computational models of DBS with Cicerone v1.2 software, a freely available academic DBS research tool [19]. In the first step, preoperative MRI, CT (with stereotaxic frame fiducials), intraoperative microelectrode recordings, postoperative CT (with electrode), and a volumetric atlas containing thalamus and basal ganglia are co-registered, to give an estimate of electrode location in relation to those structures. Image registration in Cicerone is performed using a previously published mutual-information algorithm [20] which is used extensively in many commercial and open-source image imaging programs. In this case, each patient's pre-operative MRI and post-operative CT were coregistered, along with registration of the patient MRI and the atlas MRI. Next, based on a finite-element model of the electrically conductive tissue surrounding the electrode, an estimate is computed of the electric field in spatial relation to the neuroanatomical structures surrounding the electrode, using the stimulation parameters (electrode contacts, voltage, pulse width, and frequency) for each patient. Finally, based on a multicompartment-model of excitable neuronal elements, with detailed simulation of ion channel dynamics using Hodgkin-Huxley formalism, a volume of tissue activated (VTA) is computed [21], estimating the region within which stimulation produces action potentials (Figure 2).

Atlas Registration

The brain atlas used in Cicerone provides surface representations of the thalamus and STN, but lacks representations of other smaller anatomical regions that were of interest for the present study. To address this limitation we coregistered each patient with a detailed anatomical atlas of Mai et al [14] that delineated zona incerta (ZI), fields of Forel (FF) and other nearby structures. We extracted the following structures from each applicable page of the Mai et al atlas [14]: thalamus, H1, H2, STN, ZI, anterior commissure, posterior commissure. First, distinct grayscale values were assigned to the nuclei in each slice using Photoshop (Adobe Systems Inc, USA). Then outlines of each nucleus in each slice were imported into Mimics (Materialise HQ, Leuven, Belgium) at

Table 1. Patient characteristics.

Patient	Dominant hand	Age (years)	Disease duration (months)	UPDRS motor OFF	Pre-operative levodopa equivalent	% Levodopa reduction	Time since surgery (months)
A	right	62	27	28	1954	−47%	28
B	right	65	13	*	2148	−41%	74
C	right	58	19	50	1275	−57%	5
D	right	53	18	16	935	−6%	75
E	right	63	16	29	1250	−100%	70
F	right	72	9	28	0	0%	26
G	left	52	7	30	1239	−76%	11
H	right	69	12	13	1150	−58%	8
I	right	54	15	39	1193	−48%	16
J	right	64	12	43	1439	−48%	8
K	right	64	11	33	650	−54%	9
L	right	61	13	21	706	−60%	7
M	right	67	10	25	542	+29%	9
N	right	62	19	47	863	−77%	25

Dominant hand: right or left (all patients were tested with the dominant hand and contralateral STN stimulator). Age (years), at time of testing. Disease duration: time (years) from onset of Parkinson's symptoms to time of testing. UPDRS motor OFF: UPDRS motor section total score in the off-medication, DBS-naive state. Preoperative levodopa equivalent: total daily levodopa equivalent (mg) preoperatively. % Levodopa Reduction: Percent change in daily levodopa equivalent from preoperatively to time of testing. Time since surgery: time of testing in months since electrode implantation. Missing data indicated by "*".

Table 2. Stimulation Characteristics.

Patient	Electrode	Contacts	Frequency	Pulse width	Voltage
A	3389	1−,2−,3+	130	90	4.0
B	3387	1−,3+	135	90	3.5
C	3389	1−,C+	130	60	3.1
D	3387	1−,3+	185	90	3.6
E	3387	1−,C+	145	90	2.9
F	3387	2−,C+	185	90	2.8
G	3389	1−,3+	130	60	3.6
H	3389	2−,C+	130	60	2.8
I	3389	1−,C+	130	60	2.0
J	3389	1−,C+	130	60	2.8
K	3389	1−,3+	185	90	3.3
L	3389	2−,3+	135	60	3.6
M	3389	3−,2+	130	60	2.9
N	3389	1−,3+	185	90	3.5

Electrode Model: type of electrode implanted (Medtronic model 3387 or 3389). Contacts: electrode contacts stimulated (0–3, and "C" for "Case"). Frequency: stimulation frequency, in Hz. Pulse width: stimulation pulse width setting, in microseconds. Voltage: stimulation amplitude, in volts. These values represent each patient's clinically optimized DBS settings which were chosen prior to, and independently of this study.

relative positions determined from the slice thicknesses specified in the atlas (e.g. see figure 3B). We then used the outlines of each nucleus to create a closed polygonal surface, and loaded the surfaces and the original atlas slices into SCIRun (SCI Institute, University of Utah), which also contained the original nuclei surfaces from Cicerone. To register the two atlases, we first confirmed the alignment of both groups of nuclei (x-direction = -medial-lateral, y-direction = anterior-posterior, z-direction = dorsal-ventral), and scaled the Mai-Paxinos atlas slightly in the anterior-posterior direction to provide precise alignment of the anterior and posterior commissures. Next we used a previously-published [21] minimum least squares method in Matlab (Mathworks Inc, Natick, MA) to align the STN and thalamus from the Mai et al and Cicerone atlases (these nuclei were chosen because they were common to both atlases). This method allows translation and rotation (shear and scaling were not permitted) of one set of nuclei relative to another set of nuclei in order to minimize the total "error distance" between the pairs of thalamus and STN surfaces. The distance was measured from the normal vector from each surface point in the Cicerone atlas to the location where it intersected the analogous surface in the Mai-Paxinos atlas. Once this transformation matrix was determined, it was applied to all surfaces and slices from the Mai-Paxinos atlas to position them in the Cicerone atlas space. These registration steps were necessary for integration of all patients' VTAs into a common atlas space that included ZI, FF, and STN boundaries.

Probabilistic Stimulation Atlas (PSA) [15,16]

Finally, we combined all 14 patients' bradykinesia wash-out data into the common anatomical space. This was done by creating a 3D lattice that was large enough to contain the VTAs from all patients. The lattice was constructed from 1 mm^3 voxels with overall dimensions of 30 mm×30 mm×30 mm. Each VTA was used to mask the voxels contained within it, and each of those voxels was assigned values for %STEP. From these individual scores, average values were computed for voxels that were contained within two or more VTA. This analysis was performed using Matlab (Mathworks Inc, Natick, MA).

Results

Figure 1, shows how we quantified the amount of abrupt decrease in stimulation effect, relative to the subsequent slow-decay with the %STEP parameter. Large values of %STEP (predominantly the fast-decaying process) occurred with laterally located electrodes and small values (predominantly the long-lasting process) with medial ones.

Figure 2 shows VTAs for the 7 patients with highest (A,B, seen from two different angles) vs. 7 lowest (C,D, from the same two angles) values of %STEP. VTAs for patients with predominantly slow-decaying effect are clustered medial to the STN, while VTAs for patients with predominantly fast-decaying effect are centered on the STN proper. Some VTAs extend dorsally into the thalamus, apparently following the path of pallidothalamic fibers located medial to STN to their thalamic terminations. On the other hand, this may reflect bipolar stimulation (see Table 2). When a patient is stimulated with a ventral cathode and a dorsal anode, the VTA will include activation by *both* contacts, and cannot determine whether the more dorsal contact contributes to that patient's %STEP value, *vs.* %STEP being wholly determined by the ventral contact, with no contribution from more dorsal activation in thalamus.

Whereas the most slow-decaying VTAs were confined to a medial zone, the fastest-decaying VTAs included both lateral and medial regions. Consistent with this observation, none of the patients in our sample exhibited a pure fast-decaying effect whereas a pure slow-decaying effect was seen in some cases. That is, some patients in our sample had a %STEP value of 0% (zero percent fast, 100% slow), whereas even the most fast-decaying patients had a %STEP value of 85% (85% fast, 15% slow). This asymmetry is likely explained by the lack of far-laterally located electrodes in our sample. Far-laterally located electrodes activate corticospinal and corticobulbar fibers, causing side effects, and such patients were rare in our study, because we enrolled only

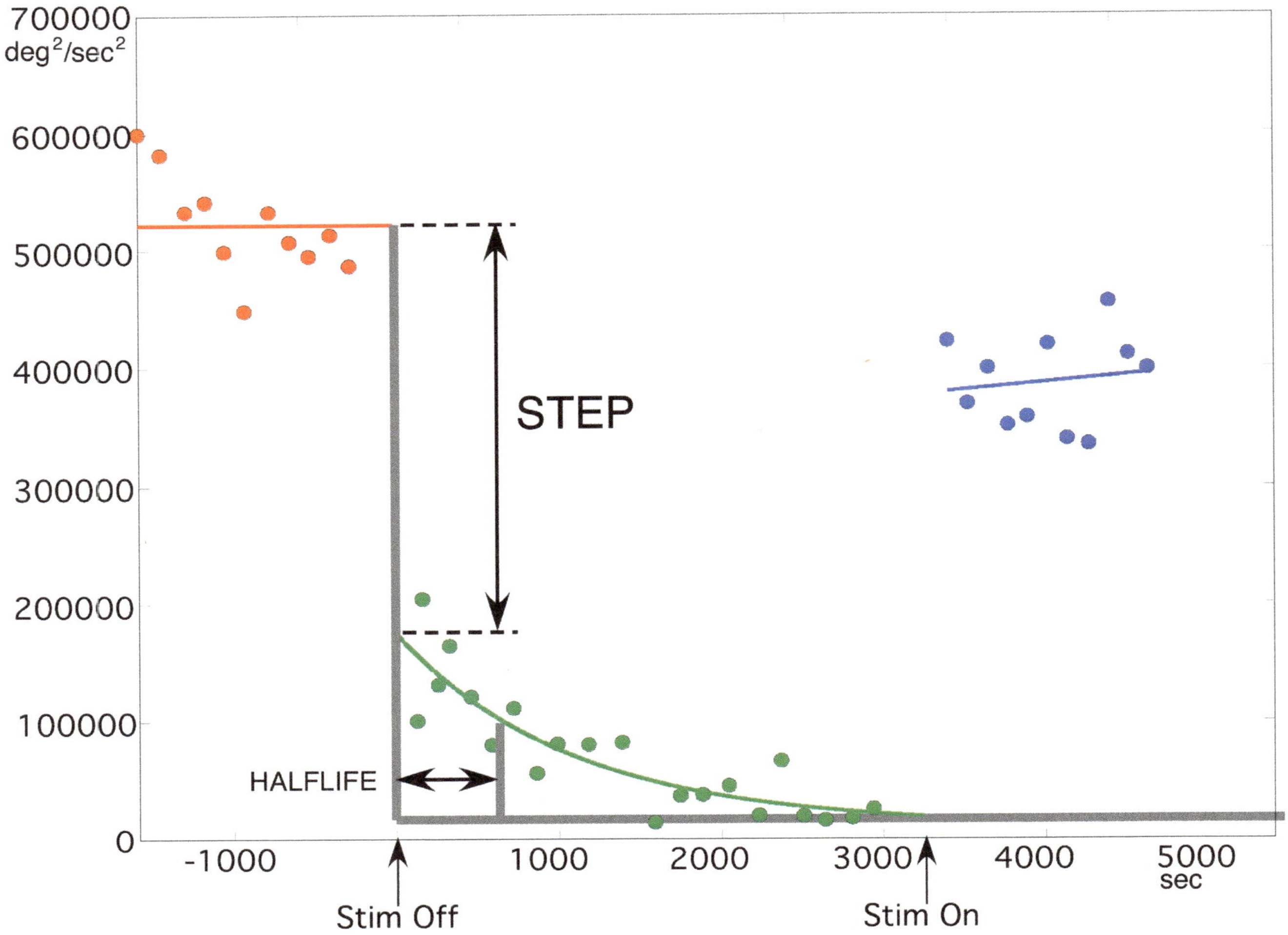

Figure 1. Data from one patient, showing the decaying exponential fit to bradykinesia measurements after DBS was turned off, and the abrupt change in bradykinesia quantified by %STEP, followed by further slow washout of residual therapeutic effect. In this patient, about two-thirds of the total bradykinesia returned abruptly, while the remaining one-third washed out slowly, giving a value for %STEP of 67%.

patients with good clinical response to the surgery. Therefore, in our sample, whenever a VTA included lateral STN, the electrode tended to be located in central or medial STN, with activation spreading to lateral STN. Since, with increasing stimulation amplitude, activation spreads both medially and laterally, such VTAs tend to encompass a large mediolateral range. In contrast, medial electrode placement was less constrained by side effects, and so our sample includes patients with relatively selective medial stimulation and pure slow-decaying effect.

In order to provide a more detailed identification of stimulation targets we generated a PSA that averaged data across VTAs from all patients (Figure 2 E,F). The resulting scalar field is represented as a regular grid, with size and color of each grid point representing the average value of %STEP for all patients whose VTA included that point. The lowest values of %STEP (the most slow-decaying DBS effect) are located medial to the STN (large blue grid points), while higher values (more fast-decaying effect) occur in STN proper (small red grid points).

Figure 3 shows the scalar field in the space of the detailed anatomical atlas [14]. We found that the slow-decaying region (lower values of %STEP: blue) is centered in the vicinity of posterior zona incerta and fields of Forel, extending dorsally into ventrolateral thalamic nucleus (VLA). In contrast, larger values of %STEP (red) occur in STN proper.

Could the %STEP gradient (blue to red gradient in Figure 3) have arisen under the null hypothesis that %STEP is unrelated to which neuroanatomical structures are stimulated? To answer that question, we performed the regression analysis in Figure 4. In this analysis, each data point is a single grid point in Figure 2 E, F. As shown in Figure 4, there was a strong dependence on mediolateral location of stimulation (Fig. 4 A, Bonferroni-corrected $p<0.001$), and on anteroposterior location of stimulation (Fig. 4B, Bonferroni-corrected $p<0.01$), and no dependence on the dorsoventral axis (Fig. 4C, $p>0.5$). Thus, our observations have very low likelihood under the null hypothesis. A closer examination of the data shows that the effect is driven by mediolateral (X) location. This may be seen by direct comparison of Fig. 4A with Fig 4B, as well as by the following procedure, shown in Fig. 4 D, E: When variance predicted by Y is partialed out of %STEP, and the residual regressed on X the relationship remains clear (Fig. 4D), whereas, with the inverse procedure (variance predicted by X partialed out, and residual regressed on Y) the relationship is lost (Fig. 4E).

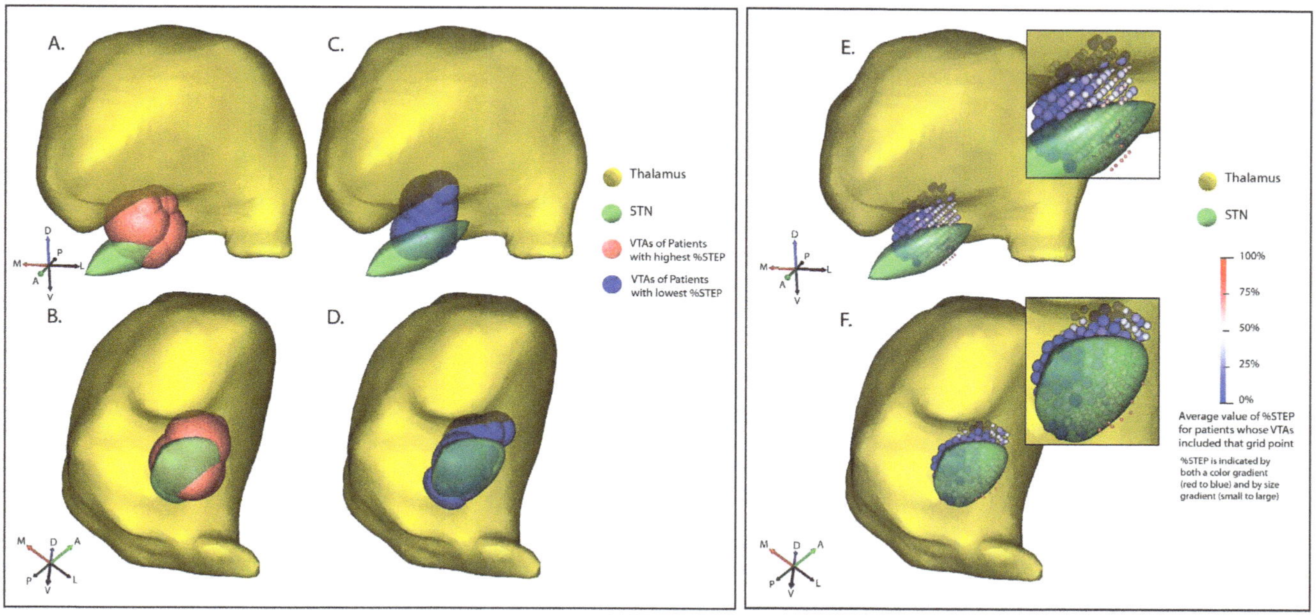

Figure 2. Estimated volumes of tissue activated (VTA) for the 7 patients with the most rapidly-decaying DBS effect, i.e. highest %STEP (mean ± sd 58±21% A, B; viewed from two different angles) and the 7 with the most slowly-decaying DBS effect, i.e. lowest %STEP (mean ± sd −8±28%; C, D, from the same two angles). E–F Spatial average of data from all 14 patients. Size and color of each grid point represent the average value of %STEP for all patients whose VTA included that point.

This analysis significantly extends our earlier result in which %STEP was shown to be related to electrode contact locations [12]. In that analysis, contacts stimulated at low or high voltage, with positive or negative polarity were treated the same: no allowance was made for the difference between anodal vs. cathodal stimulation or the differential spread of current with higher vs. lower amplitude stimulation. In the present analysis, these factors are taken into account by the VTA calculation, and the %STEP gradient is again seen.

Discussion

Clinical Implications

A growing number of publications suggest that DBS clinical outcomes reflect subtle differences of targeting in and around the STN. The classical target is the dorsolateral-anterior STN, where neuronal activity is related to passive and active limb movement [22], and related anatomically (in animal models) to motor cortex [23]. However, different locations of stimulation may give difference in side effects [10] differential effectiveness for different symptoms [22,24,15], or difference in both respects [25]. The present study distinguishes between medial (Zona incerta/Fields of Forel, ZI/FF) and lateral (STN proper) targets based on rates of washout, but does not attempt to assess their relative clinical merits: we do not conclude that one target is better than the other; neither do we conclude that they are equally good. Other studies address this: Clinical [5–8] and postmortem [26,27] studies suggest that stimulation just outside the STN proper in ZI/FF may give clinical outcomes as good as or better than stimulation within the nucleus. One potentially useful conclusion suggested by our results is that intermittent stimulation may be more effective with the medial target. Existing DBS implantable pulse generators (IPGs) can be programmed to deliver stimulation alternating with "stimulation-off" periods (and the newest generation of IPGs approved for DBS in the United States allows this without safety concerns related to charge imbalance). If the "off" intervals are short, relative to the washout halflife, this could give similar clinical benefit to continuous stimulation, but with lower power consumption, prolonging battery life. Our results suggest a more medial target, if such a strategy is attempted.

What does seem clear, though, is that DBS targeting has progressed beyond the stage of aiming for a visually conspicuous histological or atlas feature, and is now concerned with finding the best target within an anatomically complex region. The strength of this view derives from the variety of different techniques supporting it: in-vivo reconstruction of contact locations in comparatively large series, post-mortem histological location of contact locations in individual cases, and computation of volumes of tissue activated (VTAs).

Potential DBS mechanisms

Can we associate particular physiological processes with our fast- and slow- decaying processes? The current state of knowledge leaves wide scope for speculation: for example a recent review [28] lists 11 hypothetical mechanisms whereby DBS may alleviate symptoms, arranged according to the time scale on which their effects would occur. The bulk of research on Parkinson's STN DBS mechanisms has focused on stimulation's ability to directly depolarize neurons, overriding the spontaneous, pathological pattern of activity [29]. Such a mechanism would be expected to have very rapid onset/offset, on the order of milliseconds, hence fits well with our "fast" mechanism. According to the classical view, this mechanism operates orthodromically, exciting action potentials via the glutamatergic subthalamopallidal synapse [30], while, according to a novel view supported by optogenetics [31] see also [32] it operates antidromically exciting cortex via the hyperdirect pathway [23]. In either case, the effect would be evoked from STN proper, which is where we find our "fast" effect.

Less research exists on possible DBS mechanisms whose washout might fit our "slow" process; however, Lee [33] has

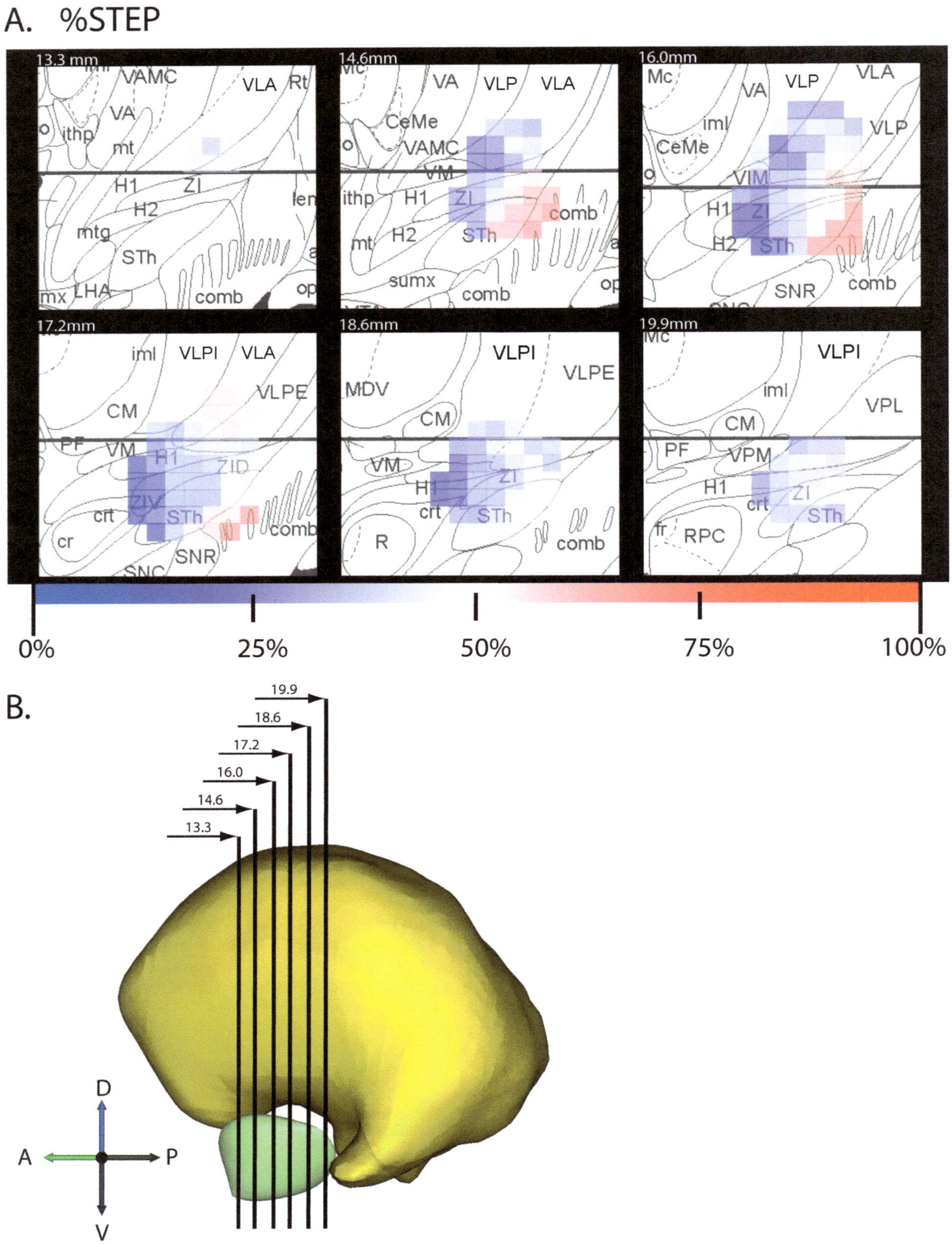

Figure 3. A) Slices corresponding to Mai et al [15] atlas sections were taken through the 3-dimensional field representing the average value of %STEP over the 14 patients. B) Average value of %STEP is shown in false-color, in relation to the structures delineated in the atlas.

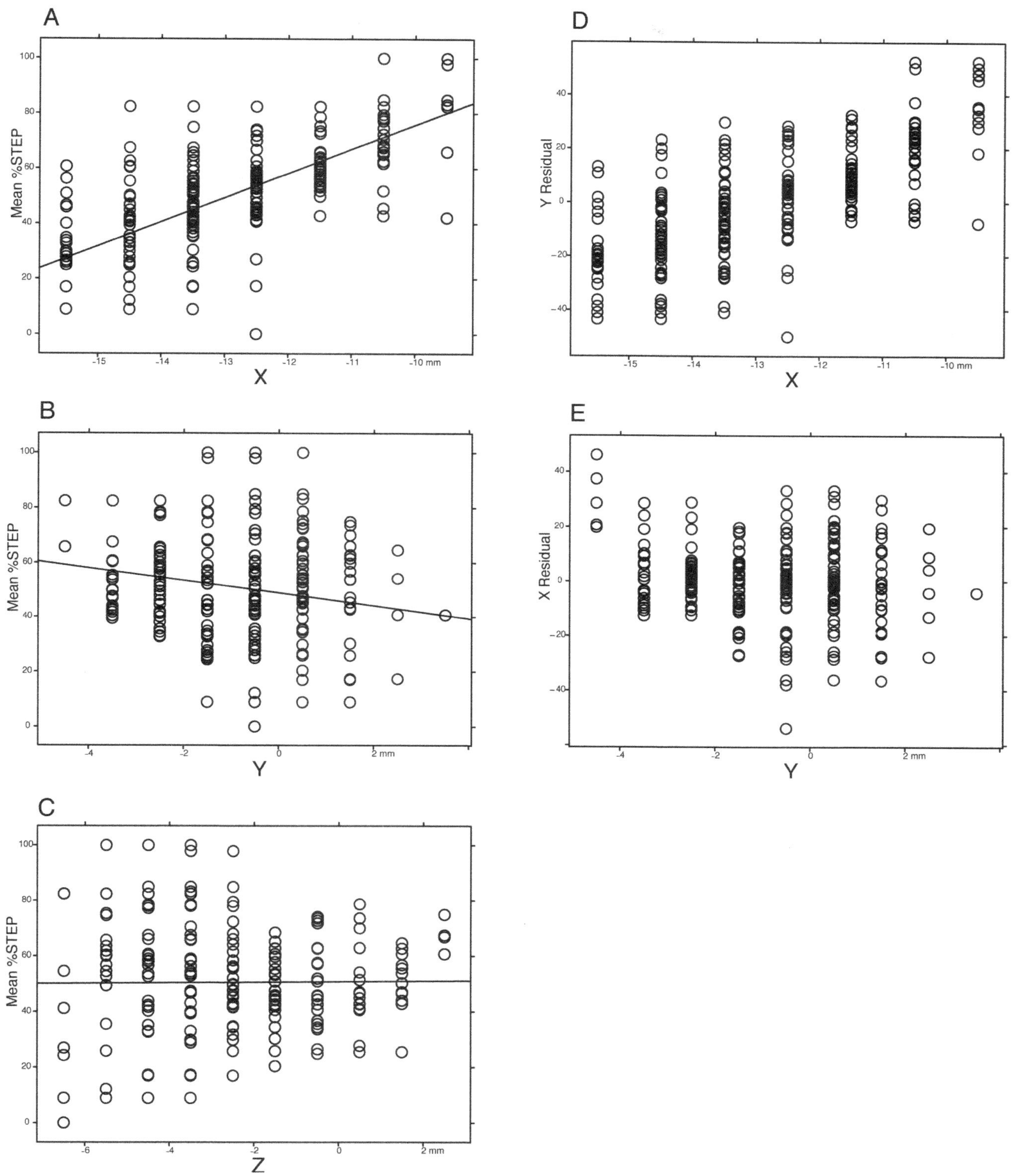

Figure 4. Mean %STEP vs stereotaxic coordinate in stereotaxic space. Each point is a grid point as shown in Fig. 2 E, F. Figure 4 A, B, C: simple regressions on X (mediolateral), Y (anteroposterior), & Z (dorsoventral) coordinate. Figure 4 D, E: residual variances. Fig. 4 D shows the effect of X coordinate when Y is partialed out, and Fig. 4 E shows the effect of Y when X is partialed out. Note that %STEP is related to both X and Y, however, the effect of X is independent of Y, whereas the converse is not true.

proposed extracellular neurotransmitter accumulation as a DBS mechanism, and this appears [34] to exhibit washout on the correct time scale for our slow process. Our slow process originates from a zone in the vicinity of posteroventral ZI, H1, and H2. Forel's fields H1 and H2 are fiber tracts, carrying pallidal efferents; in contrast, ZI is a nucleus with wide projections, including to thalamus, substantia nigra, and spinal cord [35]. Since direct stimulation of GPi improves PD symptoms [36], Parent & Parent [37] have suggested that stimulation of pallidothalamic fibers in the fields of Forel may have a similar therapeutic effect; this may explain why the zone of long-lasting DBS effects extends into ventrolateral thalamus where pallidothalamic fibers terminate. Hypothetically, extracellular neurotransmitter accumulation and reuptake at pallidothalamic synapses, incerto-thalamic synapses, or in ZI proper might produce the slow-washout effect, but available data do not allow us to do more than speculate.

Limitations

Our findings must be interpreted in the context of known limitations in our approach. First, no perfect or universally-accepted method exists for determination of electrode locations. We used Cicerone software [19] to define the electrode location relative to the individual patient anatomy. This particular technique has proven to be effective in numerous previous studies e.g. [10,12,37–40], nonetheless uncertainty is associated with each patient. These types of errors or uncertainty exist for all forms of DBS electrode location estimation in human brains [41,42]. However, a new addition from this study was the integration of the Mai et al. atlas within the context of Cicerone. This allowed us to visualize additional anatomical structures, but required an additional registration step which introduced an additional degree of error into our analysis. Direct quantification of this error is impossible, because no ground truth point exists for the dataset; however, we did attempt to minimize the error by using a least squares optimization algorithm to fit the Mai et al. atlas to each patient's Cicerone model.[10,12,38–40].

Second, since VTAs cannot be imaged directly, estimation of VTAs requires computational models, which introduce uncertainty. The methods we used to generate VTAs have been tested in prior studies [21]. Finally, we have attempted to locate our estimated VTAs in relation to anatomical structures which are quite small, and whose spatial relationship to each other is complex. We chose the atlas of Mai et al because it provides a high level of detail for the fields of Forel and zona incerta, and coregistered VTAs to that atlas using common landmarks (thalamus and STN). Nonetheless, this procedure must be regarded as approximate at best. The complex interdigitation of ZI, H1, and H2 in the slow-decaying target zone makes it unlikely that VTA studies alone can tell us which of them is responsible for therapeutic DBS effects evoked from that region, although, in future fiber tract activation modeling [40] may offer a way to disentangle them.

Acknowledgments

Portions of the analysis were performed using SCIRun, an open-source problem solving environment that was developed through grants from the National Center for Research Resources (5P40R012553-15) and the National Institute of General Medical Sciences (8 P41 GM103545-15) from the National Institutes of Health.

Author Contributions

Conceived and designed the experiments: SC. Performed the experiments: SC. Analyzed the data: SC KD AN CM CB. Wrote the paper: SC KD CB. Edited the manuscript: SC KD AN CM AM CB. Interpreted the data: SC KD AM CB.

References

1. Deuschl G, Schade-Brittinger C, Krack P, Volkmann J, Schafer H, et al. (2006) A randomized trial of deep-brain stimulation for Parkinson's disease. New England Journal of Medicine 355(9): 896–908.
2. Ostrem JL, Racine CA, Glass GA, Grace JK, Volz MM, et al. (2011) Subthalamic nucleus deep brain stimulation in primary cervical dystonia. Neurology 76(10): 870–878.
3. Lind G, Schechtmann G, Lind C, Winter J, Meyerson BA, et al. (2008) Subthalamic stimulation for essential tremor. Short- and long-term results and critical target area. Stereotact Funct Neurosurg 86(4): 253–258.
4. Mallet L, Polosan M, Jaafari N, Baup N, Welter ML, et al. (2008) Subthalamic nucleus stimulation in severe obsessive-compulsive disorder. New England Journal of Medicine 359(20): 2121–2134.
5. Voges J, Volkman J, Allert N, Lehrke R, Koulousakis A, et al. (2002) Bilateral high-frequency stimulation in the subthalamic nucleus for the treatment of Parkinson disease: correlation of therapeutic effect with anatomical electrode position. Journal of Neurosurgery 96(2): 269–279.
6. Hamel W, Fietzek U, Morsnowski A, Schrader B, Weinert D, et al. (2003) Subthalamic nucleus stimulation in Parkinson's disease: correlation of active electrode contacts with intraoperative microrecordings. Stereotactic and Functional Neurosurgery 80(1–4): 37–42.
7. Godinho F, Thobois S, Magnin M, Guenot M, Polo G, et al. (2006) Subthalamic nucleus stimulation in Parkinson's disease: anatomical and electrophysiological localization of active contacts. Journal of Neurology 253(10): 1347–1355.
8. Plaha P, Ben-Shlomo Y, Patel NK, Gill SS (2006) Stimulation of the caudal zona incerta is superior to stimulation of the subthalamic nucleus in improving contralateral parkinsonism. Brain 129(Pt 7): 1732–1747.
9. Anheim M, Batir A, Fraix V, Silem M, Chabardes S, et al. (2008) Improvement in Parkinson disease by subthalamic nucleus stimulation based on electrode placement: effects of reimplantation. Archives of Neurology 65(5): 612–616.
10. Frankemolle AM, Wu J, Noecker AM, Voelcker-Rehage C, Ho JC, et al. 2010 Reversing cognitive-motor impairments in Parkinson's disease patients using a computational modelling approach to deep brain stimulation programming. Brain 133(Pt 3): 746–761.
11. McNeely ME, Hershey T, Campbell MC, Tabbal SD, Karimi M, et al. (2011) Effects of deep brain stimulation of dorsal versus ventral subthalamic nucleus regions on gait and balance in Parkinson's disease. J Neurol Neurosurg Psychiatry 82(11): 1250–1255.
12. Cooper SE, Noecker AM, Abboud H, Vitek JL, McIntyre CC (2011) Return of bradykinesia after subthalamic stimulation ceases: relationship to electrode location. Exp Neurol 231(2): 207–213.
13. McIntyre CC, Mori S, Sherman DL, Thakor NV, Vitek JL (2004) Electric field and stimulating influence generated by deep brain stimulation of the subthalamic nucleus. Clin Neurophysiol 115(3): 589–595.
14. Mai JK, Assheuer J, Paxinos G (2007) Atlas of the Human Brain. San Diego: Academic Press.
15. Butson CR, Cooper SE, Henderson JM, Wolgamuth B, McIntyre CC (2011) Probabilistic analysis of activation volumes generated during deep brain stimulation. Neuroimage 54(3): 2096–2104.
16. Nowinski WL, Belov D, Pollak P, Benabid AL (2005) Statistical analysis of 168 bilateral subthalamic nucleus implantations by means of the probabilistic functional atlas. Neurosurgery 57(4 Suppl): 319–30;
17. Goetz CG, Tilley BC, Shaftman SR, Stebbins GT, Fahn S, et al. (2008) Movement Disorder Society-sponsored revision of the Unified Parkinson's Disease Rating Scale (MDS-UPDRS): scale presentation and clinimetric testing results. Movement Disorders 23(15): 2129–2170.
18. Jones E, Oliphant T, Peterson P (2001) SciPy: Open Source Scientific Tools for Python.
19. Miocinovic S, Noecker AM, Maks CB, Butson CR, McIntyre CC (2007) Cicerone: stereotactic neurophysiological recording and deep brain stimulation electrode placement software system. Acta Neurochir Suppl 97(Pt 2): 561–567.
20. Viola P Wells WMI (1997) Alignment by maximization of mutual information. International Journal of Computer Vision 24: 137–154.
21. Butson CR, Cooper SE, Henderson JM, McIntyre CC (2007) Patient-specific analysis of the volume of tissue activated during deep brain stimulation. NeuroImage, 34(2), 661–70.
22. Saint-Cyr JA, Hoque T, Pereira LC, Dostrovsky JO, Hutchison WD, et al. (2002) Localization of clinically effective stimulating electrodes in the human subthalamic nucleus on magnetic resonance imaging. Journal of Neurosurgery 97(5): 1152–1166.
23. Nambu A, Tokuno H, Takada M (2002) Functional significance of the cortico-subthalamo-pallidal' 'hyperdirect' pathway. Neuroscience Research 43(2): 111–117.
24. Hilliard JD, Frysinger RC, Elias WJ (2011) Effective subthalamic nucleus deep brain stimulation sites may differ for tremor, bradykinesia and gait disturbances

in Parkinson's disease Stereotactic and Functional Neurosurgery, 89(6): 357–364.
25. Plaha P, Khan S, Gill SS (2008) Bilateral stimulation of the caudal zona incerta nucleus for tremor control. J Neurol Neurosurg Psychiatry 79(5): 504–513.
26. Henderson JM, Pell M, O'Sullivan DJ, McCusker EA, Fung VS, et al. (2002) Postmortem analysis of bilateral subthalamic electrode implants in Parkinson's disease. Mov Disord 17(1): 133–137.
27. Guehl D, Vital A, Cuny E, Spampinato U, Rougier A, et al. (2008) Postmortem proof of effectiveness of zona incerta stimulation in Parkinson disease. Neurology 70(16 Pt 2): 1489–1490.
28. Lozano AM, Lipsman N (2013) Probing and regulating dysfunctional circuits using deep brain stimulation. Neuron 77: 406–424.
29. Jenkinson N, Brown P (2011) New insights into the relationship between dopamine, beta oscillations, and motor function. Trends in Neurosciences 34(12): 611–618.
30. Hashimoto T, Elder CM, Okun MS, Patrick SK, Vitek JL (2003) Stimulation of the subthalamic nucleus changes the firing pattern of pallidal neurons. Journal of Neuroscience 23(5): 1916–1923.
31. Gradinaru V, Mogri M, Thompson KR, Henderson JM, Deisseroth K (2009) Optical deconstruction of parkinsonian neural circuitry. Science 324: 354–359.
32. Li Q, Ke Y, Chan DCW, Qian Z-M, Yung KKL, et al. (2012) Therapeutic deep brain stimulation in parkinsonian rats directly influences motor cortex. Neuron 76: 1030–1041.
33. Lee KH, Chang S-Y, Jang D-P, Kim I, Goerss S, et al. (2011) Emerging techniques for elucidating mechanism of action of deep brain stimulation. 33rd annual International Conference of the IEEE EMBS. 2011: 677–680.
34. Lee KH, Kristic K, van Hoff R, Hitti FL, Blaha C, et al. (2007) High-frequency stimulation of the subthalamic nucleus increases glutamate in the subthalamic nucleus of rats as demonstrated by in vivo enzyme-linked glutamate sensor. Brain Research 1162: 121–129.
35. Mitrofanis J (2005) Some certainty for the "zone of uncertainty"? Exploring the function of the zona incerta. Neuroscience 130(1): 1–15.
36. Follett KA, Weaver FM, Stern M, Hur K, Harris CL, et al. (2010) Pallidal versus subthalamic deep-brain stimulation for Parkinson's disease. New England Journal of Medicine 362(22): 2077–2091.
37. Parent M, Parent A (2004) The pallidofugal motor fiber system in primates. Parkinsonism Relat Disord 10(4): 203–211.
38. Mikos A, Bowers D, Noecker AM, McIntyre CC, Won M, et al. (2011) Patient-specific analysis of the relationship between the volume of tissue activated during DBS and verbal fluency. Neuroimage 54 Suppl 1 (S238–46).
39. Zhang J, Wang ZI, Baker KB, Vitek JL (2012) Effect of globus pallidus internus stimulation on neuronal activity in the pedunculopontine tegmental nucleus in the primate model of Parkinson's disease. Exp Neurol 233(1): 575–580.
40. Lujan JL, Chaturvedi A, Malone DA, Rezai AR, Machado AG, et al. (2012) Axonal pathways linked to therapeutic and nontherapeutic outcomes during psychiatric deep brain stimulation. Human Brain Mapping 33(4): 958–968.
41. Bardinet E, Bhattacharjee M, Dormont D, Pidoux B, Malandain G, et al. (2009) A three-dimensional histological atlas of the human basal ganglia. II. Atlas deformation strategy and evaluation in deep brain stimulation for Parkinson disease. J Neurosurg 110(2): 208–219.
42. Videen TO, Campbell MC, Tabbal SD, Karimi M, Hershey T, et al. (2008) Validation of a fiducial-based atlas localization method for deep brain stimulation contacts in the area of the subthalamic nucleus. J Neurosci Methods 168(2): 275–281.

8

Pressure Pain Thresholds Increase after Preconditioning 1 Hz Repetitive Transcranial Magnetic Stimulation with Transcranial Direct Current Stimulation

Tonya M. Moloney*, Alice G. Witney

Department of Physiology, Trinity College Institute of Neuroscience and Trinity Centre for BioEngineering, Trinity College, Dublin, Ireland

Abstract

Background: The primary motor cortex (M1) is an effective target of non-invasive cortical stimulation (NICS) for pain threshold modulation. It has been suggested that the initial level of cortical excitability of M1 plays a key role in the plastic effects of NICS.

Objective: Here we investigate whether transcranial direct current stimulation (tDCS) primed 1 Hz repetitive transcranial magnetic stimulation (rTMS) modulates experimental pressure pain thresholds and if this is related to observed alterations in cortical excitability.

Method: 15 healthy, male participants received 10 min 1 mA anodal, cathodal and sham tDCS to the left M1 before 15 min 1 Hz rTMS in separate sessions over a period of 3 weeks. Motor cortical excitability was recorded at baseline, post-tDCS priming and post-rTMS through recording motor evoked potentials (MEPs) from right FDI muscle. Pressure pain thresholds were determined by quantitative sensory testing (QST) through a computerized algometer, on the palmar thenar of the right hand pre- and post-stimulation.

Results: Cathodal tDCS-primed 1 Hz-rTMS was found to reverse the expected suppressive effect of 1 Hz rTMS on cortical excitability; leading to an overall increase in activity ($p<0.001$) with a parallel increase in pressure pain thresholds ($p<0.01$). In contrast, anodal tDCS-primed 1 Hz-rTMS resulted in a corresponding decrease in cortical excitability ($p<0.05$), with no significant effect on pressure pain.

Conclusion: This study demonstrates that priming the M1 before stimulation of 1 Hz-rTMS modulates experimental pressure pain thresholds in a safe and controlled manner, producing a form of analgesia.

Editor: Andrea Antal, University Medical Center Goettingen, Germany

Funding: This study was supported by the Department of Physiology, Trinity College, Dublin [http://www.tcd.ie/Graduate_Studies/prospectivestudents/awards/studentships/]. The funders had no role in study design, data collection and analysis, decision to publish, or preparation of the manuscript.

Competing Interests: The authors have declared that no competing interests exist.

* E-mail: molonet@tcd.ie

Introduction

Pain perception and modulation have become crucial topics of exploration within the scientific community due to increasing numbers seeking treatment for pain and the current inadequacy of available therapies. Chronic, persistent pain is a complex condition that has been identified as one of the most disabling and costly afflictions in North America, Europe, and Australia with a lifetime prevalence of up to 55.2% in the adult population [1].

In particular, musculoskeletal pain is a cause of long term pain and disability associated with common disorders such as rheumatoid arthritis, osteoarthritis and fibromyalgia. Algometry is used for the assessment of pressure pain thresholds in these patients with chronic musculoskeletal pain. Measurement of these pressure pain thresholds and assessment of the defined 18 tender points forms part of the American College of Rheumatology (ACR) guidelines for the diagnosis of fibromyalgia [2]. Testing pressure pain thresholds at both these tender points and control sites in healthy participants in concert with novel therapies will be important to increase the understanding of alterations in pain processing in these patients.

One method of therapy has been realized in the form of non-invasive cortical stimulation (NICS) with the primary motor cortex (M1) being the most effective target for the modulation of both experimental and chronic pain [3,4]. Particular efficacy for NICS has been found in patients with musculoskeletal pain [5–8]. However a lack of understanding of the underlying physiological mechanisms has limited these techniques progress in clinical applications.

In this study we investigate the physiological mechanism of a novel NICS protocol in healthy adults. Pressure pain thresholds were used as an index of pain sensitivity so as to aid translation of our findings to a musculoskeletal pain population in future studies. There are currently very few studies assessing the efficacy of NICS on this clinically useful pain modality, which needs to be addressed [3].

Non-invasive Cortical Stimulation (NICS)

There are two main methods of NICS; transcranial direct current stimulation (tDCS) and repetitive transcranial magnetic stimulation (rTMS) which are safe, easy to use and associated with relatively negligible side effects [3]. Both techniques can produce bidirectional after-effects on cortical excitability but depend on different stimulation parameters and physiological mechanisms [9]. tDCS has been hypothesized to modulate the resting membrane potentials of axons, altering the endogenous excitability of the target cortical area. It is primarily a modulatory technique with effects dependent on the polarity of stimulation used. In action, cathodal tDCS diminishes cortical excitability through the hyperpolarisation of neurons whereas anodal leads to neuronal depolarisation and increased cortical excitability [10]. However, the underlying mechanisms of tDCS require further research as recent studies have found that tDCS may not only modulate neurons but could also manipulate glial cells. Calculations indicated that transmembrane potential change is of similar magnitude as observed physiologically in astrocytes during neuronal activation [11]. In contrast rTMS is a stimulatory technique as it can generate propagated action potentials leading to the activation of neural circuits [3]. rTMS is frequency dependent with low frequencies (1 Hz or less) associated with decreased cortical excitability and high frequencies (20–50 Hz) associated with increased excitability. It is this mode of high frequency rTMS which has been established as a method of pain treatment with frequencies $\geq$10 Hz necessary to significantly modulate pain thresholds [3,12]. Yet, high frequency rTMS can produce unpleasant scalp sensations which can be uncomfortable. Some patients in rTMS clinical trials have been unable to tolerate this sensation and have dropped out, which can hinder the use of rTMS as a form of pain management [13].

Combined Paradigm (tDCS-rTMS)

It has been suggested that the initial state of the motor cortex may play a key role in the plastic effects of rTMS. Siebner *et al.*, demonstrated how a combined paradigm using tDCS to "prime" or "precondition" motor cortex can successfully shape the conditioning effects of subsequent rTMS [14]. Results show that facilitatory preconditioning via anodal tDCS led to an overall inhibition of cortical excitability after subsequent stimulation by low frequency 1 Hz-rTMS and of particular note, inhibitory preconditioning via cathodal tDCS reverses the expected suppressive effects of low frequency 1 Hz-rTMS leading to an overall increase in cortical excitability. Thus, primed 1 Hz-rTMS can effectively simulate the result of high frequency rTMS on the human motor cortex. Similar studies suggest that this effect is mediated by homeostatic mechanisms whereby the human motor cortex stabilizes corticospinal excitability within a physiologically useful range [14–16]. tDCS-primed rTMS may also prove a more robust protocol as tDCS alone has recently been found to induce highly variable responses [17]. These discoveries prompted the use of a combined paradigm in our pain modulation research.

Pain Modulation

Previous work revealed that tDCS-primed 1 Hz-rTMS can be applied to enhance the modulation of experimental thermal pain thresholds [18]. Inhibitory preconditioning via cathodal tDCS successfully produced increased thermal pain thresholds after subsequent stimulation of 1 Hz rTMS, simulating the physiological effects of high frequency rTMS whilst being a better tolerated method of intervention.

In our present study the technique of tDCS-primed 1 Hz rTMS is applied to pressure pain thresholds. Pressure pain has been proposed as a particularly useful modality, in that it is more directly related to a variety of clinical outcomes in a diverse range of pain patients [19,20]. In the past, manual pressure pain assessment using traditional algometers has been documented to suffer from numerous limitations. This is predominantly due to human error of the operator as they were originally required to manually generate accurate and repeatable force profiles involving controlled ramp rate, consistent stimulus duration and inter-stimulus intervals. This experiment employs a computerized algometer (Medoc, Ramat Yishai, Israel) which acts to standardize the testing procedure and avoid operator-related error. This may allow pain researchers to attain accurate and repeatable force profiles which would be suitable for integration into a clinical setting, particularly in rheumatology patients.

Here, this preconditioning protocol is used to investigate the modulation of both cortical excitability and mechanical pressure pain which may prove useful in the translation of NICS effects between experimental and chronic pain groups.

Materials and Methods

Ethics Statement

The study was performed in accordance with the Declaration of Helsinki and approved by the Faculty of Health Sciences Research Ethics Committee, Trinity College Dublin. All participants provided written informed consent to participate in the study.

Participants

Fifteen healthy male volunteers (mean age, 24.5 years $\pm$3.4 SD, 12 right handed) were recruited to take part in the research study, by advertisement. Participants were approved to partake in the project once they completed a medical questionnaire which was deemed suitable by a qualified medical professional. Subjects with any previous or concomitant psychiatric or neurological disease, any conditions associated with acute or chronic pain or with somatosensory abnormalities were excluded. All participants were able to understand the QST protocol instructions and gave their written informed consent. All were completely naïve to the purpose of the experimental procedures.

Quantitative Sensory Testing (QST)

In order to determine pressure pain thresholds (PPT), a QST protocol was conducted using a standard digital algometer (FDIX; Wagner Instruments, Greenwich, CT) computer-controlled through The Medoc Pathway System (Medoc, Ramat Yishai, Israel). The algometer comprised of a pressure gauge and a 1 cm^2 rubber plunger tip with a digital display of force in increments of 0.01 KPa. Real-time, visual and auditory feedback allowed the investigator to control and monitor applied pressure rates. The computerized algometer applied pressure stimuli according to the method of limits algorithm within the Pathway software and simultaneously recorded thresholds via a push-button response unit (Figure 1).

PPT was defined as the amount of force required to elicit a sensation of pain distinct from pressure or discomfort or in other terms; the point at which pressure transitioned to discomfort or pain [21]. In measuring PPTs, the algometer was applied perpendicularly to the skin and lowered at a rate of approximately 30 KPa/s until PPT was reached. The palmar thenar eminence of the hand was targeted for PPT measurement due to its ease of

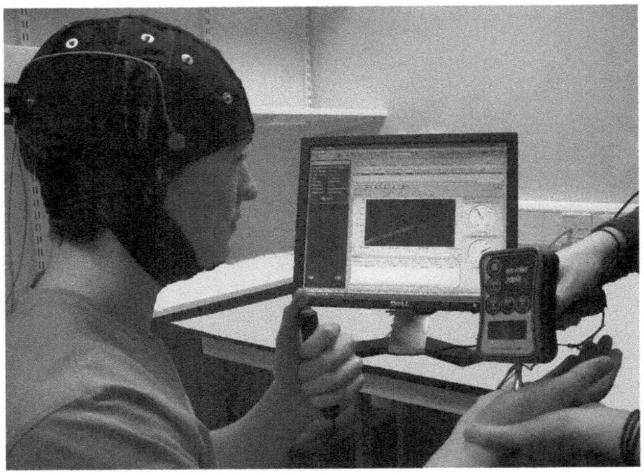

Figure 1. Pressure Pain Assessment Set-up. Handheld algometer used to determine pressure pain thresholds (PPT) of the right palmar thenar eminence via the Medoc Pathway System. The algometer was held perpendicular to the target site and applied according to computer controlled audio and visual prompts, with PPT detection reported via push-button response unit. tDCS was applied using the fitted MindCap with electrodes fixed in the C3/F8 position.

accessibility and proximity to the stimulated FDI. The palmar thenar eminence has also been used in clinical assessments in patients with musculoskeletal pain as a designated control site, distant from defined tender points [22]. The threshold was tested 4 times with an interval of ~5 s between each successive trial, as illustrated in Figure 2A. Each trial lasted 20–25 s in duration, thus a full QST cycle required a solitary moment of focused, direct testing. QST was performed both prior to (PRE) and immediately after (POST) the combined neurostimulation intervention.

Electromyograms and determination of stimulation parameters

Motor evoked potentials (MEPs) were recorded using surface electromyography (EMG) from the right first dorsal interosseous (FDI) muscle using conductive adhesive Ag/AgCl electrodes (Tyco Healthcare, Mansfield, UK) in a belly tendon montage. EMG signals were amplified, band-pass filtered (10–50 Hz) and sampled at 1,000 Hz using an Octal BioAmp (AD Instruments, Oxford, UK). The peak-to-peak amplitudes of the MEPs were then analysed off-line using custom-written software. The optimal placement for stimulation was defined as the site where single pulse TMS resulted in the largest MEP in a consistent fashion. These biphasic pulses were provided using a Magstim Rapid^2 stimulator (Magstim Company Limited, Whitland, Wales, UK) connected to a figure of eight double coil (70 mm). The coil was placed tangentially to the scalp, with the handle pointing backward and laterally at a 45° angle to the sagittal plane, inducing a posteroanterior current in the brain [23] The resting motor threshold (RMT) is defined as the minimum TMS intensity which achieved peak-to-peak MEP amplitude of ≥50 μV in the resting FDI muscle, in 3 out of 5 stimulations. The measured RMT was used to set the output for subsequent rTMS protocols.

Measurement of Motor System Excitability

To detect current-driven changes of excitability, motor-evoked potentials (MEPs) of the right FDI following stimulation of its motor-cortical representational field were recorded. A train of ~20 TMS-evoked MEPs were recorded at 3.5 s intervals at an intensity of 120% of each individual's RMT. This train of MEPs was carried out prior to (PRE), in between (INTER) and immediately after stimulation (POST).

Preconditioning the left M1 using tDCS

The application of tDCS was performed to the hand area of the left motor cortex; C3 according to the international 10–20 EEG system, through the use of a HDC kit (Magstim Company Limited, Whitland, Wales, UK). Direct currents were applied through a pair of saline soaked (0.89%NaCl) synthetic buckskin electrodes (25 cm^2) with the active electrode placed over C3 and the reference electrode positioned contralaterally above the right orbit. These electrodes were held in place with use of the MindCap (Magstim Company Limited, Whitland, Wales, UK). Each of the four experimental conditions involved the continuous application of a current of 1 mA intensity for a duration of 10 minutes, as these parameters proved successful in priming the motor cortex in previous experiments [14]. Most subjects were aware of the current flow as an itching/burning sensation was reported upon stimulation with both polarities. For sham stimulation, placement of the electrodes was identical to both cathodal and anodal conditions. Here, current flow increased gradually over a 5 s interval reaching the designated 1 mA to mimic the initial itching sensation of real tDCS. The stimulation was then terminated after 10 s, so that a conditioning effect on cortical excitability would not be induced [24].

Stimulation of left M1 with 1 Hz –rTMS

Using each participant's individual RMT, the TMS protocol was set to produce repetitive TMS (rTMS) at the designated 90% of a participant's individual RMT. This sub threshold intensity was chosen for two reasons: First, the intensity is likely to activate the corticospinal neurons trans-synaptically avoiding direct activation of these neurons [25]. Second, it was reasoned that sub threshold intensity may produce a relatively "weak" after-effect that would be more susceptible to the effects of pre-conditioning [14]. rTMS was then carried out at a frequency of 1 Hz with a train of 900 pulses, each of 1 s duration with a 1 s wait period (15 min total duration). Sham rTMS was administered with the coil tilted at a 45° angle from the surface of the head, discharging the same number of stimuli at the same rate as real rTMS. All subjects were naive to TMS, hence accepted the explanation that differences in scalp sensation between sham and real rTMS were due to stimulation at different intensity levels [26]. All rTMS protocols were carried out in accordance with the outlined safety guidelines [27].

Experimental Protocol

A sham-controlled, single-blind study was conducted, consisting of four separate experiments, to determine how priming the motor cortex using tDCS may enhance the effects of rTMS on the modulation of pressure pain thresholds in healthy volunteers. The four conditions consisted of;

1) Sham tDCS – Sham rTMS
2) Sham tDCS – Real rTMS
3) Cathodal tDCS – Real rTMS
4) Anodal tDCS – Real rTMS

Each treatment was performed on the same day, at the same time over a period of 3 weeks in order to avoid any potential issues regarding a variation of pain thresholds due to circadian rhythms.

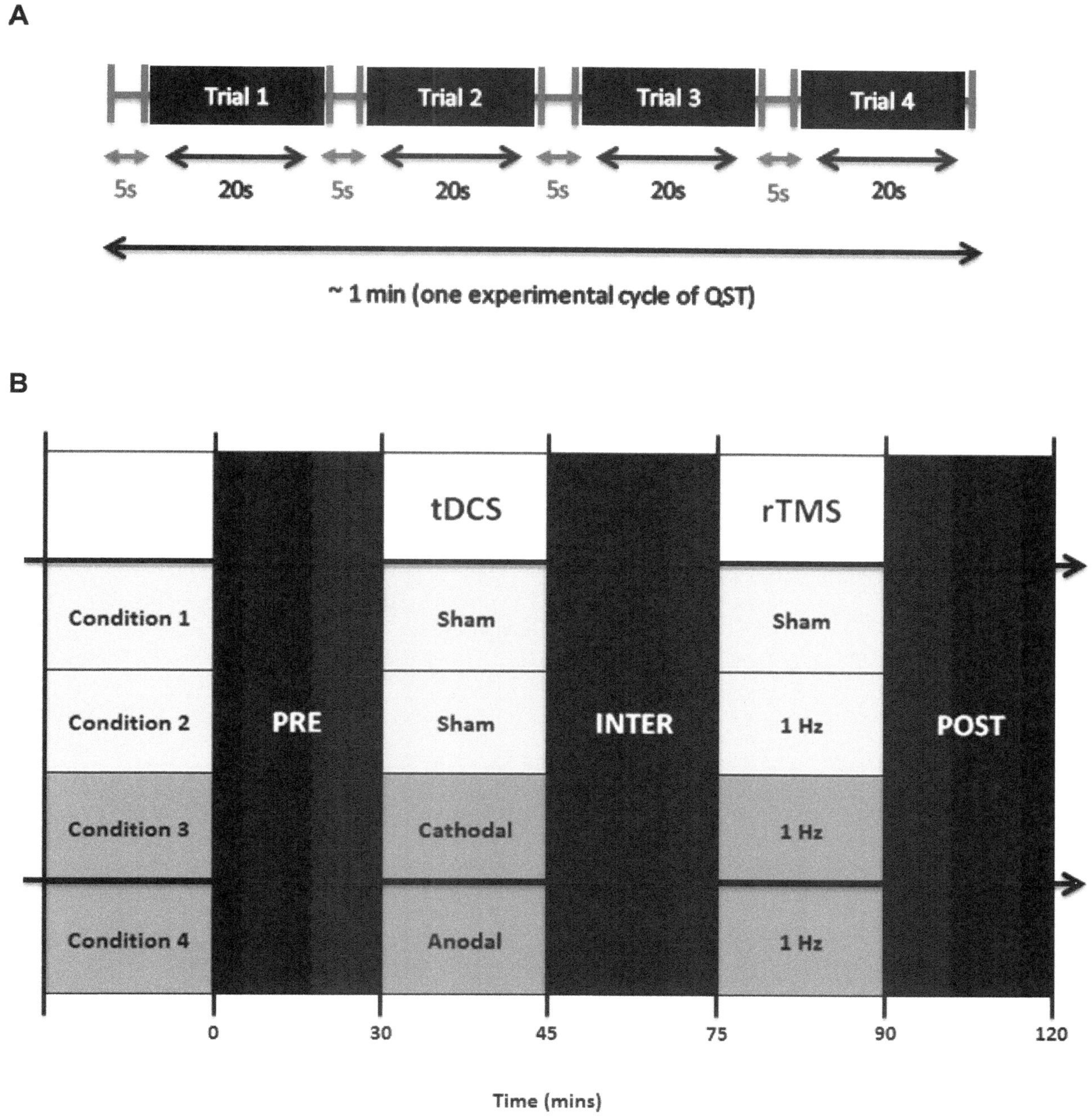

Figure 2. Experimental Approach. Panel A illustrates one cycle of pressure pain threshold (PPT) measurement using quantitative sensory testing (QST). Panel B depicts the timeline of the experimental sessions over the testing period. Experiments were conducted on the same day at the same time, every week, for experimental accuracy in data collection.

Figure 2B illustrates a simple timeline of the treatment order and the time involved in each section. Overall, each experimental treatment takes approximately 2 hours in duration.

Each experiment was performed by the same, trained female examiner and at the same time of day. Sessions lasted approximately 2 hours for each condition, with participants kept conscious and alert by being addressed by the examiner during breaks from stimulation. An interval of one week was required between active testing conditions to avoid any interference that could be caused by the after-effects of stimulation. Treatment 1 and 2 acted as control sessions and were therefore suitable to be performed on the same day without risk of interference. Sham, cathodal and anodal tDCS-primed – 1 Hz rTMS interventions were presented in a pseudo randomized sequence and participants were unaware of the presented condition.

Statistical Analysis

Collected data was first tested for normality of distribution using the Shapiro-Wilk's test within the SPSS statistical package (Version 20, IBM, New York, US). MEP data required transformation to square root in order to address moderate positive skew. All analyses were carried out using normally distributed data.

Test-retest reliability of PPT baseline measurements for each condition was calculated using SPSS based on a single rating, absolute agreement, 2-way mixed effect model ($ICC_{2,\ 1}$). This statistic was used a measure of internal consistency and reproducibility across all conditions.

A two-way repeated measure (4×2) ANOVA was carried out to test the effects of Condition (Anodal, Cathodal, Control 1 and Control 2) and Time (Pre and Post) on the PPT data. A separate two-way repeated measure (4×3) ANOVA was used to assess the effects of Condition (Anodal, Cathodal, Control 1 and Control 2) and Time (Pre, Inter and Post) on MEP values. Planned contrasts were employed to assess statistical significance within each model. Values are presented as the mean of each participant's mean ± the standard error of the mean (SEM). A confidence level of 0.05 was set for all statistical tests.

Results

Fifteen healthy male participants completed all protocols designed to determine if preconditioning the left M1 using tDCS (anodal, cathodal, sham) can modulate baseline cortical excitability and thereby shape the subsequent effects of low frequency rTMS (1 Hz) on pressure pain thresholds. None of the participants experienced any adverse side effects during or after the neurostimulation sessions.

Quantitative Sensory Testing (QST) Analysis

Pressure pain threshold testing was found to be reliable on a test-retest basis across all conditions with an average baseline of 360±3.7 KPa, an intraclass correlation coefficient (ICC) value of 0.9 and a 95% confidence interval of 0.798–0.960. This indicates test-retest reliability to be highly consistent, allowing for greater statistical power in further analysis.

Raw QST results revealed a main effect for both Condition ($F(2, 28) = 3.42$, $p<0.05$, $\eta^2_p = 0.196$) and Time ($F(1,14) = 5.02$, $p<0.05$, $\eta^2_p = 0.264$), however the respective interactions were not statistically significant ($F(3,42) = 2.17$, $p = 0.105$, $\eta^2_p = 0.135$). Planned contrasts demonstrated cathodal tDCS-primed 1 Hz-rTMS produced a significant increase in PPT from a baseline threshold of 365.73±90.92 KPa to 405.07±97.44 KPa post neurostimulation in regards to both the effects of Condition ($F(1,14) = 10.68$, $p<0.01$, $\eta^2_p = 0.433$) and Time ($F(1,14 = 5.02$, $p<0.05$, $\eta^2_p = 0.264$) (as seen in Figure 3). There was no statistical difference detected for any of the other conditions.

Cortical Excitability (MEP) Analysis

The ANOVA revealed a significant main effect for the interaction of the factors Condition x Time ($F(2,29) = 12.06$, $p<0.001$, $\eta^2_p = 0.463$) showing that this priming protocol did indeed have an effect on cortical excitability. However no significance was evident for the individual main effects of Condition ($F(2,24) = 1.07$, $p = 0.35$, $\eta^2_p = 0.071$) or Time ($F(2,28) = 1.03$, $p = 0.371$, $\eta^2_p = 0.068$).Within subject contrasts indicated a significant initial increase in MEP amplitude from a baseline of 0.6±0.34 mA (PRE) to 0.75±0.45 mA (INTER) after anodal tDCS priming ($F(1,14) = 17.64$, $p<0.001$, $\eta 2p = 0.558$) and alternatively induced a significant decrease in amplitude ranging from 0.75±0.45 mA (INTER) to 0.6±0.47 mA (POST) due to the subsequent effects of 1 Hz rTMS ($F(1,14) = 8.66$, $p<0.05$, $\eta^2_p = 0.382$). Cathodal tDCS-primed 1 Hz-rTMS resulted in an opposite response of cortical activity as displayed in Figure 4. Cathodal tDCS priming produced an initial decrease in cortical excitability from a baseline of 0.56±0.32 mA (PRE) to 0.39±0.28 mA (INTER)($F(1,14) = 61.96$, $p<0.001$, $\eta^2_p = 0.816$) and an equally significant increase in excitability from 0.39±0.28 mA (INTER) to 0.68±0.44 mA (POST) immediately after 1 Hz rTMS ($F(1,14) = 25.93$, $p<0.001$, $\eta^2_p = 0.649$). In comparing controls (Control 1: Sham tDCS-Sham rTMS vs Control 2: Sham tDCS-1 Hz rTMS) significant change was only seen INTER vs POST with a decrease in MEP size from 0.62±0.3 mA to 0.55±0.25 mA ($F(1,\ 14) = 9.56$, $p<0.01$, $\eta^2_p = 0.406$).

Discussion

In this study we demonstrate that cathodal tDCS-primed 1 Hz-rTMS of the M1 can increase pain thresholds resulting in decreased sensitivity to experimentally provoked pressure pain. Further, cathodal tDCS-primed 1 Hz-rTMS was found to significantly increase cortical excitability, between the modified baseline levels (INTER) and final measurements (POST). Contrastingly, anodal tDCS-primed 1 Hz-rTMS produced a significant decrease in cortical excitability INTER vs POST with no effect on pain thresholds. These changes in excitability may provide a physiological basis for the observed pain modulatory effect.

tDCS-primed 1 Hz-rTMS Alters Cortical Excitability Modulation

Prior to our exploration of homeostatic plasticity and pain threshold modulation, 1 Hz-rTMS had been found ineffective in pain relief and unworthy of further research in the field [28]. As a general rule, low frequency rTMS (<5 Hz) is thought to facilitate a depression in neuronal excitability whilst high frequency rTMS (>5 Hz) has been shown to increase neuronal excitability and consequently lead to a parallel increase in pain thresholds [26]. However, our investigation has found tDCS-primed 1 Hz-rTMS successful in enhancing the effects of low frequency rTMS and the modulation of pressure pain thresholds.

Our findings suggest that rTMS-induced plastic changes depend on the functional state of the motor cortex, which can be modified using tDCS, consistent with previous research [14,15,29]. These have been interpreted in the context of "homeostatic plasticity". This concept of brain plasticity refers to the negative feedback mechanisms in place to regulate the activity of neural circuitry and prevent them from becoming hyper- or hypoactive [30]. The original model of homeostatic plasticity was formalized as the Bienenstock-Cooper-Munro (BCM) rule of bidirectional synaptic plasticity [31], where the threshold for long term potentiation(LTP)/depression(LTD) induction is not constant, but instead varies as a function of previous activity of the post synaptic neuron. Bienenstock, Cooper and Munro proposed the existence of a sliding modification threshold for synaptic plasticity, in that; the threshold for LTP induction increases if the previous level of post synaptic neuronal activity was high, but decreases if it was low, and vice versa for LTD induction where; the threshold for LTD induction decreases if post synaptic activity was high and increases if it was low.

Current preconditioning techniques seek to manipulate these homeostatic mechanisms. In effect, tDCS is used to augment background motor cortical excitability and thus enhance the cortical plastic changes induced by subsequent low-frequency rTMS. In the present study; we used the mean MEP amplitude as an index of the changes in primary motor cortex excitability. Of particular importance, participants displayed an increase in cortical activity in response to 1 Hz rTMS when previously

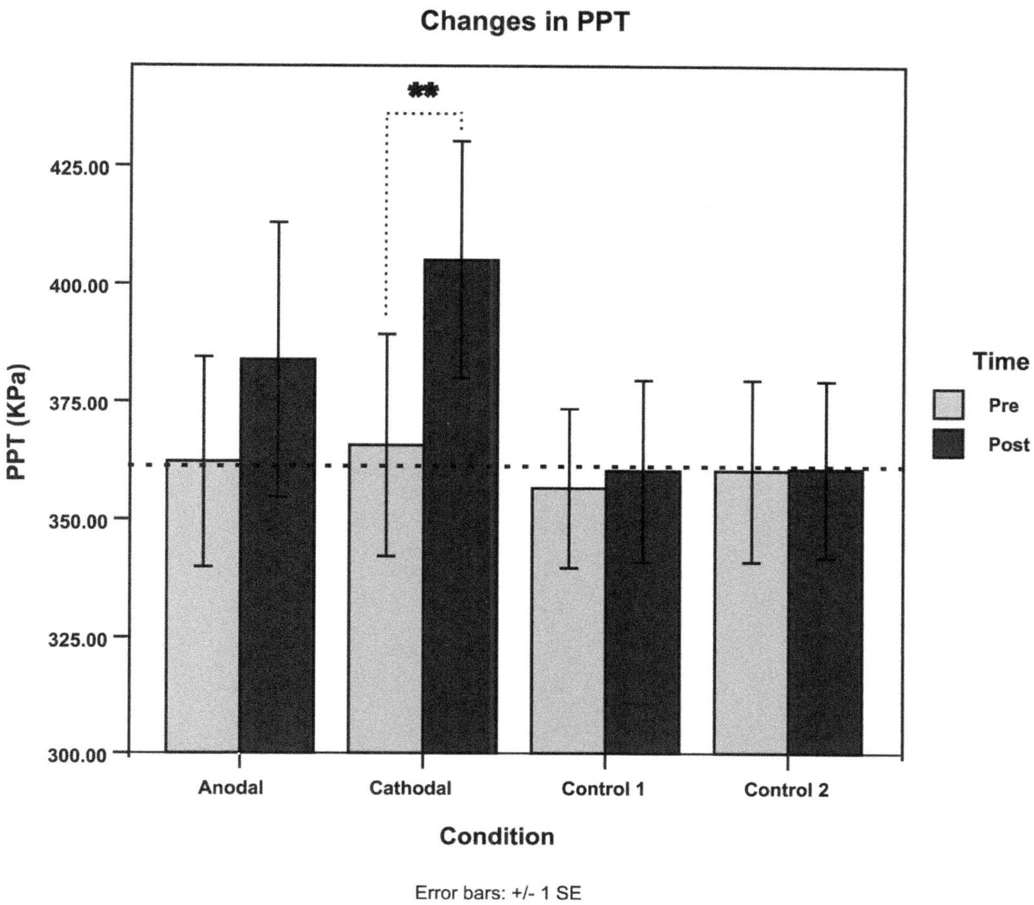

Figure 3. Changes in Pressure Pain Thresholds (PPT). Raw pressure pain thresholds (PPT) averaged and presented across all conditions, prior to stimulation (PRE) and immediately after stimulation (POST). Dotted line represents the average baseline of PPTs across all participants ~361.25 KPa. (*Denotes significance, ** $p<0.01$ within the 4x2 ANOVA as a main effect of the factor Condition)

inhibited by cathodal tDCS, successfully reversing the expected suppressive effects of 1 Hz rTMS. Contrastingly, the same 1 Hz rTMS protocol decreased the excitability of the motor cortex back to baseline levels after cortical excitability had been enhanced by a preceding anodal tDCS.

The level of homeostatic regulation appears to be dependent on the intensity of the stimulation applied. A study using tDCS to precondition the motor cortex before subsequent stimulation via high frequency 5 Hz-rTMS reported effects in agreement with our findings [15]. Healthy participants were found to demonstrate a decrease in cortical excitability in response to 5 Hz-rTMS when the motor cortex had been previously enhanced via facilitatory anodal tDCS priming. In effect, this may have resulted in a destabilizing potentiation of neuronal activity which required an increased level of homeostatic regulation leading to an ultimate depression of cortical excitability. In line with this theory, an equal level of homeostatic regulation would be appropriate in the case of our protocol comprised of cathodal tDCS-primed low frequency 1 Hz-rTMS, which would result in an overall extreme depotentiation of neuronal activity if it were not for the action of negative-feedback mechanisms eliciting an overall increase in cortical excitability.

Conversely, the same 5 Hz-rTMS protocol induced a rise in cortical excitability to return to baseline values after the motor cortex had been inhibited by a preceding session of cathodal tDCS [15]. Therefore combinations such as cathodal tDCS-primed 5 Hz-rTMS and our anodal tDCS-primed 1 Hz-rTMS did not provoke an equal level of homeostatic regulation and merely resulted in the return of MEP amplitudes to baseline. The nature of the biological mechanisms that generate this stability have yet to be elucidated, but in a recent paper Turrigiano et al, discusses how neuronal firing arises from the interplay between synaptic currents and the intrinsic firing properties of a neuron, providing two clear modes by which neurons could homeostatically regulate excitability [32].

Pain Modulation

The present study reinforces the results of our previous work [18], in providing new evidence for the modulation of pressure pain thresholds using tDCS-primed 1 Hz-rTMS. However using the modality of pressure pain as an index and the same neurostimulation intervention, an increase in thresholds was seen post anodal and cathodal primed 1 Hz-rTMS, with significance present only for cathodal effects. This did not compare with the modulation of thermal thresholds as reported effects were significantly polarity dependent, demonstrating a decrease in thresholds post anodal tDCS-primed 1 Hz-rTMS and an increase post cathodal tDCS-primed 1 Hz-rTMS. While the physiological pathways underlying the perception of thermal stimuli are relatively understood within the scientific community [33,34],

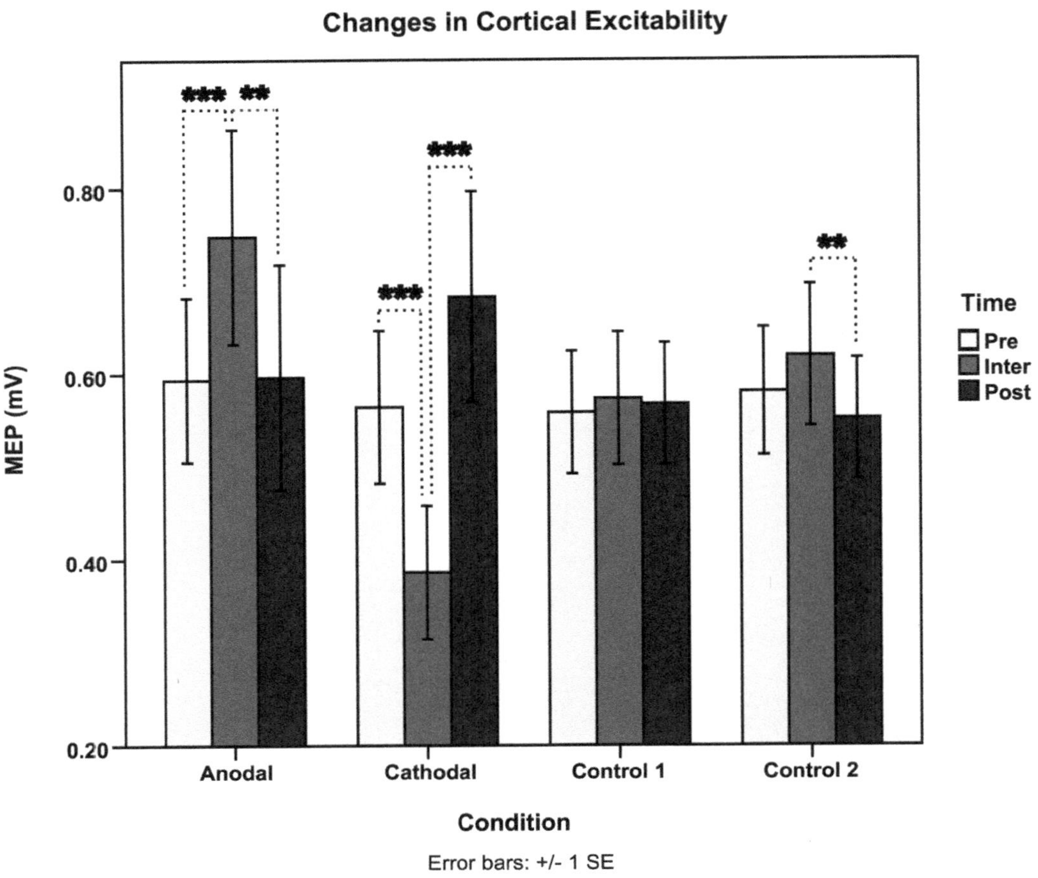

Figure 4. Changes in Cortical Excitability. Changes in cortical excitability were indexed using motor-evoked potentials (MEPs). Here MEP amplitudes are averaged and presented across all conditions, prior to stimulation (PRE), in-between stimulations (INTER) and immediately after stimulation (POST). (*Denotes significance. *(blue) infers significance PRE vs INTER, *(purple) INTER vs POST.

those of mechanical stimuli such as pressure pain, have not yet been elucidated. Variations in the molecular mechanisms and related pathways between the perception and modulation of these two modalities may explain the contrasting effects seen within our studies.

How these forms of neurostimulation act on the M1 to modulate pain thresholds is also not yet fully understood. However many brain imaging studies have been carried out in relation to motor cortex stimulation (MCS), a technique comprised of an invasive, surgical procedure whereby electrodes are implanted onto the surface of the motor cortex. Results reveal activity changes in all neural structures involved in pain processing, such as the thalamus, anterior cingulate cortex (ACC), orbitofrontal cortex, insula, second somatosensory cortex (S2) or the periaqueductal grey matter (PAG) [35–38]. It has been hypothesized that part of the pain relief afforded by stimulation of the motor cortex could be through influencing thalamic activity, as the thalamus acts as the main relay centre for sensory information to the cortex. High frequency rTMS may directly activate the thalamus via corticothalamic projections and thereby suppress the transmission of sensory information via the spinothalamic pathway [39].Alternatively, it has been suggested that M1 stimulation may alter intracortical motor circuitry. According to Lefaucheur et al., high frequency rTMS (10 Hz) was found to re-establish intracortical inhibition in parallel with pain relief [40].

The molecular mechanisms underlying NICS-induced pain modulation also remain speculative. Lefaucheur et al., hypothesized that these analgesic effects may be mediated by the inhibitory GABAergic system [40]. This hypothesis has been supported by a recent study investigating an animal model of central pain due to spinal cord lesion [41]. It indicated that M1 stimulation produces its analgesic effects by enhancing GABAergic activity in the zona incerta, resulting in an increased inhibition of thalamic neurons involved in nociceptive processing.

We hypothesize that in altering the functional state of the M1 using cathodal tDCS before subsequent stimulation via 1 Hz rTMS, the resulting increase of pain thresholds mirror those of high frequency rTMS. This suggests the need for further research into the state dependent effects of rTMS in both healthy and patient populations with the aim of determining optimal protocols for clinical integration.

Limitations

However the strength of our conclusions may be limited by our small, gender-specific sample size. Previous work in NICS and pain modulation have mainly used male participants due to stable hormone levels throughout testing periods with the aim of reducing inter-subject variability. A recent report outlined the presence of this strong male-orientated bias in experimental subject choice to date and issued a call for all experiments to be performed on both sexes [42]. Women are also greatly overrepresented among patients with chronic pain, with pain syndromes such as fibromyalgia occurring far more often in the female population [42]. Thus future studies would benefit from the extension of this work with the inclusion of female volunteers and a larger sample size to control for the increased variability. However, for initial insights into the physiological mechanisms underlying the efficacy of tDCS-primed 1 Hz rTMS, it is beneficial to reduce variability by selecting a healthy male cohort.

Future in Clinical Practice

Future studies relating to clinical integration of these techniques must take into consideration the disease state of the individual. Pathophysiology is likely to alter the functional state of the cortex and lead to a different response pattern provoked by rTMS compared with healthy control subjects [43,44]. Studies have demonstrated complete opposite results of this priming technique when performed on pain patients, suggesting a dysregulation in the inhibitory homeostatic mechanisms in various neurological disorders [45]. This knowledge can aid us in the progressive development of these preconditioning protocols seeking to amend these malfunctions in the neuronal circuitry and help to uncover novel, effective means of pain relief.

Conclusion

Our study has found clear evidence to support the use of this tDCS-primed 1 Hz rTMS technique as a novel method in the modulation of pain. In line with current literature on metaplasticity, our results have shown cathodal tDCS-primed 1 Hz rTMS can increase cortical excitability and further, lead to a parallel increase of pressure pain thresholds, successfully producing a form of analgesia. These combined neurophysiological treatments have the potential to be beneficial in both experimental and clinical settings as a safe, non-invasive and innovative approach to pain modulation.

Acknowledgments

We particularly thank David Fletcher, Aidan Kelly, Sophia Karok and Colm Bhandal of Trinity College and Tom Broughton of AD Instruments in regards to their expert technical advice and assistance throughout the project.

Author Contributions

Conceived and designed the experiments: TMM AGW. Performed the experiments: TMM. Analyzed the data: TMM. Contributed reagents/materials/analysis tools: AGW. Wrote the paper: TMM. Designed the program used in analysis: AGW.

References

1. Harstall C, Ospina M (2003) How prevalent is chronic pain. Pain Clinical Updates 11: 1–4.
2. Wolfe F, Smythe HA, Yunus MB, Bennett RM, Bombardier C, et al. (1990) The American College of Rheumatology 1990 Criteria for the Classification of Fibromyalgia. Report of the Multicenter Criteria Committee. Arthritis Rheum 33: 160–172.
3. Mylius V, Borckardt JJ, Lefaucheur JP (2012) Noninvasive cortical modulation of experimental pain. Pain 153: 1350–1363.
4. Fregni F, Freedman S, Pascual-Leone A (2007) Recent advances in the treatment of chronic pain with non-invasive brain stimulation techniques. Lancet Neurology: 188–191.
5. Antal A, Terney D, Kuhnl S, Paulus W (2010) Anodal transcranial direct current stimulation of the motor cortex ameliorates chronic pain and reduces short intracortical inhibition. J Pain Symptom Management 39: 890–903.
6. Valle A, Roizenblatt S, Botte S, Zaghi S, Riberto M, et al. (2009) Efficacy of anodal transcranial direct current stimulation (tDCS) for the treatment of fibromyalgia: results of a randomized, sham-controlled longitudinal clinical trial. J Pain Manag 2: 353–361.
7. Marlow NM, Bonilha HS, Short EB (2013) Efficacy of transcranial direct current stimulation and repetitive transcranial magnetic stimulation for treating fibromyalgia syndrome: a systematic review. Pain Pract 13: 131–145.
8. Villamar MF, Wivatvongvana P, Patumanond J, Bikson M, Truong DQ, et al. (2013) Focal modulation of the primary motor cortex in fibromyalgia using 4x1-ring high-definition transcranial direct current stimulation (HD-tDCS): immediate and delayed analgesic effects of cathodal and anodal stimulation. J Pain 14: 371–383.
9. Zaghi S, Heine N, Fregni F (2009) Brain stimulation for the treatment of pain: a review of costs, clinical effects, and mechanisms of treatment for three different central neuromodulatory approaches. Journal of Pain Mangement 2: 339–352.
10. Nitsche MA, Paulus W (2000) Excitability changes induced in the human motor cortex by weak transcranial direct current stimulation. J Physiol 527 Pt 3: 633–639.
11. Ruohonen J, Karhu J (2012) tDCS possibly stimulates glial cells. Clin Neurophysiol 123: 2006–2009.
12. Borckardt JJ, Reeves ST, Beam W, Jensen MP, Gracely RH, et al. (2011) A Randomized, Controlled Investigation of Motor Cortex Transcranial Magnetic Stimulation (TMS) Effects on Quantitative Sensory Measures in Healthy Adults Evaluation of TMS Device Parameters. Clinical Journal of Pain 27: 486–494.
13. Borckardt JJ, Smith AR, Hutcheson K, Johnson K, Nahas Z, et al. (2006) Reducing pain and unpleasantness during repetitive transcranial magnetic stimulation. J ECT 22: 259–264.
14. Siebner HR, Lang N, Rizzo V, Nitsche MA, Paulus W, et al. (2004) Preconditioning of low-frequency repetitive transcranial magnetic stimulation with transcranial direct current stimulation: evidence for homeostatic plasticity in the human motor cortex. J Neurosci 24: 3379–3385.
15. Lang N, Siebner HR, Ernst D, Nitsche MA, Paulus W, et al. (2004) Preconditioning with transcranial direct current stimulation sensitizes the motor cortex to rapid-rate transcranial magnetic stimulation and controls the direction of after-effects. Biological Psychiatry 56: 634–639.
16. Cosentino G, Fierro B, Paladino P, Talamanca S, Vigneri S, et al. (2012) Transcranial direct current stimulation preconditioning modulates the effect of high-frequency repetitive transcranial magnetic stimulation in the human motor cortex. Eur J Neurosci 35: 119–124.
17. Wiethoff S, Hamada M, Rothwell JC (2014) Variability in response to transcranial direct current stimulation of the motor cortex. Brain Stimulation. In Press. DOI: 10. 1016/j.brs.2014.02.003
18. Moloney TM, Witney AG (2013) Transcranial direct current stimulation (tDCS) priming of 1 Hz repetitive transcranial magnetic stimulation (rTMS) modulates experimental pain thresholds. Neurosci Lett 534: 289–294.
19. Harte SE, Mitra M, Ichesco EA, Halvorson ME, Clauw DJ, et al. (2013) Development and validation of a pressure-type automated quantitative sensory testing system for point-of-care pain assessment. Medical & biological engineering & computing: 1–12.
20. Treede RD, Rolke R, Andrews K, Magerl W (2002) Pain elicited by blunt pressure: neurobiological basis and clinical relevance. Pain 98: 235–240.
21. Fischer AA (1987) Pressure algometry over normal muscles. Standard values, validity and reproducibility of pressure threshold. Pain 30: 115–126.
22. Carli G, Suman AL, Biasi G, Marcolongo R (2002) Reactivity to superficial and deep stimuli in patients with chronic musculoskeletal pain. Pain 100: 259–269.
23. Nitsche MA, Seeber A, Frommann K, Klein CC, Rochford C, et al. (2005) Modulating parameters of excitability during and after transcranial direct current stimulation of the human motor cortex. 568 1: 291–303.
24. Bachmann CG, Muschinsky S, Nitsche MA, Rolke R, Magerl W, et al. (2010) Transcranial direct current stimulation of the motor cortex induces distinct changes in thermal and mechanical sensory percepts. Clinical Neurophysiology 121: 2083–2089.
25. Di Lazzaro V, Oliviero A, Profice P, Insola A, Mazzone P, et al. (1999) Effects of voluntary contraction on descending volleys evoked by transcranial electrical stimulation over the motor cortex hand area in conscious humans. Exp Brain Res 124: 525–528.
26. Summers J, Johnson S, Pridmore S, Oberoi D (2004) Changes to cold detection and pain thresholds following low and high frequency transcranial magnetic stimulation of the motor cortex. Neuroscience Letters 368: 197–200.
27. Rossi S, Hallett M, Rossini PM, Pascual-Leone A, Group TSoTC (2009) Safety, ethical consideration, and application guidelines for the use of transcranial magnetic stimulation in clinical practice and research. Clinical Neurophysiology 120: 2008–2039.
28. O'Connell NE, Wand BM, Marston L, Spencer S, Desouza LH (2010) Non-invasive brain stimulation techniques for chronic pain. Cochrane Database Syst Rev: CD008208.
29. Ziemann U, Siebner HR (2008) Modifying motor learning through gating and homeostatic metaplasticity. Brain Stimul 1: 60–66.
30. Turrigiano GG, Nelson SB (2004) Homeostatic plasticity in the developing nervous system. Nat Rev Neurosci 5: 97–107.
31. Bienenstock EL, Cooper LN, Munro PW (1982) Theory for the development of neuron selectivity: orientation specificity and binocular interaction in visual cortex. The Journal of Neuroscience 2: 32–48.
32. Turrigiano G (2011) Too many cooks? Intrinsic and synaptic homeostatic mechanisms in cortical circuit refinement. Annu Rev Neurosci 34: 89–103.

33. Caterina MJ, Julius D (2001) The vanilloid receptor: a molecular gateway to the pain pathway. Annu Rev Neurosci 24: 487–517.
34. Schepers RJ, Ringkamp M (2010) Thermoreceptors and thermosensitive afferents. Neurosci Biobehav Rev 34: 177–184.
35. Garcia-Larrea L, Peyron R (2007) Motor cortex stimulation for neuropathic pain: From phenomenology to mechanisms. Neuroimage 37 Suppl 1: S71–79.
36. Garcia-Larrea L, Peyron R, Mertens P, Gregoire MC, Lavenne F, et al. (1999) Electrical stimulation of motor cortex for pain control: a combined PET-scan and electrophysiological study. Pain 83: 259–273.
37. Peyron R, Faillenot I, Mertens P, Laurent B, Garcia-Larrea L (2007) Motor cortex stimulation in neuropathic pain. Correlations between analgesic effect and hemodynamic changes in the brain. A PET study. Neuroimage 34: 310–321.
38. Tamura Y, Okabe S, Ohnishi T, D NS, Arai N, et al. (2004) Effects of 1-Hz repetitive transcranial magnetic stimulation on acute pain induced by capsaicin. Pain 107: 107–115.
39. Pleger B, Jansenn F, Schwenkreis P, Volker B, Maier C, et al. (2004) Repetitive transcranial magnetic stimulation of the motor cortex attenuates pain perception in complex regional pain syndrome type I. Neuroscience Letters 356: 87–90.
40. Lefaucheur JP, Drouot X, Menard-Lefaucheur I, Keravel Y, Nguyen JP (2006) Motor cortex rTMS restores defective intracortical inhibition in chronic neuropathic pain. Neurology 67: 1568–1574.
41. Lucas JM, Ji Y, Masri R (2011) Motor cortex stimulation reduces hyperalgesia in an animal model of central pain. Pain 152: 1398–1407.
42. Mogil JS (2012) Sex differences in pain and pain inhibition: multiple explanations of a controversial phenomenon. Nat Rev Neurosci 13: 859–866.
43. Siebner HR, Auer C, Conrad B (1999) Abnormal increase in the corticomotor output to the affected hand during repetitive transcranial magnetic stimulation of the primary motor cortex in patients with writer's cramp. Neurosci Lett 262: 133–136.
44. Siebner HR, Tormos JM, Ceballos-Baumann AO, Auer C, Catala MD, et al. (1999) Low-frequency repetitive transcranial magnetic stimulation of the motor cortex in writer's cramp. Neurology 52: 529–537.
45. Antal A, Lang N, Boros K, Nitsche M, Siebner HR, et al. (2008) Homeostatic metaplasticity of the motor cortex is altered during headache-free intervals in migraine with aura. Cereb Cortex 18: 2701–2705.

9

Transplantation of Induced Pluripotent Stem Cells Improves Functional Recovery in Huntington's Disease Rat Model

Shuhua Mu[1,2]☯, Jiachuan Wang[2]☯, Guangqian Zhou[2], Wenda Peng[1], Zhendan He[2], Zhenfu Zhao[2], CuiPing Mo[2], Junle Qu[1]*, Jian Zhang[1,2]*

1 College of Optoelectronics Engineering, Shenzhen University, Shenzhen, China, **2** School of Medicine, Shenzhen University, Shenzhen, China

Abstract

The purpose of this study was to determine the functional recovery of the transplanted induced pluripotent stem cells in a rat model of Huntington's disease with use of ^{18}F-FDG microPET/CT imaging.

Methods: In a quinolinic acid-induced rat model of striatal degeneration, induced pluripotent stem cells were transplanted into the ipsilateral lateral ventricle ten days after the quinolinic acid injection. The response to the treatment was evaluated by serial ^{18}F-FDG PET/CT scans and Morris water maze test. Histological analyses and Western blotting were performed six weeks after stem cell transplantation.

Results: After induced pluripotent stem cells transplantation, higher ^{18}F-FDG accumulation in the injured striatum was observed during the 4 to 6-weeks period compared with the quinolinic acid-injected group, suggesting the metabolic recovery of injured striatum. The induced pluripotent stem cells transplantation improved learning and memory function (and striatal atrophy) of the rat in six week in the comparison with the quinolinic acid-treated controls. In addition, immunohistochemical analysis demonstrated that transplanted stem cells survived and migrated into the lesioned area in striatum, and most of the stem cells expressed protein markers of neurons and glial cells.

Conclusion: Our findings show that induced pluripotent stem cells can survive, differentiate to functional neurons and improve partial striatal function and metabolism after implantation in a rat Huntington's disease model.

Editor: Dinender K. Singla, University of Central Florida, United States of America

Funding: This research was supported by the National Science Foundation of China (No. 81301063), which URL is http://www.nsfc.gov.cn/. The funders played no role in study design, data collection and analysis, decision to publish, or preparation of the manuscript.

Competing Interests: The authors have declared that no competing interests exist.

* Email: jlqu70@gmail.com (JQ); jzhanghappy@163.com (JZ)

☯ These authors contributed equally to this work.

Introduction

Huntington's disease (HD) is characterized by the expansion of CAG repeats in the huntingtin gene and the loss of medium spiny neurons in the striatum, resulting in progressive cognitive impairment, neuropsychiatric symptoms, and involuntary choreiform movements [1]. The neuropathological changes in HD are selective and progressive degeneration of striatal GABAergic medium spiny projection neurons [2]. Intrastriatal injection of an excitotoxin such as quinolinic acid (QA) mimics some of the pathology of HD, including the loss of projection GABAergic neurons with a relative preservation of interneurons, and allows for the study of therapeutics, such as transplantation [3,4]. Currently, there is no proven medical therapy to alleviate the onset or progression of Huntington's disease [5].

The clinical uses of cell replacement therapy in neurodegenerative diseases have been investigated for the last 20 years. Although the procedures are theoretically feasible, some limitations of the therapy still give cause for concern [6]. The transplantation of fetal striatal tissue to the striatum to modify HD progression in humans has been investigated, and some favorable effects have been found [7,8], but it does not alter the toxic effects of mutant huntingtin and has difficulties in tissue availability and viability, high risk of rejection, ethical arguments and concerns about contamination and heterogeneity of the tissues [9].

One solution to above problems may be to use induced pluripotent stem cells (iPSCs). The projected use of iPSC derivative cell types in cell-based therapies offers unique advantages over the use of many adult stem cell types with respect to limited proliferation capacity and donor availability, and where patient matched cells may overcome the vexing issues of immune rejection associated with human cell transplantation treatments [6,10]. iPSCs can be generated by transduction of defined transcription factors from adult somatic cells through reprogramming and have been differentiated in vitro into the early neural stem cell stage or the neural lineage, including neurons and glial cells [11]. More recently, iPSCs have been applied to a variety of nervous system disease, including stroke [11,12], spinal cord injury [13,14] and Parkinson disease [15,16]. However, to better understand the in vivo behavior and efficacy of iPSCs, a noninvasive, sensitive, and clinically applicable approach for tracking the transplanted iPSCs and monitoring the therapeutic response in living subjects needs to be developed.

PET is one of the best-suited modalities to evaluate stem cell therapy, since it can be used in patients clinically for both cell trafficking and monitoring the response to therapy [17,18]. PET studies of patients with HD demonstrate a dramatic loss of striatal glucose metabolism, even in presymptomatic stages [19,20]. PET can also be used to detect the subtle changes of glucose metabolism in vivo after stem cell therapy in various neurologic disease models, including traumatic brain injury [21], Parkinson disease [22], and Huntington disease [4]. To highly precise measurement of the FDG uptake in injured striatum, PET imaging in combination with contrast-enhanced CT was used in this study.

The aims of the present study were to investigate whether transplanted iPSC migrated and survived in QA-injured striatum of rats, improving functional and metabolic deficits of striatum, and whether ^{18}F-FDG PET imaging can monitor the improvement of cerebral energy metabolism in the striatum of rat model of HD.

Materials and Methods

1. Experimental design and animal groups

All animal procedures were performed according to the National Institutes of Health Guide for the Care and Use of Laboratory Animals and were approved by the Guangdong Medical Laboratory Animal Center Institutional Animal Care and Use Committee. Sprague-Dawley rats were housed with a 12-h light/dark cycle and *ad libitum* access to food and water. 24 adult Sprague-Dawley male rats (body weight, 250–280 g) were randomly assigned to one of the following three experimental groups (eitht per group): the iPSC transplantation group (rats received both QA injection and iPSC transplantation, QA+iPSC), the QA injection group (rats received both QA injection and PBS transplantation, QA+PBS), and the control group (rats received only saline injection). The stem cell transplantation or PBS injection was performed 10 d after QA lesions. The Morris water maze task was performed at 5 weeks after cell transplantation. ^{18}F-FDG small-animal PET/CT scans were performed before stem cell transplantation and at weeks 1, 2, 4, and 6 after cell transplantation. Animals were then sacrificed for histological, immunohistochemical (n = 4) and Western blot (n = 4) analysis.

2. Striatal quinolinic acid lesions

Unilateral lesions of the left striatum were achieved by intrastriatal injection of QA. Rats were anesthetized with a solution of ketamine (75 mg/kg) and xylazine (12.5 mg/kg). QA (Sigma) injections were made with the help of a Kopf stereotactic apparatus. Each rat was injected with 100 nmol of QA dissolved in 1 μl of saline into the left striatum at the following coordinates: 1.2 mm anterior, 2.5 mm lateral to bregma, and 5.0 mm below the dura surface. The control group received only vehicle. Injections were performed with a Hamilton syringe. The liquid was injected over a 5-min period, after which the needle was left in place for additional 15 min and then slowly removed. After surgery, rats were allowed to recover for at least 10 days before stem cell transplantation. There is no immune depressant being used during the experiment.

3. Stem Cell Preparation

Enhanced green fluorescent protein (EGFP)–labeled mouse iPSCs was bought from SiDan Sai Biotechnology Co., Ltd (China). The iPSCs was derived from the fibroblast of C57BL/6 mouse and was engineered to express green fluorescent protein (GFP) via stable transfection with a lentivirus construct containing EGFP gene under the control of the constitutive promoter from the elongation factor 1α. The iPSCs was cultured as described previously [10]. Briefly, mouse iPSCs was maintained on a mitotically inactivated mouse embryonic fibroblast feeder layer in knockout Dulbecco modified Eagle medium (Invitrogen) containing 10% fetal bovine serum (Invitrogen), 10% knockout serum replacement (Invitrogen), 2 mML-glutamine (Invitrogen), ×100 nonessential amino acids (Invitrogen), ×1000 β-2-mercaptoethanol (Invitrogen), 50 units of penicillin and a 50 mg/mL dose of streptomycin (Invitrogen), and mouse leukemia inhibitory factor (Invitrogen). Before stem cell transplantation, iPSC colonies were passaged up to 4 times without feeder cells on 60-mm culture dishes coated with 0.1% gelatin to eliminate contamination of the mouse embryonic fibroblasts.

4. Transplantation Procedure

Rats were anesthetized with a solution of ketamine (75 mg/kg) and xylazine (12.5 mg/kg) and placed in a stereotactic instrument. About 1.0×10^6 suspended iPSCs or PBS was stereotactically injected into the left lateral ventricle (0.92 mm anterior to the bregma, 1.2 mm lateral to the midline, and 3.1 mm beneath the dura) in a volume of 20 μl over 10 min with the use of a Hamilton microsyringe. The needle was left in place for an additional 10 min and then removed slowly. All surgical procedures were conducted under aseptic conditions. There is no immune depressant being used during the exprement.

5. Morris water maze task

As there is evidence that huntington's disease in rodents cause impairments when animals are tested in the Morris water maze [23], we used the Morris water maze for the current experiments. The Morris water maze task was performed according to our previous study [24] and the other [25]. Briefly, the rats were trained for 5 consecutive days, followed by the probe trial on day 6. The rats were let down in four random places (N, S, E, W) in the pool. The order of these was changed daily in a random manner. The rats were trained four times per day (120 sec/trial or until they found the platform). After the 120-sec swim, they were allowed to stay on the platform for 30 sec before the next swim trial. Single probe trials to test reference memory were conducted 1 day after the last training session. Rats were released at a random start position, and were allowed to swim during 120 sec in the absence of the platform. The tracks were recorded using video camera and Ethovision software (Noldus). Owing to different swim speeds in the different groups, the latencies of training days 1–5 were compared with the average latency for each day. For the analysis of the probe tests, the number of target annulus crossovers was compared.

6. MicroPET/CT scans and Image analysis

Lesion-induced deficits and changes after transplantation were assessed in vivo using microPET/CT scanning of [^{18}F] fluorodeoxyglucose (^{18}F-FDG) uptake to image metabolic activity, as described previously [26]. Briefly, for the first set of animals, 10 days after striatal lesion as well as 1, 2, 4 and 6 weeks after transplantation, rats were injected with 450 μCi of ^{18}F-FDG in the tail vein, in a maximum volume of 0.5 ml of sterile saline. After injection, they were returned to their cages for a 45-min uptake period in a dark and quiet environment. After the uptake period each animal was anesthetized with a solution of ketamine (75 mg/kg) and xylazine (12.5 mg/kg). The PET data were acquired at 60 min after intravenous injection in 3-dimensional mode, with emission scans of 10 min per bed position. Imaging started with a low-dose CT scan (30 mA), immediately followed by a PET scan. The CT scan was used for attenuation correction and localization of the lesion site. The coronal, transaxial, and sagittal views of PET imaging and MIP (maximum intensity projection) of the model rats were obtained after image reconstruction with a slice thickness of two-micrometer. The average radioactivity concentration within the lesion area was obtained from the mean pixel values. The lesion-to-normal homologous contralateral ratio was used for semiquantitative analysis.

7. Histology and Immunohistochemistry

Animals were anesthetized with a solution of ketamine (75 mg/kg) and xylazine (12.5 mg/kg) and perfused first with 400 ml of saline and then 400 ml of 4% paraformaldehyde (in 0.1 M phosphate buffer, pH 7.4). Brains were then removed and postfixed in the same fixative, and then coronal sections (30 μm) were cut on a vibratome (VIBRATOME, #053746). Sections were stained with Nissl according to conventional staining methods.

For immunohistochemistry, sections were pretreated with 0.3% H_2O_2 in 0.01 M PBS at 37°C for 30 min. To carry out conventional single-label immunohistochemistry, separate series of sections were incubated overnight at 4°C in mouse anti-neuronal nuclei (NeuN) (1:1000, Millipore), rabbit anti-Dopamine- and cAMP-regulated neuronal phosphoprotein (Darpp32) (1:500, Millipore), mouse anti-glial fibrillary acidic protein (GFAP) (1:1000, Santa Cruz Biotechnology), and rabbit anti- ionized calcium binding adaptor molecule 1 (Iba-1) (1:1000, Millipore). Sections were then rinsed and incubated in anti-mouse IgG or anti-rabbit IgG (1:200, Sigma), followed by incubating in the appropriate mouse or rabbit PAP complex (1:200, Sigma) at room temperature for 2 h. The DAB-peroxidase reaction (0.05% in 0.01 M PBS, pH 7.4, Sigma) was carried out for 2–8 min and mounted onto gelatin-coated slides, dried, dehydrated, cleared with xylene, and covered with neutral balsam.

To follow up on the fate of the EGFP-labeled transplanted stem cells, immunofluorescent detection was performed. NeuN was used as a mature neuronal marker, Darpp32 as the medium-sized striatal projection neurons marker, GFAP as the mature astrocyte marker, and Iba-1 as the microglia marker. Sections were blocked and incubated overnight at 4°C with primary antibodies as mentioned above. After washing in PBS, sections were incubated with fluorescence-conjugated secondary antibodies (Alexa Fluor 594, 1:500; Invitrogen) for 2 h at room temperature. Sections were washed and counterstained with the nuclear dye hoechst33258 (1:1000, Sigma) for 15 min. Fluorescence-labeled sections were viewed and images captured with a confocal microscope (Olympus).

8. Western blot

Western blotting was carried out for the marker proteins for each cell type examined. Rats were killed by decapitation after being anesthetized, and the striatum was extracted and homogenized in a lysis buffer to which protease inhibitors had been freshly added. The homogenate was centrifuged at 1500 g for 25 min, and protein concentration was determined by using a Bio-Rad DC protein assay (Bio-Rad, Hercules, CA). Samples were separated by sodium dodecyl sulfate-polyacrylamide gel electrophoresis (1% SDS-PAGE) and transferred to PVDF membranes (Millipore). Membranes were incubated in blocking buffer (5% skim milk in TBST), then with mouse anti- NeuN (1:2000, Millipore), rabbit anti- Darpp32 (1:1000, Millipore), mouse anti-GFAP (1:2000, Santa Cruz Biotechnology), and rabbit anti- Iba-1 (1:2000, Millipore), or rabbit anti -β-actin (1:2000, Millipore) in TBST overnight at 48°C. Incubated membranes were then treated with secondary antibody conjugated with horseradish peroxidase in TBST for 2 hr at 37°C. Blots were developed by enhanced chemiluminescence and digitally scanned. The optical density of each resulting labeled band was measured in an image analysis program (Image pro-Plus 6.0).

9. Data collection and statistical analysis

Histologic analysis of rat-brain volumes was performed as previously described [27]. Continuous 50 μm coronal brain sections were taken from levels corresponding approximately to the interaural plane from 10.70 to 8.74 mm [according to the atlas of [28]] and were used for volumetric analysis. The areas of the striatum as determined by Nissl staining were calculated from each continuous section and total volumes were measured by integrating each section area and depth using Image-Pro Plus 6.0 software.

For immunohistochemistry analysis, eight sections for each rat were analyzed per neuron type. Quantitative analysis of the number of positively stained cells with NeuN, Darpp32, GFAP and Iba-1 was performed on adjacent coronal sections of the striatum. For NeuN and Darpp32, the number of labeled perikarya was counted in six randomly selected areas (0.01 mm^2 for each) in striatum for each section. For GFAP and Iba-1, the integral optical density (IOD) of positive cells in six randomly selected areas (0.01 mm^2 for each) in striatum was measured with an image analysis program (Image pro-Plus 6.0).

Comparisons were performed using one-way ANOVA and unpaired t-test. Data are presented as mean±SD, and differences considered significant at $p<0.05$.

Results

1. Transplantation of iPSC improves recovery of learning and memory deficits induced by QA

In the Morris water maze task, the QA treated rats moved more along the wall of the pool and were significantly slower than controls in locating the hidden platform. However, in the iPSC-transplanted group, the animals could find the platform more quickly than the QA-treated rats (Fig. 1A). On the first day of testing, most of the animals in these three groups could not find the platform. After the initial trial, QA-treated rats showed consistently longer latencies in locating the hidden platform during the 5 days of testing, but, compared with the first day of testing, the iPSC-transplanted animals showed to find the platform sooner on Day 2 to Day 5. Analyses of the escape latency for hidden platform trials showed a significant difference among the three groups (compared between control and QA-treated groups on Day 2 to Day 5, $p<0.05$; compared between QA-treated and iPSC-transplanted groups on Day 4 to Day 5, $p<0.05$; compared between control and iPSC-transplanted groups on Day 2 to Day 5, $p<0.05$, Fig. 1B, Table S1A in File S1).

On the following probe test without the platform, the control rats spent more time in the target quadrant, and the number of the animals crossing the target annulus was nearly 8; whereas the QA treated rats swam mainly in the periphery of the pool, and the mean crossover was only 2. In the iPSC-transplanted group,

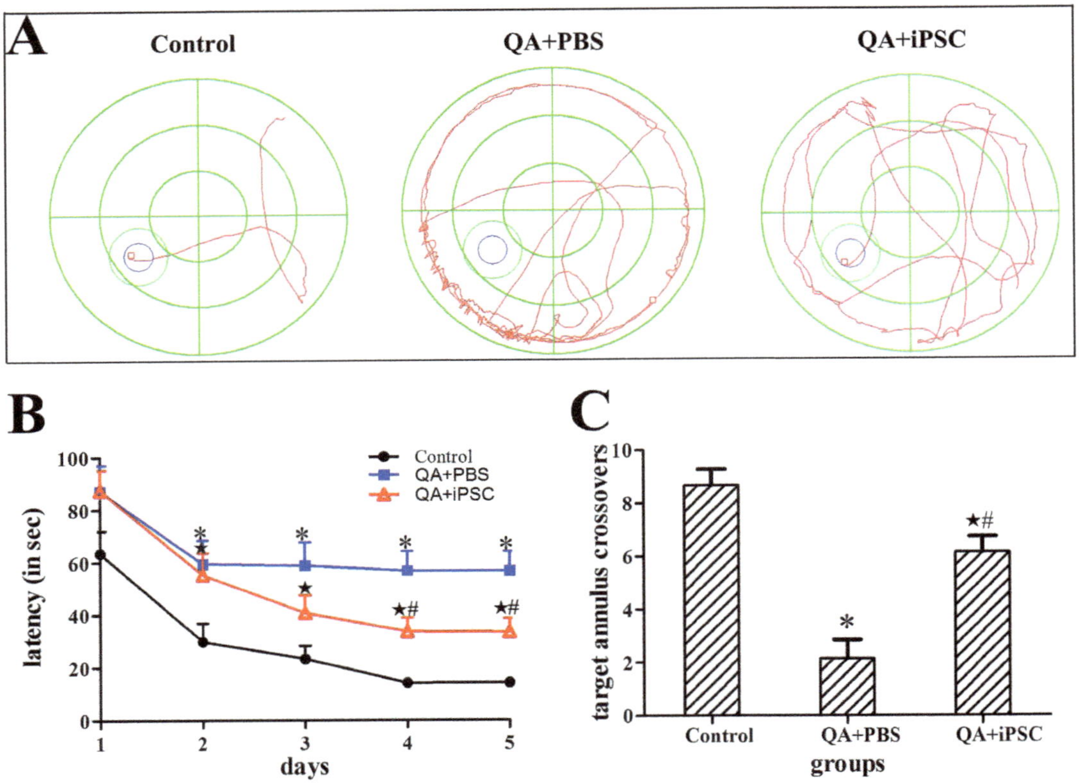

Figure 1. Transplanted iPSC improved functional recovery by Morris water maze testing. (A) The swim tracks of the rats during Morris water maze testing. The QA+iPSC rat obviously spent less time searching for the platform than the QA+PBS rat. (B) Comparison of the latency to find the platform among the three groups in Morris water maze testing. (C) Comparison of the crossovers among the three groups in probe test of Morris water maze testing. The 3 groups are presented as control (saline injection), QA+PBS (QA injection with PBS transplantation); and QA+iPSC (QA injection with iPSC transplantation) groups. Error bars represent SD, and * $P<0.05$, compared between control and QA+PBS groups; ★ $P<0.05$, compared between control and QA+iPSC groups; # $P<0.05$, compared between QA+PBS and QA+iPSC groups.

the mean crossovers could be up to 6 times. Statistical analysis showed a significant difference of the crossovers among the three groups (compared between the control and QA-treated groups, $p<0.001$; compared between QA-treated and iPSC-transplanted groups, $p<0.001$; compared between the control and iPSC-transplanted groups, $p<0.05$, Fig. 1C, Table S1B in File S1).

2. iPSC transplantation results in enhanced glucose metabolism of the lesioned striatum

To document that the iPSC implant corresponds to enhanced glucose metabolic activity, ^{18}F-FDG small-animal PET/CT scans were performed sequentially at 0, 1, 2, 4 and 6 weeks after iPSC transplantation. The ^{18}F-FDG PET/CT scans allowed the visualization and quantification of glucose metabolism throughout the brain at each time point (Fig. 2). For the animals included in this study, the lesion-to-normal homologous contralateral radioactivity ratio was used for semiquantitative analysis. In rats that were injected with QA into the left striatum and imaged 10 days later, there was a marked asymmetry of FDG uptake in the striatum, compared to the non-lesioned right hemisphere (Fig. 2A). From 1 week to 6 weeks after transplantation, glucose metabolism in the striatum of QA-treated animals remained unchanged. In contrast, the glucose metabolism in iPSC-transplanted rats showed a slight increase, resulting in a growth of the radioactivity ratio (Figs. 2A, 2B). This growth persisted through the four-week scan, suggesting that the transplant protected the ipsilateral striatum from metabolic decline. Analysis of the radioactivity ratios demonstrated no significant differences between the QA-treated and iPSC-transplanted groups at either 1 or 2 weeks after transplantation ($p>0.05$, Fig. 2B). However, the radioactivity ratios were significantly increased in the iPSC-transplanted group at both 4 and 6 weeks after stem cell transplantation ($p<0.001$, Fig. 2B, Table S2 in File S1), indicating that transplantation of iPSC increased glucose metabolism in the lesioned area.

In addition, there was no focal abnormal increase in glucose metabolism in the cerebral lesioned area, thus indicating no tumor or teratoma formation at 6 weeks after stem cell transplantation.

3. iPSC transplantation improves striatum volume after QA-induced excitotoxicity

At 10th day after injection of QA, the striatal atrophy and lateral veniricle dilation were severe in the QA-injection side compared with the contra-lateral side. Nissl staining showed that a clear lesion was located in the striatum and neuronal loss was observed in the lesion area. Striatum volumes were calculated by Nissl staining to evaluate the effects of iPSC transplantation. Six weeks after surgery, striatum volumes were not changed in the control group, but were obviously decreased in the QA-lesioned and iPSC-transplanted groups (Fig. 2C). However, striatum volumes in iPSC-transplanted group were partially

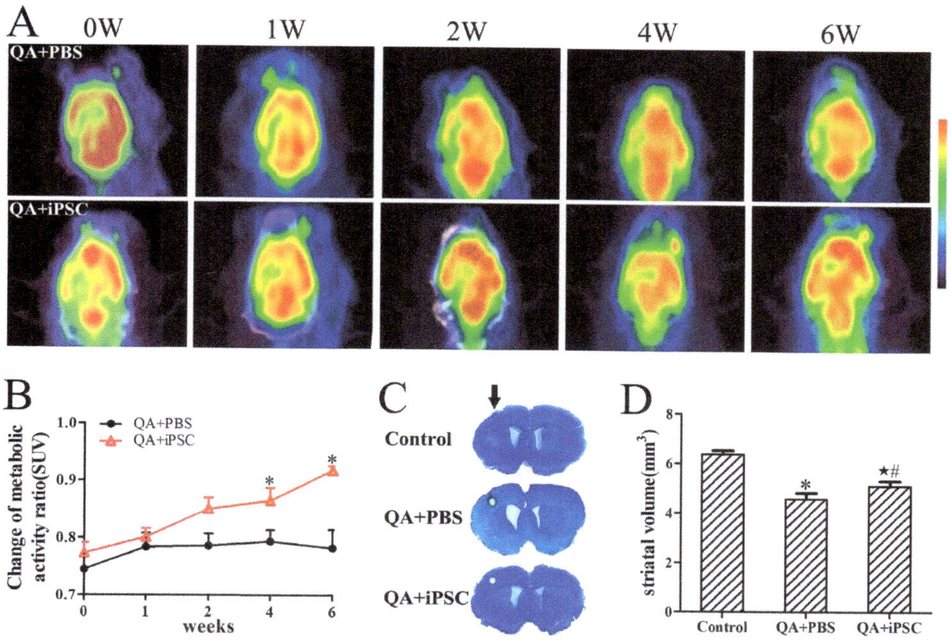

Figure 2. Enhanced glucose metabolism and decreased striatal atrophy following iPSC transplantation. (A) Serial PET images demonstrating metabolism recovery after stem cell treatment for QA-treated rats. Images are shown in axial view. Scale was set according to signal intensity. (B) Semiquantitative analysis of variance of glucose metabolism after stem cell transplantation in each group. (C) Photomicrographs show the difference in striatal volumes in unilateral lesion rat. There was no striatal atrophy in the control group, but the striatal volumes in the lesion side of QA+PBS and QA+iPSC groups were significantly decreased compared with the contralateral side. Arrow indicates surgery sites in each group. (D) Quantification of striatal volumes show increased volumes in the QA+iPSC group. The 3 groups are presented as control (saline injection), QA+PBS (QA injection with PBS transplantation); and QA+iPSC (QA injection with iPSC transplantation) groups. Error bars represent SD, and * $P<0.05$, compared between control and QA+PBS groups; ★ $P<0.05$, compared between control and QA+iPSC groups; # $P<0.05$, compared between QA+PBS and QA+iPSC groups.

recovered in comparison with QA-lesioned group (Fig. 2D). The striatum volume of the control group was approximately 6.37 ± 0.15 mm^3, while in the QA-lesioned and iPSC - transplanted groups striatum volume was 4.57 ± 0.25 mm^3 and 5.10 ± 0.20 mm^3, respectively. The statistical analysis showed a significant difference among these three groups ($P<0.001$ for control and QA groups, $P<0.05$ for QA and iPSC-transplanted groups, $P<0.05$ for control and iPSC-transplanted groups, Fig. 2D, Table S3 in File S1).

4. Histological confirmation of neural protection after iPSC transplantation

4.1 Neural loss and gliosis induced by QA injection. To evaluate QA-induced striatal lesion, immunohistochemical (NeuN, Darpp32, GFAP and Iba-1) methods were used. NeuN was used as a mature neuronal marker, and Darpp32 as the medium-sized striatal projection neurons marker. In QA-treated rats, a clear lesion area was obviously located in the striatum. NeuN and Darpp32 immunolabeling confirmed a serious loss of neurons in the lesion core (Fig. 3B, 3D). Quantitative data showed that the number of striatal neurons in the QA group was $93.5\pm10.4/0.01$ mm^2 (NeuN) and $74.9\pm8.6/0.01$ mm^2 (Darpp32), respectively, corresponding to $170.2\pm3.9/0.01$ mm^2 (NeuN) and $149.5\pm7.8/0.01$ mm^2 (Darpp32) in the control. The statistical analysis showed a significant difference between the two groups ($P<0.001$ for NeuN, $P<0.001$ for Darpp32, Fig. 3I, Table S4 in File S1). Furthermore, histological detection in astrocyte and microglia were carried out using GFAP and Iba-1 immunohistochemistry. In the control group, astrocyte and microglia were scattered in striatum uniformly. After QA treatment, there were numerous glial cell proliferations in the lesion core (Fig. 3F, 3H). Statistical analysis showed that in the QA group, the optical density of GFAP and Iba-1 in striatum was $27045\pm1093/0.01$ mm^2 and $25137\pm1359/0.01$ mm^2, respectively, which showed a significant difference compared with the controls for Iba-1 ($19456\pm1453/0.01$ mm^2, $P<0.05$) but not for GFAP ($24560\pm1203/0.01$ mm^2, $P>0.05$, Fig. 3J, Table S5 in File S1).

4.2 Transplanted cells survive and differentiate into neurons and astrocytes in lesioned striatum. We next investigated the distribution and differentiation of the transplanted iPSC in QA-lesioned striatum. As labeled by EGFP, transplanted iPSC could be identified under fluorescence microscope. A number of transplanted iPSC appeared to have migrated from lateral ventricle to the lesioned striatum, and the cells spread out into the lesioned area (Fig. 4). While, there is no EGFP-marked cell can be detected in contra-lateral side.

Furthermore, we determined the cell types of differentiated iPSC surviving in the QA impaired striatum. Confocal microscope images showed a larger number of GFP-labeled cells in the QA-lesioned striatum co-expressing NeuN (Fig. 5A), Darpp32 (Fig. 5B), GFAP (Fig. 5C) and Iba-1 (Fig. 5D). Then, we counted the number of NeuN- and Darpp32-expressing cell in striatum. In the iPSC-transplanted animals, the number of NeuN-positive cells was significantly higher than that in the QA-injected group ($119.8\pm9.3/0.01$ mm^2 vs $93.5\pm10.4/0.01$ mm^2; $P<0.05$, Fig. 3I). The number of Darpp32-expressing cells in the iPSC-transplanted group was more than that in

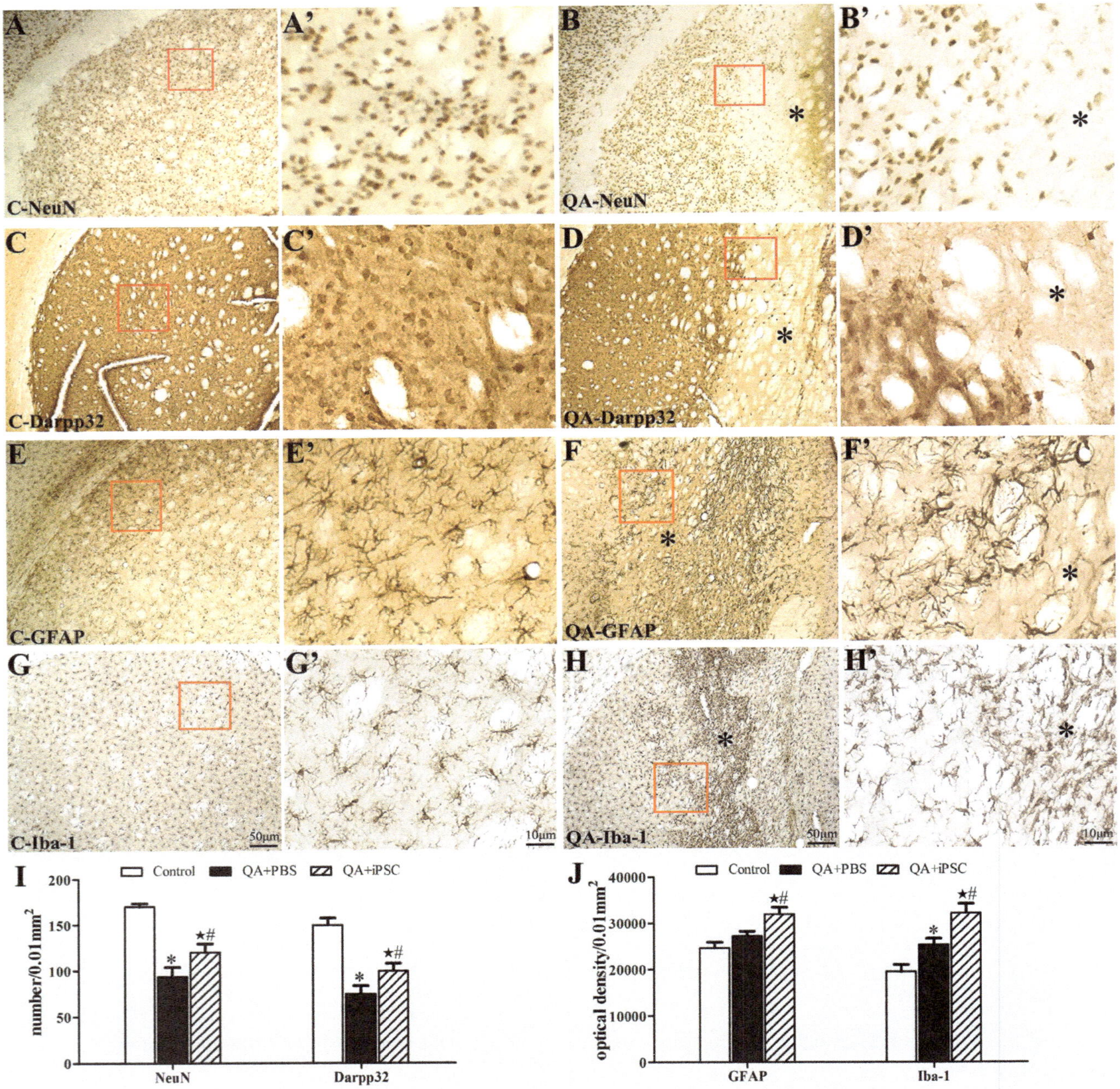

Figure 3. Neuronal loss and gliosis in striatum induced by QA injection. (A, C, E, G and A′, C′, E′, G′) Immunohistochemical staining for NeuN (A–A′), Darpp32 (B–B′), GFAP (C–C′), Iba-1 (D–D′) in striatum in the control rats. (B, D, F, H and B′, D′, F′, H′) Immunohistochemical staining for NeuN (B–B′), Darpp32 (D–D′), GFAP (F–F′), Iba-1 (H–H′) in striatum in the QA-treated rats, which showed the loss of NeuN- and Darpp32-positive neurons and proliferations of astrocyte and microglia in the lesion area. A–H were the same magnification; A′–H′ were the same magnification; A′–H′ were the higher magnification views of the red box in A–H. (I) Comparison of the number of NeuN- and Darpp32-positive neurons in striatum among the three groups. (J) Comparison of the optical density of GFAP- and Iba-1-positive glial cells in striatum among the three groups. The 3 groups are presented as control (saline injection), QA+PBS (QA injection with PBS transplantation); and QA+iPSC (QA injection with iPSC transplantation) groups. Error bars represent SD, and * $P<0.05$, compared between control and QA+PBS groups; ★ $P<0.05$, compared between control and QA+iPSC groups; # $P<0.05$, compared between QA+PBS and QA+iPSC groups.

the QA-treated group ($99.4\pm8.3/0.01\ mm^2$ vs $74.9\pm8.6/0.01\ mm^2$) and there was statistically significant difference between the two groups ($P<0.05$, Fig. 3I, Fig. 3J). The IOD of GFAP and Iba-1 in striatum was also quantified. Expression of GFAP in the iPSC-transplanted striatum was significantly higher than that in the QA-treated group ($31934\pm1493/0.01\ mm^2$ vs $27045\pm1093/0.01\ mm^2$; $P<0.05$). Meanwhile, the IOD of Iba-1 in the iPSC-transplanted group was significantly higher than that of the QA-injected group ($332143\pm2019/0.01\ mm^2$ vs $25137\pm1359/0.01\ mm^2$; $P<0.001$, Fig. 3J). Analyses of the four cell types between the control and iPSC-transplanted groups also showed a significant

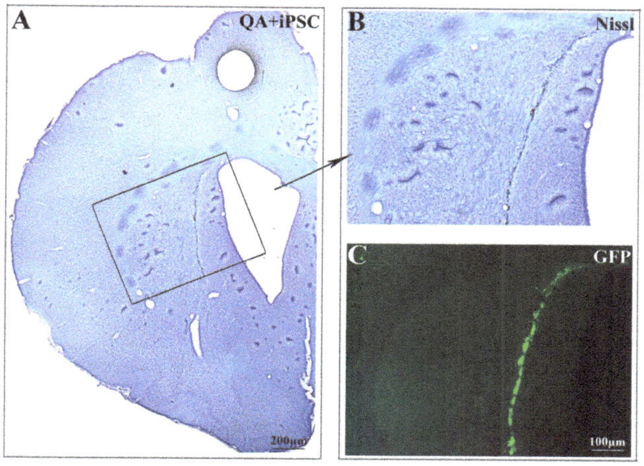

Figure 4. Transplanted iPSC migrated into the lesioned striatum after QA injection. (A, B) Nissl staining of striatum after iPSC transplantation. B was the higher magnification views of the black box in A. (C) Migration and distribution of the transplanted iPSC in QA-lesioned striatum were observed under fluorescence microscope. B and C were the same magnification.

difference ($P<0.05$ for NeuN and Darpp32, $P<0.001$ for GFAP and Iba-1, Fig. 3I, Fig. 3J, Table S4 and S5 in File S1).

5. Changes of protein marker in striatal neuron and gliocyte after iPSC transplantation

We then examined the protein expression of NeuN, Darpp32, GFAP and Iba-1 in striatum after iPSC transplanted for six weeks. Western blotting revealed that treated with QA significantly decreased NeuN and Darpp32 protein in rat striatum, but iPSC-transplanted rat had higher levels of these molecules than the QA-treated rat ($p<0.05$; Fig. 6). QA-treated rat expressed increased levels of both GFAP and Iba-1 in striatum compared with the control animals, and iPSC transplantation could enhance their expression more significantly than the QA-treated rats ($p<0.05$; Fig. 6), indicating that iPSC activated the proliferation of gliocyte. Statistical analysis also showed a significant difference between the control and iPSC-transplanted groups for NeuN, GFAP and Iba-1, but not Darpp32 ($p<0.05$ for NeuN; $p<0.001$ for GFAP and Iba-1; $p>0.05$ for Darpp32, Fig. 6, Table S6 in File S1).

Discussion

In the present study, we found that transplantation of iPSCs reduced learning and memory dysfunction in QA-lesioned rat, as determined by Morris water maze. Within the damaged striatum, a large number of iPSCs could migrate into the damaged striatal region and underwent differentiation, as shown by the expression

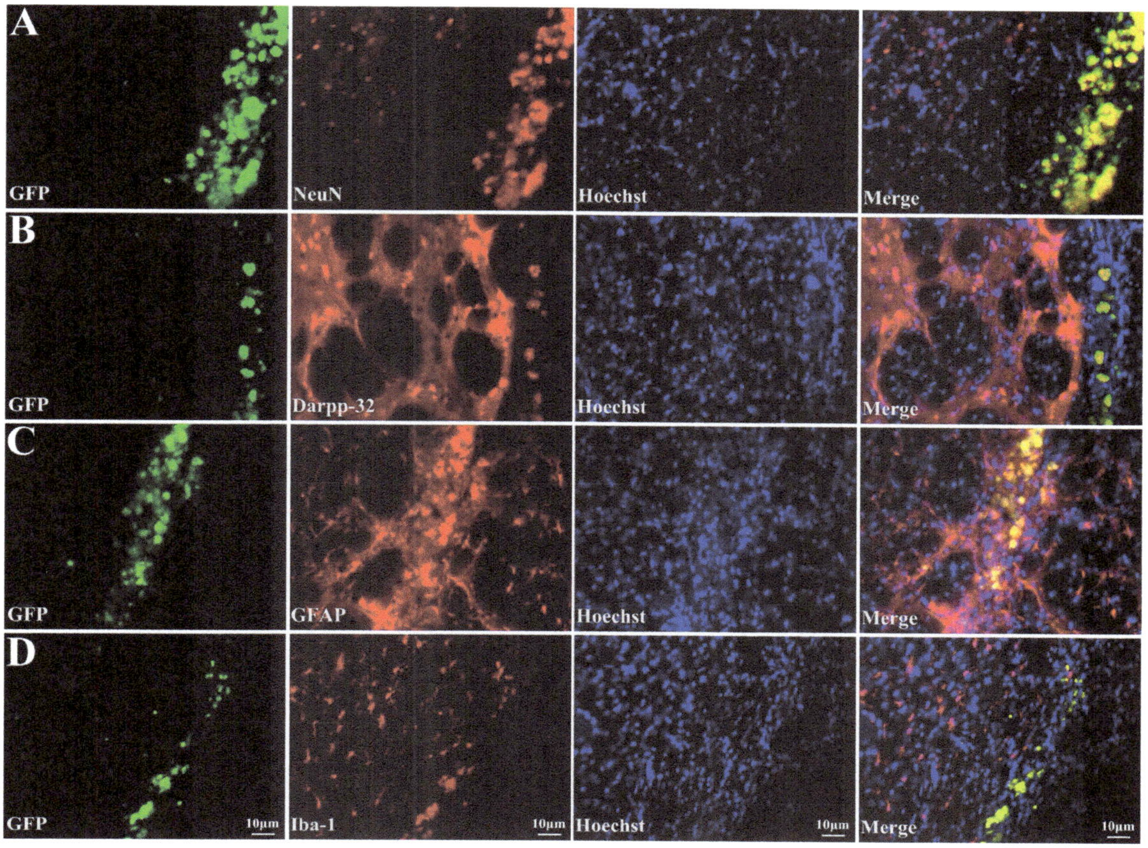

Figure 5. Transplanted cells differentiate into neurons and astrocytes in lesioned striatum. Transplanted iPSCs show green fluorescence; immunostaining with antibodies against NeuN (A), Darpp32 (B), GFAP (C) and Iba-1 (D) show red fluorescence; nuclei stained with Hoechst 33258 show blue fluorescence; and merged images show that engrafted iPSC express neuron, projection neuron, astrocyte, or microglia features.

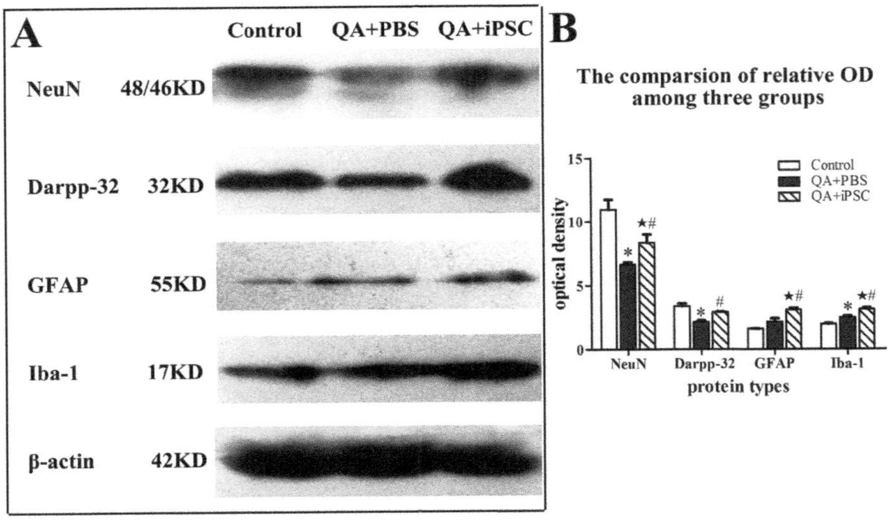

Figure 6. Increased protein expression of neurons and glia cell in striatum after iPSC transplantation. (B) was the semiquantitative analysis of (A) expressed as relative optical density, which showed that the levels of NeuN, Darpp32, GFAP and Iba-1 proteins increased after iPSC transplantation. The 3 groups are presented as control (saline injection), QA+PBS (QA injection with PBS transplantation); and QA+iPSC (QA injection with iPSC transplantation) groups. Error bars represent SD, and *$P<0.05$, compared between control and QA+PBS groups; ★ $P<0.05$, compared between control and QA+iPSC groups; # $P<0.05$, compared between QA+PBS and QA+iPSC groups.

markers for mature neurons, striatal medium spiny projection neurons, astrocytes and microglia. Moreover, the potential therapeutic effect of iPSCs was evaluated by serial ^{18}F-FDG PET/CT scans.

Elevated cerebral glucose uptake reflects a higher synaptic activity in the brain if no inflammatory or malignant process is present [29]. Reduction of the cerebral glucose metabolism, observed by PET imaging, is confirmed a well-known feature in symptomatic HD and the preclinical gene carrier state [30]. Therefore, monitoring glucose utilization in animal models of HD, and also in patients, can provide useful information about neuronal functional deficit before and after therapeutic interventions. It has reported that cystamine-induced neuroprotection in R6/2 transgenic mice can be monitored by micro PET-[^{18}F] FDG in the striatum, cortex and cerebellum [31]. Here, we used micro ^{18}F-FDG PET imaging to investigate whether iPSC transplantation can ameliorate the cerebral energy metabolism in the striatum of rat model of HD. The similar study has been verified in the cerebral ischemia. Wang et al reported that serial ^{18}F-FDG small-animal PET demonstrated metabolic recovery after iPSC and ESC transplantation in a rat model of cerebral ischemia [12]. Clinically, a previous study demonstrated enhanced glucose metabolism in some patients that had undergone transplantation of fetal striatum. Although the sample size was small, the metabolic rates, observed by PET appeared to correlate with improved clinical status [7]. In the present study, by using a rat model of Huntington's disease, we were able to find increased glucose metabolic activity in the striatum-lesioned area during the 6-wk period after iPSC transplantation under serial ^{18}F-FDG PET scans. Thus, PET seems likely to be one of the best-suited modalities to evaluate stem cell therapy, and it can be used in patients clinically for both cells trafficking and monitoring the response to therapy.

In the injured brain, some upregulated environmental elements may account for the migration of endogenous neural stem cells or transplanted immortalized, neonate-derived neural precursor cells to the lesioned region and their differentiation into neurons [32]. In previous studies, brain injury induced neurogenesis and enhanced neuronal migration to the lesioned region to enhance proliferation of correct cell types, such as Dcx-expressing neuroblasts, to reconstruct the damaged cell architecture, as seen after stroke [33] and HD [34]. In the present study, immunohistochemical analyses indicated that many transplanted cells survived and integrated close to the injured striatum and that most of the cells expressed protein markers for parenchymal cells such as neurons and astrocytes. What are the mechanisms or factors that promote reduced deficits with iPSC transplantation after HD? One possibility is that the transplanted stem cells integrate into the tissue, replace damaged cells, and reconstruct the neural circuitry. Previous reports demonstrated that human induced PSC-derived dopaminergic neurons have been shown to survive and improve behavioural impairments after intrastriatal transplantation in an animal model of Parkinson's disease [16]. Another reasonable explanation is that changes in the microenvironment may contribute to tissue protection and repair [35] or that the interaction of grafted stem cells with the host brain may lead to production of trophic factors [36]. For example, increased neurogenesis and neuroprotection by neurotrophic or growth factors, and new synapse formation with reorganization, have been suggested by stroke models [37]. The decreased striatal atrophy, the increased glucose metabolic activity and the improved functional recovery of the HD model in our study also suggest that iPSC transplantation protects the host brain from further destruction.

Recently, the role of glial cells in integrity of the central nervous system had been well elucidated, and accumulating evidence suggested that glial cells were critical to neuronal survival [38,39]. Gliocyte populations in different brain regions have been shown to have important roles in neurogenic support [40]. A recent report revealed a surprising outcome where SVZ-mediated astrogenesis may be beneficial over neurogenesis in a period after cortical injury, in agreement with potentially protective roles for astrocytes during recovery process in the spinal cord [41]. In both cultured astrocytes and HD mouse brains, mutant huntingtin reduces glial glutamate uptake and glial cells protected neurons against mutant htt-mediated neurotoxicity [42], suggesting that dysfunction of glial cell may critically contribute to neuronal excitotoxicity in HD. In addition, in injured striatum, mutant huntingtin may affect the production of chemokines and neurotrophic factors such as tumor necrosis factor alpha (TNF-a) [43], glial-derived neurotrophic factor (GDNF) [44] and nerve growth factor (NGF) [45] from glial cells. In our present study, a large number of iPSCs that differentiated into astrocyte and microglia may contribute to chemokine secretion and iPSCs transplantation may provide a beneficial environment that attracts glial cell activation and proliferation. Once the numbers of activated glial cells are boosted, their trophic support will slow the excitotoxic damage to GABAergic neurons in the striatum.

Conclusion

In summary, we have demonstrated that iPSCs survive, migrate into injured striatum and differentiate into neurons and glial cells after transplantation in the QA-induced HD model, accompany with the decreased striatal atrophy, the increased glucose metabolic activity and the improved functional recovery. Furthermore, we have demonstrated that ^{18}F-FDG PET scan seems likely to be a feasible modality to evaluate stem cell therapy in HD. Collectively, this study demonstrates the therapeutic potential of iPSCs for cell replacement therapy and indicates that iPSCs may provide an alternative cell source for transplantation therapy in the treatment of HD and other neurodegenerative diseases.

Supporting Information

File S1 This file contains Tables S1–S6. Table S1–S6 showed the raw data of this study. Table S1 showed the raw data of Morris water maze testing, A is the latency and B is the target annulus crossovers. Table S2 showed the raw data of SUV of PET/CT. Table S3 showed the raw data of the striatal volume (mm^3). Table S4 showed the raw data of the number of NeuN and Darpp32/0.01 mm^2 in striatum. Table S5 showed the raw data of the optical density of GFAP and Iba-1/0.01 mm^2 in striatum. Table S6 showed the raw data of the optical density of Western blot.

Author Contributions

Conceived and designed the experiments: SHM GQZ JLQ JZ. Performed the experiments: SHM JCW CPM. Analyzed the data: SHM WDP. Contributed reagents/materials/analysis tools: SHM ZDH ZFZ. Contributed to the writing of the manuscript: SHM JZ.

References

1. Landles C, Bates GP (2004) Huntingtin and the molecular pathogenesis of Huntington's disease. Fourth in molecular medicine review series. EMBO Rep, 5(10): p. 958–63.
2. Vonsattel JP, Myers RH, Stevens TJ, Ferrante RJ, Bird ED, et al. (1985) Neuropathological classification of Huntington's disease. J Neuropathol Exp Neurol, 44(6): p. 559–77.
3. Freeman TB, Hauser RA, Sanberg PR, Saporta S (2000) Neural transplantation for the treatment of Huntington's disease. Prog Brain Res, 127: p. 405–11.
4. Visnyei K, Tatsukawa KJ, Erickson RI, Simonian S, Oknaian N, et al. (2006) Neural progenitor implantation restores metabolic deficits in the brain following striatal quinolinic acid lesion. Exp Neurol, 197(2): p. 465–74.
5. Ramaswamy S, Shannon KM, Kordower JH (2007) Huntington's disease: pathological mechanisms and therapeutic strategies. Cell Transplant, 16(3): p. 301–12.
6. Payne NL, Sylvain A, O'Brien C, Herszfeld D, Sun G, et al. (2014) Application of human induced pluripotent stem cells for modeling and treating neurodegenerative diseases. N Biotechnol.
7. Bachoud-Levi AC, Remy P, Nguyen JP, Brugieres P, Lefaucheur JP, et al. (2000) Motor and cognitive improvements in patients with Huntington's disease after neural transplantation. Lancet, 356(9246): p. 1975–9.
8. Keene CD, Sonnen JA, Swanson PD, Kopyov O, Leverenz JB, et al. (2007) Neural transplantation in Huntington disease: long-term grafts in two patients. Neurology, 68(24): p. 2093–8.
9. Bjorklund A (1993) Neurobiology. Better cells for brain repair. Nature, 362(6419): p. 414–5.
10. Takahashi K, Yamanaka S (2006) Induction of pluripotent stem cells from mouse embryonic and adult fibroblast cultures by defined factors. Cell, 126(4): p. 663–76.
11. Tornero D, Wattananit S, Gronning Madsen M, Koch P, Wood J, et al. (2013) Human induced pluripotent stem cell-derived cortical neurons integrate in stroke-injured cortex and improve functional recovery. Brain.
12. Wang J, Chao F, Han F, Zhang G, Xi Q, et al. (2013) PET demonstrates functional recovery after transplantation of induced pluripotent stem cells in a rat model of cerebral ischemic injury. J Nucl Med, 54(5): p. 785–92.
13. Tsuji O, Miura K, Okada Y, Fujiyoshi K, Mukaino M, et al. (2010) Therapeutic potential of appropriately evaluated safe-induced pluripotent stem cells for spinal cord injury. Proc Natl Acad Sci U S A, 107(28): p. 12704–9.
14. Nori S, Okada Y, Yasuda A, Tsuji O, Takahashi Y, et al. (2011) Grafted human-induced pluripotent stem-cell-derived neurospheres promote motor functional recovery after spinal cord injury in mice. Proc Natl Acad Sci U S A, 108(40): p. 16825–30.
15. Sundberg M, Bogetofte H, Lawson T, Jansson J, Smith G, et al. (2013) Improved cell therapy protocols for Parkinson's disease based on differentiation efficiency and safety of hESC-, hiPSC-, and non-human primate iPSC-derived dopaminergic neurons. Stem Cells, 31(8): p. 1548–62.
16. Hargus G, Cooper O, Deleidi M, Levy A, Lee K, et al. (2010) Differentiated Parkinson patient-derived induced pluripotent stem cells grow in the adult rodent brain and reduce motor asymmetry in Parkinsonian rats. Proc Natl Acad Sci U S A, 107(36): p. 15921–6.
17. Zhang Y, Ruel M, Beanlands RS, deKemp RA, Suuronen EJ, et al. (2008) Tracking stem cell therapy in the myocardium: applications of positron emission tomography. Curr Pharm Des, 14(36): p. 3835–53.
18. Jiang H, Cheng Z, Tian M, Zhang H (2011) In vivo imaging of embryonic stem cell therapy. Eur J Nucl Med Mol Imaging, 38(4): p. 774–84.
19. Kuwert T, Lange HW, Langen KJ, Herzog H, Aulich A, et al. (1990) Cortical and subcortical glucose consumption measured by PET in patients with Huntington's disease. Brain, 113 (Pt 5): p. 1405–23.
20. Antonini A, Leenders KL, Spiegel R, Meier D, Vontobel P, et al. (1996) Striatal glucose metabolism and dopamine D2 receptor binding in asymptomatic gene carriers and patients with Huntington's disease. Brain, 119 (Pt 6): p. 2085–95.
21. Zhang H, Zheng X, Yang X, Fang S, Shen G, et al. (2008) 11C-NMSP/18F-FDG microPET to monitor neural stem cell transplantation in a rat model of traumatic brain injury. Eur J Nucl Med Mol Imaging, 35(9): p. 1699–708.
22. Shyu WC, Li KW, Peng HF, Lin SZ, Liu RS, et al. (2009) Induction of GAP-43 modulates neuroplasticity in PBSC (CD34+) implanted-Parkinson's model. J Neurosci Res, 87(9): p. 2020–33.
23. Lione LA, Carter RJ, Hunt MJ, Bates GP, Morton AJ, et al. (1999) Selective discrimination learning impairments in mice expressing the human Huntington's disease mutation. J Neurosci, 19(23): p. 10428–37.
24. Mu S, OuYang L, Liu B, Zhu Y, Li K, et al. (2011) Preferential interneuron survival in the transition zone of 3-NP-induced striatal injury in rats. J Neurosci Res, 89(5): p. 744–54.
25. Vorhees CV, Williams MT (2006) Morris water maze: procedures for assessing spatial and related forms of learning and memory. Nat Protoc, 1(2): p. 848–58.
26. Araujo DM, Cherry SR, Tatsukawa KJ, Toyokuni T, Kornblum HI (2000) Deficits in striatal dopamine D(2) receptors and energy metabolism detected by in vivo microPET imaging in a rat model of Huntington's disease. Exp Neurol, 166(2): p. 287–97.
27. Lee ST, Chu K, Jung KH, Im WS, Park JE, et al. (2009) Slowed progression in models of Huntington disease by adipose stem cell transplantation. Ann Neurol, 66(5): p. 671–81.
28. Paxinos G, Watson (1986) The Rat Brain in Stereotaxic Coordinates.
29. Jueptner M, Weiller C (1995) Review: does measurement of regional cerebral blood flow reflect synaptic activity? Implications for PET and fMRI. Neuroimage, 2(2): p. 148–56.
30. Feigin A, Leenders KL, Moeller JR, Missimer J, Kuenig G, et al. (2001) Metabolic network abnormalities in early Huntington's disease: an [(18)F]FDG PET study. J Nucl Med, 42(11): p. 1591–5.
31. Wang X, Sarkar A, Cicchetti F, Yu M, Zhu A, et al. (2005) Cerebral PET imaging and histological evidence of transglutaminase inhibitor cystamine induced neuroprotection in transgenic R6/2 mouse model of Huntington's disease. J Neurol Sci, 231(1–2): p. 57–66.
32. Gaura V, Bachoud-Levi AC, Ribeiro MJ, Nguyen JP, Frouin V, et al. (2004) Striatal neural grafting improves cortical metabolism in Huntington's disease patients. Brain, 127(Pt 1): p. 65–72.

33. Arvidsson A, Collin T, Kirik D, Kokaia Z, Lindvall O (2002) Neuronal replacement from endogenous precursors in the adult brain after stroke. Nat Med, 8(9): p. 963–70.
34. Lin YT, Chern Y, Shen CK, Wen HL, Chang YC, et al. (2011) Human mesenchymal stem cells prolong survival and ameliorate motor deficit through trophic support in Huntington's disease mouse models. PLoS One, 6(8): p. e22924.
35. Feng M, Zhu H, Zhu Z, Wei J, Lu S, et al. (2011) Serial 18F-FDG PET demonstrates benefit of human mesenchymal stem cells in treatment of intracerebral hematoma: a translational study in a primate model. J Nucl Med, 52(1): p. 90–7.
36. Sadan O, Shemesh N, Barzilay R, Dadon-Nahum M, Blumenfeld-Katzir T, et al. (2012) Mesenchymal stem cells induced to secrete neurotrophic factors attenuate quinolinic acid toxicity: a potential therapy for Huntington's disease. Exp Neurol, 234(2): p. 417–27.
37. Emerich DF, Thanos CG, Goddard M, Skinner SJ, Geany MS, et al. (2006) Extensive neuroprotection by choroid plexus transplants in excitotoxin lesioned monkeys. Neurobiol Dis, 23(2): p. 471–80.
38. Chung WS, Clarke LE, Wang GX, Stafford BK, Sher A, et al. (2013) Astrocytes mediate synapse elimination through MEGF10 and MERTK pathways. Nature, 504(7480): p. 394–400.
39. Borlongan CV, Yamamoto M, Takei N, Kumazaki M, Ungsuparkorn C, et al. (2000) Glial cell survival is enhanced during melatonin-induced neuroprotection against cerebral ischemia. Faseb J, 14(10): p. 1307–17.
40. Dusart I, Marty S, Peschanski M (1991) Glial changes following an excitotoxic lesion in the CNS – II. Astrocytes. Neuroscience, 45(3): p. 541–9.
41. Benner EJ, Luciano D, Jo R, Abdi K, Paez-Gonzalez P, et al. (2013) Protective astrogenesis from the SVZ niche after injury is controlled by Notch modulator Thbs4. Nature, 497(7449): p. 369–73.
42. Shin JY, Fang ZH, Yu ZX, Wang CE, Li SH, et al. (2005) Expression of mutant huntingtin in glial cells contributes to neuronal excitotoxicity. J Cell Biol, 171(6): p. 1001–12.
43. Acarin L, Gonzalez B, Castellano B (2000) Neuronal, astroglial and microglial cytokine expression after an excitotoxic lesion in the immature rat brain. Eur J Neurosci, 12(10): p. 3505–20.
44. Marco S, Canudas AM, Canals JM, Gavalda N, Perez-Navarro E, et al. (2002) Excitatory amino acids differentially regulate the expression of GDNF, neurturin, and their receptors in the adult rat striatum. Exp Neurol, 174(2): p. 243–52.
45. Strauss S, Otten U, Joggerst B, Pluss KVolk B (1994) Increased levels of nerve growth factor (NGF) protein and mRNA and reactive gliosis following kainic acid injection into the rat striatum. Neurosci Lett, 168(1–2): p. 193–6.

10

Suppression of Motor Cortical Excitability in Anesthetized Rats by Low Frequency Repetitive Transcranial Magnetic Stimulation

Paul A. Muller[1], Sameer C. Dhamne[1], Andrew M. Vahabzadeh-Hagh[1,2], Alvaro Pascual-Leone[2,3], Frances E. Jensen[4], Alexander Rotenberg[1,2]*

1 Department of Neurology, Boston Children's Hospital, Harvard Medical School, Boston, Massachusetts, United States of America, **2** Berenson-Allen Center for Noninvasive Brain Stimulation, Beth Israel Deaconess Medical Center, Harvard Medical School, Boston, Massachusetts, United States of America, **3** Institut Universitari de Neurorehabilitació Guttmann, Universidad Autónoma de Barcelona, Badalona, Spain, **4** Department of Neurology, Perelman School of Medicine, University of Pennsylvania Health System, Philadelphia, Pennsylvania, United States of America

Abstract

Repetitive transcranial magnetic stimulation (rTMS) is a widely-used method for modulating cortical excitability in humans, by mechanisms thought to involve use-dependent synaptic plasticity. For example, when low frequency rTMS (LF rTMS) is applied over the motor cortex, in humans, it predictably leads to a suppression of the motor evoked potential (MEP), presumably reflecting long-term depression (LTD) – like mechanisms. Yet how closely such rTMS effects actually match LTD is unknown. We therefore sought to (1) reproduce cortico-spinal depression by LF rTMS in rats, (2) establish a reliable animal model for rTMS effects that may enable mechanistic studies, and (3) test whether LTD-like properties are evident in the rat LF rTMS setup. Lateralized MEPs were obtained from anesthetized Long-Evans rats. To test frequency-dependence of LF rTMS, rats underwent rTMS at one of three frequencies, 0.25, 0.5, or 1 Hz. We next tested the dependence of rTMS effects on N-methyl-D-aspartate glutamate receptor (NMDAR), by application of two NMDAR antagonists. We find that 1 Hz rTMS preferentially depresses unilateral MEP in rats, and that this LTD-like effect is blocked by NMDAR antagonists. These are the first electrophysiological data showing depression of cortical excitability following LF rTMS in rats, and the first to demonstrate dependence of this form of cortical plasticity on the NMDAR. We also note that our report is the first to show that the capacity for LTD-type cortical suppression by rTMS is present under barbiturate anesthesia, suggesting that future neuromodulatory rTMS applications under anesthesia may be considered.

Editor: Guglielmo Foffani, Hospital Nacional de Parapléjicos, Spain

Funding: This work was supported by the Boston Children's Hospital Translational Research Program (AR), NIH K08 NS055895 (AR), NIH 5R01NS031718 (FEJ), IDDRC P30-HD18655 (AR, FEJ). The funders had no role in study design, data collection and analysis, decision to publish, or preparation of the manuscript.

Competing Interests: Paul A. Muller, Sameer C. Dhamne, Andrew M. Vahabzadeh-Hagh, report no financial interest or potential conflicts of interest. Alvaro Pascual-Leone serves on the scientific advisory board for Codman-Johnson & Johnson, Nexstim, Neuronix, Starlab, and Neosync. Alvaro Pascual-Leone, Frances E. Jensen and Alexander Rotenberg are listed as inventors on issued and pending patents integrating TMS with brain imaging and neurophysiology. The authors confirm that the patent does not pose any conflict of interest. The patent focuses on EEG-coupled methods of use in epilepsy, and on particular coil configurations relevant only to humans. The present translational experiments do not directly relate to the patent. The details of the patent are as follows: Transcranial magnetic stimulation (TMS) methods and apparatus; US20100210894 A1.

* E-mail: alexander.rotenberg@childrens.harvard.edu

Introduction

Transcranial magnetic stimulation (TMS) is a well-tolerated method for noninvasive stimulation and modulation of regional cortical excitability in humans. TMS is based on the principles of electromagnetic induction where small intracranial electrical currents are induced by a powerful fluctuating extracranial magnetic field. In common clinical and experimental practice, TMS is applied unilaterally over the motor cortex, and coupled with surface electromyography (EMG) such that reliable unilateral motor evoked potentials (MEP) can be recorded from the subject's contralateral hand muscles. MEP measures can then be used as markers of cortico-spinal excitability [1,2].

Repetitive transcranial magnetic stimulation (rTMS) of the human motor cortex induces a durable change in cortico-spinal excitability as reflected by a lasting change in the MEP size and appears mediated, at least in part, by intracortical mechanisms [3,4]. Such capacity to modulate cortical excitability is thought to critically contribute to the therapeutic effects of rTMS in several neuropsychiatric diseases, including major depression, chronic pain and epilepsy [5–10].

The mechanisms by which rTMS alters cortico-motor excitability are not sufficiently understood. Human data and experimental work in animals suggest that the lasting effects of high ($\geq$ 10 Hz) or low ($\leq$1 Hz) rTMS on cortico-spinal excitability rely on synaptic plasticity mechanisms similar to those of long-term-potentiation (LTP) and long-term depression (LTD) [11–18]. Specifically, rTMS resembles classical LTD and LTP plasticity in that rTMS effects are frequency dependent, cause an immediate change in excitability, outlast stimulation, and appear to be dependent on activation of the N-methyl-D-aspartate glutamate receptor (NMDAR) [3].

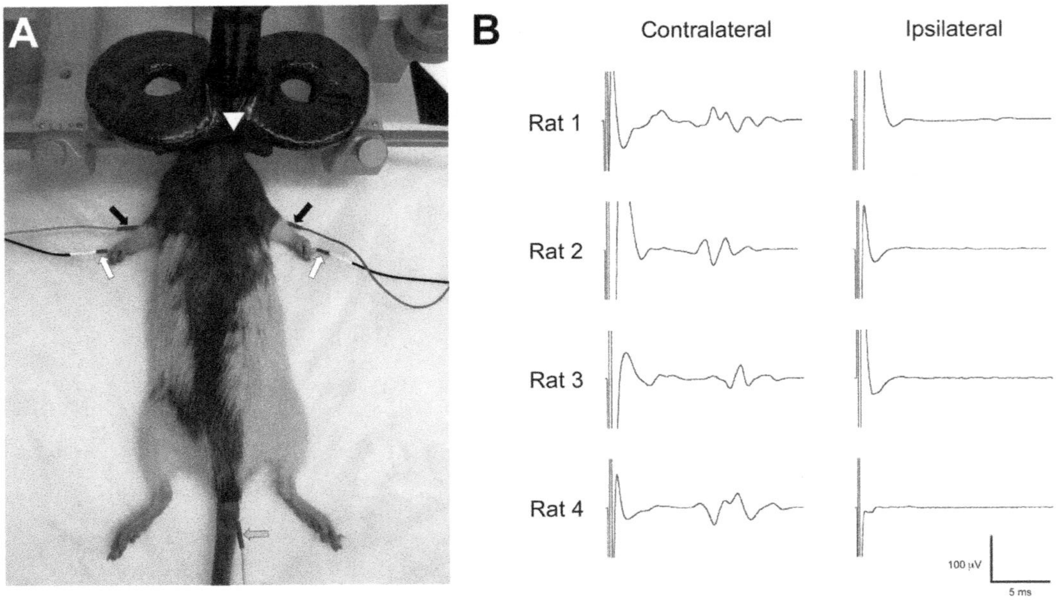

Figure 1. (A) EMG-rTMS rat setup. Photograph shows rat in stereotaxic frame. Monopolar stainless steel needle electrodes are placed into the brachioradialis of each forelimb and between the third and fourth digit in the footpad (arrows). A ground electrode is inserted in the tail. A 40 mm figure-of-eight coil is fixed to a micromanipulator arm and positioned over the left or right hemisphere. **(B) Demonstration of contralateral activation by TMS in rat.** Representative brachioradialis MEPs (average of ten consecutive sweeps) are shown. Note, at motor threshold, lateralized TMS elicits isolated MEP in the contralateral forelimb.

To approximate human protocols in translational (rat) TMS research, our group has developed methods for lateralized single pulse TMS (spTMS) and paired-pulse TMS (ppTMS) to enable focal cortical stimulation and provide a measure of regional cortical excitability [19–22]. Here, we establish an rTMS model that will enable mechanistic studies of LF rTMS protocols that are currently used in the clinical arena [23,24] and anticipate this as a step toward valuable insights at the cellular and molecular level that can be obtained from animal models to improve therapeutic clinical LF rTMS protocols. Specifically, we demonstrate that a lasting reduction in motor excitability can be induced by LF rTMS in anesthetized rats, and examine whether and to what extent the rTMS-induced change in excitability depend on stimulation frequency and the NMDAR.

Methods

Ethics Statement

All animal procedures were in accordance with the guidelines of the National Institutes of Health's *Guide for the Care and Use of Laboratory Animals*. The protocol was approved by the Animal Care and Use Committee at Boston Children's Hospital (protocol number: 10-03-1633R).

Animals

48 adult male Long-Evans rats (231 g ±20.7 g) were used. All efforts were made to minimize the number of rats used in the present experiments.

Anesthesia

Animals were anesthetized with intraperitoneal (i.p.) sodium pentobarbital at 65 mg/kg (50 mg/ml solution). Ten minutes later a second dose, equal to approximately 20% of the primary injection, was given i.p. This pentobarbital dosing protocol was adapted from previously described methods and enabled sufficient anesthesia for the 70-minute experiment [19,20]. Once anesthetized, rats were placed into a stereotaxic frame (Stoelting Wood Dale, Illinois). The frame was electrically grounded. The stereotaxic frame's points of contact with the animal (ear bars and nose clamp) were covered with several layers of paraffin film to avoid potential conductance of induced electrical current between the rat and the metal frame, and the rat torso was isolated from the frame base by plastic padding [19].

Pharmacology

Two separate groups, both stimulated with 1 Hz rTMS, (n = 6 rats/group) received MK801 3 mg/kg (2 mg/ml) or AP5 5 mg/kg (5 mg/ml) dissolved in 0.9% saline by i.p. injection. These doses were based on published methods for systemic administration of the NMDAR antagonists AP5 [25–29] and MK801 [30–33]. NMDAR antagonists were administered 20 minutes before sodium pentobarbital. Note: due to the sedating effects of MK801, the second dose of pentobarbital was not administered in this group.

Electromyography

MEPs were recorded with monopolar uninsulated 28 G stainless steel needle electrodes (Chalgren Enterprises Inc., Gilroy, CA) inserted into each brachioradialis muscle (Fig. 1a) [19,20]. Brachioradialis location was determined by palpation of the extended forelimb. A reference electrode was positioned distally in the paw between the 3rd and 4th digit. Each animal was electrically grounded by one needle electrode placed in the tail (Fig. 1a). EMG signal was band pass filtered 100–1000 Hz, amplified X1000 (AM Systems Model 1700; Sequim, WA), digitized with 40 kHz sampling, and stored for post hoc analysis (AD Instruments Colorado Springs, CO).

Repetitive Transcranial Magnetic Stimulation

A MagStim Rapid stimulator and a customized 70 mm figure-of-eight coil (40 mm external diameter of each lobe; Magstim Company, Wales, U.K.) were used to apply rTMS over the motor cortex (coil center 9.0±0.9 mm lateral and 3.3±1.0 mm anterior to bregma). The coil position was adjusted to produce unilateral MEPs in the brachioradialis muscle contralateral to the site of stimulation and no MEPs in the ipsilateral brachioradialis at motor threshold (MT) (Fig. 1b). By visual inspection, such lateralized TMS produced a twitch only in the contralateral forepaw and shoulder. An exclusive unilateral MEP response was the inclusion criterion for the study.

TMS intensity was recorded as percent machine output (% MO), with 100% corresponding to the maximal electrical current in the coil with corresponding maximal magnetic field. Bregma was located by measurement of the interaural line [34]. MT was defined as the minimum stimulus intensity to obtain MEPs of ≥ 20 μV peak-to-peak amplitude in at least 5 of 10 trials [20].

To stay within a relatively narrow steady-state anesthesia time window, a pre-rTMS recruitment curve, similar to our previous publication, was rapidly generated by adjusting the stimulator intensity in steps of 5% MO from 55% to 95% MO with a 7 sec inter-stimulus interval for a total of 630 seconds [19]. 10 stimuli were repeated at each step in the recruitment curve. Following baseline and MT acquisition, the stimulator was set to either 100% MT for active stimulation or 5% MO for sham stimulation (n = 6 rats per treatment condition). Stimulation was performed at one of three frequencies; 1 Hz, 0.5 Hz, or 0.25 Hz such that total number of pulses delivered was 300, resulting in 5, 10, and 20 minutes of stimulation for 1, 0.5, and 0.25 Hz, respectively.

For the purposes of timing, we designated end of rTMS as minute "0". Thereafter, two additional recruitment curves were obtained at 8 and 35 minutes following rTMS (Fig. 2a). The time to the first post-rTMS recruitment curve was limited by the stimulator and coil temperature as pilot runs indicated that a 7-minute cooling period was required for the coil to be functional after 300 rTMS pulses. Therefore, the 8-minute time point was selected as the earliest start point for the recruitment curve used to assess immediate rTMS effects. The second post-rTMS recruitment curve was started 15 minutes after the end of the first post-stimulation curve (lasting 12 minutes), making it the 35th minute of the experiment.

Statistical Analysis

Absolute integrated voltage from ten consecutive sweeps was averaged for comparison of MEP voltages at each TMS intensity [19,20]. Means of derived MEP amplitudes were analyzed at each timepoint after LF rTMS as a ratio relative to matched MO from the baseline recruitment curve for each animal. All data expressed as ratios were log-transformed prior to analysis. Group and stimulation intensity contributions to differences between recruitment curves were evaluated by two-way ANOVA with corresponding post hoc paired t-test.

For purposes of analysis, comparisons between multiple groups were made using integrated MEP voltage ratios and their log transformation at 80% MO, an intensity that was the lowest MO value that was suprathreshold for MEP activation in all test animals. We note also that we chose the 80% MO intensity, somewhat arbitrarily, given the relatively coarse MT approximation in 5% MO steps, and absent EMG-based definition of MT in rats.

Results

MEP Suppression by LF rTMS

Following 1 Hz rTMS (LF rTMS), the integrated MEP voltage is reduced at all suprathreshold TMS intensities for the duration of the experiment, up to 47 minutes post-rTMS (Fig. 2a). Representative traces demonstrate the reduction seen in MEP amplitude for active 1 Hz stimulation as compared to its sham counterpart (Fig. 2c). Two-way ANOVA comparison of the integrated MEP voltages between groups indicates that recruitment curve is significantly depressed at both the 8-minutes [stimulation effect: $F(1,90) = 28.35$, $p<0.0001$] and 35-minutes [stimulation effect: $F(1,90) = 30.29$, $p<0.0001$] timepoints following the 300-pulse rTMS train (Fig. 2b). Post hoc t-tests show that the difference is largely attributable to significant suppression at the 8-minutes timepoint for 75, 80, 85 and 90% MO ($p<0.01$, $p<0.001$, $p<0.01$, $p<0.05$, respectively) when comparing baseline and post-stimulation absolute integrated MEP voltages. For the 35-minutes timepoint, we note a significant decrease in values relative to sham at 75, 80 and 85% MO ($p<0.05$, $p<0.01$, $p<0.01$).

rTMS Effect is Frequency-dependent

We also find that the suppressive LF rTMS effect is strongly dependent on the rTMS frequency. Specifically, there is no significant difference between sham and active stimulation for either 0.25 Hz or 0.5 Hz at either timepoint after the LF rTMS train. This is illustrated in figure 3 which shows a comparison of the effects of rTMS trains over a short range of frequencies at 80% MO. In contrast, after 1 Hz active rTMS the MEPs are significantly suppressed to 55% (±18%; $p<0.004$) and 69% (±27%; $p<0.04$) of the baseline integrated voltage, at the 8-minutes and 35-minutes timepoints, respectively. The time effect not significant for either group, but the frequency effect of frequency was significant for both sham [$F(2,30) = 4.43$, $p<0.021$] and active [$F(2,30) = 6.20$, $p<0.0056$] by two-way ANOVA. Furthermore, two-way ANOVA analysis of frequency versus stimulation condition at both 8 minute and 35 minutes identified significant contributions of both time points respectively [frequency effect: $F(2,30) = 4.88$, $p<0.015$; sham/active effect: $F(1,30) = 7.95$, $p<0.0084$] [frequency effect: $F(2,30) = 4.31$, $p<0.023$; sham/active effect: $F(1,30) = 4.33$, $p<0.046$].

1 Hz rTMS Effect is Dependent on NMDAR Activation

To test whether MEP modulation by LF rTMS is dependent on NMDAR activation, we treated separate groups of rats (n = 6 rats per group) with either the non-competitive NMDA antagonist MK801 or the competitive antagonist AP5. Motor threshold (MT) was unchanged following either MK801 or AP5 administration. MT comparison among treatment conditions showed no significant difference among groups when evaluated by one-way ANOVA (Fig. 4a). Average MT across all groups was 73.5±2.5% MO. Following active rTMS, at 80% MO, we find 48.2% ($p<0.01$) and 53% ($p<0.05$) reduction of the MEP integrated voltage at 8 and 35-minutes after the rTMS train, respectively, when compared to their individual pre-rTMS baseline. However, there is no significant difference between sham, MK801, and AP5 conditions (Fig. 4b).

Discussion

LTD-like Forelimb MEP Suppression in Anesthetized Rats

As a step toward establishing a mechanistic rTMS model and enabling further trasnslational rTMS research, we show for the first time a long-term depression of the lateralized forelimb MEPs

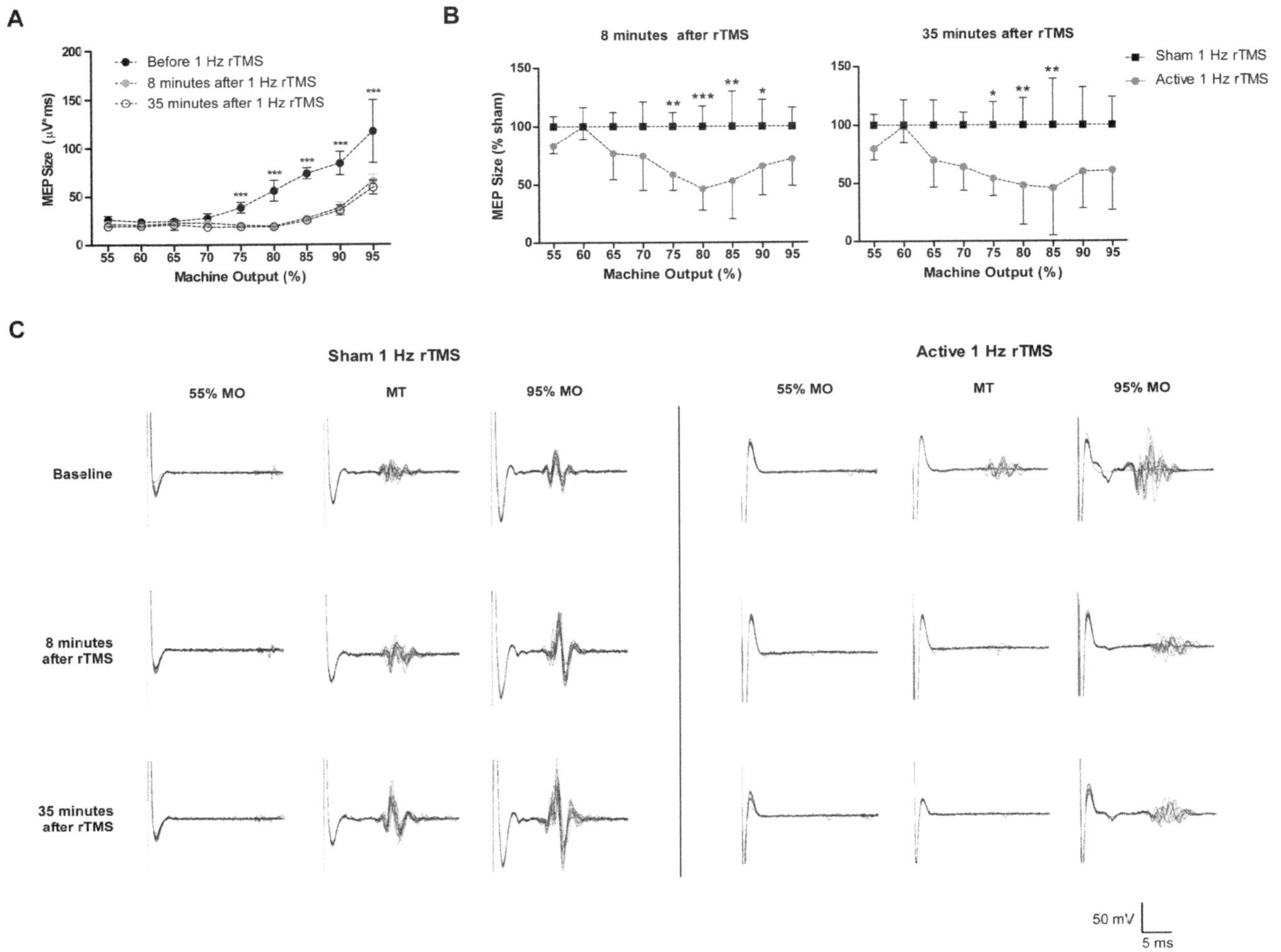

Figure 2. (A) Representative recruitment curves. Averaged integrated voltage (uV*s) for the baseline recruitment acquisition from all animals is compared to post-stimulation values at both the 8 and 35-minutes timepoints after rTMS. By 2-way ANOVA, there is a significant reduction in the integrated MEP size following 1 Hz stimulation at both 8-minutes [stimulation effect: $F(1,162) = 294.3$, $p < 0.0001$; MO effect: $F(8,162) = 127.5$, $p < 0.0001$; interaction effect: $F(8,162) = 25.86$, $p < 0.0001$] and the 35-minutes [stimulation effect: $F(1,162) = 355.6$, $p < 0.0001$; MO effect: $F(8,162) = 118.2$, $p < 0.0001$; interaction effect: $F(8,162) = 27.23$, $p < 0.0001$] timepoints. Significance is confirmed by post-hoc t-test from 75–95% MO. Error bars indicate SD. ***$p < 0.001$. **(B) MEP changes following 1 Hz rTMS.** All values are normalized to sham rTMS control. The difference between active and sham rTMS recruitment curves is significant by 2-way ANOVA at the 8-minute [stimulation effect: $F(1,90) = 28.35$, $p < 0.0001$] and 35-minutes [stimulation effect: $F(1,90) = 30.29$, $p < 0.0001$] timepoints. At individual stimulator intensities, using post-hoc t-test, there is a significant suppression at 75, 80, 85 and 90% MO ($p < 0.01$, $p < 0.001$, $p < 0.01$, $p < 0.05$, respectively) at the 8-minutes timepoint, and significant suppression at 75, 80 and 85% MO ($p < 0.05$, $p < 0.01$, $p < 0.01$) at the 35-minutes timepoint. Error bars indicate SD. *$p < 0.05$; **$p < 0.01$; ***$p < 0.001$. **(C) Representative MEPs following 1 Hz active or sham rTMS.** Ten consecutive MEP sweeps at 55% MO, 100% MT, and 95% MO from one animal per condition, active or sham rTMS, are shown. Baseline traces are followed by MEPs generated at the same MO at the 8-minutes and 35-minutes timepoints.

in rats by low frequency rTMS. This lasting modulation of corticospinal excitability after rTMS has several essential features of LTD-type plasticity: (1) Frequency dependence with preferential response to 1 Hz stimulation, (2) immediate (within 8 minutes) and durable (up to 35 minutes) modulation of post-stimulation excitability, and (3) NMDAR dependence. Notably, the magnitude and duration of MEP suppression by LF rTMS in our study approximates the 20–50% MEP reduction reported in humans 15–30 minutes after 1 Hz rTMS [13,35,36]. We also demonstrate that other aspects of forelimb MEP modulation by LF rTMS are in line with human studies, including frequency dependence and NMDAR involvement. We appreciate that other research groups have also produced analogous results in different experimental rTMS settings [37–39], and underscore that the present report adds to the literature results specific to plasticity of a lateralized motor evoked response, akin to that which is seen in humans [19].

Frequency Dependent Effect of LF rTMS

1 Hz rTMS elicits a greater reduction in motor excitability than either 0.5 Hz or 0.25 Hz stimulation. This is consistent with published LTD data suggesting a preferential response to 1.0 Hz stimulation when compared to other low frequencies [40]. These results also approximate frequency-dependent effects seen in low-frequency rTMS in humans, whereby 1.0 Hz stimulation has the most prominent effect on MEP size [35,41]. While sub-1.0 Hz stimulation appears to have little to no effect on the MEP in our setup, a depression of the MEP by lower frequencies has been shown in humans [42] and LF rTMS below 1.0 Hz has

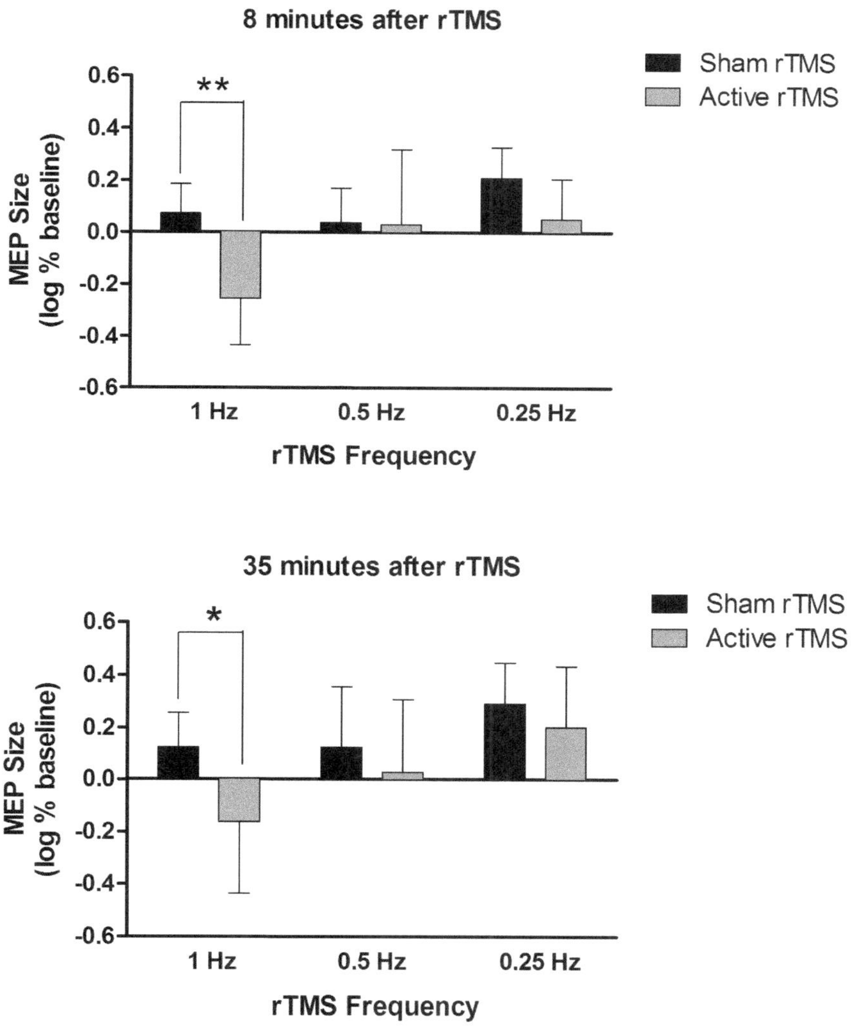

Figure 3. MEP change as a function of rTMS frequency. All conditions are shown at 80% MO. All ratios of average MEP integrated voltage relative to pre-rTMS baseline were log transformed. Compared to its baseline, 1 Hz active rTMS is the only condition where the MEP size was suppressed at both the 8-minues ($p<0.01$) and 35-minutes ($p<0.05$) timepoints. Error bars indicate SD. *$p<0.05$, **$p<0.01$.

therapeutic promise in epilepsy (0.3 Hz [43], 0.5 Hz [24]) and tinnitus (0.5 Hz [44]), among other disease states [45,46]. Plausibly, this discrepancy is due to the physiologic differences between our rat setup and human rTMS, or to the the physiologic effects of anesthesia, or to the relatively short train duration (300 pulses) which is 3–6 times shorter than many human rTMS protocols (reviewed in [42]). Yet an additional and intriguing explanation is perhaps a fundamental difference in physiologic sequelae of 1 Hz rTMS as compared to lower frequencies as suggested in limited human work [41]. Further examination of rodent LF rTMS, particularly if coupled with molecular neuroscience techniques that are available only in preclincal studies, could provide valuable insight into the mechanism of action these sub-1.0 Hz frequencies in neurological disorders. Although detailed study of a large range of stimulation protocols as has been done in humans (reviewed in [42]) is beyond the scope of this experiment, our anticipation is that the present report will facilitate such mechanistic studies with methods for lateralized rTMS in anesthetized rats [19].

NMDA Dependent Mechanism of Neuronal Modulation by rTMS

Our data provide further insight into LF rTMS mechanism by testing the hypothesis that LF rTMS mediated motor suppression is dependent on NMDAR activation. In human studies, the role of NMDARs in high frequency (potentiating) rTMS has been studied extensively [47,48]. However, human studies of the NMDAR contribution to motor cortex plasticity with LF rTMS are limited in number, and also limited to only one noncompetitive NMDA antagonist, dextromethorphan, which likely acts on the NMDAR indirectly via active metabolites and may have off-target effects [48,49]. Similar future human rTMS work with healthy volunteers will also, for ethical reasons, be very likely limited to sub-anesthetic doses of NMDAR antgonists such as ketamine or synthetic opioids. Thus the rat model here provides an explicit validation for the LF rTMS mechanism, as we demonstrate a similar NMDAR dependence in rats as is suggested in human studies, but with more selective NMDAR competitive and noncompetitive NMDAR antagonism.

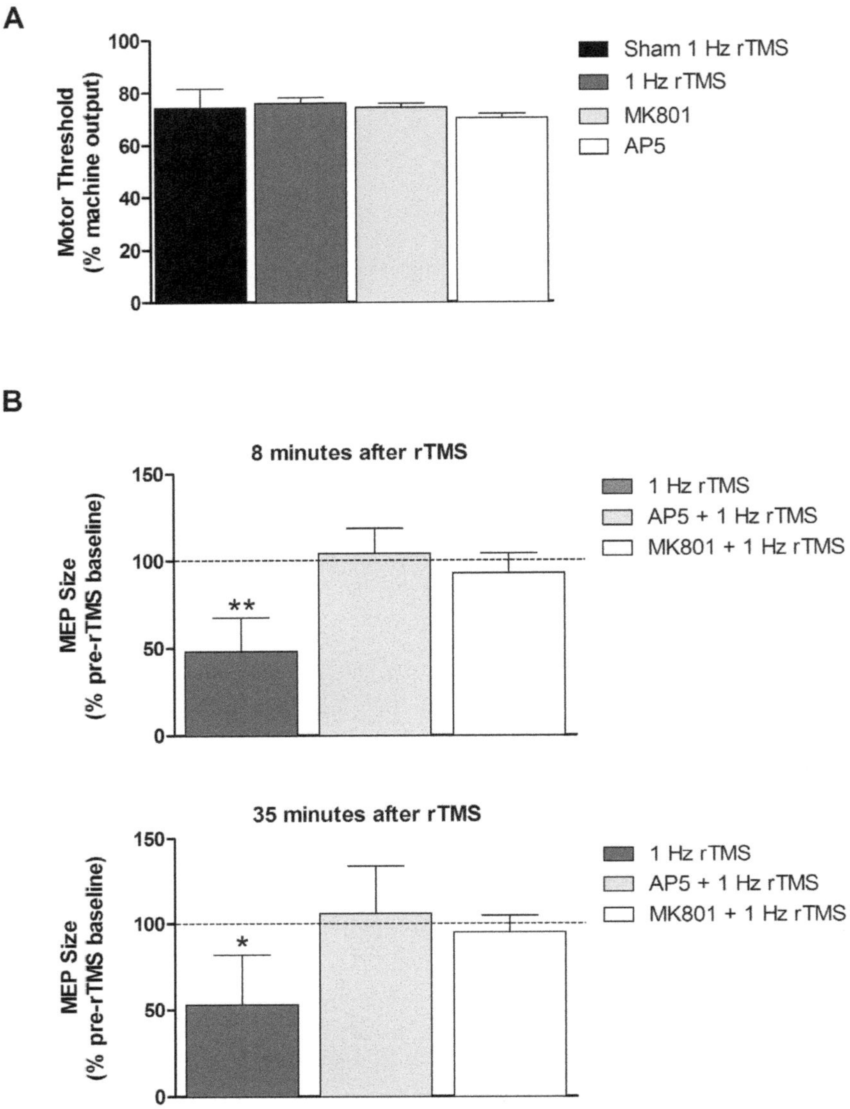

Figure 4. (A) Average motor threshold per treatment group. Percent machine output needed to achieve motor thresholds across sham 1 Hz rTMS, 1 Hz rTMS, MK801, and AP5 (74.2%MO ±7.3%MO, 75.8%MO ±4.9%MO, 74.2%MO ±3.8%MO, 70%MO ±4.5%MO respectively). No significant difference between groups was detected. Error bars indicate SD. **(B) Effects of NMDAR antagonists on MEP suppression by 1 Hz rTMS.** Integrated MEP voltage (uV*s) is measured at 80% MO. Statistics per treatment pair were obtained by comparison with the corresponding sham condition. For the 1 Hz rTMS group, there is a 48.2% ($p<0.01$) and 53% ($p<0.05$) reduction at the 8-minutes and 35-minutes timepoints after rTMS, respectively. There is no significant change from pre-rTMS baseline after pretreatment with MK801 or AP5 conditions. Error bars indicate SD.*$p<0.05$, **$p<0.01$.

We chose two common NMDAR antagonists, MK801 and AP5, and found that application of either antagonist prevents MEP depression by 1 Hz rTMS. Notably, in classic in vitro LTD experimental setups, in isolated hippocampal slices, AP5 has been shown to inhibit LTD [50–52], but MK801 has not [53,54]. Thus we find a small discrepancy between the pharmacology of the 1 Hz focal electrical stimulation *in vitro* and 1 Hz rTMS *in vivo*. We underscore this discrepancy as such distinctions in the biochemistry of rTMS effects and those of classic LTD data will need to be reconciled if we are to apply information from the vast LTD literature toward experimental design and clinical rTMS protocols. It is ultimately not surprising that rTMS effects, which could follow from simultaneous electromagnetic stimulation of all components of a cortical volume (principal neurons, interneurons, etc.), may not be fully predicted by data from experimental protocols that involve precise electrical stimulation of a single afferent pathway and focal recording from its target; for instance, where the Schaffer collaterals are stimulated to evoke a post-synaptic response in CA1 in classic LTD experimental setups.

rTMS in an Anesthetized Subject

Our data are the first to show LTD-type MEP suppression by 1 Hz rTMS in rats under pentobarbital anesthesia. For extension of the present experiment toward further studies, the finding of motor pathway plasticity under anesthesia is valuable, as anesthesia will likely be needed for future rodent rTMS experiments and the interaction between anesthesia and rTMS will require further exploration [20,55].

An interesting translational extension of the data may be toward testing whether rTMS-mediated cortical plasticity is preserved in humans who are under barbiturate sedation or another anesthetic state. Such scenarios may be of clinical relevance for patient populations, such as children or adults with developmental disabilities, who may benefit from rTMS, but who may not tolerate rTMS in the awake state. Our results demonstrating that cortical excitability can be modulated by rTMS in the anesthetized state also raise the prospect for rTMS in patients treated with high barbiturate doses for management of an acute medical condition such as status epilepticus, as supported by recent case reports [56,57].

Study Limitations

We note limitations to the present study that warrant further investigation. Among these, is the confound of anesthesia. As most data in humans are obtained in the waking state, the value of the current findings as a model for human LF rTMS is compromised. The anesthetized state and specific choice of anesthetic likely affect mechanisms of synaptic plasticity as suggested by rodent rTMS results published by Gersner et al. [55]and discussed by Benali et al. [37], and limit extension of the present findings to human rTMS. Along these lines, we cautiously anticipate that the establishment of LTD-like motor depression in rats will enable our lab and others to test the effects of specific anesthetics on rTMS plasticity mechanisms in rodents, in vivo. While the magnitude direction and duration of MEP change after LF-rTMS in rats, as well as its frequency and NMDAR dependence, suggest some mechanistic overlap with human LF rTMS physiology, further experiments to validate these early results, perhaps by ex vivo tissue analysis that follows stimulation of unanesthetized rodents will be needed [38,58].

Another pharmacologic confound of our experiment, also common to human rTMS studies, is the systemic administration of NMDAR antagonists. While we cautiously infer that the NMDAR dependence of the LTD-like motor phenomenon is cortical, we recognize that systemic drug treatment may affect the corticomotor response at numerous sites between the cortex the neuromuscular junction, as well as at cortical and subcortical motor regulatory systems. Although beyond the scope of this project, further delineation of the contribution of region-specific neurotransmitter receptor populations to rTMS-related cerebral plasticity, as can be accomplished by transgenic or optogenetic methods, or by site-specific microinjections, will be helpful in advancing the value of translational rTMS research [59–61].

Last, a necessary limitation of rodent rTMS research is the reduction in TMS spatial resolution. The reduced focality of the electromagnetic stimulus adds to the complexity of the interpretation of TMS effects on distinct neuronal populations that has been discussed in prior translational rTMS studies [37]. Here, as in our prior work, we addressed the problem by eccentric positioning of the coil center relative to the rat's scalp midline, such that the major coil conductive components are non-tangential to the scalp and thus produce poor electromagnetic coupling between the rat brain and the coil [19,20,62,63]. With this setup, we note that the brachioradialis response was strongly lateralized. However, we recognize that physiologic markers of cortical activation outside the motor areas are absent in our results, and thus interpretation of MEP modulation as resultant from selective motor cortex stimulation should be with caution.

Conclusion

We provide the first in-vivo electrophysiologic demonstration of LTD-like modulation of motor cortex excitability by low frequency rTMS in anesthetized rats. Consistent with human data, we show effects that outlast stimulation, frequency-dependent cortico-spinal plasticity, as well as a further demonstration of LF rTMS NMDAR-dependence. While limitations of rodent rTMS methods will be essential to address, we are hopeful that our results will facilitate future mechanistic studies, at the cellular and molecular level. Such work is already in progress and that can be best completed in translational rTMS models [37,55]. We suggest a concerted effort to standardize rTMS studies in animals, with emphasis on specialized coil development. We believe the present study most closely approximates human rTMS findings to this point and expansion of this model will be valuable to uncovering basic rTMS mechanisms as well as to the development of therapeutic rTMS protocols.

Author Contributions

Conceived and designed the experiments: PAM SCD AR. Performed the experiments: PAM SCD AMVH. Analyzed the data: PAM SCD AR. Contributed reagents/materials/analysis tools: APL FEJ AR. Wrote the paper: PAM SCD FEJ APL AR.

References

1. Kobayashi M, Pascual-Leone A (2003) Transcranial magnetic stimulation in neurology. Lancet Neurol 2: 145–156.
2. Hallett M (2007) Transcranial magnetic stimulation: a primer. Neuron 55: 187–199.
3. Hoogendam JM, Ramakers GM, Di Lazzaro V (2010) Physiology of repetitive transcranial magnetic stimulation of the human brain. Brain Stimul 3: 95–118.
4. Kobayashi M (2010) Effect of slow repetitive TMS of the motor cortex on ipsilateral sequential simple finger movements and motor skill learning. Restor Neurol Neurosci 28: 437–448.
5. Fregni F, Pascual-Leone A (2005) Transcranial magnetic stimulation for the treatment of depression in neurologic disorders. Curr Psychiatry Rep 7: 381–390.
6. Patrizi F, Freedman SD, Pascual-Leone A, Fregni F (2006) Novel therapeutic approaches to the treatment of chronic abdominal visceral pain. ScientificWorldJournal 6: 472–490.
7. Padberg F, George MS (2009) Repetitive transcranial magnetic stimulation of the prefrontal cortex in depression. Exp Neurol 219: 2–13.
8. Rotenberg A, Bae EH, Takeoka M, Tormos JM, Schachter SC, et al. (2009) Repetitive transcranial magnetic stimulation in the treatment of epilepsia partialis continua. Epilepsy Behav 14: 253–257.
9. Rosen AC, Ramkumar M, Nguyen T, Hoeft F (2009) Noninvasive transcranial brain stimulation and pain. Curr Pain Headache Rep 13: 12–17.
10. Rotenberg A (2010) Prospects for clinical applications of transcranial magnetic stimulation and real-time EEG in epilepsy. Brain Topogr 22: 257–266.
11. Siegelbaum SA, Kandel ER (1991) Learning-related synaptic plasticity: LTP and LTD. Curr Opin Neurobiol 1: 113–120.
12. Maeda F, Keenan JP, Tormos JM, Topka H, Pascual-Leone A (2000) Modulation of corticospinal excitability by repetitive transcranial magnetic stimulation. Clin Neurophysiol 111: 800–805.
13. Rizzo V, Siebner HR, Modugno N, Pesenti A, Munchau A, et al. (2004) Shaping the excitability of human motor cortex with premotor rTMS. J Physiol 554: 483–495.
14. Peinemann A, Reimer B, Loer C, Quartarone A, Munchau A, et al. (2004) Long-lasting increase in corticospinal excitability after 1800 pulses of subthreshold 5 Hz repetitive TMS to the primary motor cortex. Clin Neurophysiol 115: 1519–1526.
15. Esser SK, Huber R, Massimini M, Peterson MJ, Ferrarelli F, et al. (2006) A direct demonstration of cortical LTP in humans: a combined TMS/EEG study. Brain Res Bull 69: 86–94.
16. Khedr EM, Rothwell JC, Ahmed MA, Shawky OA, Farouk M (2007) Modulation of motor cortical excitability following rapid-rate transcranial magnetic stimulation. Clin Neurophysiol 118: 140–145.
17. Aydin-Abidin S, Trippe J, Funke K, Eysel UT, Benali A (2008) High- and low-frequency repetitive transcranial magnetic stimulation differentially activates c-Fos and zif268 protein expression in the rat brain. Exp Brain Res 188: 249–261.

18. Pell GS, Roth Y, Zangen A (2011) Modulation of cortical excitability induced by repetitive transcranial magnetic stimulation: influence of timing and geometrical parameters and underlying mechanisms. Prog Neurobiol 93: 59–98.
19. Rotenberg A, Muller PA, Vahabzadeh-Hagh AM, Navarro X, Lopez-Vales R, et al. (2010) Lateralization of forelimb motor evoked potentials by transcranial magnetic stimulation in rats. Clin Neurophysiol 121: 104–108.
20. Vahabzadeh-Hagh AM, Muller PA, Pascual-Leone A, Jensen FE, Rotenberg A (2011) Measures of cortical inhibition by paired-pulse transcranial magnetic stimulation in anesthetized rats. J Neurophysiol 105: 615–624.
21. Vahabzadeh-Hagh AM, Muller PA, Gersner R, Zangen A, Rotenberg A (2012) Translational neuromodulation: approximating human transcranial magnetic stimulation protocols in rats. Neuromodulation 15: 296–305.
22. Rotenberg A, Muller P, Birnbaum D, Harrington M, Riviello JJ, et al. (2008) Seizure suppression by EEG-guided repetitive transcranial magnetic stimulation in the rat. Clin Neurophysiol 119: 2697–2702.
23. Muller PA, Pascual-Leone A, Rotenberg A (2012) Safety and tolerability of repetitive transcranial magnetic stimulation in patients with pathologic positive sensory phenomena: a review of literature. Brain Stimul 5: 320–329 e327.
24. Sun W, Mao W, Meng X, Wang D, Qiao L, et al. (2012) Low-frequency repetitive transcranial magnetic stimulation for the treatment of refractory partial epilepsy: a controlled clinical study. Epilepsia 53: 1782–1789.
25. Loeb C, Patrone A, Besio G, Balestrino M, Mainardi P (1990) The excitatory amino acid antagonist amino-phosphono-valeric acid (APV) provides protection against penicillin-induced epileptic activity in the rat. Epilepsy Res 6: 249–251.
26. Loeb C, Patrone A, Besio G, Balestrino M, Mainardi P (1993) The antiepileptic effect of low-dose amino-phosphono-valeric acid (APV) is not enhanced by phosphatidylserine association. Seizure 2: 309–310.
27. Kent S, Kernahan SD, Levine S (1996) Effects of excitatory amino acids on the hypothalamic-pituitary-adrenal axis of the neonatal rat. Brain Res Dev Brain Res 94: 1–13.
28. Guerrini L, Molteni A, Wirth T, Kistler B, Blasi F (1997) Glutamate-dependent activation of NF-kappaB during mouse cerebellum development. J Neurosci 17: 6057–6063.
29. McGuire M, Liu C, Cao Y, Ling L (2008) Formation and maintenance of ventilatory long-term facilitation require NMDA but not non-NMDA receptors in awake rats. J Appl Physiol (1985) 105: 942–950.
30. Bouras R, Chapman CA (2003) Long-term synaptic depression in the adult entorhinal cortex in vivo. Hippocampus 13: 780–790.
31. de Olmos S, Bender C, de Olmos JS, Lorenzo A (2009) Neurodegeneration and prolonged immediate early gene expression throughout cortical areas of the rat brain following acute administration of dizocilpine. Neuroscience 164: 1347–1359.
32. Han RZ, Hu JJ, Weng YC, Li DF, Huang Y (2009) NMDA receptor antagonist MK-801 reduces neuronal damage and preserves learning and memory in a rat model of traumatic brain injury. Neurosci Bull 25: 367–375.
33. Lai MC, Lui CC, Yang SN, Wang JY, Huang LT (2009) Epileptogenesis is increased in rats with neonatal isolation and early-life seizure and ameliorated by MK-801: a long-term MRI and histological study. Pediatr Res 66: 441–447.
34. Whishaw IQ, Cioe JD, Previsich N, Kolb B (1977) The variability of the interaural line vs the stability of bregma in rat stereotaxic surgery. Physiol Behav 19: 719–722.
35. Chen R, Classen J, Gerloff C, Celnik P, Wassermann EM, et al. (1997) Depression of motor cortex excitability by low-frequency transcranial magnetic stimulation. Neurology 48: 1398–1403.
36. Muellbacher W, Ziemann U, Boroojerdi B, Hallett M (2000) Effects of low-frequency transcranial magnetic stimulation on motor excitability and basic motor behavior. Clin Neurophysiol 111: 1002–1007.
37. Benali A, Trippe J, Weiler E, Mix A, Petrasch-Parwez E, et al. (2011) Theta-burst transcranial magnetic stimulation alters cortical inhibition. J Neurosci 31: 1193–1203.
38. Funke K, Benali A (2011) Modulation of cortical inhibition by rTMS - findings obtained from animal models. J Physiol 589: 4423–4435.
39. Wang F, Geng X, Tao HY, Cheng Y (2010) The restoration after repetitive transcranial magnetic stimulation treatment on cognitive ability of vascular dementia rats and its impacts on synaptic plasticity in hippocampal CA1 area. J Mol Neurosci 41: 145–155.
40. Nakano M, Yamada S, Udagawa R, Kato N (2004) Frequency-dependent requirement for calcium store-operated mechanisms in induction of homosynaptic long-term depression at hippocampus CA1 synapses. Eur J Neurosci 19: 2881–2887.
41. Cincotta M, Borgheresi A, Gambetti C, Balestrieri F, Rossi L, et al. (2003) Suprathreshold 0.3 Hz repetitive TMS prolongs the cortical silent period: potential implications for therapeutic trials in epilepsy. Clin Neurophysiol 114: 1827–1833.
42. Fitzgerald PB, Fountain S, Daskalakis ZJ (2006) A comprehensive review of the effects of rTMS on motor cortical excitability and inhibition. Clin Neurophysiol 117: 2584–2596.
43. Brasil-Neto JP, de Araujo DP, Teixeira WA, Araujo VP, Boechat-Barros R (2004) Experimental therapy of epilepsy with transcranial magnetic stimulation: lack of additional benefit with prolonged treatment. Arq Neuropsiquiatr 62: 21–25.
44. Lee SL, Abraham M, Cacace AT, Silver SM (2008) Repetitive transcranial magnetic stimulation in veterans with debilitating tinnitus: a pilot study. Otolaryngol Head Neck Surg 138: 398–399.
45. Dragasevic N, Potrebic A, Damjanovic A, Stefanova E, Kostic VS (2002) Therapeutic efficacy of bilateral prefrontal slow repetitive transcranial magnetic stimulation in depressed patients with Parkinson's disease: an open study. Mov Disord 17: 528–532.
46. Sokhadze EM, El-Baz A, Baruth J, Mathai G, Sears L, et al. (2009) Effects of low frequency repetitive transcranial magnetic stimulation (rTMS) on gamma frequency oscillations and event-related potentials during processing of illusory figures in autism. J Autism Dev Disord 39: 619–634.
47. Stefan K, Kunesch E, Benecke R, Cohen LG, Classen J (2002) Mechanisms of enhancement of human motor cortex excitability induced by interventional paired associative stimulation. J Physiol 543: 699–708.
48. Wankerl K, Weise D, Gentner R, Rumpf JJ, Classen J (2010) L-type voltage-gated Ca2+ channels: a single molecular switch for long-term potentiation/long-term depression-like plasticity and activity-dependent metaplasticity in humans. J Neurosci 30: 6197–6204.
49. Fitzgerald PB, Benitez J, Oxley T, Daskalakis JZ, de Castella AR, et al. (2005) A study of the effects of lorazepam and dextromethorphan on the response to cortical 1 Hz repetitive transcranial magnetic stimulation. Neuroreport 16: 1525–1528.
50. Manahan-Vaughan D (1997) Group 1 and 2 metabotropic glutamate receptors play differential roles in hippocampal long-term depression and long-term potentiation in freely moving rats. J Neurosci 17: 3303–3311.
51. Watanabe K, Kamatani D, Hishida R, Kudoh M, Shibuki K (2007) Long-term depression induced by local tetanic stimulation in the rat auditory cortex. Brain Res 1166: 20–28.
52. Kourrich S, Glasgow SD, Caruana DA, Chapman CA (2008) Postsynaptic signals mediating induction of long-term synaptic depression in the entorhinal cortex. Neural Plast 2008: 840374.
53. Wohrl R, von Haebler D, Heinemann U (2007) Low-frequency stimulation of the direct cortical input to area CA1 induces homosynaptic LTD and heterosynaptic LTP in the rat hippocampal-entorhinal cortex slice preparation. Eur J Neurosci 25: 251–258.
54. Rodriguez-Moreno A, Paulsen O (2008) Spike timing-dependent long-term depression requires presynaptic NMDA receptors. Nat Neurosci 11: 744–745.
55. Gersner R, Kravetz E, Feil J, Pell G, Zangen A (2011) Long-term effects of repetitive transcranial magnetic stimulation on markers for neuroplasticity: differential outcomes in anesthetized and awake animals. J Neurosci 31: 7521–7526.
56. Thordstein M, Constantinescu R (2012) Possibly lifesaving, noninvasive, EEG-guided neuromodulation in anesthesia-refractory partial status epilepticus. Epilepsy Behav 25: 468–472.
57. Liu A, Pang T, Herman S, Pascual-Leone A, Rotenberg A (2013) Transcranial magnetic stimulation for refractory focal status epilepticus in the intensive care unit. Seizure 22: 893–896.
58. Ghiglieri V, Pendolino V, Sgobio C, Bagetta V, Picconi B, et al. (2012) Theta-burst stimulation and striatal plasticity in experimental parkinsonism. Exp Neurol 236: 395–398.
59. Rogan SC, Roth BL (2011) Remote control of neuronal signaling. Pharmacol Rev 63: 291–315.
60. Ting JT, Feng G (2013) Development of transgenic animals for optogenetic manipulation of mammalian nervous system function: progress and prospects for behavioral neuroscience. Behav Brain Res 255: 3–18.
61. Tostes JG, Medeiros P, Melo-Thomas L (2013) Modulation of haloperidol-induced catalepsy in rats by GABAergic neural substrate in the inferior colliculus. Neuroscience 255: 212–218.
62. Tofts PS, Branston NM (1991) The measurement of electric field, and the influence of surface charge, in magnetic stimulation. Electroencephalogr Clin Neurophysiol 81: 238–239.
63. Zheng J, Li L, Huo X (2005) Analysis of Electric Field in Real Rat Head Model during Transcranial Magnetic Stimulation. Conf Proc IEEE Eng Med Biol Soc 2: 1529–1532.

11

Real-Time Dopamine Measurement in Awake Monkeys

Erik W. Schluter[1], Andrew R. Mitz[1], Joseph F. Cheer[2], Bruno B. Averbeck[1]*

1 Laboratory of Neuropsychology, Division of Intramural Research, National Institute of Mental Health, National Institutes of Health, Bethesda, Maryland, United States of America, **2** Department of Anatomy and Neurobiology, University of Maryland School of Medicine, Baltimore, Maryland, United States of America

Abstract

Fast-scan cyclic voltammetry (FSCV) is often used to measure real-time dopamine (DA) concentrations in awake, behaving rodents. Extending this technique to work in monkeys would provide a platform for advanced behavioral studies and a primate model for preclinical research. The present study demonstrates the feasibility of DA recordings in two awake monkeys (*Macaca mulatta*) using a mixture of techniques adapted from rodent, primate and brain slice work. We developed a long carbon fiber electrode to operate in the larger primate brain. This electrode was lowered into the striatum each day using a recording chamber and a detachable micromanipulator system. A manipulator also moved one or more tungsten stimulating electrodes into either the nearby striatum or the ventral tegmental area/substantia nigra pars compacta (VTA/SNc). We developed an electrical stimulation controller to reduce artifacts during electrical stimulation. We also introduce a stimulation-based methodology for estimating distances between electrodes in the brain. Dopamine responses within the striatum were evoked by either stimulation of the striatum near the FSCV electrode, or stimulation within the VTA/SNc. Unexpected juice rewards also evoked dopamine responses in the ventral striatum. Thus, we demonstrate that robust dopamine responses can be recorded from awake, behaving primates with FSCV. In addition, we describe how a stimulation technique borrowed from the neuroprosthetics field can activate the distributed monkey midbrain dopamine system in a way that mimics rodent VTA stimulation.

Editor: Xiaoxi Zhuang, University of Chicago, United States of America

Funding: This work was supported by the Intramural Research Program of the US National Institute of Mental Health (http://www.nimh.nih.gov). The funders had no role in study design, data collection and analysis, decision to publish, or preparation of the manuscript.

Competing Interests: The authors have declared that no competing interests exist.

* E-mail: bruno.averbeck@nih.gov

Introduction

The dopamine (DA) projection of the brain originates from the ventral tegmental area (VTA), substantia nigra pars compacta (SNc) and retrorubral area (RRA) [1], and projects to broad swaths of cortex and basal ganglia [2,3], with a smaller presence in the cerebellum [4,5]. Prior to the discovery of this neuromodulatory system, DA had been implicated in the potent reinforcer effect of median forebrain bundle (MFB) electrical stimulation [6]. The effects of rodent MFB stimulation were traced to VTA neurons and DA release through a series of pharmacological, anatomical and electrophysiological studies (see [7]). Compelling models have emerged, emphasizing a putative role for DA in reward prediction [8,9]. Validating or refuting these models has become a major focus in the study of reward-driven behavior (e.g., [10]).

In vivo real-time DA measurement with fast-scan cyclic voltammetry (FSCV) has been developed over the past two decades as a tool for unraveling the role of DA in goal-directed behavior. FSCV is an electrochemical technique for measuring the concentration of an electrolyte in solution using a wide bandwidth two-electrode sweeping voltage clamp. This technique has been extensively developed in rodents [11] where a thin (e.g., 7 μm) strand of carbon fiber is used as the working electrode. It is often used to record DA concentration in the striatum, where norepinephrine (electrochemically indistinguishable from DA), is in sufficiently low concentrations as to not interfere with DA measurements (e.g., [12]). FSCV has important advantages over other *in vivo* techniques for measuring DA concentration because of its ionic specificity, and its temporal and spatial resolutions. Constant potential amperometry is a similar method, but it does not provide information about the ionic species contributing to the current being measured [13]. Optical measurements of DA are not well suited for deep brain use because of the probe size and light dispersion properties of the brain [14]. Positron emission tomography (PET) can be used to estimate DA concentration in voxels of a few cubic centimeters. However, PET has a time course on the order of minutes rather than milliseconds (e.g., [15]). Likewise, although high-performance liquid chromatography (HPLC) offers higher spatial resolution and better selectivity than PET, the sampling time course is typically from 5 to 30 min (e.g., [12]). It is important to note that slower measures of DA capture the tonic levels, typically in the order of 10 s of nM/L, whereas phasic DA release can exceed 1 μM/L (see [11]). FSCV is a high-speed subtraction method; its measurements are localized to the region of the carbon fiber electrode and measurements are taken every 100 ms. Data from FSCV provides localized real-time phasic characteristics that can capture DA release, diffusion and clearance.

Although FSCV has emerged as a staple in rodent research (i.e., [11,16,17]), it is not routinely used in primates. Attempts to record FSCV in awake, behaving monkeys [18] or humans [19] have had limited success. From an experimental standpoint, successful FSCV in monkeys would allow one to work in a species with sophisticated behavior and increased anatomical homology with humans. From a clinical standpoint, preclinical success with a monkey model could open the door to on-line, closed-loop monitoring and control of deep brain stimulation (DBS) for treatment of Parkinson's disease (PD), neuropsychiatric and other neurological disorders [20]. However, because of the anatomy of the primate brain, FSCV in monkeys presents challenges not seen in rodent work. Monkeys have a much larger and more diffuse tegmental DA projection to the striatum. Some of the most basic tenets in the rat, like broad activation of this projection with localized VTA stimulation, do not hold in the monkey.

The goal of the present study is to demonstrate the feasibility of using FSCV to measure real-time changes in striatal DA in monkeys. As a prerequisite, we developed a carbon fiber electrode that can reach several cm into the brain while meeting other requirements: easy to reproduce, minimum damage to the brain, accurate targeting, resistance to electrical noise and high sensitivity. In rodents, the primary tool for validating FSCV recordings throughout the striatum is electrical stimulation of VTA, either directly or via the MFB. In monkeys, VTA projects to a small proportion of the ventral striatum [3]. The majority of the midbrain dopamine neurons are spread across ~6 mm of substantia nigra pars compacta (SNc). Local electrical stimulation anywhere along the VTA/SNc axis leads to restricted activation of DA in the striatum. Finding the restricted area of release in a monkey can be a major challenge in a striatum ~8 times larger than that of a rat. MFB stimulation does not seem to provide a viable alternative in the monkey. The monkey MFB is apparently not a spatially restricted bundle [21,22], although groups of MFB fibers can be activated with high currents [23]. Thus, it is not possible to activate the bulk of midbrain DA neurons in a monkey using techniques common in rodents. To address these issues, we employed a mixture of rodent and monkey techniques. This allowed us to survey sites in both the VTA/SNc and the striatum. In addition, we borrowed the technique of local electrical stimulation from brain slice work to expand our ability to survey DA release sites. We were able to demonstrate that FSCV is an effective method for recording DA release from monkey striatum. We also recommend modifications to this hybrid method that will greatly enhance the utility of VTA/SNc stimulation in monkeys.

Materials and Methods

Unless otherwise stated, the FSCV methods discussed here are similar to those used for rodent recordings by Robinson and Wightman [24].

Ethics Statement

All experimental procedures were performed in accordance with the National Institutes of Health Guide for the Care and Use of Laboratory Animals and were approved by the Animal Care and Use Committee of the National Institute of Mental Health. Procedures adhered to applicable United States federal and local laws, regulations and standards, including the Animal Welfare Act (AWA 1990) and Regulations (PL 89-544; USDA 1985) and Public Health Service (PHS) Policy (PHS 2002).

Two rhesus monkeys (*Macaca mulatta*) served as subjects in this project, monkey B (9 kg male) and monkey N (7 kg male). Animals were obtained through an approved government source. They were tested for TB and Herpes B twice per year, and received regular dental checks.

Each animal was pair housed with a compatible partner using joining cages in a temperature and automatic lighting controlled (12-hr cycle) animal facility along with other housed conspecifics and no other species. No bedding was in the cage. Environmental enrichment included a toy, most often a chew toy, outside of the cage that could be readily pulled through the bars. Most days, including weekends, animals on study received fruit pieces, often just before or after an experiment. Animals were otherwise fed 12 monkey chow biscuits twice each day at 7 a.m. and 2 p.m. When not on water control, animals had unlimited access to water through a bottle attached to the outside of the cage or a spigot at the rear of the cage. When on fluid control, animals received water every day regardless of performance. Body weight was measured at least once each week and the animal was taken off study if this dropped below 15% of the fully hydrated and fully nourished weight.

Implantation surgeries were conducted in a surgical theater set up specifically for primates. Surgeries were done under a full anesthesia regimen shown effective and safe with non-human primates (ketamine HCl 10–20 mg/kg, i.m. induction followed by isoflurane gas, 1% to 4%, to effect, inhalation) and with sterile technique directed by individuals with appropriate training. Animals were closely monitored prior to, during and after surgery until they could safely sit upright on their own. Postoperative analgesics were administered based on consultation with attending or central facility veterinarian. The regimen most commonly used was ketoprofen (1–2 mg/kg BID x 3 days) followed by ibuprofen (100 mg PO BID x 4 days).

Structural MRI scans were used initially to guide implantation and multiple additional times for health monitoring. For each scan, the animal was sedated or anesthetized, depending upon the duration of the procedure, and monitored throughout the scan and during recovery from anesthesia. The endpoint of the experiment was the first of 1) sufficient data to achieve the stated goal of the experiments, 2) concern that damage from repeated electrode tracks might interfere with recordings (based on MRI scans), or 3) a health issue, including damage from electrodes. Monkey B developed a paralysis after 53 deep electrode tracks. That animal was euthanized using Ketamine sedation followed by deep anesthesia and then transcardial perfusion. Monkey N finished this series of experiments after 32 deep electrode tracks. That animal was subsequently assigned to a different experimental study under the same protocol (animal study protocol number LN-23).

Both animals were naive before the study. They were each gradually adapted to transitions from cages to adjustable primate chairs using a pole-and-collar system and positive (food) reinforcement. Studies took place in either a light and acoustic attenuating chamber designed for non-human primate experiments, or a similar custom-designed inner laboratory room. Animals were adapted to each new environment for days before testing. Likewise, after implantation of a post for head restraint, adaptation to its use was gradual and encouraged with food rewards.

Implants

Each subject received a custom, plastic 14×30 mm recording chamber (Fig. 1) implanted with the long edge over the midline in a sterile surgery. The rostro-caudal position of the chamber was centered on approximately AP 4, based on the Saleem and Logothetis atlas [25] and a T_1-weighted structural MRI of each animal prior to surgery. A Titanium head post was positioned posterior to the chamber in the same surgery. After recovery from surgery, a grid matrix was filled with Betadine gel and placed in the chamber just before a second structural MRI (Fig. 2). Candidate grid sites and depth measurements were determined using the free MRIcro software package (http://www.mccauslandcenter.sc.edu/mricro/mricro/mricro.html). Gadolini-

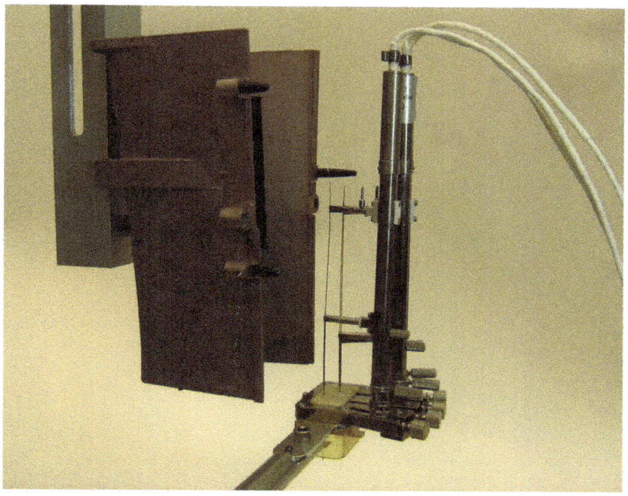

Figure 1. Electrode positioner, shield and chamber arrangement. Electrodes and guide cannulas were back loaded through a 1 mm×1 mm grid and gripped by electrically isolated clamps. Lower clamps could be raised and lowered by hand. Upper clamps were raised and lowered by remotely operated screw-driven stepper motors. The larger component of the Faraday shield has been mounted on a holder for illustration purposes. Normally the smaller component is held fixed (see Fig. 3). Its height and contours snugly fit the recording apparatus, with room near the top to accommodate electrode connections. The arm and plastic recording chamber in this picture are part of the preparation stand. After preparation, the micropositioner and grid are transferred to an equivalent plastic chamber affixed to the monkey's head.

um was also injected into the brain at defined coordinate positions, and imaged with structural MRI to verify the coordinate system.

Carbon Fiber Electrode Fabrication and Conditioning

Carbon fiber microelectrodes constructed for rodents (e.g., [11]) are too short for deep structures in larger brains. The specific resistance of carbon fiber used for FSCV is in the order of 1500 μΩ-cm, or about 4.5 KΩ per cm for a 7 μm diameter fiber. This high resistance requires providing a conductive wire electrical connection near the electrode tip. Therefore, we developed a two-stage fused silica design that could be manipulated with a microdrive typically used for single-unit recording. The design is similar to previous electrode designs [26–28].

The electrode is schematized in Fig. 3A and pictured in Fig. 3B–C. A 4 cm length of carbon fiber, 7 μm diameter (Type C 005722, Tex #795, Goodfellow, Oakdale, PA), is threaded through a 1.5 cm length of polyimide-coated silica capillary tubing (150 μm O.D., 75 μm I.D., Type TSP075150, Polymicro Technologies, Phoenix, AZ, USA). The carbon fiber and silica tube are submerged in a Petri dish of isopropanol during this step. This step is aided by a dissection microscope illuminated from below. Tapping the silica tube against the bottom of the Petri dish dislodges air bubbles in the lumen of the tube and allows the tube to fill completely. The fiber is then pushed into the tube with a cotton-tipped applicator while the tube is stabilized with fine forceps.

Once threaded, the tube with inserted fiber is removed from the isopropanol and mounted with tape on a small platform. The protruding carbon fiber is allowed to hang over the edge of the platform. A scrap piece of tubing is placed underneath the opposite end of the tube to lift it from the platform. The fiber protruding out the elevated end can then be pulled through the tube. The fiber is glued at one end of the silica tube with two-part epoxy gel (Devcon 14240, ITW Devcon, Danvers, MA) using a stainless steel wire to apply the mixed gel. Care is necessary to limit the epoxy contact with the fiber near the entry point of the tube. The fiber is then pulled slightly into the tube as the epoxy is applied, so that some of the epoxy joint is inside the tubing and the epoxy outside the tube tapers smoothly (Fig. 3C). The epoxy cures in about two hours. After curing, the assembly is taped to a flat surface. The exposed carbon fiber on the glued end is cut to a length between 125–150 μm with iridectomy scissors. This completes the first stage of the assembly.

A second stage "shaft" is necessary because: 1) the overall length of the electrode needs to be about 10 cm, 2) the small capillary tubing is not stiff enough to track a straight trajectory in the brain, and 3) the carbon fiber is a poor conductor. The second stage is constructed using larger capillary tubing with internal stainless steel wire. This larger polyimide-coated silica capillary tubing (350 μm O.D., 180 μm I.D., Type TSP180350, Polymicro Technologies, Phoenix, AZ) is cut to length as necessary (typically 95 mm). A 0.051 mm diameter stainless steel wire (part number 792600, 0.002 in, half-hard, 155–185 kPSI, A–M Systems, Sequim, WA) is threaded through the larger capillary tubing. The wire is cut so about 2 cm extends beyond each end. The carbon fiber assembly is taped flat onto an opaque surface under the dissecting microscope; here, the assembly is illuminated from above. The stainless steel wire is coated on one end with conductive silver paint (05002-AB, SPI Supplies, West Chester, PA). The next steps must be done quickly while the silver paint is still wet. The painted stainless steel wire is inserted into the back of the carbon fiber/silica tube assembly, which pushes the carbon fiber deep into the assembly. Care must be taken to ensure the carbon fiber does not fold too sharply and break. The large tube is slipped over the small tube, leaving about 8–10 mm of the small tube protruding from the large one. The two capillary tubes are sealed together with cyanoacrylate (KG585, Krazy Glue, Columbus, OH). The stainless steel wire extending from the back of the large capillary tubing is also sealed with cyanoacrylate and trimmed to about 2 cm. This wire provides an electrical contact for the voltammetry head stage. The full assembly is allowed to sit overnight before use.

Carbon fiber microelectrodes were cycled at 60 Hz for approximately 30 min in aCSF solution just prior to use to condition the carbon surface and thus raise sensitivity for recording stability [29]. We monitored stability by quantifying baseline shifts during every 2-min voltammetry recording, both in the flow cell and *in vivo*. Electrodes that could not maintain a stable baseline (less than 5 nA change in any 10 s epoch) in the flow cell were rejected. Those that could not maintain a stable baseline in the brain were removed and recordings were usually terminated for that day. Background noise of the electrode was an equally important factor, because it established the minimum resolution of the background-subtracted DA measurements. Electrodes with subtracted noise levels above 0.5 nA were rejected. When excessive electrode noise developed during an experiment, recordings were terminated. Electrodes were fabricated in batches of 10 to 20 electrodes. About half met criteria for use after flow cell testing. The shelf life of an electrode was from 3 to 7 days.

Reference Electrode Fabrication

Ag/AgCl electrodes were used to reference the voltammetry signals. A length of high purity 30 gauge silver wire (AG10X, Sigmund Cohn/Medwire, Mt. Vernon, NY) was cut and electrolytically coated with chloride using a regulated power

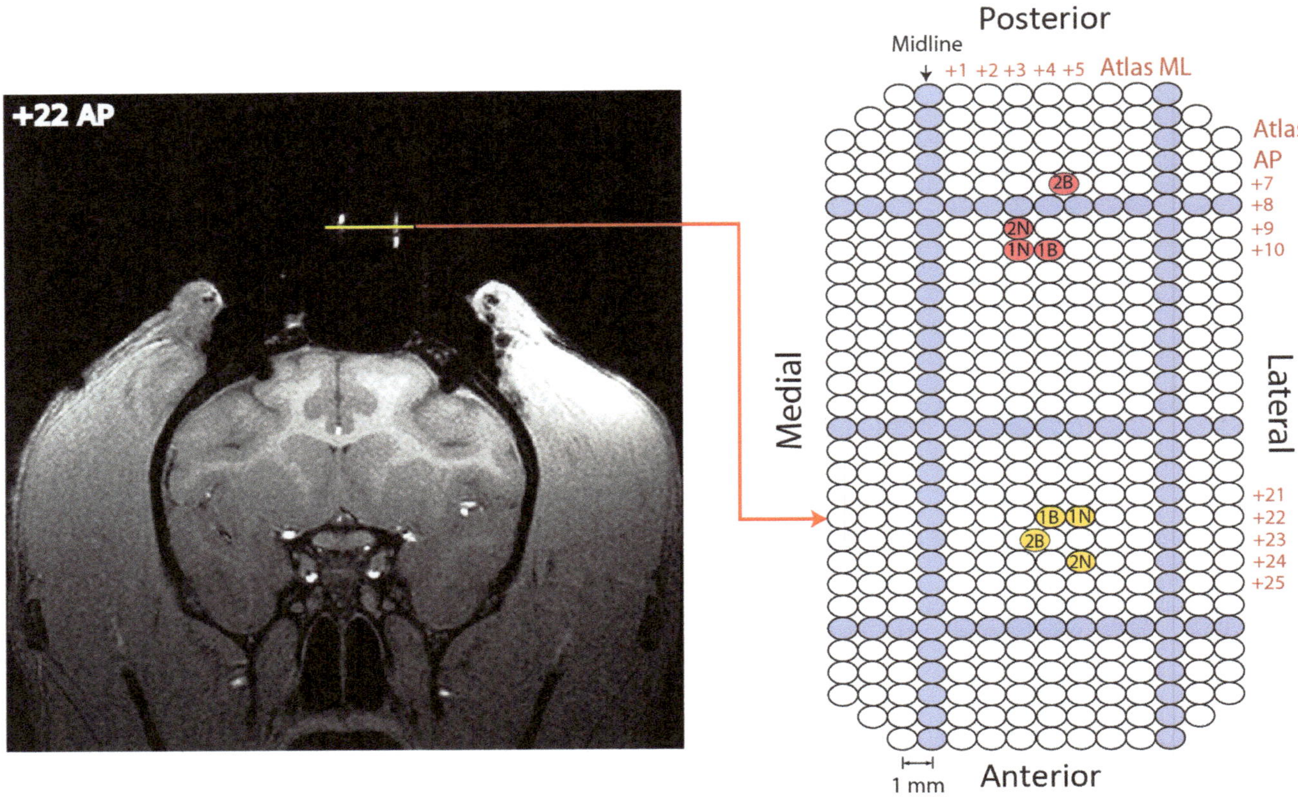

Figure 2. Location of stimulation and recording sites. A grid with 1 mm×1 mm spacing (see Fig. 1) was filled with a contrast agent to align T1-weighted structural MRIs with the coordinate system of the recording chamber. The same grid could be offset by 0.5 mm in the mediolateral (ML) axis, so some penetrations occurred half way between adjacent ML holes in this figure. Left: Frontal MRI section that best matches atlas coordinate AP 22 in monkey B. The horizontal line above the brain is parallel to the plane of the recording chamber. It intersects with two of the filled grid holes, which appear as vertical lines. The distance between the filled grid holes is 8 mm. Right: Map of grid holes used for recording and stimulation. Darker rows indicate holes filled with contrast agent for MRI in monkey B. An arrow shows best AP correspondence with MRI to the left. The AP and ML atlas coordinates of each hole are shown alongside the grid for select grid locations, so that results from both monkeys can be shown here on a common grid map. Example VTA/SNc stimulation (posterior group) and matching FSCV recording (anterior group) sites are plotted on the grid. Matching sites have the same letter/number designation. Letter designates monkey B or N. Table 1 shows the depths of the labeled sites.

supply set to 9 V DC. The silver wire was connected to the positive terminal via a clip-lead and dipped 1 to 2 cm deep into 0.1 N HCl solution for 10 s. A submerged stainless steel ground wire served as the return lead for the 9 V power source. The coated silver wire was threaded through a 95 mm length of large silica capillary tubing, as used in the carbon fiber electrode fabrication. The coated end was extended 7 mm from one end of the tube and glued in place with cyanoacrylate. The other end was also sealed with cyanoacrylate and trimmed to a convenient length for electrical connection.

Electrical Stimulation

Electrical stimulation was used to produce large, time-locked DA release. Stimulation-evoked DA release provides a strong DA signal to test electrodes *in vivo*, helps locate regions of the striatum where DA signals are present, and provides a tool to monitor the effects of pharmacological agents in awake primates.

We tested two different approaches to electrical stimulation: local stimulation near the carbon fiber electrode in the striatum and VTA/SNc stimulation aimed at the cell bodies or perhaps axons of midbrain DA neurons. VTA/SNc stimulation was effective in 3 of 12 attempts from monkey N and in 2 out of 20 attempts from monkey B. Local stimulation was effective in 10 out of 14 attempts in monkey N. In either case, Epoxylite coated 250 μm diameter sharpened Tungsten electrodes (FHC Inc., Bowdoin, ME) were used both for single unit recording and monopolar electrical stimulation. For stimulation, insulation near the tip of stock electrodes was removed with a sharp scalpel to increase the surface area. We selected 10–90 kΩ impedance (Z, measured at 1 KHz in saline using a sinusoidal waveform) electrodes for local stimulation and Z = 50–140 kΩ electrodes for VTA/SNc stimulation. The differences in these ranges reflect the evolution of our methods more than any systematic choice based on the region being stimulated. Low impedance electrodes are appropriate for the currents used in this study. The electrodes with Z near 100 kΩ have ~1000 μm^2 surface area and relatively blunt tips. These electrode characteristics are preferred for repeated electrical stimulation deep in the brain [30]. The distribution of current spread beyond ~50 μm from the electrode tip resembles that of a point source [30], so it is easier to make estimates of current spread compared to bipolar electrodes. Bipolar electrodes are, by necessity, larger. We chose to avoid the larger electrodes because our experiment used repeated entry into different parts of the VTA/SNc and striatum. Bipolar electrodes would have caused substantially more damage.

We kept most stimulation currents below 400 μA and all stimulation was symmetric biphasic to minimize the negative

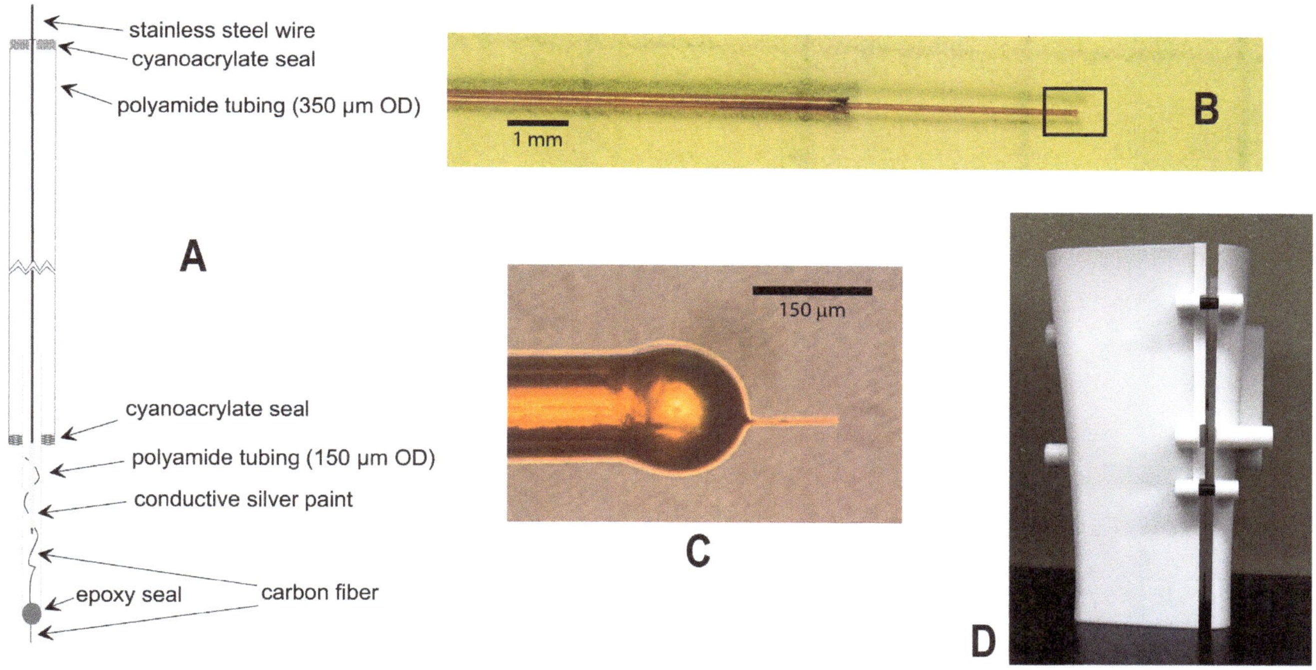

Figure 3. Carbon fiber electrode and printed Faraday shield. (A) Schematic of carbon fiber electrode construction. The 7 μm carbon fiber is electrically connected to a 51 μm (.002 in) diameter stainless steel wire using silver paint. Cyanoacrylate and epoxy provide seals for the two different size polyimide-coated silica capillary tubing. (B) Photograph of the carbon fiber electrode centered near junction of large and small tubes. (C) Expanded region of the black outlined square in tile B is a photomicrograph of exposed carbon fiber and epoxy seal. (D) Two-part Faraday shield. Each side of the clamshell shield was printed on a plastic printer. Plastic alignment pins (in black) and retaining screws (not shown) were added after printing. Base of shield closely fits the dimensions of the microdrive base and chamber (see Fig. 1), providing clearance for the posterior head post. The upper portion is wider to accommodate connections to the microdrive towers. The smaller section is held fixed and the larger section is removable. Photo taken before the application of conductive paint.

effects of charge density and net charge transfer. These characteristics are in line with other studies of stimulation evoked DA release (e.g., [10,31]). When higher currents were tested, they never exceeded 3 times the threshold for a nearby response. Given the long-term, e.g., hours, of stable evoked DA responses we observed in this study and our extensive experience using the same stimulation method mapping cortical motor areas [22,32], it is evident that our electrodes and stimulation parameters are effective and sufficiently benign.

The timing of electrical stimulation was controlled by a custom-built circuit that generated the number and frequency of stimulation pulses (Appendix S1). It tracked the FSCV sweeps and avoided these sweeps to assure electrical stimulation did not produce artifacts in the voltammograms. Optionally, it was often programmed to interfere with just the first stimulus pulse to provide a timing marker on the voltammogram. Once the stimulation timing pulses were generated, these pulses were delivered to a Master-8-vp (AMPI, Jerusalem, Israel) to provide cathode-first biphasic rectangular pulses of varying amplitudes in the ±2 V range. In the last step, these biphasic voltage pulses drove a biphasic linear isolation unit (LSIU-01, Cygnus Technology, Delaware Water Gap, PA) connected to the stimulation electrode and referenced to the same electrode's stainless steel guide cannula. The isolation unit has an electrode shorting input to assure no current can flow between stimulus trains. The shorting circuit was managed by the microprocessor-based controller. The internal calibration of the Master-8-vp output voltage range was readjusted to match the isolation unit range (±2 V), which permitted finer resolution of the delivered current. Stimulation was delivered as symmetric biphasic pulses, 500 μs/phase, cathodal first. Stimulation trains were delivered at 120 PPS and lasted for approximately 1 s, unless otherwise noted. Stimulation was delivered starting 20 s into each 40 s voltammetry recording. Unless otherwise noted, a minimum of 5 min separated each stimulation pulse train.

Microstimulation

On a few occasions, we observed and noted evoked movements in response to microstimulation in the midbrain. For these tracks, 100 ms pulse trains were delivered through tungsten electrodes (Z = 15 kΩ) at 300 PPS. Stimulation was delivered as symmetric biphasic pulses, 500 μs/phase, cathodal first. There was no specific wait time imposed between these stimulation trains. All stimulation was delivered using the guide cannula of the stimulation electrode as the reference electrode.

Voltammetry

Electrode selection. Voltammetry was carried out using a version of the Tar Heel CV recording system developed at the University of North Carolina, and updated and supplied by Dr. Scott Ng-Evans (Seattle, WA). A matching system was used for flow-cell testing and electrode selection. Flow cell components were provided by the same vendor. This system uses a syringe infusion pump (Model 22, Harvard Apparatus, Holliston, MA) to deliver a constant flow of 1.5 ml/min through a 250 μL sample loop, switched in-line by a 2-way injection valve (V-1451-DC,

Upchurch/IDEX, Oak Harbor, WA). Carbon fiber electrodes were fabricated with target flow-cell sensitivity between 10 and 25 nA/μM (Fig. 4A).

The goal of FSCV is to measure the concentration of a chemical species in the brain by measuring current flow during oxidation. The voltage between a working electrode and suitable reference is swept through the peak oxidation potential, and then swept back through the reduction potential, for the chemical species being measured [11]. During these sweeps, the current flow through the working electrode is converted to a voltage with a high-gain gyrator circuit, and then digitized. When subtracted from background current, the current measured during a sweep provides a signature for the chemical species and an estimate of the change in concentration of that species in solution. The rising voltage sweep passes through the peak oxidation potential of DA (+0.6 V versus Ag/AgCl reference), and current differences of about 1 to 50 nA reflect interstitial concentration changes of DA. The very small surface area of the working electrode permits rapid measurements in a small volume of tissue and produces small oxidation/reduction currents.

Calibration of electrode sensitivity (nA/μM) is necessary to estimate DA concentration. Calibration requires bathing the electrode in known concentrations of the electrolyte in a flow cell. These are idealized conditions, however. Voltage scanning parameters [11], electrode conditioning [33] and environmental factors limit in vivo accuracy based upon flow cell electrode calibration. Environmental factors affecting current response to intracerebral DA include local calcium (Ca^{2+}) and magnesium (Mg^{2+}) concentrations [34], interference by pH and O_2 changes [18], fouling of the carbon fiber surface by extracellular metabolites [35] and the difference between flow-cell temperatures and body temperatures [36].

The flow cell was used to select candidate electrodes. On each recording day, the sensitivity of each available electrode was estimated by a single flow cell measurement at 1.0 μM DA concentration. An example is shown in Fig. 4A. Only electrodes that produced stable recordings, low noise, and current values nearest to 20 nA, were selected for use.

To correlate this single measurement with electrode sensitivity, we ran a complete calibration on a single sample electrode using 5 different test concentrations (0.5 μM, 0.75 μM, 1.0 μM, 1.5 μM, 2.0 μM) of DA solution (Fig. 4B). All test solutions were prepared from a 2.0 mM stock solution of DA mixed the day of calibration. First, a 20.0 μM solution was made from the 2.0 mM stock, then a 2.0 μM solution was created from the 20.0 μM solution. Test solutions were mixed in amber vials wrapped in foil to prevent light exposure and kept over ice prior to flow cell loading. Electrode calibration began with the smallest test concentration (0.5 μM) followed by increasing concentrations. The injection circuit was flushed with DI water and cleared with air between concentrations. Recording files were 20 s in duration with a 1–5 s DA injection during the recording. Each concentration was tested 4–5 times. The average peak current at the oxidation potential of DA (near +0.6 V) was plotted at each concentration (Fig. 4B). The slope of the regression line is 13.1 nA/μM, which is taken to be the actual sensitivity of the electrode in aCSF. The first value at each concentration was higher than subsequent values. At 1.0 μM DA concentration, the first value was 17.4 nA. We note that taking an average of 5 measurements at 1.0 μM provides a substantially better estimate (Fig. 4B). Thus, we presume that relying on a single flow cell test tends to overestimate the electrode sensitivity in aCSF.

Shielding and microdrive system. Faraday shielding for single unit and voltammetry recording was provided by a custom

Table 1. VTA/SNc evoked dopamine responses.

Site	Stimulation AP	Stimulation ML	Stimulation EBZ	FSCV Recording AP	FSCV Recording ML	FSCV Recording EBZ	Current
1N	10.0	3.0	9.0	22.0	5.0	17.0	11.0 nA
2N	9.0	3.0	8.0	24.0	5.0	17.5	1.5 nA
1B	10.0	4.0	11.4	22.0	4.0	16.1	11.5 nA
2B	7.0	4.5	9.5	23.0	3.5	9.5	10.0 nA

Site designations match those in Fig. 2. AP, ML and EBZ (ear bar zero) are atlas coordinates [25]. Current is the largest dopamine current evoked at the site.

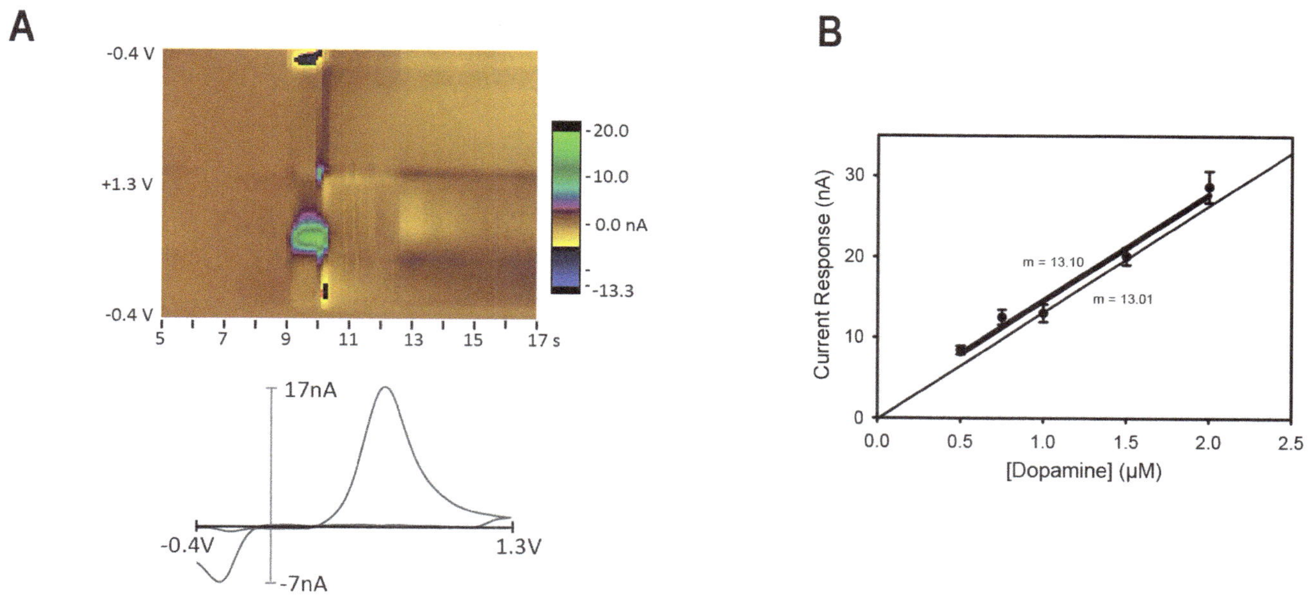

Figure 4. Electrode selection. Electrodes were selected for low noise, stability and reasonable sensitivity. Just prior to recording, available electrodes were tested by injecting a single 1.0 μM, 1–5 s bolus of DA at 1.5 ml/min in a flow-cell apparatus. (A) Pseudo-color plot and corresponding voltammogram response to single bolus at 1.0 μM. The measured peak value is 16.9 nA at 0.62 V. (B) Thick line: complete calibration of another electrode calculated by averaging 4–5 samples of each concentration from the series 0.5, 0.75, 1.0, 1.5 and 2.0 μM (sensitivity = 13.1 nA/μM). Error bars are SEM. Thin line: simplified calibration using only the values collected at 1 μM and the origin (sensitivity = 13.0 nA/μM).

two-part plastic encasement printed on a Fortus 360 mc 3D plastic printer (Stratasys, Eden Prairie, MN), using ABS-M30 material (Figs. 1, 3D). All plastic surfaces were coated with CuPro-Cote conductive paint (Less EMF Inc, Latham, NY) using a paintbrush. The encasement was air dried for 48 hours before use. The voltammetry, reference and recording/stimulation electrodes were each mounted on a stepper motor-driven multi-electrode microdrive (NAN-S4 with custom base, NAN Instruments, Nazareth, Israel), and each was guided by a sharpened 22 gauge standard-wall stainless steel cannula (Fig. 1). Each microdrive tower provides manual movement of a guide cannula and precision movement of an electrode along the same axis. The shield was designed to provide a snug fit to the base of the recording chamber and a loose fit near the electrode wire connections. The shield can be opened and closed without disturbing the electrical connections. The shield height matched the stepper motor tower heights. The posterior, smaller component of the encasement was shaped to avoid the Titanium head post. To determine the shape, a model was first molded using many layers of aluminum foil with all the recording components mounted on the subject's head. The 3D aluminum foil structure was then cut along the long axis for removal and rejoined with thermal glue. Additional glue helped stabilize the model. The final design was drawn as a straight-line segment approximation of the model. The split between the two shield components was located for maximum access to electrodes when the larger component was removed.

Electrode mounting was performed prior to recordings on a support arm (Fig. 1). Cannulae were inserted into a grid array of holes and a microdrive tower was adjusted to align with each cannula. The grid could be inserted in two different orientations, providing a 0.5 mm medial-lateral offset between the orientations. After insertion, cannulae were clamped to a lower, manual positioner and remained electrically isolated from the tower and base. Electrodes, one of each type, were inserted into each cannula and clamped to the upper, stepper motor positioner, also electrically isolated from the other components. The electrodes were then carefully aligned to the lower margin of a 30 mm×14 mm grid array of drilled guide holes using the positioning motors. After loading and alignment, the assembly was transferred to the recording chamber on the monkey. The guide cannulas were carefully lowered through the dura by hand, each to a predetermined depth. The reference electrode cannula was placed just below the dura. The other two cannulas were lowered to within 3–5 mm above the electrode final target positions. The Faraday shield was closed as the electrodes were automatically lowered to the bottom of their respective guide cannulas. The reference electrode was inserted into the brain first, followed by the carbon fiber electrode. The stimulation electrode was then lowered to its starting position in the brain. All electrodes were lowered at a maximum rate of 0.1 mm/s while still in the guide tube, and 0.01 mm/s in the brain until reaching the initial recording and stimulation sites. Once the electrodes were in position, the carbon fiber electrode was cycled at 10 Hz for up to 45 min. Electrodes were then moved at 0.001 mm/s between recording and stimulation sites.

During local stimulation, voltammetry recordings were often made after electrode movement, but before stimulation, to assess the stability and noise characteristics of the carbon fiber electrode. The stimulation electrode was advanced in 0.1 mm steps and stimulation was tested at every depth until finding a strong response without an overwhelming artifact. Stimulus trains were always separated by at least 5 min following a DA response. After choosing a final position for the electrode, the time of the first stimulation train at this depth was assigned time = 0 for the purpose of testing response stability.

Recording sessions. During setup, the carbon fiber electrode microdrive tower was positioned over a grid hole above the striatum. When used for local stimulation, the stimulation

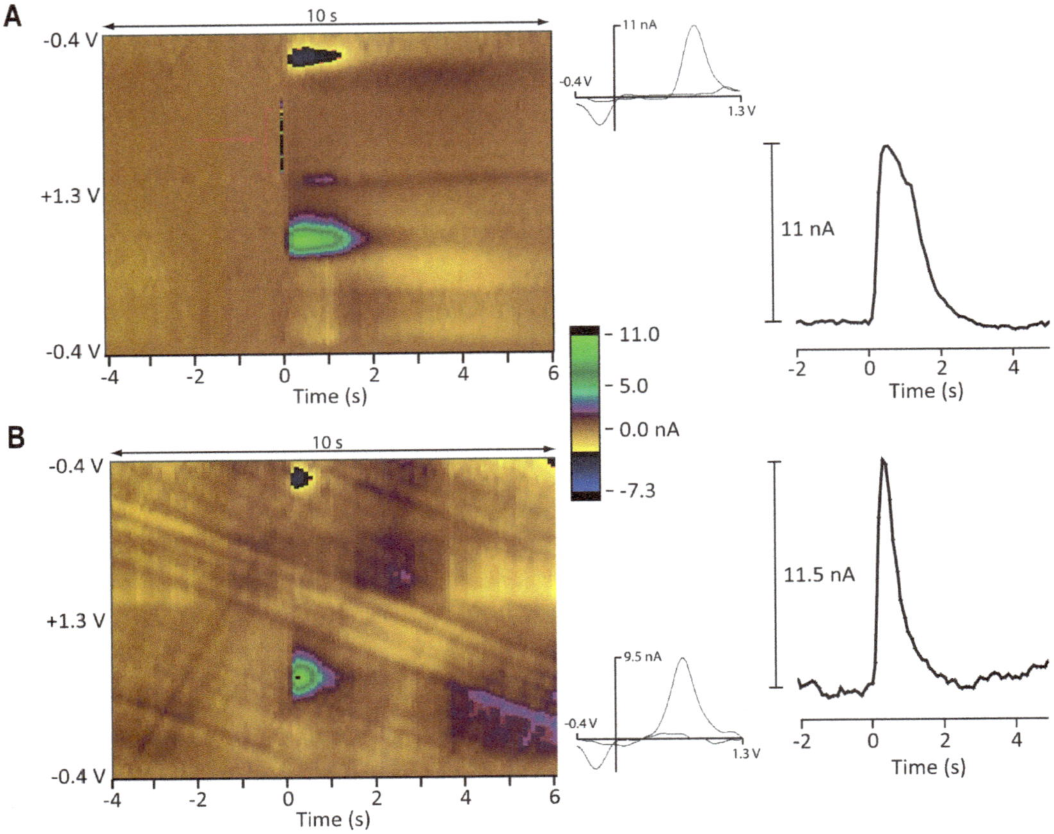

Figure 5. VTA/SNc stimulation-evoked response in two subjects. VTA/SNc stimulation-evoked dopamine response recorded from the ventral striatum of two monkeys. (A) Monkey N. Stimulation parameters: 400 μA, 120 PPS, 1 s train. Left: background subtracted color plot corresponding to the pair of sites designated 2N in Fig. 2 and Table 1. DA release follows rapidly after stimulation at time 0. The red arrow and bracket point to the intentional stimulation artifact that marks onset of stimulation. Right: Small inset graph shows the voltammogram at maximum DA release. Larger plot shows the current response at peak oxidation potential. (B) Monkey B. Stimulation parameters: 200 μA, 120 PPS, 2 s train. Left: background subtracted color plot corresponding to the pair of sites 1B in Fig.2 and Table 1. DA release following stimulation at time 0. Right: Same plots as in A. Vertical color bar shows pseudocolor calibration for both color plots.

electrode tower was positioned over a grid hole 1 mm posterior to the carbon fiber electrode in the same ML plane. Alternatively, for VTA/SNc stimulation, the stimulation tower was placed over a grid hole positioned above the VTA/SNc. The reference electrode tower was placed above the primary motor cortex, 7–10 mm lateral to the midline. Stimulation and recording tracks were chosen based on whether or not the track had been explored previously, whether DA had been found along that track, or whether multiple electrodes broke along the track. We chose, initially, to explore most of the available tracks throughout the ventral striatum before returning to previously explored tracks, even though we were successful in evoking DA from previously explored tracks. When we were able to record DA release and did not move the stimulation electrode, the stimulation-evoked response remained consistent throughout the recording session. During these recording sessions, stimulation evoked DA was recorded every 5 min until the end of the experimental protocol.

The stimulation controller (Appendix S1) could be programmed to deliver single microstimulation stimuli during the next FSCV sweep following a button press. The size of the "artifact" recorded by the voltammetry system provides a relative measure of distance between the stimulation and carbon fiber electrodes. We used these artifacts to evaluate the accuracy of our electrode positioning measurements by estimating the distance between electrodes as a function of normalized current strength. Current measurements as a function of electrode position were fitted to:

$$i_N = r_0^2/\left(r_0^2 + x^2\right)$$

where i_N is normalized current, x is the distance between electrodes and r_0 is the nearest approach. Derivation and application of this approach is provided in Appendix S2. Errors in nearest distance measurements and in depth measurements were estimated separately after fitting the equation. This technique provides measurements separate from the microdrive system, which is subject to the flexible nature of the carbon fiber electrode and the long distances traveled by both electrodes.

With each new animal, single unit recordings, usually in the first week of recording, helped locate deep structures in the region of the VTA and substantia nigra. Unit recordings were made with one of two Tucker-Davis Technologies RZ series recording systems (RZ2 and RZ5, Tucker-Davis Technologies, Alachua, FL). A custom remote-switching head stage permitted recording and stimulation through a single electrode in monkey B.

Results

FSCV Response to VTA/SNc Stimulation

We carried out experiments in which a stimulation electrode was introduced into the VTA/SNc and a carbon fiber electrode was introduced into the ventral striatum. Electrode locations were verified with MRI (see Implants section). Example stimulation and recording sites from both monkeys are shown in Fig. 2 with atlas coordinates and peak evoked currents in Table 1. Fig. 5A shows an example of evoked DA release in the striatum of monkey N when the stimulation electrode was in the ventromedial aspect of the SNc (Fig. 2 and Table 1 grid position 1N). The red arrow in the color plot shows where the first pulse of the stimulator intentionally interfered with the first voltammetry scan cycle of the stimulation period, providing a marker 20 s into the recording period (see Appendix S1). The maximum stimulation evoked response in this example was about 11 nA, using a 400 μA stimulation current. DA release was rapid (latency <100 ms) and the response persisted throughout the entire 1 s stimulation train period. We also evoked dopamine release by stimulating DA neuron cell bodies in monkey B (Fig. 5B, grid position 1B in Fig. 2 and Table 1) and, in this case, the largest peak response was over 11 nA. VTA/SNc evoked dopamine oxidation peaks in the brain were higher than oxidation peaks recorded in the flow cell, typically by about 160 mV.

Our stimulation covered much of the SNc that projects to the caudate and ventral striatum and a portion of the VTA (Fig. 6). The medial most part of VTA was inaccessible with our microdrive arrangement because it would have risked damage to the superior sagittal sinus. This part of the VTA projects to the most medial and most ventral regions of the striatum [3]. The most ventral regions of the striatum were explored sparingly during the stimulation experiments to limit damage to the remainder of the striatum.

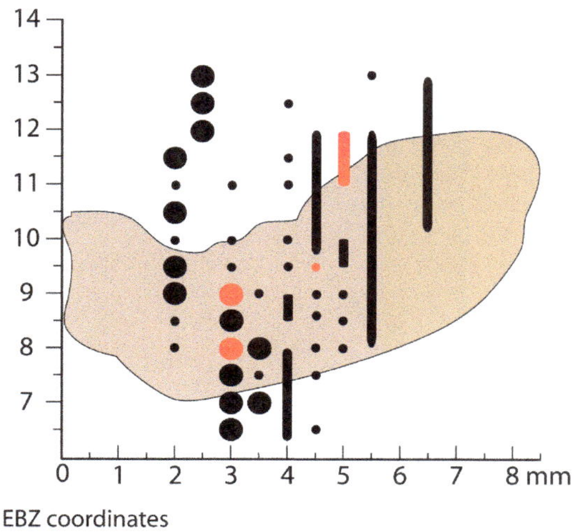

Figure 6. Distribution of stimulation sites in the VTA/SN. Outline of VTA/SN from all AP levels projected onto a single AP plane. The origins of the remaining axes are relative to ear bar zero (EBZ, see description in [25]). Black circles represent all stimulation sites where no dopamine release was observed. Red circles represent all stimulation sites where dopamine release was recorded. Small circles indicate stimulation currents ≤300 μA. Large circles indicate application of a > 300 μA, typically 400 μA current. The vertical columns represent a series of stimulation sites along the rostral-caudal axis separated by less than 250 μm. In these columns, color and size codes remain the same.

Larger stimulation currents may have allowed us to evoke DA release more consistently in the striatum. However, it was rarely possible to employ large (>400 μA) currents when stimulating in VTA or SNc. Electrical stimulation within the VTA/SNc can evoke movements from the nearby magnocellular division of the red nucleus (RN) and the cerebral peduncles. The rostral tip of RN is just lateral to VTA. Further, SNc is sandwiched by RN dorsally and the cerebral peduncle ventrally [25]. Unwanted evoked movements mechanically disturb the carbon fiber electrode and thereby produce voltammetry recording artifacts. We observed stimulus evoked movement latencies in the voltammetry recordings as brief as 200 ms (two voltammetry cycles). We decided to map the somatotopy of stimulation-evoked movement along two tracks to verify that current spread to known motor structures was the source of evoked movements. Fig. 7 shows the two electrode tracks where microstimulation evoked movements using short stimulus trains (50 ms duration, 30 pulses) and relatively low currents (50 μA). The results from these two tracks suggest that large movement artifacts were caused by current spread to the RN [37] or to corticospinal fibers passing through the cerebral peduncles [38], but not to thalamic sites; thalamic stimulation sites at this AP level did not produce movements or movement artifacts.

FSCV Response to Local Stimulation

We also carried out local stimulation in the striatum, near the carbon-fiber electrode (<1 mm). This approach is commonly used in rodent brain slice preparations of striatal tissue. The distance between the stimulation electrode and the carbon fiber electrode is generally 100 to 400 μm in brain slice experiments [10,39,40]. The mechanism of DA release in striatum is consistent with axonal depolarization by the stimulation current [40]. These studies use bipolar electrodes and stimulus currents in the hundreds of microamperes. In the present study, monopolar stimulation was used deep in the brain to prevent the additional damage caused by inserting a larger bipolar electrode each day. Fig. 8A shows a representative phasic DA release event in the ventral striatum evoked by local electrical stimulation at 50 μA. We applied local stimulation in monkey N at sites in both the ventral striatum and more dorsal-laterally in the putamen.

Voltammetry recordings made after electrode movement, but before stimulation, did not show any transient DA release attributable to movement of the stimulation electrode. However, we did not attempt to measure changes in the background level of DA that may have resulted from movement of the stimulation electrode.

In 6 of the days that we were able to evoke release, we tested the stability of the DA recording for at least 20 min. On those days, we continued to record stimulation-evoked DA responses every 5 min over a 20 min period. On 4 of 6 days testing was continued for at least 5 more min. Fig. 8B shows the time course averages for these stability tests. The first two measurements (at times 0 and 5 min) on each day are averaged to define the baseline for that day. All points are plotted as a percent change from baseline averaged across days.

Based upon depth measurements, the clearest examples of recorded DA did not seem to occur when the two electrodes were adjacent. When the electrodes were at their closest point, the DA oxidation potential was often obscured by other signals on the voltammogram (not shown), presumably related to shifts in pH or Ca^{2+} ions [18,21]. However, when the electrodes were farther apart (>2 mm), we were not able to evoke a DA response. To verify these distance observations, we examined the accuracy of electrode position measurements by artifact analysis (see Appendix

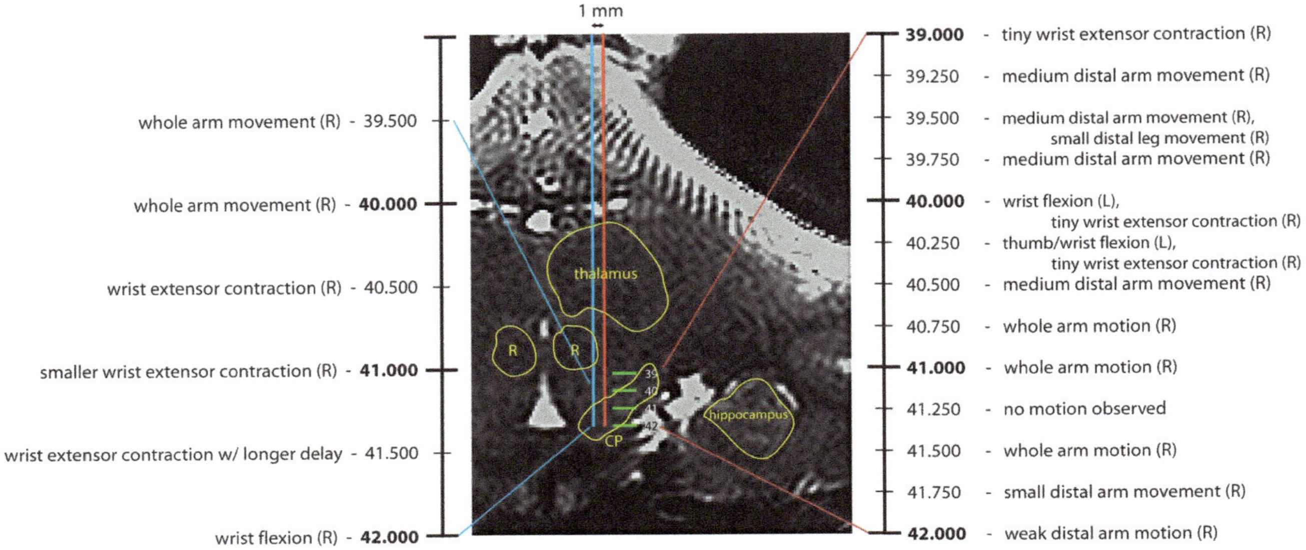

Figure 7. Microstimulation mapping of movements evoked near VTA/SNc. Microstimulation was used to map observed limb movements evoked along two tracks in Monkey N. 100 μA was used for the more medial track (ML 4.5), 50 μA was used 1 mm more laterally (ML 5.5) in the same AP (+9) plane. Stimulus trains were 100 ms at 300 PPS. Actual depths (below cortical surface) are denoted on the scan image. Expanded scales on the left and right indicate observed movements. All movements were brief and time-locked to the stimulation. Anatomical landmarks are outlined on the image (CP – cerebral peduncle; R – red nucleus).

S2). Measured errors in electrode position were within ±0.5 mm along the XY plane of the microdrive (Fig. 9A). Relative depth readings were accurate and stimulation electrode positions were systematically a little more superficial than expected (Fig. 9B). We confirm that a separation of 200–500 μm was beneficial for observing DA.

Juice Reward

In monkeys and rodents, DA neurons increase their firing rates, or DA is released when the animal receives an unexpected rewarding stimulus [41,42], which can depend upon the behavioral state [43]. To examine responses to unexpected rewards, apple juice was delivered with a precision pressure driven liquid delivery system [44]. We manually delivered three ~0.5 ml squirts of juice in rapid succession to the monkey. We were able to evoke reward-related DA during 4 of 10 experiments over a 7-week period. In two experiments, DA was evident after every reward trio (15/15 over 98 min and 7/7 over 28 min). In one experiment, DA was evoked only about half the time (6/13 over 177 min). In the last case, DA was evoked only once (1/4 over 70 min). Fig. 10 shows two example responses from one experiment. The responses were relatively small (<1 nA) compared to stimulation-evoked responses, but occurred with all 15 trios of rewards over 98 min. The response amplitudes are consistent with those observed in rodent studies.

Discussion

We have demonstrated that FSCV can be used to measure transient DA release in monkey striatum using three different methods: recording DA responses time-locked with electrical stimulation in VTA/SNc (Fig. 5), by recording DA responses time-locked with local electrical stimulation in the striatum (Fig. 8), and by recording DA responses time-locked to unexpected rewards (Fig. 10). As expected from the rat literature (e.g., [31]), the responses to behaviorally evoked DA in the monkey were about an order of magnitude smaller than electrically evoked responses. Electrical stimulation helps locate DA rich sites in the striatum, providing a method to position an electrode prior to behavioral experiments [32]. Stimulation is also an aid for observing some pharmacological manipulations since it provides a robust DA signal. Both targets of electrical stimulation are helpful for validating our method, but each has its own benefits. Local stimulation was a more reliable way to achieve putative evoked DA release. Reliability is important for pharmacological manipulations that will further validate that DA is the source of the signal being measured. For now, VTA/SNc stimulation provides the best demonstration that DA is the chemical species being measured, because its projection to the striatum comes specifically from DA-containing neurons.

Compared to rats [11,31,45], finding effective stimulation sites in monkeys VTA/SNc is more difficult. We found active sites of DA release paired with VTA/SNc sites 10–25% of the time in our two monkeys. This relatively low yield is best understood by comparing the anatomical differences between species. Fig. 11 charts the relative sizes of striatum and VTA/SNc in the two species on a common scale by comparing representative coronal sections. DA cell bodies are distributed throughout the VTA/SNc in both the rat [23] and monkey [3]. In the rat, the VTA/SNc is readily activated with 100–350 μA of current (e.g., [16,31,45]). Although bipolar electrodes are most commonly used, current spread to (DA-containing) cell bodies near the electrode tips will be comparable to monopolar stimulation when balanced pulses are used [30,46]. More importantly, the whole of the rat VTA/SNc can be activated at these currents because the DA neurons are all within 2 mm of each other (Fig. 11B, [47]). In the monkey, DA neurons are distributed over the entire 7–8 mm long axis of the VTA/SNc (Fig. 11A, [3]). The current strengths used in rats can activate only a fraction of the DA-containing neurons in monkeys. Larger currents (e.g., [23]) spread outside the VTA/SNc before an

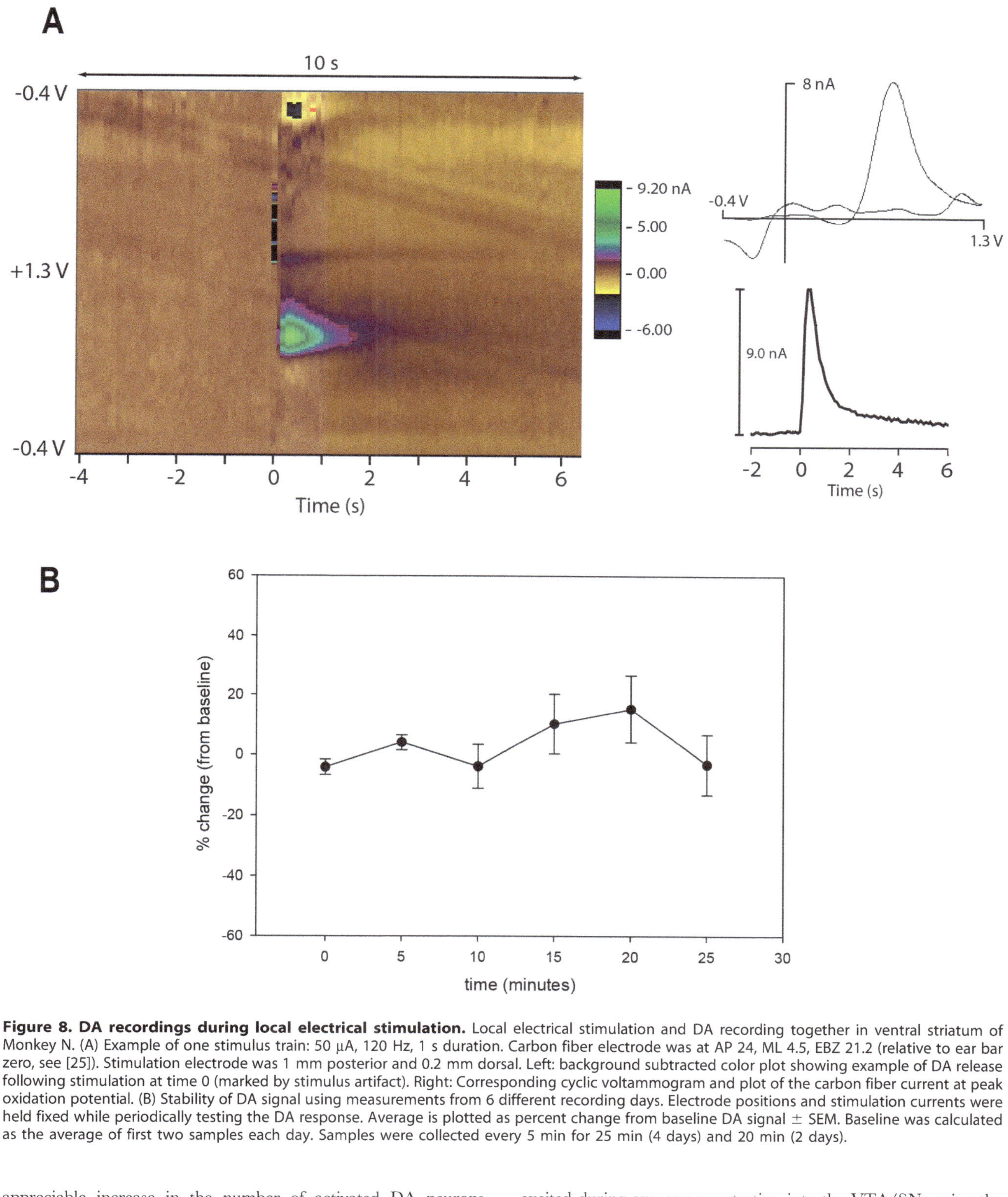

Figure 8. DA recordings during local electrical stimulation. Local electrical stimulation and DA recording together in ventral striatum of Monkey N. (A) Example of one stimulus train: 50 µA, 120 Hz, 1 s duration. Carbon fiber electrode was at AP 24, ML 4.5, EBZ 21.2 (relative to ear bar zero, see [25]). Stimulation electrode was 1 mm posterior and 0.2 mm dorsal. Left: background subtracted color plot showing example of DA release following stimulation at time 0 (marked by stimulus artifact). Right: Corresponding cyclic voltammogram and plot of the carbon fiber current at peak oxidation potential. (B) Stability of DA signal using measurements from 6 different recording days. Electrode positions and stimulation currents were held fixed while periodically testing the DA response. Average is plotted as percent change from baseline DA signal ± SEM. Baseline was calculated as the average of first two samples each day. Samples were collected every 5 min for 25 min (4 days) and 20 min (2 days).

appreciable increase in the number of activated DA neurons owing to the elongated shape of the VTA/SNc (Fig. 11A, bottom) and the high input resistances of the lightly myelinated DA fibers. This current spread outside VTA/SNc evoked movements from the RN and/or cerebral peduncle (Fig. 7). Movements interfered with recordings and even higher currents would likely be noxious to the animal. Thus, only a fraction of the DA neurons can be excited during any one penetration into the VTA/SNc using the angle of penetration we employed. Concomitantly, only a restricted region of the striatum will experience evoked DA release. Searching for the region of striatum experiencing the DA release is hampered by the large territory of the monkey striatum (Fig. 11A, top), especially compared to the rat striatum (Fig. 11B, top). In these illustrative sections, the monkey striatum is

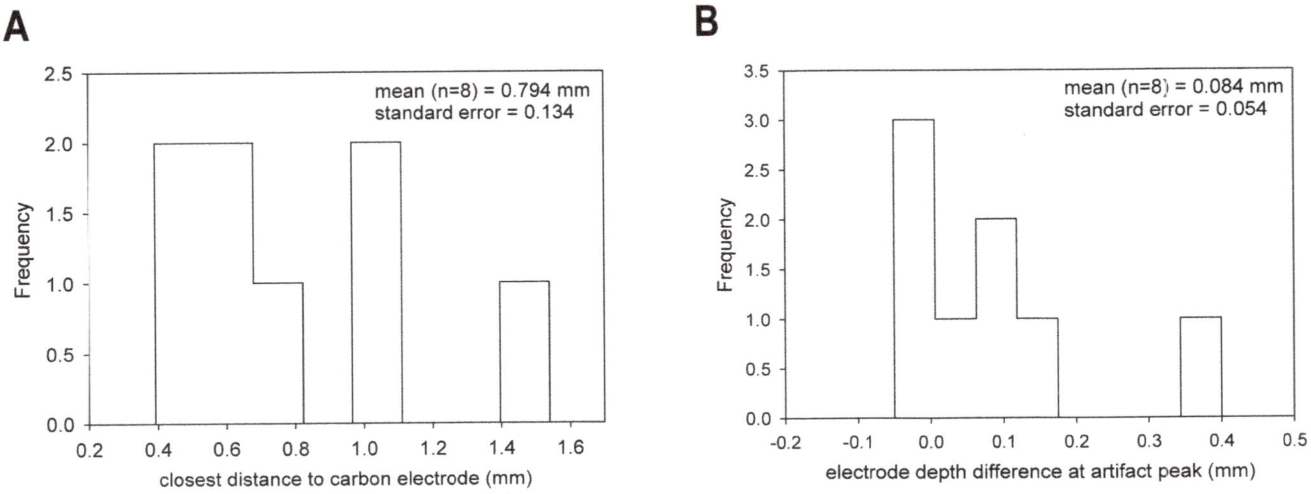

Figure 9. Accuracy of electrode positioning. Errors in drive position along different dimensions as estimated by using the stimulus artifact. (A) Distribution of nearest points between electrodes when using grid holes with 1 mm separation. (B) Distribution of differences between depth of peak artifact and point where both electrodes have the same depth reading. Positive values indicate the stimulation electrode was more superficial than expected.

approximately 8.6 times the size of the rat striatum. The actual search territory is, of course, volumetric across the anterior-posterior dimension.

We chose to use new voltammetry electrodes and make new penetrations with our microdrive each recording day rather than using long-term recording from a single location [27]. This

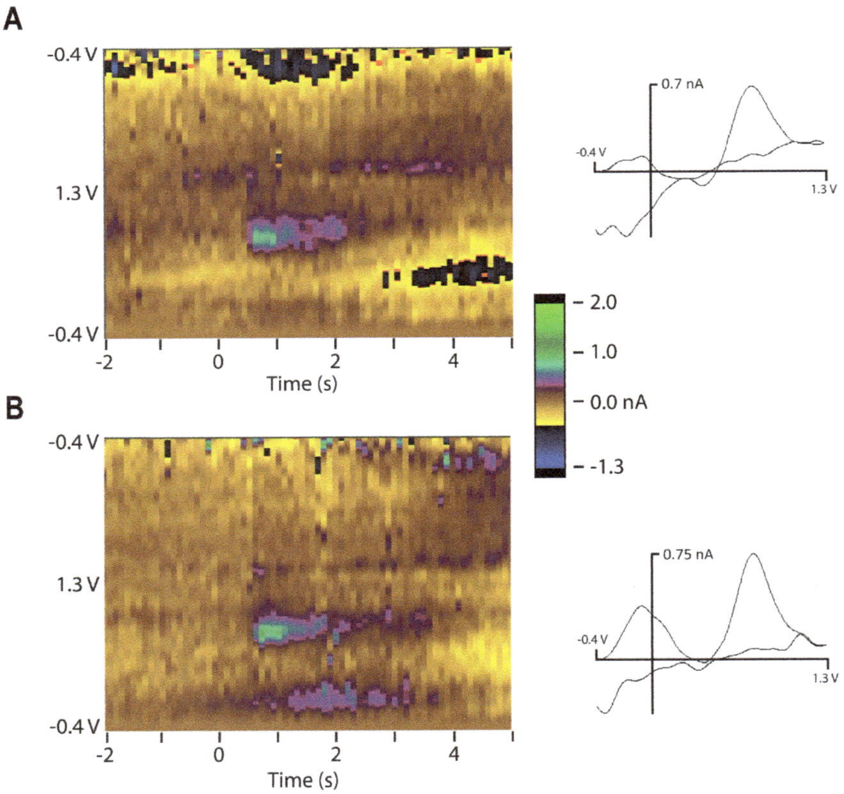

Figure 10. Reward related DA release in the ventral striatum. Triplets of juice rewards were delivered unexpectedly to monkey B, repeated 15 times over the course of 98 min. Carbon fiber electrode was at AP 21, ML 3.0, EBZ 16.1 (relative to ear bar zero, see [25]). Small, but constant dopamine responses occurred with every triplet. Example color plot and accompanying cyclic voltammograms for unexpected juice triplets delivered (A) 69.5 min after the first juice delivery and (B) 30 s later. Dopamine oxidation peaks are about 0.82 V.

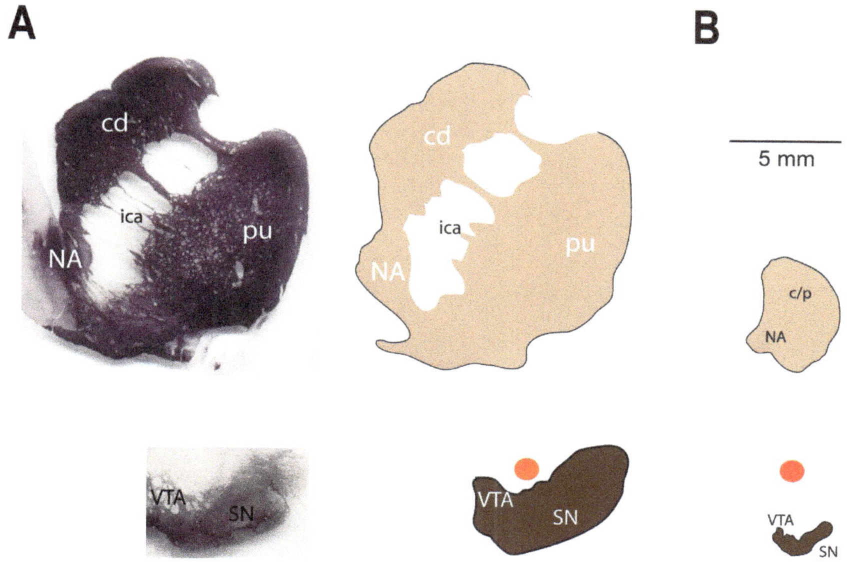

Figure 11. Monkey and rat striatum and VTA/SNc drawn to the same scale. Outlines of representative frontal sections from monkey and rat, striatum and VTA/SN. (A) Photomicrographs (left) of monkey tyrosine hydroxylase (TH) stained sections sized to the scale bar dimensions in B. Territory of monkey (right) striatum and VTA/SN based upon TH sections. (B) Outlines of dopamine neuron cell bodies and terminals in the rat VTA/SN (bottom, plate 43) and striatum (top, plate 17) from Paxinos and Watson atlas [50] estimated using the AChE stains. Circles above VTA/SN are each 1 mm diameter. Approximate area ratios (monkey:rat): striatum including ica = 8.6:1, VTA/SN = 11.2:1. NA - nucleus accumbens, cd - caudate, pu - putamen, ica - internal capsule, c/p - combined caudate/putamen.

allowed us to search broadly for sites where DA release could be evoked by the stimulation electrode, to investigate the distribution of active release sites in the large primate brain and to evaluate the condition of the electrode each day after moving it through cm of brain. The disadvantage of this approach is the cumulative damage incurred by daily tracks. Future work would benefit from a low-profile microdrive that could leave the electrode implanted for weeks, permit electrode movement and allow insertion of a new electrode from time-to-time.

Our microdrive system did not reach into the center of the VTA (Fig. 6), because our chamber was mounted in the horizontal plane. Reaching the center of VTA would have required breaching the superior sagittal sinus with a guide cannula, a risky procedure. As just discussed, although electrical stimulation centered in the VTA will activate the vast majority of midbrain dopamine neurons in the rat, in monkeys it has a restricted projection, primarily to the nucleus accumbens [3]. Using a moveable electrode in monkeys offers an opportunity to explore micro-domains of DA release that may be governed by different regions of the VTA/SNc. During our stimulation experiments, we explored nucleus accumbens less than other parts of striatum because each penetration into that region was accompanied by damage to the more dorsal striatum, and because the center of VTA was difficult to reach. Exploration of nucleus accumbens in concert with VTA stimulation would likely yield additional DA release sites.

There are a number of ways to improve the yield of FSCV DA recordings during VTA/SNc stimulation in monkeys. The evoked DA release shown in Fig. 5A was found in the ventral striatum during stimulation of the ventromedial aspect of the SNc, in rough correspondence with the general topographic organization described by Haber [3]. A detailed map of the VTA/SNc projection could guide electrode placement. This might be accomplished by more fine-grained analysis of existing tracer data or through electrical stimulation mapping with fMRI. Even without additional information, it would be possible to reach more of the VTA and striatum, including medial portions, with a more lateral approach of the stimulating electrode. In this arrangement, a chamber could be tilted along the long axis of the VTA/SNc. A different approach was used by Shon et al. [48] in another large mammal. They evoked DA release over a wide area of the striatum using high levels of stimulation centered on the subthalamic nucleus. To activate such a large area, the animal had to be anesthetized and movements inhibited with additional muscle relaxants.

We propose an alternative strategy for increasing the number of VTA/SNc stimulation-evoked DA responses in awake monkeys. The long axis of the monkey VTA/SNc is well suited for implantation of a passive linear array electrode (e.g., V-Probe, Plexon, Inc., Dallas, TX). Available contact sizes include a diameter of 40 µm, which yields a nearly ideal surface area for stimulation (1257 μm^2). Using 32 contacts spaced 200 µm apart, most of the midbrain dopamine neuron cell bodies would be within 2 to 3 mm of a stimulation contact. Given a suitable switching circuit, electrical stimulation could be tested at each site with monopolar stimulation, or at each pair of sites with bipolar stimulation. The entire VTA/SNc could be activated simultaneously using continuous interleaved sampling, a methodology developed for auditory prosthetics [39]. In this scheme, only one contact receives a stimulation pulse at any given moment, but all contacts receive a complete stimulus train nearly contemporaneously. Readily available electrophysiology equipment can generate these stimuli and synchronize with voltammetry (e.g., AlphaLab SnR, Alpha-Omega USA, Inc., Alpharetta, GA).

Local stimulation was a more reliable method for locating sites of DA release in the monkey. The optimal position for the stimulation electrode was near the carbon fiber electrode, but at least a few hundred µm away. Stimulating either too close to the carbon fiber electrode or with too high currents caused large artifacts that interfered with DA recordings. These observations are consistent with the distances most commonly used for brain slices (e.g., [10,40]). The greater ease of finding DA responses with local stimulation provides utility in multiple ways. Local stimulation can be used to test pharmacological manipulations, as others have done (e.g., [11]). Because local stimulation can produce a large DA signal, it can be used to locate local DA rich areas.

The present work lays the foundation for studying DA activity in awake, behaving monkeys, essential for understanding the influence of DA upon complex behavior. Non-human primates are critical to pre-clinical studies towards human voltammetry applications, e.g., voltammetric recordings in concert with deep brain stimulation [20,49]. We have addressed key methodological challenges associated with navigating a larger brain in an awake primate model. We have shown that stimulating DA terminals directly, and the cell bodies in the VTA/SNc, can each evoke phasic DA release.

Supporting Information

Appendix S1 Microprocessor-based stimulation controller. A microprocessor circuit was used to control electrical stimulation pulse timing. The device synchronizes with the FSCV clock signal to avoid interfering with voltammetry recordings. A best-effort heuristic algorithm interleaves stimulation pulses with FSCV cycles over a wide range of pulse rates and durations. One option overlaps the first pulse of a pulse train with a FSCV cycle to display the timing of that event as an artifact on the voltammogram.

Appendix S2 Estimating the accuracy of electrode trajectories in the brain. The distance between two electrodes in the brain can be estimated using stimulation artifacts as long as one electrode is movable. We describe the geometry, application and a simplified method to estimate distance.

Acknowledgments

The authors wish to thank Dr. Paul E. M. Phillips for his consultation early in this project. We thank Drs. Kendall Lee and Paul Min for their frequent consultations, aid with methodological issues, and for open sharing of unpublished data. We thank Dr. Elizabeth Murray for providing the monkey histological sections stained for tyrosine hydroxylase and Dr. Kadharbatcha Saleem for his guidance with several anatomical issues. We are indebted to Ms. Shannon Gallagher whose energy and hard work were essential to this project. We also thank Ms. Laura Kennerly for her invaluable help with later versions of the manuscript.

Author Contributions

Conceived and designed the experiments: BBA. Performed the experiments: EWS ARM JFC BBA. Analyzed the data: EWS ARM BBA. Contributed reagents/materials/analysis tools: EWS ARM JFC BBA. Wrote the paper: EWS ARM JFC BBA.

References

1. Dahlstroem A, Fuxe K (1964) Evidence for the existence of monoamine-containing neurons in the central nervous system. I. Demonstration of monoamines in the cell bodies of brain stem neurons. Acta Physiol Scand Suppl: SUPPL 232:231–255.
2. Fuxe K, Dahlstrom AB, Jonsson G, Marcellino D, Guescini M, et al. (2010) The discovery of central monoamine neurons gave volume transmission to the wired brain. Prog Neurobiol 90: 82–100.
3. Haber SN, Fudge JL, McFarland NR (2000) Striatonigrostriatal pathways in primates form an ascending spiral from the shell to the dorsolateral striatum. J Neurosci 20: 2369–2382.
4. Giompres P, Delis F (2005) Dopamine transporters in the cerebellum of mutant mice. Cerebellum 4: 105–111.
5. Ikai Y, Takada M, Shinonaga Y, Mizuno N (1992) Dopaminergic and non-dopaminergic neurons in the ventral tegmental area of the rat project, respectively, to the cerebellar cortex and deep cerebellar nuclei. Neuroscience 51: 719–728.
6. Wise RA (2005) Forebrain substrates of reward and motivation. J Comp Neurol 493: 115–121.
7. Olds ME, Fobes JL (1981) The central basis of motivation: intracranial self-stimulation studies. Annu Rev Psychol 32: 523–574.
8. Glimcher PW (2011) Understanding dopamine and reinforcement learning: the dopamine reward prediction error hypothesis. Proc Natl Acad Sci U S A 108 Suppl 3: 15647–15654.
9. Schultz W, Dayan P, Montague PR (1997) A neural substrate of prediction and reward. Science 275: 1593–1599.
10. Apawu AK, Maina FK, Taylor JR, Mathews TA (2013) Probing the ability of presynaptic tyrosine kinase receptors to regulate striatal dopamine dynamics. ACS Chem Neurosci 4: 895–904.
11. Robinson DL, Venton BJ, Heien ML, Wightman RM (2003) Detecting subsecond dopamine release with fast-scan cyclic voltammetry in vivo. Clin Chem 49: 1763–1773.
12. Panin F, Cathala A, Piazza PV, Spampinato U (2012) Coupled intracerebral microdialysis and electrophysiology for the assessment of dopamine neuron function in vivo. J Pharmacol Toxicol Methods 65: 83–92.
13. Kawagoe KT, Wightman RM (1994) Characterization of amperometry for in vivo measurement of dopamine dynamics in the rat brain. Talanta 41: 865–874.
14. Silva L, Duarte K, Freitas AC, Panteleitchouk TSL, Rocha-Santos TAP, et al. (2012) A fluorescence-based optical fiber analyzer for catecholamine determination. Analytical Methods 4: 2300–2306.
15. Thompson JL, Urban N, Slifstein M, Xu X, Kegeles LS, et al. (2012) Striatal dopamine release in schizophrenia comorbid with substance dependence. Mol Psychiatry.
16. Cheer JF, Aragona BJ, Heien ML, Seipel AT, Carelli RM, et al. (2007) Coordinated accumbal dopamine release and neural activity drive goal-directed behavior. Neuron 54: 237–244.
17. Stamford JA (1986) In vivo voltammetry: some methodological considerations. J Neurosci Methods 17: 1–29.
18. Ariansen JL, Heien ML, Hermans A, Phillips PE, Hernadi I, et al. (2012) Monitoring extracellular pH, oxygen, and dopamine during reward delivery in the striatum of primates. Front Behav Neurosci 6: 36.
19. Mitz AR, Godschalk M, Wise SP (1991) Learning-dependent neuronal activity in the premotor cortex: activity during the acquisition of conditional motor associations. J Neurosci 11: 1855–1872.
20. Lee KH, Chang SY, Jang DP, Kim I, Goerss S, et al. (2011) Emerging techniques for elucidating mechanism of action of deep brain stimulation. Conf Proc IEEE Eng Med Biol Soc 2011: 677–680.
21. Jones SR, Mickelson GE, Collins LB, Kawagoe KT, Wightman RM (1994) Interference by pH and Ca2+ ions during measurements of catecholamine release in slices of rat amygdala with fast-scan cyclic voltammetry. J Neurosci Methods 52: 1–10.
22. Godschalk M, Mitz AR, van Duin B, van der Burg H (1995) Somatotopy of monkey premotor cortex examined with microstimulation. Neurosci Res 23: 269–279.
23. Domesick VB (1988) Neuroanatomical organization of dopamine neurons in the ventral tegmental area. Ann N Y Acad Sci 537: 10–26.
24. Robinson DL, Wightman RM (2007) Rapid Dopamine Release in Freely Moving Rats. In: Michael AC, Borland LM, editors. Electrochemical Methods for Neuroscience. Boca Raton FL: Taylor & Francis Group, LLC.
25. Saleem KS, Logothetis N (2012) A Combined MRI and Histology Atlas of the Rhesus Monkey Brain in Stereotaxic Coordinates. London: Academic Press.
26. Swiergiel AH, Palamarchouk VS, Dunn AJ (1997) A new design of carbon fiber microelectrode for in vivo voltammetry using fused silica. J Neurosci Methods 73: 29–33.
27. Clark JJ, Sandberg SG, Wanat MJ, Gan JO, Horne EA, et al. (2010) Chronic microsensors for longitudinal, subsecond dopamine detection in behaving animals. Nat Methods 7: 126–129.
28. Kishida KT, Sandberg SG, Lohrenz T, Comair YG, Saez I, et al. (2011) Sub-second dopamine detection in human striatum. PLoS One 6: e23291.
29. Roberts JG, Moody BP, McCarty GS, Sombers LA (2010) Specific oxygen-containing functional groups on the carbon surface underlie an enhanced sensitivity to dopamine at electrochemically pretreated carbon fiber microelectrodes. Langmuir 26: 9116–9122.
30. McIntyre CC, Grill WM (2001) Finite element analysis of the current-density and electric field generated by metal microelectrodes. Ann Biomed Eng 29: 227–235.
31. Roitman MF, Stuber GD, Phillips PE, Wightman RM, Carelli RM (2004) Dopamine operates as a subsecond modulator of food seeking. J Neurosci 24: 1265–1271.
32. Mitz AR, Wise SP (1987) The somatotopic organization of the supplementary motor area: intracortical microstimulation mapping. J Neurosci 7: 1010–1021.

33. Heien ML, Phillips PE, Stuber GD, Seipel AT, Wightman RM (2003) Overoxidation of carbon-fiber microelectrodes enhances dopamine adsorption and increases sensitivity. Analyst 128: 1413–1419.
34. Kume-Kick J, Rice ME (1998) Dependence of dopamine calibration factors on media Ca2+ and Mg2+ at carbon-fiber microelectrodes used with fast-scan cyclic voltammetry. J Neurosci Methods 84: 55–62.
35. Hashemi P, Dankoski EC, Petrovic J, Keithley RB, Wightman RM (2009) Voltammetric detection of 5-hydroxytryptamine release in the rat brain. Anal Chem 81: 9462–9471.
36. Zen JM, Hsu CT, Hsu YL, Sue JW, Conte ED (2004) Voltammetric peak separation of dopamine from uric acid in the presence of ascorbic acid at greater than ambient solution temperatures. Anal Chem 76: 4251–4255.
37. Gibson AR, Houk JC, Kohlerman NJ (1985) Magnocellular red nucleus activity during different types of limb movement in the macaque monkey. J Physiol 358: 527–549.
38. Ghosh S, Porter R (1988) Corticocortical synaptic influences on morphologically identified pyramidal neurones in the motor cortex of the monkey. J Physiol 400: 617–629.
39. Heien ML, Johnson MA, Wightman RM (2004) Resolving neurotransmitters detected by fast-scan cyclic voltammetry. Anal Chem 76: 5697–5704.
40. Iravani MM, Muscat R, Kruk ZL (1996) Comparison of somatodendritic and axon terminal dopamine release in the ventral tegmental area and the nucleus accumbens. Neuroscience 70: 1025–1037.
41. Schultz W (1998) Predictive reward signal of dopamine neurons. J Neurophysiol 80: 1–27.
42. Wightman RM, Robinson DL (2002) Transient changes in mesolimbic dopamine and their association with 'reward'. J Neurochem 82: 721–735.
43. Brown HD, McCutcheon JE, Cone JJ, Ragozzino ME, Roitman MF (2011) Primary food reward and reward-predictive stimuli evoke different patterns of phasic dopamine signaling throughout the striatum. Eur J Neurosci 34: 1997–2006.
44. Mitz AR (2005) A liquid-delivery device that provides precise reward control for neurophysiological and behavioral experiments. J Neurosci Methods 148: 19–25.
45. Garris PA, Christensen JR, Rebec GV, Wightman RM (1997) Real-time measurement of electrically evoked extracellular dopamine in the striatum of freely moving rats. J Neurochem 68: 152–161.
46. Zhang TC, Grill WM (2010) Modeling deep brain stimulation: point source approximation versus realistic representation of the electrode. J Neural Eng 7: 066009.
47. Ranck JB Jr (1975) Which elements are excited in electrical stimulation of mammalian central nervous system: a review. Brain Res 98: 417–440.
48. Shon YM, Lee KH, Goerss SJ, Kim IY, Kimble C, et al. (2010) High frequency stimulation of the subthalamic nucleus evokes striatal dopamine release in a large animal model of human DBS neurosurgery. Neurosci Lett 475: 136–140.
49. Van Gompel JJ, Chang SY, Goerss SJ, Kim IY, Kimble C, et al. (2010) Development of intraoperative electrochemical detection: wireless instantaneous neurochemical concentration sensor for deep brain stimulation feedback. Neurosurg Focus 29: E6.
50. Wise SP, Moody SL, Blomstrom KJ, Mitz AR (1998) Changes in motor cortical activity during visuomotor adaptation. Exp Brain Res 121: 285–299.

12

Mechanical Ventilation for Comatose Patients with Inoperative Acute Intracerebral Hemorrhage: Possible Futility of Treatment

Toru Fukuhara*, Mizuho Aoi, Yoichiro Namba

Department of Neurological Surgery, National Hospital Organization Okayama Medical Center, Okayama, Japan

Abstract

Background: Comatose patients with acute intracerebral hemorrhage (ICH) diagnosed as inoperative due to their severe comorbidity will be treated differently between countries. In certain countries including Japan, aggressive medical care may be performed according to the patients' family requests although the effects on the outcome are obscure. For respiratory distress in comatose patients with inoperative acute ICH, the role of mechanical ventilation on the outcome is unknown. We speculated that the efficacy of a ventilator in such a specific condition is limited and possibly futile.

Methods: We retrospectively evaluated the in-hospital mortality and further outcome of 65 comatose patients with inoperative ICH. Among the patients, 56 manifested respiratory distress, and the effect of the ventilator was evaluated by comparing the patients treated with and without the ventilator.

Results: The in-hospital mortality was calculated as 80%. A statistically significant parameter affecting the mortality independently was the motor subset on the Glasgow Coma Scale ($P = 0.015$). Among the patients who manifested respiratory distress, 7.7% of patients treated with a ventilator and 14.0% of patients not treated with a ventilator survived; an outcome is not significantly different. The mean survival duration of patients treated with a ventilator was significantly longer than the mean survival duration of patients not treated with a ventilator ($P = 0.021$). Among the surviving 13 patients, 7 patients died 5 to 29 months after onset without significant consciousness recovery. Another 6 patients suffered continuous disablement due to prolonged severe consciousness disturbances.

Conclusion: The current results indicate that treating comatose patients resulting from inoperative acute ICH may be futile. In particular, treating these patients with a ventilator only has the effect of prolonging unresponsive life, and the treatment may be criticized from the perspective of the appropriate use of public medical resources.

Editor: Nades Palaniyar, The Hospital for Sick Children and The University of Toronto, Canada

Funding: The authors have no support or funding to report.

Competing Interests: The authors have declared that no competing interests exist.

* Email: torufk@ninus.ocn.ne.jp

Introduction

The medical care limitations associated with the do not resuscitate (DNR) order at the acute stage of intracerebral hemorrhage (ICH) is a well-recognized independent factor leading to poor prognosis [1–3]. In spite of the definition of a DNR order: "no attempt of resuscitation required in the case of cardiopulmonary arrest", a DNR obtained early leads to an overall lack of aggressive care [2]. A DNR order does not necessarily mean the withdrawal of medical efforts leading to the best possible outcome. In fact, it was reported that proper medical care even with DNR orders did not lead to a poor outcome of patients with ICH [4].

However, medical resources are limited in the rapidly aging society, and since medical resources are public in nature, the priority for using limited medical resources should be seriously discussed. This "medico-social triage," involving treatment priorities even in a non-disaster situation, will be the physicians' responsibility in the near future, in order to maximize the quality and quantity of cured lives. Especially in Japan where even the brain-dead patients are commonly managed with continuous medical care according to their family's wishes, the recognition of medical futility is the first important step to keep the medical care system functioning properly.

For the purpose of decreasing the burden on medical resources, medical care termination as early as possible has a larger impact, although early outcome prediction is frequently difficult [5,6]. In the management of ICH, the role of surgical hematoma evacuation is multifactorial and it has been difficult to establish simple guidelines [7,8]. Comparatively, the patient's condition with inoperative ICH would be less complicated and the treatment strategy limited. Although artificial support with a mechanical ventilator might be the choice in the case of respiratory distress, it often sustains unresponsive life leading to eventual death. Many patients' families refuse ventilator support to avoid sustaining unresponsive life. However, there exists a dilemma in making a decision regarding the uncertainty whether comatose patients due to ICH with respiratory distress have a chance to recover, and if they do recover, how significant their functions would be.

The aim of this study is to evaluate the efficacy of mechanical ventilator support on the outcome of comatose patients with inoperative ICH. As well as determining the factors affecting the in-hospital mortality for these patients, the effects of a ventilator on sustaining life and the final outcome are further explored. Based on these results, medical futility in neurosurgical fields is extensively discussed.

Materials and Methods

Study Population

After obtaining approval by the Institutional Review Board of National Hospital Organization Okayama Medical Center in December 2012 (H24-59), the medical records of the patients who were admitted to our hospital due to non-traumatic spontaneous ICH between July 2006 and June 2013 were retrospectively reviewed. According to the ethical guideline for clinical research, published by the Japanese Ministry of Health, Labor and Welfare (revised version on July 31, 2008), the retrospective clinical study without involving the analysis on biological samples from the patients does not require obtaining the informed consent, but does require notifying the information about the study, including the purpose and method, described on page 19 (in Japanese). Since this study is the retrospective study without utilizing any biological samples, obtaining the informed consent is not required, and no informed consent was taken for this retrospective observational study. Instead, the information of the study has been open to public through the homepage of the hospital and posting a notice in the hospital. Any identifiable information of the patients including name, birthday, address and the admission or discharge date were not extracted for the study, in order to anonymized the data prior to analysis.

During these 7 years, 471 patients (8 patients were counted twice because of different admissions with two distant attacks) were admitted to our hospital due to ICH without known organic etiologies. Among these patients, comatose patients, defined as both subsets of the Glasgow Coma Scale (GCS) on the verbal response and on the eye opening response scored at 1, diagnosed at admission or deteriorated to coma within 24 hours after admission, were extracted. In order to exclude epileptic deterioration with acute ICH onset, patients who improved within 48 hours after admission were not counted. After the exclusion of the patients to whom emergency hematoma evacuation surgery was offered, there remained 66 patients whose hematomas were considered to be inoperative due to their associated conditions. Inoperative conditions were classified into 6 categories: 1) high age over 90 years old (8 patients), 2) unstable vital signs and highly likely to die during surgery (11 patients), 3) disturbances in hematological laboratory data; defined as a platelet count of less than 80,000 and/or INR>2.5 (20 patients), 4) associated with terminal uncontrolled diseases (7 patients; 2 patients with liver cirrhosis, 2 patients with multiple myeloma, 1 patient with myelodysplasia, 1 patient with gastric cancer and 1 patient with lung cancer), 5) associated with severe active diseases (6 patients; 2 patients with acute myocardial infarction, 1 patient with severe liver dysfunction, 1 patient with progressing untreated renal failure, 1 patient with severe uncontrolled diabetes and 1 patient with lung emphysema) and 6) hematoma location on the brain stem, either primary or extending into (38 patients). Emergency surgery was not offered for these 66 patients, since they had at least one of the inoperative conditions mentioned above. One patient whose family wished discontinuation of the dialysis and died 2 days after admission was excluded from the analysis, since the mortality of this patient was strongly affected by the withdrawal of the dialysis. Patients whose dialysis continued after the admission or who died within 2 days after the admission were included so the analysis was performed with 65 patients. When the patients were comatose at admission or deteriorated to coma after the admission, we asked their families whether treatment with a mechanical ventilator was preferred in case of respiratory distress occurrence. We explained the effects of ventilators as, "it mostly sustains life for several days, but it may increase the survival rate. Surviving patients are most likely to be in a vegetative state." Families of 48 patients refused treatment with a mechanical ventilator for the patients, and the patients were managed without a ventilator in spite of 43 patients progressing to respiratory distress. Families of 9 patients required the patients to be managed with a ventilator, and 7 patients were actually managed with a ventilator, although 2 patients did not progress to respiratory distress. In 2 patients, the families were unable to decide, however respiratory distress did not occur to these patients, and they were managed without a ventilator. In 6 patients, treatment with a ventilator was initiated in the emergency room (ER) according to the regular resuscitation protocol before confirming the families will, so 13 patients in total, due to the families' requirement in 7 patients and due to the resuscitation in the ER in 6 patients, were managed with a ventilator.

Management Protocol

With diltiazem hydrochloride infusion, maintaining a systolic blood pressure of less than 150 mmHg was the first target of the treatment. In order to decrease the intracranial pressure, 20 g glycerol in 5% fructose was infused three times per day. For supratentorial hematoma, phenytoin infusions were initiated to avoid epileptic deterioration. Associated significant disorders were also treated; suspected infections such as pneumonias or urinary tract infections were treated with antibiotic infusions. Vitamin K injection was added in the case of INR>1.5. No patients became "operative" after the reversal of the coagulopathies, since other associated conditions prevented the patients from requiring evacuation surgeries (mostly too late with unstable vital signs).

Continuous monitoring of arterial oxygen saturation with transcutaneous pulse oximetry digit sensor was performed immediately after arriving at the hospital and high-flow oxygen supply up to 6 liters per minute with non-rebreather mask was initiated at SpO2 of less than 98%. Upper airway obstruction due to coma by the tongue root was treated initially with nasal cannula, and in selected cases with severe obstruction, endotracheal intubations were performed. We seldom used sedative medication for comatose patients with ICH because the usage disturbed the exact evaluation of the consciousness level. Respiratory distress, such as frequent apnea of more than 10 seconds, or ataxic breathing was the indication of the ventilator, and ventilator support was provided to patients whose families preferred that option. Any doubtful respiratory abnormalities were confirmed with an arterial blood gas examination. Other indications of the ventilator for patients with ICH include; intravenous sedative medication usage for controlling the pain after surgery or status epilepticus, and pulmonary diseases requiring ventilation support irrespective of the consciousness level, both of which were not included in the studied patient cohort. During the ventilator support, the treatment was continued, and the blood pressure reduction at the terminal stage was treated with continuous dopamine infusion. In our institution, as is common in Japan, the diagnostic procedure of brain death was not performed except for organ donation, which did not occur for these enrolled patients, so even with the patients entering a condition clinically equivalent to brain death, the treatment was continued until the heart beat stopped. For the patients whose families requested no treatment with a ventilator, even at blood pressure reduction, vasopressor infusion was not conducted.

Evaluated Parameters

The primary outcome is in-hospital mortality. Possible factors affecting the mortality were analyzed and grouped into 3 categories, which were the pre-admission parameters, the clinical parameters during coma and the initial radiological parameters at entering the coma state. The pre-admission parameters included the following 5 factors: age at admission, sex, the pre-onset ADL expressed by modified Rankin Scale (mRS), current oral antiplatelet and/or anticoagulation treatment and receiving regular dialysis. The clinical parameters during coma included the following 3 factors: motor subset on GCS (GCS-M) at the coma diagnosis (eye and verbal response were both at 1 for these enrolled patients), abnormalities of pupils at the coma diagnosis, and the further presence of respiratory distress within 5 days of onset. The initial radiological parameters at entering the coma state included the following 6 factors: locations of hematoma categorized into the supratentorial (right and left) or infratentorial (brain stem and cerebellum), the existence of midline shift, intraventricular hemorrhage, brain stem compression, and hematoma on brain stem, and the maximum diameter of hematoma on head CT scan (the IVH was not included in the hematoma size).

Another evaluation was performed on the efficacy of the ventilator, analyzed among the patients manifesting the respiratory distress. The duration of respiratory distress was calculated from the medical records, between the first description on the medical records regarding respiration abnormalities and death or recovery from respiratory distress. Recovery from respiratory distress was defined as regular respiration rhythm for patients treated without a ventilator and weaning from the ventilator for patients treated with a ventilator. Respiratory distress was defined as apnea longer than 10 seconds or ataxic breathing. In order to extract respiratory distress only from brain stem dysfunction due to ICH compression, respiratory distress occurred within 5 days after admission was counted, but respiratory distress resulting from other etiologies such as pneumonia seen at the later period was not extracted. Endotracheal intubation itself was not counted as respiratory distress, since it was often only for airway clearance. Between the two groups supported by a ventilator (the ventilator group) and not supported by a ventilator (the no-ventilator group), survival duration and in-hospital mortality were compared.

All the surviving patients were followed up after discharge until October 31, 2013. Consciousness state at the last follow-up was also obtained by referral to the physician in charge. Disturbed consciousness was divided into 3 categories. Vegetative state (VS) is unresponsive but wakeful, and minimally conscious state (MCS), originally defined by Giacino et al. in 2002 [9], is awake and aware. The better state was described by Schnakers et al. in 2009 [10] as emerged from MCS (EMCS), judged with functional communication and/or functional object use at JFK Coma Recovery Scale-Revisited [11]. In making a referral to each physician who is taking care of the patient, the meaning and the difference in the above-mentioned 3 categories was ensured. In order to grasp how much improvement can occur for these patients after discharge, we also categorized the consciousness state of these surviving patients at discharge of our hospital in the same manner and set the tentative neurological condition at discharge although this assignment was used only for comparison with the final outcome.

Statistical analysis

The 13 parameters mentioned above, possibly affecting the in-hospital mortality were analyzed univariately, then significant factors on univariate analysis were included in further multivariate analysis. The categorical parameters were evaluated using Chi-square analysis as the univariate, and the ordinal parameters (age, the pre-admission mRS, GCS-M and the maximum size of hematoma) were analyzed using Mann-Whitney U test as the univariate. Then significant parameters with these univariate analyses were included in the multivariate logistic regression model, to confirm the independently significant parameters on the in-hospital mortality.

For analysis of the ventilator effects on the prognosis, patients manifesting respiratory distress (56 patients) were examined. Both survival duration and in-hospital mortality were compared between the ventilator group (13 patients) and the no-ventilator group (43 patients). In-hospital mortality was compared with a contingency table using Chi-square analysis. The survival duration of the two groups was compared by using Man Whitney U test. Additionally, the mean survival duration was estimated using Kaplan-Meier method and the difference was compared by log-rank test. Results were considered statistically significant at $P < 0.05$, and all P values were 2 sided. All patients data used for the analysis were shown in Appendix S1, 1–4.

Results

Overall outcome

Among the enrolled 65 patients, 50 patients died due to ICH, and 2 patients were considered to have died with complications (pneumonia and myocardial infarction), so the gross in-hospital mortality was calculated as 80%. There were 13 patients who survived to discharge; however, all patients were severely disabled at 5 on mRS. Figure 1 shows overall mortality in relation to the occurrence of respiratory distress and ventilator usage.

Parameters affecting the in-hospital mortality

With the univariate analysis, there were 6 factors affecting the in-hospital mortality. Using chi-square analysis, abnormal pupillary reflex ($P = 0.001$), respiratory distress ($P < 0.001$), IVH ($P = 0.003$) and brain stem compression ($P = 0.021$) tended to be seen more frequently in the mortality group. Using Mann-Whitney U test, GCS-M tended to be low ($P < 0.001$) and the maximum diameter of hematoma tended to be larger ($P = 0.047$) in the mortality group. Multivariate analysis was performed with these 6 factors, and only GCS-M at the coma diagnosis turned out to be a significant factor independently affecting the mortality (OR 3.1, $P = 0.015$), meaning the mortality increases approximately three-fold with each reduction of the GCS-M score. Details of the effects of the examined factors on mortality are shown in Table 1.

Ventilator effect on prognosis

The enclosed area with a dotted line in Fig. 1 indicates the overall mortality of the patients manifesting respiratory distress in relation with ventilator usage. With 56 patients who manifested respiratory distress, the effect of a ventilator was evaluated. Thirteen patients were treated with a ventilator (the ventilator group), due to the families' preference in 7 patients and due to resuscitation at ER in 6 patients, on the contrary 43 patients who did not have a ventilator (the no-ventilator group) were all due to

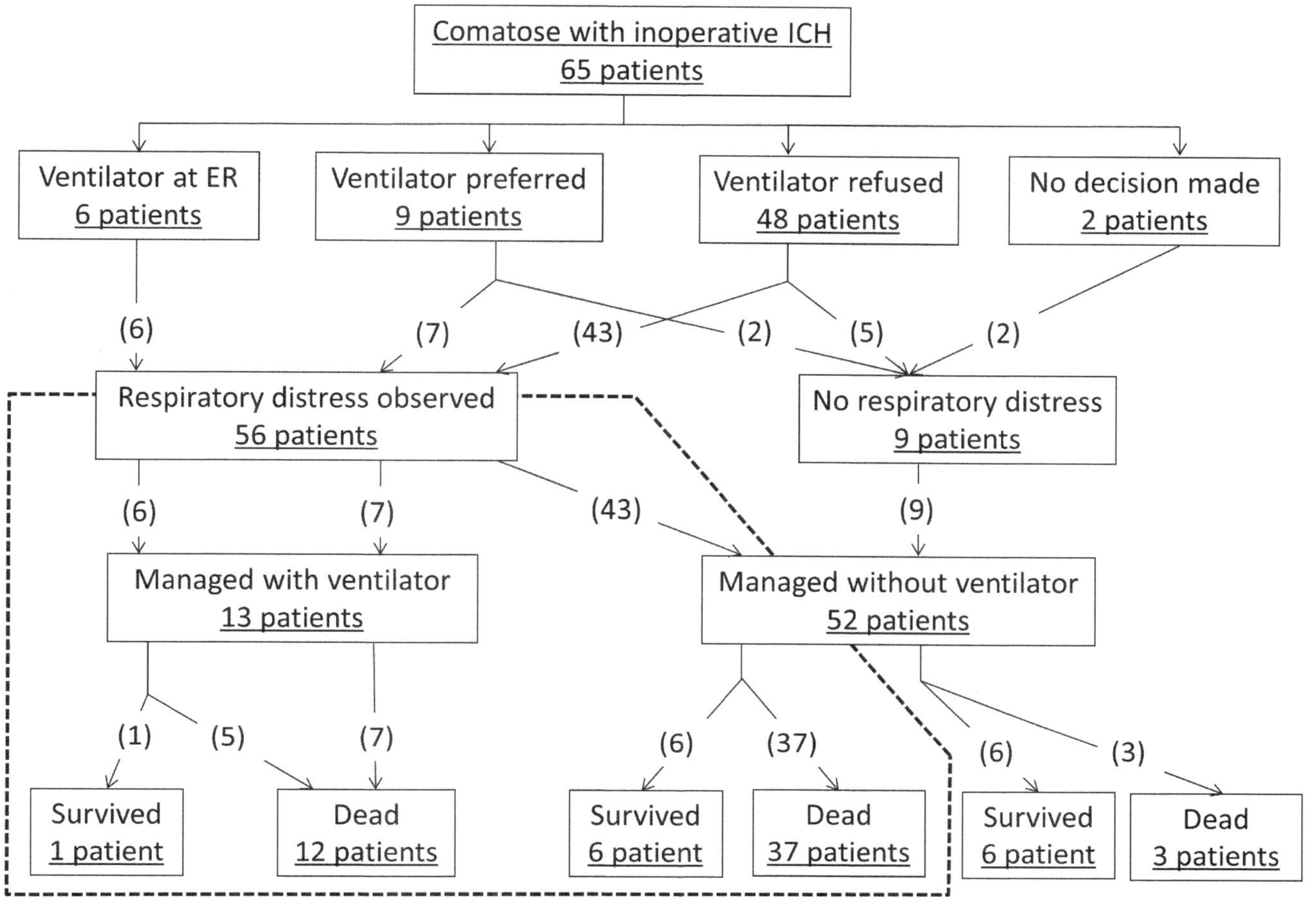

Figure 1. Flow diagram detailing the in-hospital mortality of the enrolled patients in relation to respiratory distress and ventilator usage. Enclosed area with dotted line indicates the outcome of the patients manifesting respiratory distress.

the families' wishes. In all patients in the ventilator group, the ventilator was initiated within 12 hours after ICH onset. Among the 13 patients in the ventilator group, only 1 patient (7.7%) was successfully weaned from the ventilator and survived to discharge. Among 43 patients in the no-ventilator group, 6 patients (14.0%) survived to discharge. The contingency table about the in-hospital mortality in both groups was compared by Chi-square test, and no significant frequency deviation was observed ($P = 0.72$). The survival duration in the ventilator group was 309.1±447.2 hours (mean ± standard deviation), which is significantly longer than that in the no-ventilator group (73.7±166.9 hours, $P = 0.001$) by using Man Whitney U test. The survival durations were also estimated using Kaplan-Meier method and the differences between the two groups were compared with log-rank test (Fig. 2). Again, the mean survival duration in the ventilator group (345 hours) was significantly longer than that in the no-ventilator group (115 hours, $P = 0.021$). The ventilator has an impact on prolonging survival duration although no effect was observed on in-hospital mortality.

Outcome of the surviving patients

Thirteen patients survived and were discharged from our hospital in the studied cohort. They were followed up for 5 to 50 months (mean 18.2 months). Their consciousness levels at discharge were VS in 8 patients, MCS in 2 patients and EMCS in 3 patients. Among these patients, 7 patients died at a nursing hospital between 5 and 29 months from onset. The most frequent cause of death was pneumonia (4 among 7 patients). No patients had better consciousness than EMCS, indicating all surviving patients suffered from continuously-disabled life due to prolonged consciousness disturbances. Although severely disturbed cognition remained for all patients, 4 patients had improvement in consciousness (VS to MCS in 2 patients, MCS to EMCS in 1 patient and VS to EMCS in 1 patient). On the contrary, 4 patients deteriorated after discharge (EMCS to MCS in 3 patients and MCS to VS in 1 patient), and another 5 patients were unchanged and remained at VS. The details of the surviving patient outcome are shown in Table 2.

Discussion

It is the primary responsibility of physicians to pursue the best possible outcome for the patients; however, the debate over medical futility in order to control medical costs or decrease the burden on the medical resources has been a major topic [12,13], and the advances in medical technologies unfortunately exaggerates the costly life-sustaining [12]. A conflicting mission, determining low-priority care concurrently with pursuing the better outcome, is imposed on physicians in the current "medico-social triage" era, to keep the medical care system functioning properly. Establishing concise outcome prediction models depending on the

Table 1. Clinical characteristics of sixty-five enrolled comatose patients with inoperative ICH.

Factors	Survived (n = 13)	Dead in hospital (n = 52)	Univariate Analysis*		Multivariate Analysis
			P Value	OR (95% CI)	*P* Value
Pre-admission Parameters					
Age, years (mean)	58.2–96.7 (79.7)	46.7–94.2 (77.2)	0.47		
Female	7	23	0.53		
Pre-onset mRS (median)	0–5 (2)	0–5 (1)	0.20		
Pre-onset anti-platelet and/or anti-coagulation medications	5	25	0.53		
On dialysis	1	5	0.83		
Clinical Parameters					
GCS-M (median)	2–5 (4)	1–5 (2)	<0.001#	3.1 (1.2–7.8)	0.015#
Abnormal pupillary reaction	7	48	0.001#	5.6 (0.49–63.9)	0.17
Respiratory distress	7	49	<0.001#	4.9 (0.39–60.8)	0.22
Radiological Parameters					
Supratentorial	11	42	0.75		
Midline shift	5	34	0.076		
Intraventricular hemorrhage	6	44	0.003#	2.4 (0.29–19.6)	0.42
Brain stem compression	8	46	0.021#	3.3 (0.21–50.8)	0.39
Hematoma on brain stem	7	31	0.71		
Maximum diameter of hematoma, cm (mean)	3.0–7.6 (5.1)	1.0–9.5 (6.2)	0.047#	0.55 (0.28–1.1)	0.077

*Chi-square analysis for the categorical parameters, and Mann-Whitney U test for the ordinal parameters.
#Denotes statistical significance.

various patient presentations is thus desired. Although the guidelines for managing ICH have been revised [8], the role of hematoma evacuation is uncertain [7,14]. We still believe that hematoma evacuation surgery should not be abandoned as a futile treatment since many patients who are able to return to their original lives with only limited disabilities [15]. Neurosurgeons should clarify the treatment strategies taking into account the complications of the patients' conditions, including age, etiology, lesional location and volume, consciousness levels, neurological deficits at presentation and comorbid systematic diseases [14].

Abnormal respiratory patterns are well-known symptoms for the comatose patients with ICH [16], and many comatose patients manifest respiratory distress either at presentation or in the early period after admission. Surgical evacuation of hematoma may play a role as the last resort; however, the operations often cannot be attempted due to the associated conditions of the patients, including the brain stem location of hematoma, or other comorbid significant diseases. Few options are left for these patients, and the role of artificial ventilator support may be the only the debatable issue; however, there is no description in the guidelines regarding respiration support [8]. Elliott et al. mention, "airway management, including endotracheal intubation and mechanical ventilation, is a priority in the unconsciousness patient or in those with a deteriorating conscious level" in their review article [17], although no indication of ventilation is described. The mortality rate for ventilated patients with stroke was once reported as from 57 to 90% [18], however, indications using the ventilator seem to differ between institutes. Gujjar et al. described ventilation indicated for all intubated patients [18]. In a recent article by Elmer et al., among 697 ventilated patients, 17% of the patients were with GCS score between 13 and 15, and only 20% of the patients had hypoxemia [19]. In our institute, ventilator usage for the management of patients with ICH was mostly limited for patients manifesting respiratory distress, and the studied patients were more uniform than previously reported, that is E1V1at GCS score (3–7 in total) due to inoperative ICH. Our retrospective study revealed that patients in such a specifically broken-down group would not receive significant benefits from treatment with a ventilator. The significance of this study may be specific to Japan where even brain death patients are cared for with a ventilator, and the results of this study will not be attractive at all for most western clinicians since the patients in the current study may be considered as contraindicating ventilator usage as "too much", and DNR orders for these patients will not lead to a self-fulfilling prophecy [1–4], since their medical conditions were so critical. However, it should be noted that one-third of neurologically ill patients requiring a ventilator (mixtures of different conditions) recovered fairly well (better than mRS4) [6], and self-fulfilling prophecy can be a problem in many cases with ICH. We should be clear about the danger of self-fulfilling prophecies, and the proper aggressive treatment, including the ventilator usage, and surgical intervention is to be considered for a significant amount of patients with ICH, although the self-fulfilling prophecies are not an issue for our studied subgroup.

There are several limitations in the current study. Since our study was based on a small number of patients; only 13 patients managed with ventilators, it may be too soon to draw a conclusion. However, in the comparison of the patients treated without ventilators, the survival rate did not improve at all; actually the rate was even worse (7.7% in the ventilator group versus 14.0% in the no-ventilator group), and we believe this result is worthy of remark even with the small numbers. Secondary, the policy for the

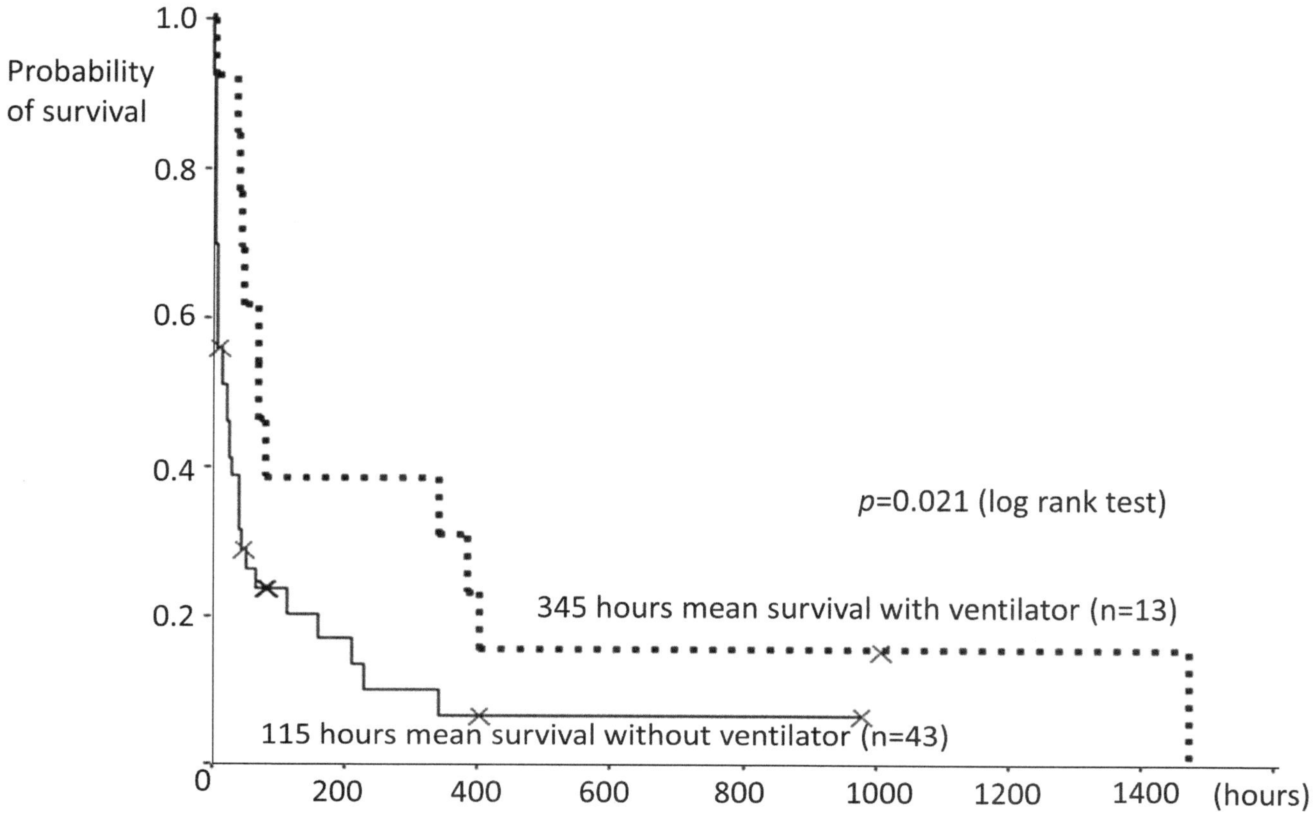

Figure 2. Graph of Kaplan-Meier survival curves after manifesting respiratory distress. The patients treated with the ventilator have longer survival duration.

management of critically-ill patients with inoperative ICH significantly differs between countries, hence, the present investigation is not necessarily extendible to the centers in other countries. In addition, there are several limitations resulting from the retrospective method. Due to the lack of prospectively-set survey sheets, pre-existing comorbidities, which should have been analyzed as the pre-admission parameters, could not be uniformly obtained, and thus were not included. As another possible limitation inherent to retrospective methods, due to the insufficient diagnostic procedures at admission for the inclusion/exclusion determination, several patients to be excluded were difficult to define from medical charts at admission, i.e., the patients manifesting epileptic respiratory arrest or abnormal respiration due to pulmonary embolism with small hematoma should be treated with a ventilator, and they are to be excluded from the current study, because their ventilator usage was medically required. Nevertheless, it was not a difficult task to distinguish respiratory distress due to ICH from that due to other etiologies by evaluating the medical course. We believe the proper inclusion/exclusion was performed in this study.

Our results indicate the outcome of the patients with inoperative ICH was uniformly poor, with 80% in-hospital mortality, and even surviving patients had severely disturbed cognition. Based on these results, treatments for comatose patients with inoperative ICH may be regarded as medically futile. However, when determining the futility of medical care, the ethical clarification regarding a "meaningful" life is prerequisite. The definition of a life worth saving by spending public costs varies among countries and may change over time even in the same country. The social attitude against the acceptance of brain death is an evident example. Although brain death is world-widely accepted concept [20], the policy on when to termination treatment with a ventilator after the diagnosis of brain death differs between countries and even between states in the US [21]. Brain death is still not accepted as "general" death in Japan, which is only diagnosed when organ donation for transplantation is attempted [22]. The withdrawal of mechanical ventilation unlikely occurs in Japan even after the confirmation of brain death, although initial refusal of ventilator support is frequently seen. And once managed with a ventilator, the clinical confirmation of brain death will not be attempted even for "clinically-assumed brain death". Among 12 patients who eventually died after being managed with the ventilator, we believe most patients resulted in the undiagnosed brain death during the course of the treatment, but medical care was continued for days. This may result from the special attitude of Japanese to death [22]: life-sustaining of brain-dead patients is not necessarily meaningless for many Japanese people [23], and such an attitude of the patient's family may be seen even in the US [24]. However, the burden on medical resources by prolonging a brain-dead patient's life is so significant and the termination of medical care for brain-dead patients should be socially accepted when establishing the guideline for the medico-social triage, otherwise no medical treatment can be judged as generally "futile".

In order to decrease the burden on public medical resources and to maintain the proper function of the healthcare system, a reasonable boundary line of medical futility should be established, and we believe that the treatment for patients fulfilling the criteria of futility should be abandoned uniformly and fairly. Study to

Table 2. Clinical characteristics and outcome of surviving patients.

Case No.	Age/Sex	Hematoma location	GCS (motor)	Diameter of hematoma (cm)	Respiratory distress	Ventilator used	Consciousness at discharge (days from onset)	Consciousness at last follow-up	Final survival/Months from onset (cause of death)
1	88.4/F	Lt supra	4	3.2	none	(no need)	MCS (25 days)	VS	alive/50 months
2	69.9/M	Lt supra	4	6.7	none	(no need)	VS (10 days)	EMCS	dead/24 months (renal failure)
3	81.5/F	Lt supra	5	6.9	observed	no	EMCS (97 days)	MCS	dead/6 months (pneumonia)
4	92.9/F	Rt supra	5	4.9	observed	no	VS (44days)	VS	dead/14 months (pneumonia)
5	76.3/M	Rt supra	4	5.0	none	(no need)	EMCS (46 days)	MCS	alive/25 months
6	80.0/M	Rt supra	3	5.2	observed	no	VS (67 days)	VS	alive/23 months
7	96.7/F	Lt supra	4	6.0	none	(no need)	EMCS (38 days)	MCS	dead/14 months (unspecified)
8	76.7/M	Lt supra	4	3.0	none	(no need)	VS (54 days)	VS	dead/29 months (pneumonia)
9	59.9/F	Rt supra	4	4.0	observed	no	MCS (60 days)	EMCS	alive/10 months
10	58.2/M	Lt supra	2	6.4	observed	yes	VS (105 days)	VS	alive/9 months
11	87.7/F	BS	4	3.8	observed	no	VS (84 days)	VS	alive/8 months
12	85.7/F	BS	5	3.1	observed	no	VS (29 days)	MCS	dead/5 months (unspecified)
13	82.1/M	Lt supra	5	7.6	none	(no need)	VS (64 days)	MCS	dead/20 months (pneumonia)

BS = brain stem; EMCS = emerged from minimally conscious state; MCS = minimally conscious state; supra = supratentorial; VS = vegetative state.

determine futile medical treatments should be recognized as medico-socially worthwhile. In many outcome studies in neurological fields, "dependent" is often seen as the boundary of a poor outcome [25,26]. Although the functional outcome; whether dependent or independent in the future is definitely a necessary observation, this boundary is not appropriate for medical futility since many dependent patients are capable of expressing their will. In fact, without the patients' advanced directives, medical care termination decided by the families because of the certainty of a functionally-dependent outcome, is ethically problematic. We propose "treatment resulting in the irreversible severely-disturbed consciousness at best" as a medical futility, and considering the perspective of this proposal, the consciousness level should be more sophisticatedly evaluated. In this report, the outcome for surviving patients was segmentalized according to their consciousness levels, which were VS, MCS and EMCS. No individual physician can define which level of the outcome is medically futile so far, and thorough national debate in each country is to be encouraged in order to establish the guidelines on how to restrict the medical care for patients with severely-disturbed consciousness. And in this debate, the recognition of the consciousness improvement, occasionally remarkable ones after a certain period [27], is essential. In fact, consciousness improvement was observed in 4 patients among our 13 surviving patients, although no patients became better than EMCS. More detailed analysis in respect of the type of the injury, the severity of the consciousness disturbance, the age of the patients and the possible expected recovery after a certain period, at least 12 months, will be needed for determining medical futility.

Conclusions

Even for neurosurgeons, determining medical futility is essential with the limited medical resources, and ventilator usage for comatose patients with inoperative ICH should be reconsidered. Further studies should be conducted with patients who have undergone hematoma evacuation for their ICH to confirm surgeries to be avoided. A reasonable boundary for medical futility should be considered in relation to the consciousness level, irrespective of functional disabilities. Detailed analysis of the consciousness outcome should be included in further studies relating to medical futility.

Supporting Information

Appendix S1 Appendix 1–4.

Author Contributions

Conceived and designed the experiments: TF MA YN. Performed the experiments: TF. Analyzed the data: TF. Contributed reagents/materials/analysis tools: TF MA YN. Contributed to the writing of the manuscript: TF.

References

1. Becker KJ, Baxter AB, Cohen WA, Bybee HM, Tirschwell DL, et al. (2001) Withdrawal of support in intracerebral hemorrhage may lead to self-fulfilling prophecies. Neurology 56: 766–772.
2. Hemphill JC 3rd, Newman J, Zhao S, Johnston SC (2004) Hospital usage of early do-not-resuscitate orders and outcome after intracerebral hemorrhage. Stroke 35: 1130–1134.
3. Zahuranec DB, Brown DL, Lisabeth LD, Gonzales NR, Longwell PJ, et al. (2007) Early care limitations independently predict mortality after intracerebral hemorrhage. Neurology 68: 1651–1657.
4. Jain A, Jain M, Bellolio MF, Schears RM, Rabinstein AA, et al. (2013) Is early DNR a self-fulfilling prophency for patients with spontaneous intracerebral hemorrhage? Neurocrit Care 19: 342–346.
5. Youngner SJ (1990) Orchestrating a dignified death in the intensive-care unit. Clin Chem 36: 1617–1622.
6. Caulfield AF, Gabler L, Lansberg MG, Eyngorn I, Mlynash M, et al. (2010) Outcome prediction in mechanically ventilated neurologic patients by junior neurointensivists. Neurology 74: 1096–1101.
7. Andaluz N, Zuccarello M (2009) Recent trends in the treatment of spontaneous intracerebral hemorrhage: analysis of a nationwide inpatient database. J Neurosurg 110: 403–410.
8. Morgenstern LB, Hemphill JC 3rd, Anderson C, Becker K, Broderick JP, et al. (2010) Guidelines for the management of spontaneous intracerebral hemorrhage: a guideline for healthcare professionals from the American Heart Association/American Stroke Association. Stroke 41: 2108–2129.
9. Giacino JT, Ashwal S, Childs N, Cranford R, Jennett B, et al. (2002) The minimally conscious state: definition and diagnostic criteria. Neurology 58: 349–353.
10. Schnakers C, Vanhaudenhuyse A, Giacino J, Ventura M, Boly M, et al. (2009) Diagnostic accuracy of the vegetative and minimally conscious state: clinical consensus versus standardized neurobehavioral assessment. BMC Neurology 9: 35.
11. Cruse D, Chennu S, Chatelle C, Fernández-Espejo D, Bekinschtein TA, et al. (2012) Relationship between etiology and covert cognition in the minimally conscious state. Neurology 78: 816–822.
12. Helft PR, Siegler M, Lantos J (2000) The rise and fall of the futility movement. N Engl J Med 343: 293–296.
13. Honeybul S, Gillett GR, Ho K (2013) Futility in Neurosurgery: A Patient-Centered Approach. Neurosurgery 73: 917–922.
14. Kelly ML, Sulmasy DP, Weil RJ (2013) Spontaneous intracerebral hemorrhage and the challenge of surgical decision making: a review. Neurosurg Focus 34: 1–7.
15. Zhang HT, Xue S, Li PJ, Fu YB, Xu RX (2013) Treatment of huge hypertensive putaminal hemorrhage by surgery and cerebrospinal fluid drainage. Clin Neurol Neurosurg 115: 1602–1608.
16. Tindall SC (1990) Level of consciousness. In: Walker HK, Hall WD, Hurst JW, editors. Clinical Methods: The History, Physical, and Laboratory Examinations. Boston: Butterworths. pp. 296–299.
17. Elliott J, Smith M (2010) The acute management of intracerebral hemorrhage: a clinical review. Anesth Analg 110: 1419–1427.
18. Gujjar AR, Deibert E, Manno EM, Duff S, Diringer MN (1998) Mechanical ventilation for ischemic stroke and intracerebral hemorrhage: indications, timing, and outcome. Neurology 51: 447–451.
19. Elmer J, Hou P, Wilcox SR, Chang Y, Schreiber H, et al. (2013) Acute respiratory distress syndrome after spontaneous intracerebral hemorrhage. Crit Care Med 41: 1992–2001.
20. Wijdicks EFM (2002) Brain death worldwide: accepted fact but no global consensus in diagnostic criteria. Neurology 58: 20–25.
21. Burkle CM, Schipper AM, Wijdicks EF (2011) Brain death and the courts. Neurology 76: 837–841.
22. Posner JB, Saper CB, Schiff ND, Plum F (2007) Diagnosis of stupor and coma. New York: Oxford Univ Press. pp.377–379.
23. Maruya J, Nishimaki K, Nakahata J, Suzuki H, Fujita Y, et al. (2008) Prolonged somatic survival of clinically brain-dead adult patient. Neurol Med Chir (Tokyo) 48: 114–117.
24. Applbaum AI, Tilburt JC, Collins MT, Wendler D (2008) A family's request for complementary medicine after patient brain death. JAMA 299: 2188–2193.
25. Rost NS, Smith EE, Chang Y, Snider RW, Chanderraj R, et al. (2008) Prediction of functional outcome in patients with primary intracerebral hemorrhage: the FUNC score. Stroke 39: 2304–2309.
26. Hemphill JC 3rd, Farrant M, Neill TA Jr (2009) Prospective validation of the ICH Score for 12-month functional outcome. Neurology 73: 1088–1094.
27. Edlow BL, Giacino JT, Hirschberg RE, Gerrard J, Wu O, et al (2013) Unexpected recovery of function after severe traumatic brain injury: the limits of early neuroimaging-based outcome prediction. Neurocrit Care 19: 364–375.

13

Increased Hippocampal Excitability in the 3xTgAD Mouse Model for Alzheimer's Disease *In Vivo*

Katherine E. Davis, Sarah Fox, John Gigg*

Faculty of Life Sciences, University of Manchester, Manchester, United Kingdom

Abstract

Mouse Alzheimer's disease (AD) models develop age- and region-specific pathology throughout the hippocampal formation. One recently established pathological correlate is an increase in hippocampal excitability in vivo. Hippocampal pathology also produces episodic memory decline in human AD and we have shown a similar episodic deficit in 3xTg AD model mice aged 3–6 months. Here, we tested whether hippocampal synaptic dysfunction accompanies this cognitive deficit by probing dorsal CA1 and DG synaptic responses in anaesthetized, 4–6 month-old 3xTgAD mice. As our previous reports highlighted a decline in episodic performance in aged control mice, we included aged cohorts for comparison. CA1 and DG responses to low-frequency perforant path stimulation were comparable between 3xTgAD and controls at both age ranges. As expected, DG recordings in controls showed paired-pulse depression; however, paired-pulse facilitation was observed in DG and CA1 of young and old 3xTgAD mice. During stimulus trains both short-latency (presumably monosynaptic: 'direct') and long-latency (presumably polysynaptic: 're-entrant') responses were observed. Facilitation of direct responses was modest in 3xTgAD animals. However, re-entrant responses in DG and CA1 of young 3xTgAD mice developed earlier in the stimulus train and with larger amplitude when compared to controls. Old mice showed less DG paired-pulse depression and no evidence for re-entrance. In summary, DG and CA1 responses to low-frequency stimulation in all groups were comparable, suggesting no loss of synaptic connectivity in 3xTgAD mice. However, higher-frequency activation revealed complex change in synaptic excitability in DG and CA1 of 3xTgAD mice. In particular, short-term plasticity in DG and CA1 was facilitated in 3xTgAD mice, most evidently in younger animals. In addition, re-entrance was facilitated in young 3xTgAD mice. Overall, these data suggest that the episodic-like memory deficit in 3xTgAD mice could be due to the development of an abnormal hyper-excitable state in the hippocampal formation.

Editor: Christian Holscher, University of Lancaster, United Kingdom

Funding: The authors are grateful for RCUK funding to KED (BBSRC PhD studentship), SF (BBSRC CASE PhD studentship) and JG (BBSRC grant BB/D011159/1; Royal Society grant RSRG 24519). The funders had no role in study design, data collection and analysis, decision to publish, or preparation of the manuscript.

Competing Interests: The authors have the following interests. JG is an in vivo electrophysiology consultant for GlaxoSmithKline Neurodegeneration, China.

* E-mail: j.gigg@manchester.ac.uk

Introduction

Alzheimer's disease (AD) is characterised phenotypically by profound declarative memory deficits. The hippocampus, vital for both the formation and retrieval of declarative memory, is one of the first areas affected by AD pathological hallmarks of amyloid-beta (Aβ), extracellular plaques and tau neurofibrillary tangles [1,2]. Interestingly, however, overt plaque burden correlates poorly with cognitive decline in AD patients [3]. A more recent hypothesis is that intracellular oligomeric amyloid species, present before the accumulation of extracellular plaque pathology, may instead play a pivotal role in disease progression [4,5]. However, despite extensive research examining the causes of AD pathology and characterising behavioural phenotypes, there is still little knowledge about the physiological basis for memory loss in pathological states such as AD [6].

The hippocampal formation is comprised of the dentate gyrus (DG), hippocampus proper (CA fields), subiculum (SUB), parasubiculum, presubiculum and entorhinal cortex (EC; medial and lateral divisions; MEC and LEC). CA1 and subiculum are the principal output structures of the hippocampus [7] and EC provides the interface between incoming and outgoing information from surrounding cortex [8]. Hippocampal output can return to surrounding neocortex via deep layers of EC and/or re-enter the hippocampal formation via projections from deep to superficial EC [9,10]. The latter reverberation (or 're-entrance') is considered to be pivotal in memory formation, possibly acting as a comparator mechanism to allow processed input to be evaluated alongside new information and/or as a memory consolidation mechanism during sleep [7,11–13]. Selective lesions to all hippocampal formation structures have profound effects on memory performance [14–18]. Functional abnormalities have also been detected in the hippocampus during memory encoding in human AD patients [19]. It is of major interest, therefore, to determine the pathophysiological profile of the hippocampal formation in AD models and to elucidate, in particular, whether reverberation (re-entrance) occurs in control and AD model mice.

The triple transgenic mouse model (3xTgAD) carries familial AD transgenes for Amyloid Precursor Protein (APP_{SWE}), Presenilin-1(M146V) and an additional tauopathy mutation (Tau_{P301L}). This model develops Aβ and tau pathology targeted to the hippocampus and other medial temporal lobe structures in a manner temporally and spatially similar to human AD [20,21]. The model develops cognitive deficits at a young age [21,22] and, as we have demonstrated recently, a specific decline in episodic-like memory from 3 months that becomes a complete deficit at 6 months of age [23,24]. 3xTgAD mice also show abnormalities in basal synaptic transmission and deficits in LTP in CA1 hippocampus *in vitro* [21]. However, to date, there have been no electrophysiological recordings *in vivo* in the 3xTgAD mouse and, to our knowledge, there is only one *in vivo* account in another AD model examining evoked responses [25]. Thus, the hippocampal system in AD mouse models has largely been examined only in the reduced brain slice preparation [21,26], that is, without the substantial bi-directional cortical connectivity that also contributes to memory processes [27]. In the 3xTgAD mouse, only CA3-CA1 connectivity has been examined directly *in vitro* [21], therefore, there is a need to examine basic synaptic transmission more widely in hippocampal formation and also hippocampal network function through examining response reverberation.

One question that arises is the extent to which cognitive deficits seen in early AD stem from abnormalities in the fibre pathways projecting to the hippocampus and/or within hippocampal subfields. Recent research has indicated the presence of early myelination abnormalities in the 3xTgAD mouse Schaffer collateral pathway, prior to the occurrence of Aβ and tau pathology [28]. In human AD, tau pathology is restricted to the stellate cells in EC layer II, and leads to degenerative changes in the perforant path [29]. In addition, afferents from CA1 and SUB to EC are major sites for Aβ pathology in human AD [16]; thus, there is a strong possibility that information flow through the hippocampal formation could become impaired in AD. However, synaptic deficits first arise in AD models *in vitro* at an age prior to overt extracellular plaque and tangle pathology, suggesting that mechanisms such as intracellular Aβ accumulation or abnormalities in calcium homeostasis are major contributing factors to early cognitive symptoms [21,26].

Here, we examined the functional state of the hippocampal formation in the 3xTgAD mouse through the recording of extracellular field potentials *in vivo*. Whereas most similar studies focus on one region of hippocampus in isolation (e.g., CA1 or DG), in this study we measured synaptic integrity and short-term plasticity at three sites simultaneously, specifically, the granule cell layer of DG, CA1 stratum radiatum (CA1sr) and CA1 stratum lacunosum-moleculare (CA1slm), using a multi-site electrode recording approach [9]. These sites were chosen as regions that receive monosynaptic input from the perforant path and, for CA1sr, polysynaptic feed forward input from DG via CA3. We measured extracellular field excitatory post-synaptic potentials (fEPSPs) in these target regions and performed current-source-density (CSD) analyses on CA1-DG axis responses. Through this we aimed to map synaptic current flow, indicative of synaptic-activity throughout the laminar structure, to test the integrity of synaptic connections within the EC-hippocampal tri-synaptic circuit.

Electrophysiological recordings conducted in AD mouse lines *in vitro* support a long-term decrease in synaptic function [21,30–32]. However, *in vivo* recordings support the presence of hyper-excitability and epileptiform activity, at least in early pathological stages, which are thought to contribute to cognitive decline [33,34]. In addition, recent findings indicate the presence of spontaneous seizure activity in the 3xTgAD model [35]. Thus, in the current study, we hoped to further examine these contradictory reports of decreased/increased synaptic function and test whether our observed decline in episodic-like memory in the 3xTgAD model [23,24] correlates with excitability changes within hippocampal circuits *in vivo*.

In contrast to *in vitro* reports, we found little evidence for decreased functional connectivity in either young or old 3xTgAD mice. Indeed, in measures of short-term plasticity we saw evidence for increased DG and CA1sr excitability in 3xTgAD mice compared to controls, particularly in young mice. This was coupled, however, with relatively less facilitated fEPSP amplitudes to a stimulus train alongside an enhanced re-entrant response into the hippocampal circuit in 3xTgAD mice. Thus, our data support increased hippocampal excitability at two loci in the 3xTgAD mouse: firstly, EC layer II input to DG and CA1sr (the latter presumably via propagation of DG output via CA3) in young and aged mice; and secondly, facilitation of hippocampal re-entrance in young 3xTgAD animals, presumably through potentiated deep-to-superficial EC connectivity.

Materials and Methods

Animals

Triple-transgenic mice (3xTgAD) carrying APP_{SWE}, $PS1_{M146V}$ and Tau_{P301L} transgenes and matched controls were bred at the University of Manchester from a colony donated by the La Ferla group [21]. Mice were housed in same-sex and genotype groups of 5–6 individuals on a 12:12 light/dark cycle with access to food and water *ad libitum*. The 3xTgAD colony was maintained through the pairing of homozygous individuals and the presence of transgenes was confirmed by genotyping a subset of 3xTgAD mice in each cage. All procedures conformed to UK Home Office licensing (project license PPL 40/3231) and were approved by the University of Manchester Ethical Review Panel. Electrophysiological data were collected from a 'young' sample of mice aged 4–6 months comprising 12 control (6 males: 6 female) and 11 3xTgAD (5 males: 6 female) mice. The age of the young group was selected to coincide with the early presence of hippocampal intracellular Aβ pathology (plaques and tangles accumulate from approximately 9 months of age in 3xTgAD mice) and hippocampal-dependent memory deficits [21–24]. A second 'old' sample of mice at 17–18 months of age comprised 5 control and 4 3xTgAD mice (all female); at this age there is extracellular plaque and tau pathology within hippocampus and subiculum. Thus, these groups allowed us to explore the additive effect of both pathology and general ageing on DG and CA1 responsiveness [20–22]. All female mice had previously experienced a battery of behavioural testing (spontaneous recognition tasks) which ceased at least a month before electrophysiological recordings were conducted. Male mice used for electrophysiology were experimentally naive. In the present experiments data from young male and female mice were combined as no sex differences were seen in either their basal input/output response, or in their CSD profiles to a 5 Hz train (data not shown).

Surgery and equipment

Mice were anaesthetised (urethane 30% w/v in dH_2O, 1.6 g/kg, i.p) and monitored until areflexia was achieved. Where reflexes remained, a small additional dose of urethane (10% w/v in dH_2O, 20–30 μl, i.p.) was given. The mouse was held in a stereotaxic frame (Kopf, 1430, USA) with lamda and bregma in the same horizontal plane to match the mouse atlas of Paxinos and Franklin [36]. A homoeothermic heating blanket (Harvard Apparatus, UK) and rectal probe maintained core body temperature at 37°C. A midline scalp incision was made and the skull exposed. Craniotomies were drilled above CA1 (B–2 mm, ML 1.5 mm) for the recording electrode and dorsal subiculum (B-3.85 mm, ML 1.5 mm) for the stimulating electrode. Recordings were made using a linear multi-electrode recording array containing either 16 contacts spaced100 μm, or 32 contacts spaced 50 μm apart (both 413 μm^2 contact area; NeuroNexus Tech, USA; there were no clear differences in response profiles between the different contact arrangements so data from different arrays were pooled.). The array was lowered vertically into the brain until the tip was approximately 2.5 mm below brain surface; at this depth recording contacts spanned the CA1-DG axis fully ([9]; see Figure 1A). A bipolar stimulating electrode (twisted 125 μm diameter Teflon-insulated stainless-steel wires; Advent RM, UK) was inserted 1.5 mm from brain surface at 30° relative to vertical into the molecular layer of the mid antero-posterior part of the subiculum (Figure 1A). At this position, stimulus pulses would activate the hippocampus both directly (via activation of perforant path (PP) fibres traversing subiculum) and indirectly (via re-entrance through subicular output to deep layers of entorhinal cortex which then activate superficial entorhinal PP output [9,10]. It was expected that upon stimulation, a characteristic pattern of current sources and sinks would be identifiable across the CA1-DG axis similar to those seen in the rat, reflecting the termination pattern of PP inputs to DG and CA1 ([9]; see Figure 1B for typical evoked laminar response and C for hippocampal circuit diagram).

Stimulation Protocols

Stimulus pulses were timed using a National Instruments card (PCI-6071E, NI, UK) controlled using LabVIEW software (8.2, NI, UK). These triggered a constant-current source (DS3, Digitimer, UK) connected to the stimulating electrode. Stimulus duration was set to 0.2 ms throughout the experiments. Stimulus protocols consisted of single pulses (0.33 Hz), paired pulses (PPulse) and trains of 20 pulses.

We first confirmed that the recording electrode spanned CA1sr, CA1slm and the superior and inferior blades of DG. This was achieved by monitoring the presence of stable evoked local field potentials (LFPs) in these regions to single-pulse stimulation at 200 μA [9,10]. In all experiments, a characteristic DG molecular layer positive-going LFP component was recorded with, in most cases, a granule cell layer population spike (PS; latter visible with high intensity PPulse or train stimulation; Figure 1B point C). The CA1slm response (presumably from activation of direct EC layer III input) was not seen in all experiments, likely due to variations in the placement of recording/stimulating electrodes (Figure 1B point B). CA1sr was characterised by a longer-latency negative-going LFP (Figure 1B point A). Due to the fixed distance between contacts in the recording array, upon identification of a typical response in one layer, those in other layers could reliably be confirmed due to the distance between contacts and LFP profile (CA1sr 100 microns dorsal to CA1slm, CA1slm approximately 100 microns dorsal to the largest DG molecular layer response; see Figure 1B for illustration of spacing).

Once a characteristic laminar LFP profile was achieved, a current-voltage (input-output) response curve was recorded for each LFP component by applying pairs of pulses at 50 ms intervals over a range of current intensities (50–600 μA). The first pulse of each pair was analysed and used to plot the curve. Thereafter, for PPulse and train protocols, the stimulus current was set to the value required to evoke a half-maximal response (i.e., 50% of the value required to elicit the maximum fEPSP in CA1sr); this was typically in the range 100–200 μA.

To examine short-term plasticity, PPulses were delivered at inter-pulse-intervals (PPI) of 25, 50, 100, 200, 500 and 1000 ms. All pairs were separated by 3 seconds and repeated 20 times. To examine the effects of repetitive stimulation and re-entrance into the hippocampal circuit, a single train of 20 pulses was applied at a frequency of 5 Hz. This frequency was chosen to provide a comparison with PPulse intervals and we predicted that 5 Hz trains would not produce any long-term plastic changes [9,10].

Upon completion of all stimulation protocols, lesions were created to mark electrode placements displaying particular response components [37]. Mice were perfused transcardially with 0.2 M sodium phosphate buffer and 4% paraformaldehyde and brains removed for fixation. Electrode placements were confirmed from 30 μm thick, Nissl-stained sagittal brain sections.

Data Acquisition and Analysis

Signals were amplified at source through an AC-coupled headstage (x20 gain) and further amplified for a total gain of 500x (Recorder64 system, Plexon, USA). Signals were filtered (0.1 Hz–6 kHz) and sampled at 10 kHz per channel (12-bit resolution).

Raw fEPSP response amplitudes to single-pulse stimulation were plotted to describe the current-response relationship (input-output; I/O) in control and 3xTgAD mice. In addition, PPulse and train data were normalised to the first pulse and results shown as a percentage change for both amplitude and latency to peak/trough to demonstrate any facilitation or depression of responses. Finally, train data were subjected to 1D CSD analysis [38] using custom Matlab software (see below).

All numerical data were analysed using Prism (v5; Graphpad). Mixed ANOVA with Bonferroni post hoc comparisons were applied for identification of pair-wise genotype differences for each of the three measures (I/O, PPulse and trains) for each response (CA1sr, CA1slm and DG). Due to sex differences in the number of animals present in each sample, young and old data sets were analysed separately to control for the small female-only older mouse group; however, young male and female data were then pooled as no sex difference was seen for any measure (data not shown). If recordings became unstable during an experiment, stimulation protocol data were excluded for that animal. Final sample sizes for each hippocampal layer in each stimulation protocol are shown in Table 1.

Amplitude, Slope and Latency measurements

Amplitude and the latency of evoked responses were extracted through custom Matlab software (Mathworks, version 7.0). In brief, each response was first visually inspected to ensure it had the expected shape with no noise or other artefacts. Five cursor points were then marked on different components of a mean response (see below) averaged over the 20 stimulus-response repeats. Thereafter, the programme used this five-point template to calculate the amplitude and latency of each original response. For train data, the waveform of each pulse was measured 'by hand' to account for the rapid changes in response profile associated with repetitive stimulation. In both cases, five points on each response were marked as follows: point 1 as the sample point before the start of the stimulus artefact; points 2 and 3 surrounded the response onset and points 5 and 6 surrounded the response peak (or trough).

For response amplitude (mV), the mean value between points 2–3 was subtracted from the corresponding maximal (response peak) or minimal (response trough) value between points 4 and 5. For latency to response peak/trough (ms), the centre timestamp between points 4 and 5 was subtracted from that for point 1. We did not attempt to measure latency to response onset, as there was seldom a defined level period in the recording between the stimulus artefact and response. All data presented in this paper are the average of 20 pulses. For DG population spikes (PS), the probability of evoking a PS was calculated out of 20 sweeps for

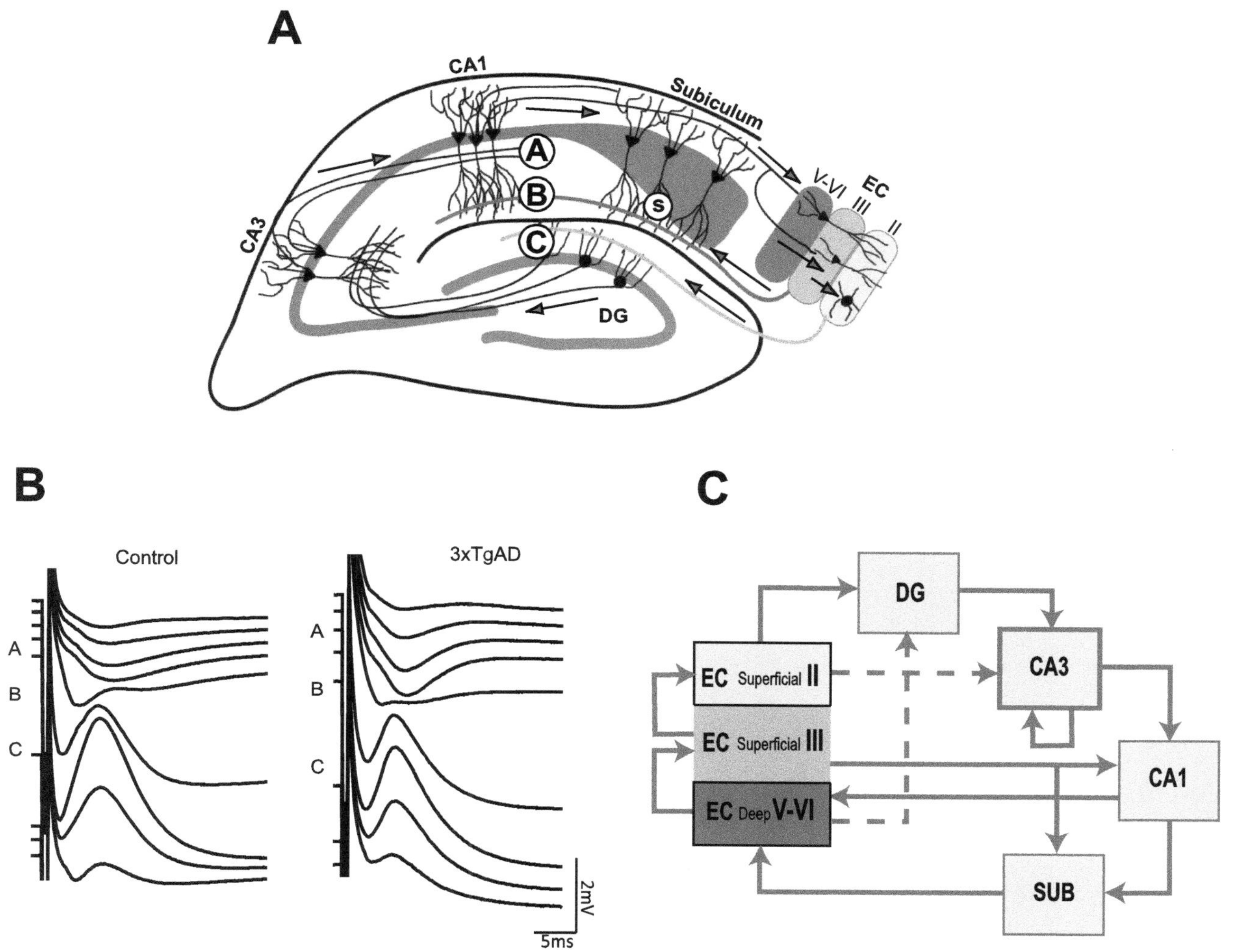

Figure 1. The hippocampal tri-synaptic circuit. A: Hippocampal formation with approximate electrode placements marked. Input and output pathways with principal direction of synaptic flow (arrows) and termination of fibre pathways from Schaffer collaterals [A], PP layer III [B] and PP layer II [C] are marked. Evoked activity at these points corresponds to CA1sr [A], CA1slm [B] and DG responses [C]. Stimulating electrode placement was in the deep dendritic layer of subiculum (S). B: Typical laminar field response to single-pulse stimulation at half-maximal current intensity. A, B and C correspond to responses recorded within regions A–F in Figure 3. C: Block diagram of the connectivity displayed in [A] for reader's clarity. Dashed lines represent the presence of sparse regional connectivity. Calibration applies to both profiles in B.

Table 1. Summary of data included in statistical analyses.

	Input/Output		Paired Pulse		Trains	
Young (4–6 months)						
	Control	**3xTgAD**	**Control**	**3xTgAD**	**Control**	**3xTgAD**
CA1sr	n = 12	n = 11	n = 12	n = 10	n = 10	n = 9
CA1slm	n = 12	n = 11	n = 12	n = 10	n = 7	n = 8
DG	n = 12	n = 11	n = 12	n = 10	n = 11	n = 9
Old (17–18 months)						
	Input/Output		**Paired Pulse**		**Trains**	
	Control	**3xTgAD**	**Control**	**3xTgAD**	**Control**	**3xTgAD**
CA1sr	n = 5	n = 4	n = 5	n = 4	n = 5	n = 3
CA1slm	n = 5	n = 4	n = 5	n = 4	n = 5	n = 3
DG	n = 5	n = 4	n = 5	n = 4	n = 5	n = 3

each PPI in animals that demonstrated PS at half-maximum stimulation.

Current Source Density Analysis

Current Source Density (CSD) analysis when applied to extracellular recordings taken from a laminar structure provides a highly detailed, anatomically aligned, spatiotemporal map of current sinks and sources produced through synaptic activity.

Single responses from train data were analysed by one-dimensional CSD analysis in a custom built Matlab programme, estimating the second-order spatial derivative using the formula of Freeman and Nicholson [38]. For this the distance between electrodes was either 100 or 50 μm and the degree of spatial smoothing applied was 2 as we analysed neighbouring contacts. It was assumed that (a) the major extracellular currents ran in parallel to the recording electrode (along the CA1-DG axis) and (b) tissue conductivity was spatially homogenous across the recording array (that is, any residual currents would represent local synaptic sinks and sources). CSD values at locations between those calculated for each electrode position were estimated by linear interpolation (20 steps) to produce a smooth and continuous mapped depiction of synaptic currents. Mapped CSD values are presented here in arbitrary units: current sources were mapped as reds, oranges and yellows; current neutral regions in light green; and regions showing current sinks as dark green to dark blue. The colour map for each CSD plot was normalised to itself (max/min) to represent the current gradient running from its maximum positive current (hot colours), to the maximum negative current (cool colours) with green equivalent to resting state or neutral.

Results

Current-response relationship

To examine the integrity of CA1 sr/slm-DG hippocampal circuitry, amplitude and latency of responses to activation of PP fibres were determined over a range of current intensities. There were no significant differences in amplitude measurements between control and 3xTgAD animals for CA1sr, CA1slm or DG responses in either young or old mice (Figure 2A–F; genotype (2) by PPI (5) mixed ANOVA). However, there was a significant effect of current intensity on all response amplitudes in all animals ($F(4,28) = 5.74–23.06$ $P<0.0001$), with higher currents eliciting larger responses as would be expected by recruitment of PP fibres with increasing current. In addition, DG population spikes developed from 200 μA stimulus current onwards in 5/12 control and 8/11 3xTgAD young mice (data not shown). In old mice, two of the four 3xTgAD animals developed DG PS at high current intensities; however, PS were not seen in old control mice (data not shown). While these observations in DG PS frequency are merely qualitative for the purpose responses to single stimuli, their occurrence was strain-dependent in 3xTgADs and controls during PPulse stimulation, as described below.

To investigate differences in response latency between 3xTgAd and control mice we compared responses from each hippocampal layer at a stimulus intensity of 200 μA (typical half-maximal stimulation current; see Table 2). The order of latencies (to response peak or trough) was consistent with our expectations for the associated synaptic delays *in vivo* of CA1sr, CA1slm and DG in response to PP stimulation as used here (i.e., fastest for DG and CA1slm; refer to Figure 1C) and no genotype differences were found (data not shown). Thus, from the similar I/O amplitude and relative response latency patterns seen with this stimulus protocol, we concluded that there were no genotype differences in functional connectivity during low-frequency activation in the PP fibre pathways from EC layers II and III traversing subiculum to the hippocampal circuit in both young and old animals.

Short-term synaptic plasticity

To assess short-term synaptic plasticity, we examined the effect of varying PPI on the amplitude and latency of responses to half-maximal stimulus current (range for all mice 100–200 μA). Measurements from the second pulse were normalised to those from the first and are presented as percentage change, such that positive values represent paired-pulse facilitation (or a decreased latency) and negative values represent paired-pulse depression (or an increased latency). CA1sr, CA1slm and DG responses were analysed in separate genotype (2) by PPI (6) mixed ANOVA with Bonferroni post-hoc comparisons.

For young animals, there was a significant effect of PPI on the amplitude of CA1sr and CA1slm responses ($F(5,100) = 7.32$, $P< 0.0001$ and $F(5,100) = 4.93$, $P<0.0005$, respectively) with maximal facilitation seen at 25 and 50 ms intervals. While there were no significant genotype differences for CA1slm responses (data not shown), for CA1sr there was an interaction ($F(5,100) = 2.54$, $P< 0.05$) and a pair-wise genotype difference at 50 ms ($t(20) = 3.27$, $P<0.01$; see Figure 3A). This was evident as 3xTgAD responses facilitating significantly more than that for controls, in stark contrast to the depression of CA1sr responses frequently seen in AD models *in vitro* during LTP protocols [21,31,32]. For the DG response, there was again a significant genotype difference ($F(1,100) = 11.80$, $P<0.005$) and an interaction ($F(5,100) = 4.88$, $P<0.001$). Furthermore, there were pair-wise genotype differences at 25 ms ($t(20) = 5.12$, $P<0.001$) and 50 ms ($t(20) = 3.54$, $P<0.01$), where response amplitudes facilitated in 3xTgAD mice and depressed in controls (Figure 3B), suggestive of DG hyper-excitability in this AD model. As expected, population spikes to the second pulse (P2) were seen in the DG granule cell layer in 4/10 3xTgAD and 6/12 controls during half-maximal amplitude PP stimulation. However, 3xTgAD mice had a higher tendency to exhibit PS at shorter PPI (25 ms–100 ms), whereas for control animals this relationship was reversed (most PS in 200 ms–1000 ms PP interval range; examples of paired-pulse responses at 50 ms and 200 ms PPI left panel Figure 3C, probability distribution across PPI for PS to P2 displayed in right panel Figure 3C).

To determine whether genotype differences in the velocity of synaptic transmission could have contributed to observed short-term amplitude differences, response latencies were examined for each hippocampal layer in response to pairs of pulses (latency of second pulse to peak/trough relative to the first). There was a significant effect of PPI on latency for CA1sr ($F(5,100) = 2.63$, $P< 0.05$) with PPI 25 ms eliciting a slightly faster response for both genotypes (3xTgAD 14.99%±3.17 SEM faster and control 5.82%±1.7 SEM faster than the first pulse). For DG, a significant effect of PPI was also seen ($F(5,100) = 7.41$, $P<0.001$), with PPI 100 ms and 200 ms eliciting a slightly slower response in both genotypes (data not shown); however, no effects of latency were observed in CA1slm. Thus, despite a significant effect of PPI on the time to peak/trough of the second pulse, there were no obvious effects of AD pathology. To summarise the data from young animals, we found an indication of increased short-term excitability in 3xTgAD mice in the form of increased LFP amplitude in CA1sr, and with DG facilitation to short interval delays; however, there was no apparent change in overt hippocampal synaptic connectivity as reflected in the absolute latencies of CA1sr and DG molecular layer LFPs.

For old animals there was a significant effect of PPI on response amplitude for CA1sr ($F(5,35) = 2.54$, $P<0.05$) and a significant

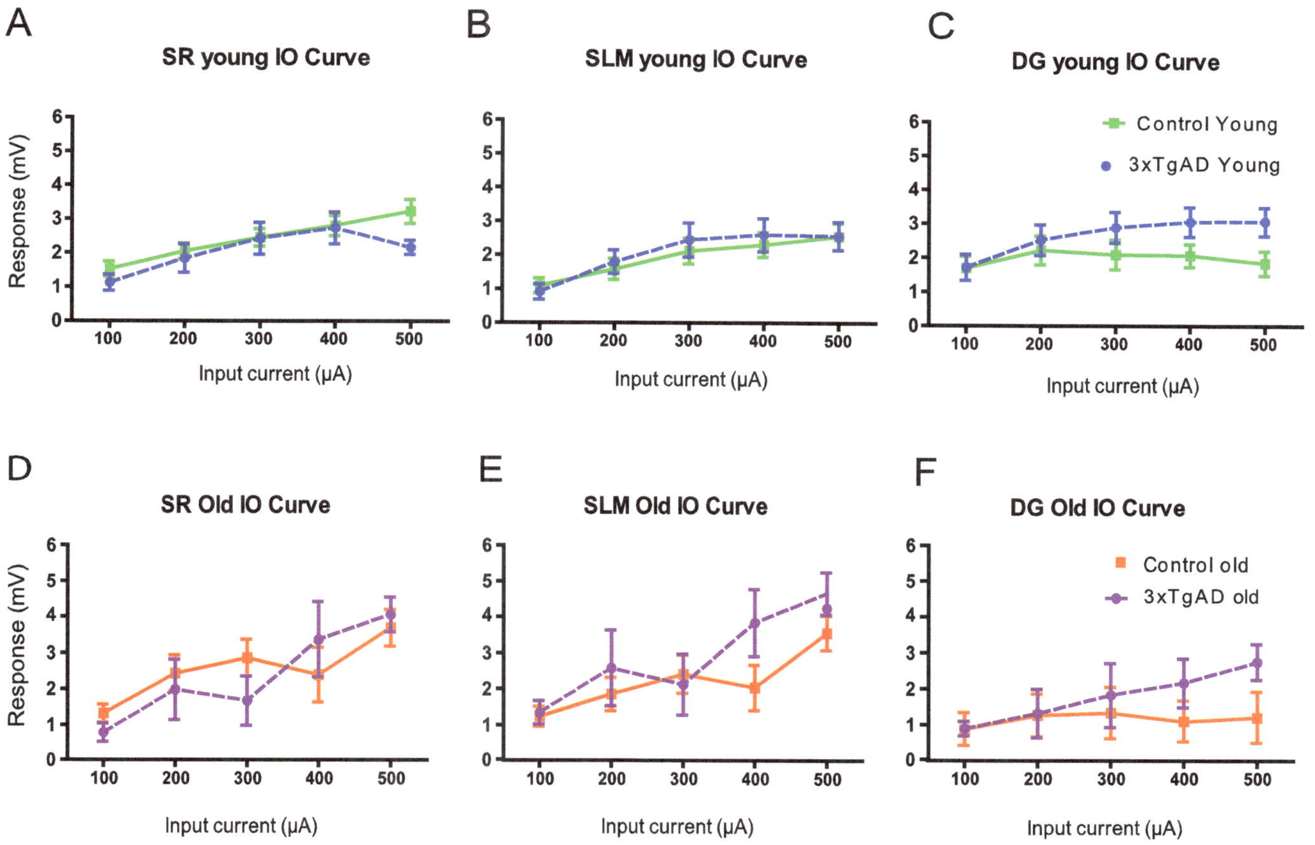

Figure 2. Input-output relationships in young and old 3xTgAD mice are similar to controls. A to F: Stimulus-response (I/O) curves in young (4–6 month) and old (17–18 months) animals in relation to increasing input current intensity at CA1sr (A and D), CA1slm (B and E) and DG (C and F). Error bars are (±SEM).

interaction ($F(5,35)=5.94$, $P<0.0005$). This manifested as a significant pair-wise genotype difference at PPI 50 ms ($t(7)=5.65, P<0.0001$; Figure 4A) where 3xTgAD animals again facilitated more than controls. There were no significant effects for CA1slm; however, there was an interaction for DG ($F(5,35)=3.46, P<0.05$) and a pair-wise genotype difference at PPI 25 ms ($t(7)=3.08$), $P<0.05$; Figure 4B), where again 3xTgAD responses facilitated in contrast to control responses which depressed. Of note, 3xTgAD DG responses tended to depress more strongly than controls at PPI of 200 ms or longer, however, these differences did not reach significance. Also of interest, control DG appeared to show little if any modulatory changes across the range of PPIs, neither depressing nor facilitating (compare Figure 3B with Figure 4B). We assume these were age-related changes in DG function, as they present a different profile to that of aged 3xTgAD animals. The implication of this reduction in paired-pulse depression for DG with normal ageing is that it may be causative in the known age-related impairment in pattern separation that may, in turn, contribute to our observed age-related deficit in episodic-like memory in older control mice ([23]; see Discussion).

For latency to peak/trough, there was a significant effect of PPI for CA1sr ($F(5,35)=2.69$, $P<0.05$), an interaction ($F(5,35)=4.23$, $P<0.005$) and a pair-wise genotype difference at PPI 50 ms ($t(7)=3.99$, $P<0.05$). In this case, 3xTgAD mice had a significantly longer latency relative to P1, whereas control mice had a slightly shorter latency (3xTgAD change 59.42% ±27.83 SEM slower, control 8.08%±3.49 SEM faster). This difference can be explained by the larger CA1sr amplitudes in 3xTgAD mice compared to controls (3xTgAD responses have a longer period from stimulus to response trough). For CA1slm, there was a significant interaction ($F(5,35)=4.35$, $P<0.01$) and a pair-wise genotype difference at PPI 50 ms ($t(7)=3.01, P<0.05$) with 3xTgAD mice showing a faster P2 response than control mice (3xTgAD 10.79%±4.28 SEM faster, control 1.47%±5.26 SEM slower). For DG, there was an effect of PPI only ($F(5,35)=3.02$, $P<0.05$). In these old animals, only one 3xTgAD mouse showed evidence of a DG PS and, as per the young animals, this was more prevalent at shorter PPI (PP25ms and PP50ms; data not shown). Thus, as per the young data, it appeared that old 3xTgAD mice demonstrate increased short-term plasticity and excitability in CA1sr and DG, albeit to a smaller degree when compared to younger mice.

To summarise the findings of the PPulse protocol, both young and old animals showed response facilitation to PPulse stimulation at short intervals in CA1sr; however, excitability in terms of increases in DG PS to short PPI was most pronounced at a young age. 3xTgAD mice had a significantly larger CA1sr response than controls and this was seen in both young and old age groups, suggesting a specific change at the CA1 level could alter excitability in this region. In addition, 3xTgAD DG responses at a short PPI were facilitated relative to controls (which depressed in young controls), indicating changes in the DG synaptic network. The DG paired-pulse depression in young controls appeared to be absent in old controls, suggesting an ageing-related shift in DG

Table 2. Response latencies in hippocampal formation.

	Control 4–6 mo			3xTgAD 4–6 mo			Control 17–18 mo			3xTgAD 17–18 mo		
	Latency	SEM	n	Latency	SEM	n	Latency	SEM	n	Latency	SEM	n
CA1sr	7.84	0.56	12	7.99	0.54	11	9.79	1.21	5	9.25	1.64	4
CA1slm	6.01	0.49	12	5.26	0.42	11	7.30	1.21	5	6.73	0.82	4
DG	8.03	0.65	12	7.46	0.36	11	6.69	2.24	5	7.81	1.26	4

Figures show peak response latencies (ms) in response to subiculum stimulation at 200 µA.

function; this attenuation may have mechanistic implications for age-related deficits in the pattern separation role carried out by DG and episodic-like memory capacity in older mice.

Train stimulation

To examine neuronal reverberation within the hippocampal formation, mice experienced low-frequency stimulation in the form of a 20-pulse train, delivered at 5 Hz. Train data were analysed in genotype (2) by pulse number (20) Mixed ANOVA as follows: raw amplitudes and peak/trough latencies were examined for each response (results labelled as 'raw') and data were also converted to a percentage change from P1, as a measure of the summated effect of train stimulation (labelled as '% change'). Data from young and old mice were also subjected to CSD analyses to identify the spatiotemporal relationships between current sources and sinks along the CA1-DG axis and to shed light on the origins and relative strength of the synaptic inputs to different laminae.

5 Hz Train analysis: Young animals at 4–6 months of age

For young animals, there was a significant effect of pulse number on the amplitude for all responses; however, for latency, there was a significant effect of pulse number only for CA1slm and DG responses and a genotype difference for CA1sr.

CA1sr ($n = 10$ control, $n = 9$ 3xTgAD) showed a significant effect of pulse number on amplitude ($F(19, 323) = 5.94$, $P<0.0001$ raw; $F(19,323) = 6.18$, $P<0.0001$%change; Figure 5A), that is, subsequent pulses facilitated with respect to pulse 1. However, despite the tendency for 3xTgAD mice to show less facilitation throughout the train this genotype difference did not reach significance. There was also no effect of pulse number on response latency, however, there was a significant genotype difference ($F(1,323) = 11.01$, $P<0.005$%change) and an interaction ($F(19,323) = 1.63$, $P<0.05$), with Bonferroni pair-wise differences at pulses 5–8 and 13 ($t(17) = 3.071–3.725$, $P<0.05/P<0.01$; Figure 5B). In this case, 3xTgAD response latencies remained the same or were slightly shorter compared to that of the first pulse, whereas control latencies increased.

CA1slm response amplitudes ($n = 7$ control, $n = 8$ 3xTgAD) showed a significant effect of pulse number only ($F(19, 247) = 5.96$, $P<0.0001$ raw; $F(19, 247) = 6.07$, $P<0.0001$, %change) as did CA1slm latencies ($F(19,247) = 3.37$, $P<0.0001$ raw; $F(19, 247) = 1.84$, $P<0.05$%change) with progressive pulses evoking a larger and slightly longer latency response (data not shown). There were no genotype differences.

DG response amplitudes ($n = 11$ control, $n = 9$ 3xTgAD) showed a significant effect of pulse number ($F(19,342) = 3.5$, $P< 0.0001$ raw; $F(19,343) = 10.36$, $P<0.0001$%change) as did response latencies ($F(19, 342) = 3.69$, $P<0.0001$ raw; $F(19, 342) = 8$, $P<0.0001$), with subsequent responses depressing slightly and latencies increasing compared to the first response. There were no genotype differences for either response amplitude or latency (data not shown).

In summary, there was a robust effect of pulse number on both the amplitude and latencies of responses. We found no significant evidence for genotype differences in the absolute amplitude of CA1 and DG responses; however, CA1sr clearly demonstrated a trend for poorer facilitation in 3xTgAD animals with an accompanying genotype difference in CA1sr latency in 3xTgAD mice.

Re-entrance into CA1 and DG: young mice

Half of the young mice from each genotype were classified as 'excitable' (5/11 control and 5/9 3xTgAD), that is, they showed increasing levels of DG population spiking for subsequent pulses in

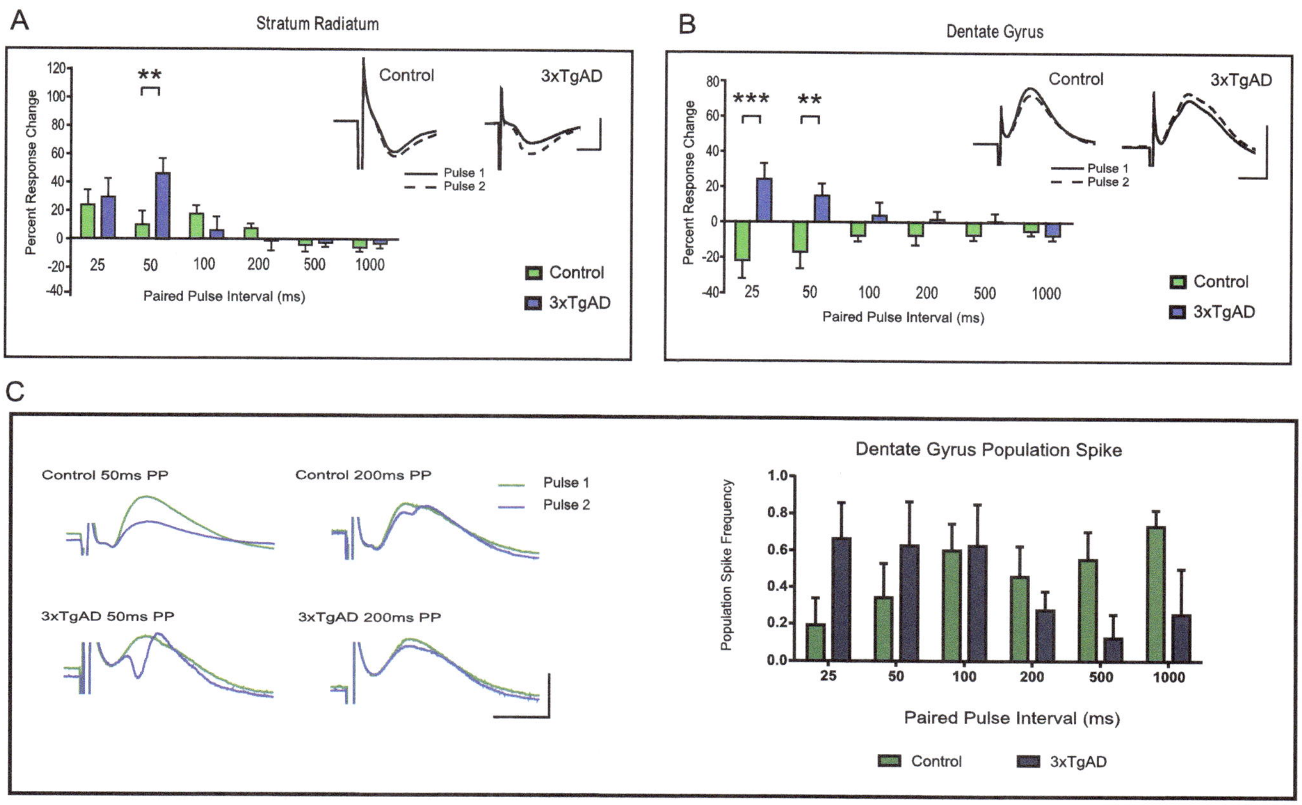

Figure 3. Increased short-term plasticity in young 3xTgAD mice. Panels A and B show fEPSP amplitude of pulse 2 normalised to pulse 1 (±SEM) for CA1sr [A], and DG [B]. No differences were observed for CA1slm (data not shown). Inserts show representative traces from single experiments with pulse 1 (black line) and pulse 2 (grey line) taken from PP50ms in all examples. Pair-wise genotype differences are evident (**P<0.01; ***P<0.0001). Calibration 12.5 ms/2 mV. C: Left panel shows examples of population spikes (PS) evoked at 50 or 200 ms in control and 3xTgAD mice (average of 20 sweeps each; calibration 10 ms/3 mV). Right panel shows the probability of evoking a PS to the second pulse of a stimulus pair versus paired-pulse interval. Note that the PS probability is highest at short intervals for 3xTgAD and longer intervals for controls. Error bars are (±SEM).

the train and, in some cases, re-entrance into the hippocampal circuit in both CA1 and DG (Figure 5 panels C and D; see arrows). This is better illustrated using 1-dimensional CSD analyses, where the evoked synaptic currents in each layer of the hippocampus can be computed and visualised over time (see next section). All animals that showed re-entrance did so by pulse 20: within the 5 excitable 3xTgAD animals, 3 showed clear re-entrance into CA1sr (at pulses 10, 17 and 20; 15.71±0.33 ms; mean latency ± SEM), 4 showed re-entrance into CA1slm (at pluses 15, 18 and twice by 20; 14.71±0.12 ms) and 3 exhibited re-entrance into DG (at pulses 7, 15 and 20 pulses; 20.69±1.98; Figure 5D). Re-entrance latencies were similar in the 5 excitable control mice; CA1sr (n = 4; 17.5±1.5 ms) and CA1slm (n = 3; 15.49±2.08 ms), whereas DG had a shorter latency re-entrance wave (n = 2; 16.32±2.22 ms). However, in contrast to 3xTgAD mice, all re-entrance was seen at pulse 20 of the train and not earlier in the sequence. It appears, therefore, that young control and 3xTgAD mice (of 4–6 months of age) can show self-sustained reverberation through the hippocampal formation following repetitive low-frequency stimulation; in addition, these responses tend to occur in 3xTgAD mice at an earlier stage in the pulse sequence.

Current Source Density analysis: young mice

Stimulation of the PP with a 5 Hz frequency train elicited a profile of current sources and sinks consistent with an electrode traversing the CA1-DG axis, with positioning parallel to the dendrites of pyramidal cells in CA1 and spanning DG [9]. Typical CSD responses in and their layers of origin are outlined in Figure 6A (control mouse response to the 5th pulse).

The CSD responses for control and 3xTgAD animals can be viewed for pulses 1, 5, 10 and 20 in Figure 6 C and D. To orientate the reader to the appearance of each synaptic component, the CSD responses to pulse 1 are referred to using the example in Figure 6A. In response to pulse 1, both 3xTgAD and control animals show an early latency current sink in CA1slm (Figure 6A: component 1) consistent with an excitatory synaptic response to activation of perforant path (EC layer III tempero-ammonic) terminals on the apical dendrites of CA1 pyramidal cells. Simultaneous with this, a sink in the molecular layer of the inferior blade of DG is seen (Figure 6A: component 2) and an accompanying current source in the granule cell layer (Figure 6A: component 3). For this control mouse, a further small current source is seen in the CA1 pyramidal cell layer, perhaps representing the passive source of a CA1slm sink-source pair (Figure 6A: component 4). In both genotypes a weak sink is visible in CA1 stratum oriens, consistent with synaptic delay from the DG mossy fibres to CA3 and output of CA3 Schaffer collaterals onto basal CA1 dendrites (Figure 6A: component 5). These CSD patterns were typical of first pulse responses for all animals, including those classified as 'excitable' (DG PS and/or re-entrance) and in those that did not show any evidence of PS in DG or CA1.

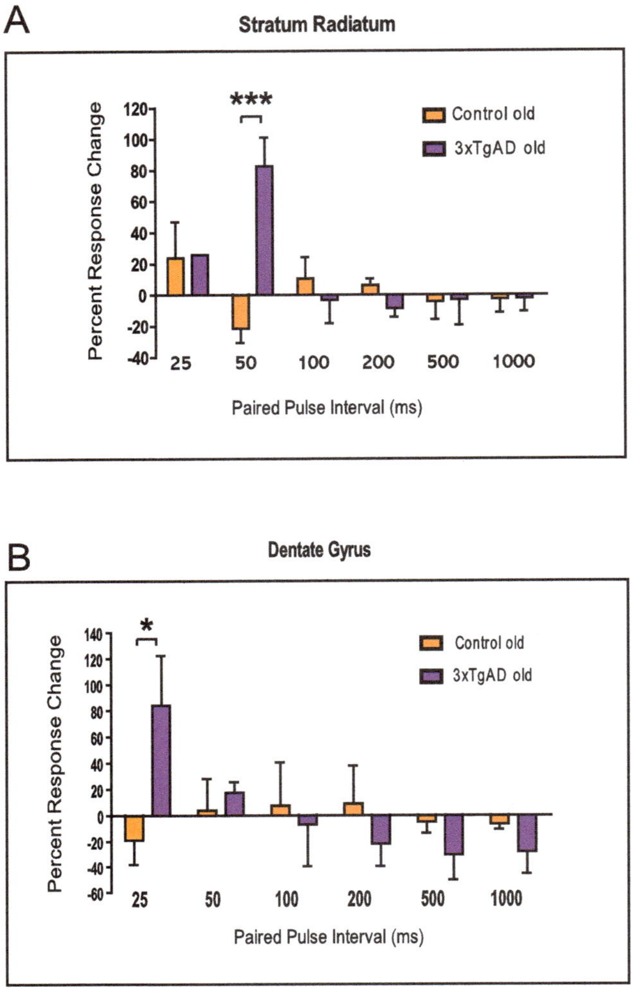

Figure 4. Increased short-term plasticity in old 3xTgAD mice. Panels A and B as per Fig 3 for CA1sr [A] and DG [B]. Pairwise genotype differences are *$P<0.05$; ***$P<0.0001$. Note lack of modulatory effect of PPI in controls for DG.

In response to pulse 5, a clear PS could be seen in the DG of the example 3xTgAD animal and this DG population spike also begins to emerge in the control animal (Figure 6, pulse 5 upward arrow). Visible in the control mouse, there was also the appearance of a slightly longer component extending the existing CA1slm sink, perhaps within the region of CA1 where CA3 Schaffer collaterals synapse onto CA1sr (also visible in Figure 6C pulses 10 and 20). It is likely that this response was also present in the selected 3xTgAD mouse; however, the sink was likely obscured by the large DG PS.

In response to pulse 10, long-latency re-entrance (presumably transferring through EC) in the 3xTgAD animal is seen in the form of a sink-source pair in CA1 cell layer at around 15 ms latency (Fig. 6D: component 6). There is still a clear early PS in DG, and there is a long-latency DG source, perhaps resulting from the inferior blade cell layer.

By pulse 20, the example control animal is also showing a clear long-latency CA1 current source; the CA1 response being accompanied by a population spike in the 3xTgAD example (Figure 6D upper black arrow). In the 3xTgAD profile the early DG cell layer response is curtailed, by a presumed inhibitory after-potential (Figure 6D: IAP); however, there is a clear re-entrant population spike in the inferior blade of DG (Figure 6D lower arrow). Figure 6B shows pulse 20 for the 3xTgAD animal in more detail, where the re-entrance of the CA1 and DG response is clearly reflected in the overlaid LFPs. Thus, the 3xTgAD animal appears to demonstrate increased excitability in DG, as indicated by a larger early response to activation of the PP.

To summarize our CSD findings in young animals, we saw a pattern of sources and sinks revealed by CSD analyses that were consistent across controls and 3xTgAD mice with the expected connectivity of the layer II and III EC inputs to the hippocampal formation. In addition, comparative excitability was increased in DG and CA1 of 3xTgADs to both the direct effect of PP activation and indirect, delayed re-entrant input, presumably also arriving via PP afferents.

5 Hz train analysis: Old animals of 17–18 months of age

For old animals, there were no significant effects on the amplitude or latency for any response (when analysed as percentage change, i.e., normalized values); however, it is likely that some effects could have been masked due to large variances in the control sample ($n=5$ control, $n=3$ AD). Nevertheless, analysing 'raw' response amplitudes did show genotype differences. In detail;

CA1sr response amplitudes showed a significant effect of genotype for raw amplitude ($F(1,114) = 6.96$, $P<0.05$), with 3xTgAD animals showing little fEPSP facilitation following the first stimulus pulse compared to controls (Figure 7A). There was a trend for controls to show facilitation over the course of the train but this effect did not reach significance. For pulse 20, the 3xTgAD fEPSP (early PP-evoked response) peaked at 9.87 ± 1.64 ms ($n=3$) and for control animals at 8.63 ± 1.45 ms ($n=5$); however, no long latency, re-entrant responses were seen in either group.

CA1slm responses showed no significant genotype differences for either fEPSP amplitude or latency (data not shown), however, there was again a trend for CA1slm amplitude to remain steady over the train in 3xTgAD mice (Figure 7B). Again, responses in controls appeared to facilitate over the course of the train but this group difference could have been masked by the large variance of the control data set. The CA1slm response to pulse 20 peaked at 6.69 ± 2.75 ms ($n=4$) in 3xTgAD and at 7.71 ± 1.26 ms ($n=5$) in control mice; however, no long-latency re-entrant responses were seen.

DG responses showed a significant effect of pulse number on response amplitude ($F(19, 114) = 4.20$, $P<0.0001$ raw; $F(19, 114) = 4.67$, $P<0.0001$% change) as pulses depressed over each subsequent trial; however, in contrast to young animals, there was little evidence of DG PS activity (except for one 3xTgAD animal: see Figure 7D). 3xTgAD early responses peaked faster than those for control animals (5.76 ± 1.17 ms ($n=3$) versus 7.47 ± 1.95 ($n=5$) respectively); however, again there was a large within group variance, perhaps due to an effect of age and sample size. Also, as there were no long-latency DG responses this again supports a lack of re-entrance in all old mice.

Laminar response profiles during pulse trains are shown in Figure 7 panels C (control) and D (3xTgAD). In contrast to the traces seen in young animals (Figure 5 panels C and D), very little facilitation was seen in any cell layer. Thus, in summary, the latencies to the initial response peak/trough in old animals were comparable, if slightly longer (c.1ms) than those in young animals; however, no long-latency response components were seen in CA1 and DG of old mice at delays that would be associated with

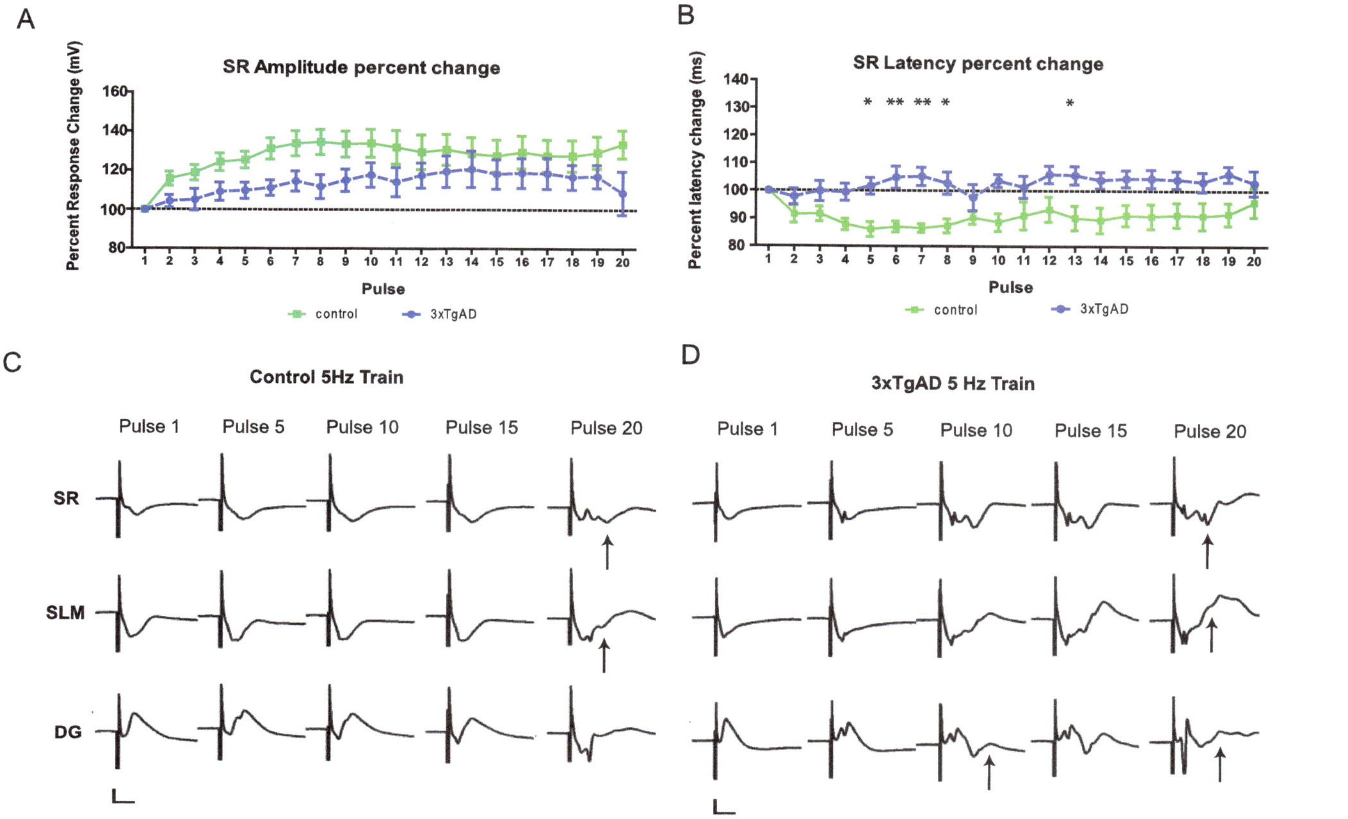

Figure 5. Changes in response latency and occurrence of hippocampal re-entrance during 5 Hz stimulus trains in young 3xTgAD animals. A & B: fEPSP amplitude [A] and latency [B] for CA1sr response, expressed as a percentage change from the response to pulse 1. Pair-wise genotype differences at *P<0.05 and **P<0.01. C & D: Example to show differential fEPSP responses to selected stimuli of a 5 Hz train in control [C] and 3xTgAD [D] mice classified as 'excitable'. Responses in 'non-excitable' animals during 5 Hz trains remained as per the response to pulse 1. Re-entrance (longer latency responses, likely propagating through EC) are shown with upward pointing black arrows for pulse 20 in both genotypes and, in this instance, by pulse 10 in [D]. Calibration bar [C,D] 2 mV by 10 ms.

hippocampal re-entrance in younger animals. The lack of an effect of pulse number in CA1 responses, and of PS activity in animals of both genotypes, likely reflects age-related changes in excitability.

Current source density analysis: old animals

Mice aged 17–18 months demonstrated a pattern of synaptic current sources and sinks consistent with activation of the EC PP from layers II and III. This profile was similar to that seen in young animals. However, whereas young 3xTgAD and control mice demonstrated increasing excitability over a pulse train, the CSD profiles of old animals remained largely unchanged (Figure 7 panels E and F). Both genotypes showed what appeared to be an inhibitory after-potential in the DG granule cell layer following the source seen in the main DG response (Figure 7 panels E and F). Control mice showed a large sink in CA1 stratum oriens (smaller in 3xTgAD) at a slightly longer latency than the CA1slm response, consistent with a synaptic delay from the CA3 Schaffer collaterals. In the example shown (Figure 7F), the 3xTgAD animal showed a current source in CA1sr/stratum pyramidale.

To summarize the results from aged animals, CSD analyses revealed that the expected synaptic components reflecting PP inputs to hippocampus were present in animals of both genotypes; however, progressive changes in excitability to 5 Hz stimulation were not observed. There was a significant effect of genotype on the absolute response amplitude evoked in CA1sr and a clear trend for a similar lack of facilitation in CA1slm (although, not significant). Thus, we found evidence for decreased short-term potentiation in the form of train responses in old 3xTgAD mice, above the general decline of amplitude seen in control mice in normal aging.

Discussion

Alzheimer's disease (AD) is characterised phenotypically by a loss of episodic memory and pathologically by the stereotypical accumulation of Aβ and tau protein. We have shown previously that the 3xTg murine model for AD exhibits a selective deficit in hippocampal-dependent, episodic-like memory at 6 months of age with intact but declining performance at 3 months [23,24]. At six months of age, 3xTgAD mice show pronounced intracellular accumulation of Aβ [20,21], strongly suggesting a causal role for this AD pathology in our observed episodic deficits. In the present study, we sought to examine whether this episodic-like memory deficit is accompanied by changes in hippocampal synaptic function through *in vivo* electrophysiological recordings in 3xTgAD and control mice. A positive outcome would provide strong evidence for a neural correlate of memory loss in early AD or MCI. To this end, we examined synaptic responsiveness to single pulses of increasing current intensity and short-term synaptic plasticity through PPF and circuit reverberation (re-entrance) in

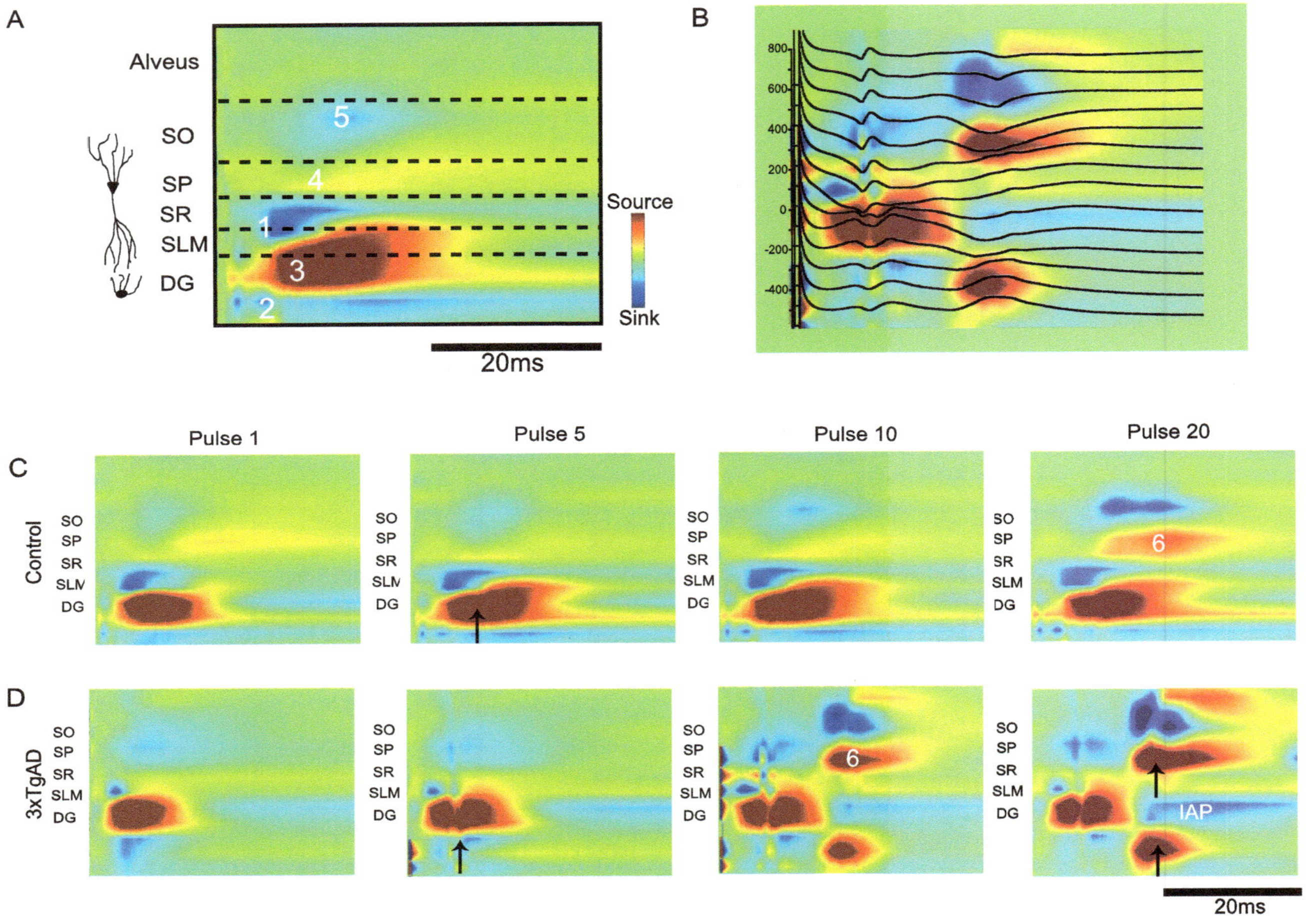

Figure 6. Laminar CSD profiles for responses to 5 Hz train stimulation in young mice. A: CSD from pulse 10 of control mouse with approximate layer boundaries indicated (SO-stratum oriens, SP-stratum pyramidale, SR-stratum radiatum, SLM-stratum lacunosum-moleculare and DG-Dentate gyrus and Alveus). Left side of all CSD panels represents point of stimulus onset. Current sources are yellow/red, current sinks light/dark blues and neutral regions are in green. The overlaid numbers 1–6 seen in [A] and in [C–D] correspond to synaptic events as follows: slm sink (1), DG molecular sink (2), DG granule cell source (3), CA1 source (4), SO sink (5) and CA1 long latency source (6). B: 3xTgAD CSD laminar profile with voltage overlay of evoked response corresponding to pulse 20 in [D]. Long-latency re-entrance and PS can be seen in CA1. CSD figures from control [C] and 3xTgAD [D] mice correspond to the field response profiles for the pulses seen in Figure 5C and D. CSD analysis of pulses 1, 5, 10, and 20 of a 20-pulse train shows progressive increases in excitability in CA1 and DG cell layers in control [C] and 3xTgAD [D] mouse. Black arrows point to short-early DG PS (pulse 5), inferior blade DG PS (pulse 20 3xTgAD) and long-latency CA1 PS that appears to propagate away from CA1 through the alveus (pulse 20 3xTgAD). Presumed inhibitory-afterpotentials labelled as IAP. Scale bar is 20 ms. CSD figures are scaled to the same parameters for each pulse and between genotypes.

response to train stimulation in 3 regions of the hippocampal circuit: CA1 stratum radiatum, CA1 stratum lacunosum-moleculare and DG.

Synaptic connectivity and the 'tri-synaptic' pathway

We found no significant genotype difference in the amplitude of evoked responses to increasing input currents in 3xTgAD and age-matched control mice at 4–6 or 17–18 months of age. This is in contrast to previous *in vitro* reports in the same model and the APP_{SWE} mouse suggesting a depression in the input/output curve upon the accumulation of intracellular Aβ [21,31] but agrees with other findings, showing no basal response change [30]. The discrepancies between reports could be due to methodological differences (*in vitro* slice recordings versus *in vivo* recordings in the present study) and/or stimulation protocol. More specifically, in the research cited above, single-pulse responses were examined through direct stimulation of a monosynaptic pathway (Schaffer collateral input to CA1 or PP input to DG [21,30,31]). In the current study, responses were generated through stimulation within the molecular layer of the subiculum, creating several discrete responses: (1) an early mono-synaptic ('direct') response in DG and CA1slm through activation of *en passage* PP fibres (the EC layer II and III inputs to DG and CA1slm, respectively); (2) di-/tri-synaptic responses in CA1sr and CA1so (presumably via propagation through CA3); and (3) a longer-latency polysynaptic ('indirect') response in DG and CA1. The latter represents 're-entrance' of synaptic activity, shown in the rat to depend on activation of subicular/CA1 output that targets deep layers of EC, from where recruitment of deep-to-superficial connectivity within EC then allows 're-entrance' of evoked activity into the DG and hippocampus via the PP [9,10]. This re-entrant response is most apparent during repetitive stimulation, suggesting that it requires substantial temporal synaptic facilitation within EC. Thus, in our *in vivo* 3xTgAD model, the combination of activating direct and

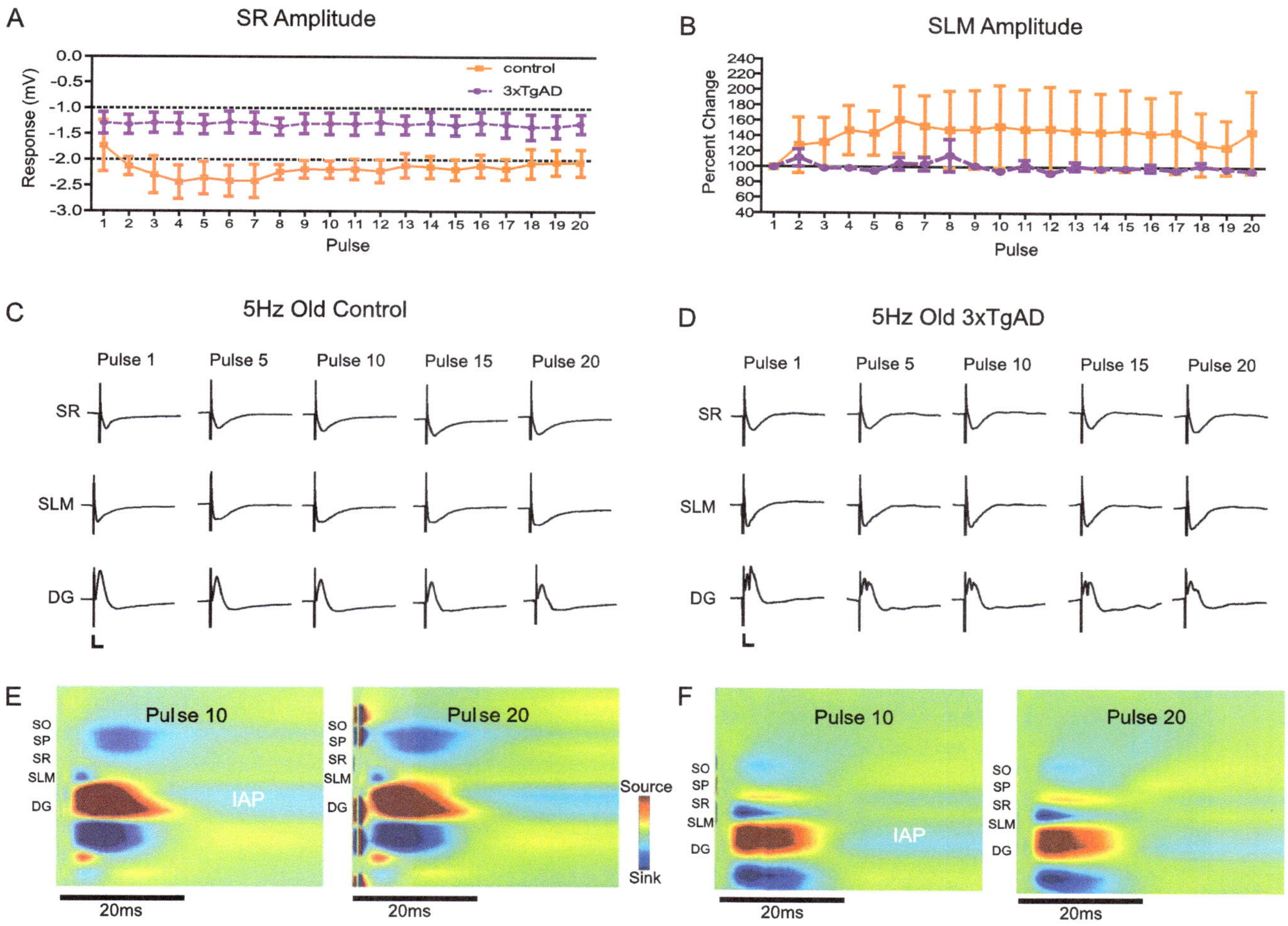

Figure 7. Train stimulation at 5 Hz in old animals. A. There is a significant genotype difference in raw fEPSP amplitude in old animals upon 5 Hz frequency stimulation in CA1sr ($P<0.05$). B. CA1 responses did not facilitate following pulse 1 in old 3xTgAD animals (data shown for CA1slm). Control [C] and 3xTgAD [D] representative responses for old animals. Note a lack of increase in response magnitude as the train progresses. 3xTgAD animal in [D] was the only old animal to show DG PS. Calibration 2 mV/10 ms. CSD analysis of pulses 10 and 20 in representative old control [E] and 3xTgAD [F] animals. CSD components are comparable to those seen in young mice at pulse 1 (Fig 6C & D; current sinks in blue, sources in red). A prolonged, facilitating afterpotential is clearly visible from 20 ms in the DG of both control and 3xTgAD animals (marked IAP).

indirect pathways could, perhaps, have offset abnormalities present in the monosynaptic CA3-CA1 pathway of the 3xTgAD as found by Oddo et al. [21]. Due to a lack of any abnormality in the basic synaptic connectivity of the 3xTgAD model shown here *in vivo*, we propose that any differences found in the current study for PPF or trains between the control and 3xTgAD mouse cannot be attributed simply to a lower capacity or conductance of damaged fibre pathways [28] as the current required to elicit a half-maximum fEPSP was not different between genotypes. Thus, in the following sections we discuss evidence for AD-specific changes in short-term synaptic plasticity that are separate from the basal synaptic abnormalities reported previously in the 3xTgAD mouse [21].

Increased synaptic facilitation in the 3xTgAD model supports the early development of hyper-excitability

To examine short-term synaptic plasticity, mice were subjected to paired-pulse stimulation over a variety of intervals [39]. In DG, the granule cell response to such short interval PPulse stimulation is modulated through a combination of: (a) feed forward, GABAa-dependent inhibition driven via PP input to local interneurons; (b) pre-synaptic metabotropic glutamate receptor activity (mGluR;[40,41]); and (c) feedback inhibition elicited from recurrent interneuron collaterals in the vicinity of the activated granule cell [41,42]. The net effect of these mechanisms is that DG responses normally show paired-pulse depression to PP activation. In the present study, control mice, as expected [42], exhibited paired-pulse depression to short PPIs (25–50 ms). This depression is presumably produced through polysynaptic GABAergic feed-back, driven by the first pulse, causing hyperpolarisation of GCs (mediated by $GABA_A$ and $GABA_B$ receptors[43,44]). This inhibitory modulation not only results in depression of the field response to PPulse stimulation, but also depresses the GC PS to the second pulse of the pair; this effect wanes as the hyperpolarising current decays during longer PPulse stimulus intervals (from 100 ms onwards; [45]). In agreement with the above mechanism, we found control mice were most likely to display a PS to the second pulse of a pair at PPIs of 100 ms or more, that is, at longer intervals where presumably inhibition has subsided. In contrast, we found the PPulse response profile of 3xTgAD mice in DG was quite different from that of controls. Young and old 3xTgAD mice showed pronounced synaptic facilitation at short PPIs (25 and

50 ms), often accompanied by a PS to the second pulse. In particular, 3xTgAD mice were more likely to display a DG PS to the second pulse at short inter-stimulus intervals with an apparent increasing suppression of PS at longer paired-pulse intervals (that in controls were more likely to elicit PS). We suggest that these results demonstrate a long-term shift to hyper-excitability in the layer II input to DG in these AD mice for high-frequency inputs. In contrast, we saw a shift to increased depression for low-frequency inputs at longer PPI and in the train stimuli. Overall, these data suggest that DG in 3xTgADs may also show a more pronounced 'late' inhibitory component compared to controls, perhaps representing a homoeostatic compensatory mechanism to ameliorate the impact of reduced 'early' inhibition. Such an increase in late inhibition may also underlie the poor facilitation shown by 3xTgADs to low-frequency train stimulation (see below).

When examining PPulse responses in CA1 sr and slm, we found no overall genotype differences in PPF, and CA1 responses facilitated relative to the first pulse at short intervals in accordance with previous reports in young AD mice [30,46]. However, we found 3xTgAD animals demonstrated significantly more facilitation in CA1sr relative to controls at a PPI of 50 ms, in accordance with the findings of Gengler et al at the same age [46]. In old animals, the CA1sr response of both genotypes was shown to facilitate at short intervals but, again, there was a significantly increased CA1sr response in old 3xTgAD animals at PPI 50 ms. Thus, it appears from examining the responses of DG (fEPSP and PS data), that there is a subtle reduction in the short-term, recurrent inhibitory feedback system in the 3xTgAD mouse at short PPIs. It is also possible that an excess of excitability in DG and subsequent polysynaptic propagation of 'overly excitatory' responses through CA3 to CA1sr could account for the facilitation that we witnessed in CA1sr. Such a mechanism could contribute to aberrant excitation and seizure-like activity, phenomena witnessed *in vivo* in other AD mouse models [33–35].

Mechanisms for increased short-term excitability

Due to the unexpected differences between control and 3xTgAD mice (i.e., the facilitation seen in 3xTgAD PPulse responses), it is worthwhile discussing mechanisms though which the AD phenotype could exert a hyper-excitable effect. There is little evidence for intra or extracellular Aβ pathology in the DG of the 3xTgAD model and no tau pathology localised to the DG in older animals [20,21]. This would suggest that any change in inhibition is separate from these signature AD pathologies. Indeed, in human AD, the DG is one of the hippocampal regions least affected by pathology [1]. Previous research in other AD mouse models (APP/PS1, APOE ε4 and hAPP J20) has demonstrated a loss of interneurons within CA1 and DG. Specifically, those expressing calcium binding proteins parvalbumin, calbindin and calretinin, resulting in alterations in GABAergic interneuron populations and paralleling interneuron loss in human AD patients [47–49]. Recently, degeneration of GABAergic interneurons in DG expressing Neuropeptide Y was seen in a novel triple-transgenic AD model (TauPS2APP mouse; [50]). Interestingly, enhanced LTP to PP stimulation was seen in this triple mutation mouse in DG (*in vitro*), therefore, it is possible that loss of GABAergic tone in this and other models could contribute to hyper-excitability originating in DG [33–35,50]. Although this could account for the excessive facilitation seen in DG and CA1sr, we know from immunohistological studies that the 3xTgAD mouse model does not experience overt cell loss [20,21]. Thus, there may be similar mechanisms present in the 3xTgAD mouse detectable through the application of antibodies sensitive to GABA interneurons expressing calcium-binding proteins. Alternative/additional factors include the abnormal calcium homeostasis linked to PS1mutations [26,51,52], a reduction in nicotinic α7 acetylcholine receptors (α7nAchRs [53]) and abnormalities in the mGluR I-III families [54,55].

3xTgAD field responses to low-frequency pulse trains are depressed; however laminar synaptic connectivity profiles appear normal and response re-entrance into the hippocampal circuit is enhanced

Alongside responses to single and PPulse stimulation, we examined the effects of low-frequency trains on presumed monosynaptic and polysynaptic/re-entrant CA1 and DG responses [7,11–13]. Young mice displayed synaptic excitability (increased DG population cell spiking) and reverberation within the hippocampal formation, in a subset of both 3xTgAD and control animals. This confirms for the first time the presence of hippocampal output and re-entrant pathways in the mouse, as seen previously in rat ([9,10]. As an effect of genotype, small changes in fEPSPs could be seen in CA1sr (and to a lesser extent in CA1slm) in young 3xTgAD mice. Over a train of 20 pulses, the fEPSP amplitude of 3xTgAD mice tended not to facilitate as much as seen in controls (although there were no significant genotype differences), further, they displayed relatively constant response latencies over the train where response latencies in control mice generally slowed. In the 3xTgAD mouse, this effect was independent of response amplitude, thus, represented a faster rise time to fEPSP peak.

CSD profiles in both 3xTgAD and control mice to train stimulation showed a pattern of current sinks and sources consistent with excitatory synapses onto DG molecular layer (GC dendrites) and apical dendrites in CA1 [9,56]. If the connectivity between subiculum, EC and hippocampus was intact in the early stages of AD we expected to see: 1) a current sink in DG, reflecting layer II EC PP inputs to the dendrites of granule cells within the molecular layer and a positive-going fEPSP (presumably a reversal of the population cell fEPSP); 2) a concomitant current sink (reflected by a fast, negative-going local field potential; LFP) within CA1slm, marking the excitatory input from layer III PP (stimulated directly by the traversing of fibres through subiculum); 3) a delayed CA1sr negative going LFP, of a latency reflecting synaptic delay through the tri-synaptic connectivity to EC, DG, CA3 and ending with the Schaffer collateral input to CA1sr [9,10].

The presence of a clear CA1slm sink was variable in both genotypes, likely due to the relative success of electrode placement within the narrow CA1slm layer, rather than an abnormality in the PP input. In all animals, a large DG current source could be seen upon population spiking, thus, synaptic transmission through PP layer II appeared intact in the 3xTgAD mouse. CSD sinks also indicated that the (presumed) Schaffer collateral input from CA3 terminated in both stratum oriens and stratum radiatum of CA1, suggesting that the connectivity of hippocampal fibre pathways are functionally intact in the 3xTgAD mouse (but see [28]). Note that we cannot discount a contribution from CA2 input to CA1 so/sr [57]. However, the CA1sr latency would appear rather too long for a di-synaptic response (EC layer III input to CA2 which then projects to CA1 so/sr). Thus, the CA1sr response is much more likely to reflect feed-forward excitation from DG via CA3 [9,10].

Animals that demonstrated response re-entrance also showed progressive DG (and CA1 in 3xTgAD) population cell spiking and, within a train of 20 pulses, there was evidence for hippocampal excitability within each layer of the CA1-DG axis. For 3xTgAD in particular, the re-entrant input to CA1 elicited PS, which could be seen within as few as ten pulses of a train. However, 3xTgAD excitatory responses were also frequently coupled with what were presumably prolonged inhibitory after potentials (also seen in non-excitable 3xTgAD mice), perhaps indicating abnormalities in the balance of inhibitory feedback within hippocampus [33]. The presence of putative inhibitory currents during a 5 Hz train is supported by the lack of a DG second PS during seen PPulse stimulation, where a 100 ms or more ISI suppressed DG PS activity in 3xTgADs.

The highly specific topographic connectivity of the hippocampal-entorhinal system [8–10,58–60] may also have meant that subtle differences in recording and stimulating placements produced a range of response profiles within each genotype; however, placement of electrodes was consistent across all animals at the targeted coordinates. Thus, the present response profiles strongly suggest that there are subtle differences in the laminar profile of hippocampal responses in 3xTgAD and control mice, in response to low-frequency stimuli.

By 17–18 months of age, we found significant differences in the size of CA1sr fEPSP amplitude generated in the 3xTgAD mouse; further, their CA1 responses did not facilitate relative to the first pulse of the train. This effect appeared to be independent of the normal ageing process, as control mice retained some degree of facilitation; therefore, we conclude that this change in the 3xTgAD mouse is due to AD-like pathological progression. The latter likely includes the appearance of extracellular plaques and hyperphosphorylated tau [20,21] in addition to a range of other pathological markers, including increase in de-myelination [28], inflammatory processes [20] and/or loss of synaptic density [32]. There was, however, a general decrease in excitability with age in both genotypes, which could be due to an age-related increase in inhibitory after-potentials, such as those after-hyperpolarisation currents seen when recording intracellularly from hippocampal slices derived from old animals [61]. The latter conclusion is supported by the CSD profiles of aged animals which appear to show: (a) a sustained sink current in DG; (b) the lack of hippocampal re-entrance; and (c) a decrease in PS probability during both PPulse and train stimulation. Due to the small numbers of animals in the old group, conclusions must be drawn with caution; nevertheless, it appears in the aged 3xTgAD mouse there is augmentation of the usual decline in synaptic facilitation associated with ageing. Of note, there is also an age-related decrease in DG paired-pulse depression in control mice, a change that may underlie the known ageing-related deficit in pattern separation (see [62] for review) and, perhaps in turn, the age-related deficit in episodic-like memory in older mice [23].

Conclusions

What do the present data contribute to our understanding of early hippocampal dysfunction in AD? We found previously that the 3xTgAD model exhibits an early deficit in episodic-like memory that develops fully by 6 months of age [23,24]. We show here that this behavioural deficit coincides with subtle abnormalities in neuronal excitability and paucity of fEPSP facilitation seen in the DG and CA1 regions, suggesting an imbalance of inhibitory feedback in the model. However, our single-pulse responses show no obvious evidence of degradation in hippocampal fibre pathways [28]. Therefore, we suggest that cellular/synaptic abnormalities (be it intracellular Aβ accumulation, abnormal calcium homeostasis or dysfunction of recurrent inhibition) are mediating the effects witnessed here, at least in young mice. These findings do not necessarily contradict deficits seen in LTP (which are likely interlinked with intracellular mechanisms) seen in this and other AD mouse models [21,25,32,46]. However, a major conclusion from the present experiments is that hippocampal synaptic integrity in the 3xTgAD model of familial human AD is largely intact (as measured through single and paired-pulse low frequency stimulation *in vivo*) but that responses to brief high-frequency activation display hyper-excitability. If the 3xTgAD model does indeed mirror the pathological progression of familial human AD (bearing in mind that no familial patient would experience multiple mutations in APP or PS1 together as in this AD model), these results provide some hope that in the early stages, the hippocampus is functionally complete. Thus, treatments that can alleviate intracellular abnormalities that underlie AD-related synaptic changes (such as chelation of excess calcium; [26] or clearance of intracellular Aβ [22]) may improve cognitive function and quality of life in individuals at the onset of AD by correcting the hippocampal hyper-excitability shown here by us and others in AD models.

Author Contributions

Conceived and designed the experiments: KED JG. Performed the experiments: KED. Analyzed the data: KED SF JG. Contributed reagents/materials/analysis tools: SF. Wrote the paper: KED SF JG.

References

1. Braak H, Braak E (1991) Neuropathological stageing of Alzheimer-related changes. Acta Neuropathol 82: 239–59.
2. Braak H, Braak E (1995) Staging of Alzheimer's disease-related neurofibrillary changes. Neurobiol Aging 16: 271–8.
3. Berg L, McKeel DW Jr, Miller JP, Storandt M, Rubin EH, et al. (1998) Clinicopathologic studies in cognitively healthy aging and Alzheimer's disease: relation of histologic markers to dementia severity, age, sex, and apolipoprotein E genotype. Arch Neurol 55: 326–35.
4. LaFerla FM, Green KN, Oddo S (2007) Intracellular amyloid-beta in Alzheimer's disease. Nat Rev Neurosci 8: 499–509.
5. Selkoe DJ (2008) Soluble oligomers of the amyloid beta-protein impair synaptic plasticity and behavior. Behav Brain Res 192: 106–13.
6. Hwang DY, Golby AJ (2006) The brain basis for episodic memory: insights from functional MRI, intracranial EEG, and patients with epilepsy. Epilepsy Behav 8: 115–26.
7. Naber PA, Witter MP, and Lopes da Silva, FH (2000) Networks of the hippocampal memory system of the rat. The pivotal role of the subiculum. Ann N Y Acad Sci 911: 392–403.
8. Van Groen T, Miettinen P, Kadish I (2003) The entorhinal cortex of the mouse: organization of the projection to the hippocampal formation. Hippocampus 13: 133–49.
9. Kloosterman F, Van Haeften T, Lopes da Silva FH (2004) Two reentrant pathways in the hippocampal-entorhinal system. Hippocampus 14: 1026–39.
10. Kloosterman F, Van Haeften T, Witter MP, Lopes da Silva FH (2003) Electrophysiological characterization of interlaminar entorhinal connections: an essential link for re-entrance in the hippocampal-entorhinal system. Eur J Neurosci 18: 3037–52.
11. Egorov AV, Hamam BN, Fransén E, Hasselmo ME, Alonso AA (2002) Graded persistent activity in entorhinal cortex neurons. Nature 420: 173–8.
12. Gerrard JL, Burke SN, McNaughton BL, Barnes CA (2008) Sequence reactivation in the hippocampus is impaired in aged rats. J Neurosci 28: 7883–90.
13. Ribeiro S, Gervasoni D, Soares ES, Zhou Y, Lin SC, et al. (2004) Long-lasting novelty-induced neuronal reverberation during slow-wave sleep in multiple forebrain areas. PLoS Biol 2: e24. doi:10.1371/journal.pbio.0020024
14. Backman L, Small BJ, Fratiglioni L (2001) Stability of the preclinical episodic memory deficit in Alzheimer's disease. Brain 124: 96–102.
15. Buckmaster CA, Eichenbaum H, Amaral DG, Suzuki WA, Rapp PR (2004) Entorhinal cortex lesions disrupt the relational organization of memory in monkeys. J Neurosci 24: 9811–25.
16. Gouras GK, Tsai J, Naslund J, Vincent B, Edgar M, et al. (2000) Intraneuronal Abeta42 accumulation in human brain. Am J Pathol 156: 15–20.
17. Reed JM, Squire LR (1997) Impaired recognition memory in patients with lesions limited to the hippocampal formation. Behav Neurosci 111: 667–75.
18. Zola-Morgan S, Squire LR, Amaral DG (1986) Human amnesia and the medial temporal region: enduring memory impairment following a bilateral lesion limited to field CA1 of the hippocampus. J Neurosci 6: 2950–67.

19. Golby A, Silverberg G, Race E, Gabrieli S, O'Shea J, et al. (2005) Memory encoding in Alzheimer's disease: an fMRI study of explicit and implicit memory. Brain 128: 773–87.
20. Mastrangelo MA, Bowers WJ (2008) Detailed immunohistochemical characterization of temporal and spatial progression of Alzheimer's disease-related pathologies in male triple-transgenic mice. BMC Neurosci 9: 81.
21. Oddo S, Caccamo A, Shepherd JD, Murphy MP, Golde TE, et al. (2003) Triple-transgenic model of Alzheimer's disease with plaques and tangles: intracellular Abeta and synaptic dysfunction. Neuron 39: 409–21.
22. Billings LM, Oddo S, Green KN, McGaugh JL, LaFerla FM (2005) Intraneuronal Abeta causes the onset of early Alzheimer's disease-related cognitive deficits in transgenic mice. Neuron 45: 675–88.
23. Davis KE, Eacott MJ, Easton A, Gigg J (2013) Episodic-like memory is sensitive to both Alzheimer's-like patholgical accumulation and normal ageing processes in mice. Behav Brain Res 254: 73–82.
24. Davis KE, Easton A, Eacott MJ, Gigg J (2013) Episodic-Like Memory for What-Where-Which Occasion is Selectively Impaired in the 3xTgAD Mouse Model of Alzheimer's Disease. J Alzheimers Dis 33: 681–698.
25. Gureviciene I, Ikonen S, Gurevicius K, Sarkaki A, Van Groen T, et al. (2004) Normal induction but accelerated decay of LTP in APP + PS1 transgenic mice. Neurobiol Dis 15: 188–95.
26. Wang Y, Greig NH, Yu QS, Mattson MP (2009) Presenilin-1 mutation impairs cholinergic modulation of synaptic plasticity and suppresses NMDA currents in hippocampus slices. Neurobiol Aging 30: 1061–8.
27. Witter MP (2003) Organization of cortico-hippocampal networks in rats related to learning and memory. International Congress Series 1250: 131–145.
28. Desai MK, Sudol KL, Janelsins MC, Mastrangelo MA, et al. (2009) Triple-transgenic Alzheimer's disease mice exhibit region-specific abnormalities in brain myelination patterns prior to appearance of amyloid and tau pathology. Glia 57: 54–65.
29. Van Hoesen GW, Hyman BT (1990) Hippocampal formation: anatomy and the patterns of pathology in Alzheimer's disease. Prog Brain Res 83: 445–57.
30. Chapman PF, White GL, Jones MW, Cooper-Blacketer D, Marshall VJ, et al. (1999) Impaired synaptic plasticity and learning in aged amyloid precursor protein transgenic mice. Nat Neurosci 2: 271–6.
31. Fitzjohn SM, Morton RA, Kuenzi F, Rosahl TW, Shearman M, et al. (2001) Age-related impairment of synaptic transmission but normal long-term potentiation in transgenic mice that overexpress the human APP695SWE mutant form of amyloid precursor protein. J Neurosci 21: 4691–8.
32. Jacobsen JS, Wu CC, Redwine JM, Comery TA, Arias R, et al. (2006) Early-onset behavioral and synaptic deficits in a mouse model of Alzheimer's disease. Proc Natl Acad Sci U S A 103: 5161–6.
33. Palop JJ, Chin J, Roberson ED, Wang J, Thwin MT, et al. (2007) Aberrant excitatory neuronal activity and compensatory remodeling of inhibitory hippocampal circuits in mouse models of Alzheimer's disease. Neuron 55: 697–711.
34. Ziyatdinova S, Gurevicius K, Kutchiashvili N, Bolkvadze T, Nissinen J, et al. (2011) Spontaneous epileptiform discharges in a mouse model of Alzheimer's disease are suppressed by antiepileptic drugs that block sodium channels. Epilepsy Res 94: 75–85.
35. Yan XX, Cai Y, Shelton J, Deng SH, Luo XG, et al. (2012) Chronic Temporal Lobe Epilepsy Is Associated with Enhanced Alzheimer-Like Neuropathology in 3xTg-AD Mice. PLoS One 7: e48782.doi:10.1371/journal.pone.0048782
36. Paxinos G, Franklin KJB (2001) The mouse brain instereotaxic coordinates. San Diego: Academic Press.
37. Townsend G, Peloquin P, Kloosterman F, Hetke JF, Leung LS (2002) Recording and marking with silicon multichannel electrodes. Brain Res Brain Res Protoc 9: 122–9.
38. Freeman JA, Nicholson C. (1975) Experimental optimization of current source-density technique for anuran cerebellum. J Neurophysiol 38: 369–82.
39. Zucker RS (1989) Short-term synaptic plasticity. Annu Rev Neurosci 12: 13–31.
40. Brown RE, Reymann KG (1995) Metabotropic glutamate receptor agonists reduce paired-pulse depression in the dentate gyrus of the rat in vitro. Neurosci Lett 196: 17–20.
41. Buzsaki G (1984) Feed-forward inhibition in the hippocampal formation. Prog Neurobiol 22: 131–53.
42. Blaise JH, Bronzino JD (2000) Modulation of paired-pulse responses in the dentate gyrus: effects of normal maturation and vigilance state. Ann Biomed Eng 28: 128–34.
43. Lambert NA, Wilson WA (1994) Temporally distinct mechanisms of use-dependent depression at inhibitory synapses in the rat hippocampus in vitro. J Neurophysiol 72: 121–30.
44. Sloviter RS (1991) Feedforward and feedback inhibition of hippocampal principal cell activity evoked by perforant path stimulation: GABA-mediated mechanisms that regulate excitability in vivo. Hippocampus 1: 31–40.
45. Bampton ET, Gray RA, Large CH (1999) Electrophysiological characterisation of the dentate gyrus in five inbred strains of mouse. Brain Res 841: 123–34.
46. Gengler S, Hamilton A, Holscher C (2010) Synaptic plasticity in the hippocampus of a APP/PS1 mouse model of Alzheimer's disease is impaired in old but not young mice. PLoS One 5: e9764.doi: 10.1371/journal.-pone.0009764.
47. Andrews-Zwilling Y, Bien-Ly N, Xu Q, Li G, Bernardo A, et al. (2010) Apolipoprotein E4 causes age- and Tau-dependent impairment of GABAergic interneurons, leading to learning and memory deficits in mice. J Neurosci 30: 13707–17.
48. Baglietto-Vargas D, Moreno-Gonzalez I, Sanchez-Varo R, Jimenez S, Trujillo-Estrada L, et al. (2010) Calretinin interneurons are early targets of extracellular amyloid-beta pathology in PS1/AbetaPP Alzheimer mice hippocampus. J Alzheimers Dis 21: 119–32.
49. Takahashi H, Brasnjevic I, Rutten BP, Van Der Kolk N, Perl DP, et al. (2010) Hippocampal interneuron loss in an APP/PS1 double mutant mouse and in Alzheimer's disease. Brain Struct Funct 214: 145–60.
50. Loreth D, Ozmen L, Revel FG, Knoflach F, Wetzel P, et al. (2012) Selective degeneration of septal and hippocampal GABAergic neurons in a mouse model of amyloidosis and tauopathy. Neurobiol Dis 47: 1–12.
51. Guo Q, Sebastian L, Sopher BL, Miller MW, Ware CB, et al. (1999) Increased vulnerability of hippocampal neurons from presenilin-1 mutant knock-in mice to amyloid beta-peptide toxicity: central roles of superoxide production and caspase activation. J Neurochem 72: 1019–29.
52. Smith IF, Hitt B, Green KN, Oddo S, LaFerla FM (2005) Enhanced caffeine-induced Ca2+ release in the 3xTg-AD mouse model of Alzheimer's disease. J Neurochem 94: 1711–8.
53. Oddo S, Caccamo A, Green KN, Liang K, Tran L, et al. (2005) Chronic nicotine administration exacerbates tau pathology in a transgenic model of Alzheimer's disease. Proc Natl Acad Sci U S A 102: 3046–51.
54. Lee HG, Zhu X, O'Neill MJ, Webber K, Casadesus G, et al. (2004) The role of metabotropic glutamate receptors in Alzheimer's disease. Acta Neurobiol Exp (Wars) 64: 89–98.
55. Phillips T, Rees S, Augood S, Waldvogel H, Faull R, et al. (2000) Localization of metabotropic glutamate receptor type 2 in the human brain. Neuroscience 95: 1139–56.
56. Leung LS, Roth L, Canning KJ (1995) Entorhinal inputs to hippocampal CA1 and dentate gyrus in the rat: a current-source-density study. J Neurophysiol 73: 2392–403.
57. Chevaleyre V, Siegelbaum SA (2010) Strong CA2 pyramidal neuron synapses define a powerful disynaptic cortico-hippocampal loop. Neuron 66: 560–72.
58. McNaughton BL, Barnes CA (1977) Physiological identification and analysis of dentate granule cell responses to stimulation of the medial and lateral perforant pathways in the rat. J Comp Neurol 175: 439–54.
59. Steward O, Scoville SA (1976) Cells of origin of entorhinal cortical afferents to the hippocampus and fascia dentata of the rat. J Comp Neurol 169: 347–70.
60. Tamamaki N (1997) Organization of the entorhinal projection to the rat dentate gyrus revealed by Dil anterograde labeling. Exp Brain Res 116: 250–8.
61. Disterhoft JF, Oh MM (2007) Alterations in intrinsic neuronal excitability during normal aging. Aging Cell 6: 327–36.
62. Yassa MA, Stark CE (2011) Pattern separation in the hippocampus. Trends Neurosci 34: 515–25.

Theta-Burst Stimulation of Hippocampal Slices Induces Network-Level Calcium Oscillations and Activates Analogous Gene Transcription to Spatial Learning

Graham K. Sheridan[1*⁹], Emad Moeendarbary[2⁹], Mark Pickering[3⁹], John J. O'Connor[4], Keith J. Murphy[5]

1 Department of Physiology, Development and Neuroscience, University of Cambridge, Cambridge, United Kingdom, **2** Hughes Hall, University of Cambridge, Cambridge, United Kingdom, **3** School of Medicine and Medical Science, Health Sciences Centre, University College Dublin, Dublin, Ireland, **4** UCD School of Biomolecular and Biomedical Science, Conway Institute, University College Dublin, Dublin, Ireland, **5** Neurotherapeutics Research Group, UCD School of Biomolecular and Biomedical Science, Conway Institute, University College Dublin, Dublin, Ireland

Abstract

Over four decades ago, it was discovered that high-frequency stimulation of the dentate gyrus induces long-term potentiation (LTP) of synaptic transmission. LTP is believed to underlie how we process and code external stimuli before converting it to salient information that we store as 'memories'. It has been shown that rats performing spatial learning tasks display theta-frequency (3–12 Hz) hippocampal neural activity. Moreover, administering theta-burst stimulation (TBS) to hippocampal slices can induce LTP. TBS triggers a sustained rise in intracellular calcium $[Ca^{2+}]_i$ in neurons leading to new protein synthesis important for LTP maintenance. In this study, we measured TBS-induced $[Ca^{2+}]_i$ oscillations in thousands of cells at increasing distances from the source of stimulation. Following TBS, a calcium wave propagates radially with an average speed of 5.2 μm/s and triggers multiple and regular $[Ca^{2+}]_i$ oscillations in the hippocampus. Interestingly, the number and frequency of $[Ca^{2+}]_i$ fluctuations post-TBS increased with respect to distance from the electrode. During the post-tetanic phase, 18% of cells exhibited 3 peaks in $[Ca^{2+}]_i$ with a frequency of 17 mHz, whereas 2.3% of cells distributed further from the electrode displayed 8 $[Ca^{2+}]_i$ oscillations at 33 mHz. We suggest that these observed $[Ca^{2+}]_i$ oscillations could lead to activation of transcription factors involved in synaptic plasticity. In particular, the transcription factor, NF-κB, has been implicated in memory formation and is up-regulated after LTP induction. We measured increased activation of NF-κB 30 min post-TBS in CA1 pyramidal cells and also observed similar temporal up-regulation of NF-κB levels in CA1 neurons following water maze training in rats. Therefore, TBS of hippocampal slice cultures *in vitro* can mimic the cell type-specific up-regulations in activated NF-κB following spatial learning *in vivo*. This indicates that TBS may induce similar transcriptional changes to spatial learning and that TBS-triggered $[Ca^{2+}]_i$ oscillations could activate memory-associated gene expression.

Editor: Christopher Mark Norris, Univ. Kentucky, United States of America

Funding: This work was supported by a research cluster award from Science Foundation Ireland (03/IN3/B403C and 07/IN.1/B1322). E. Moeendarbary is supported by University of Cambridge Herchel Smith Postdoctoral Fellowship. The funders had no role in study design, data collection and analysis, decision to publish, or preparation of the manuscript.

Competing Interests: The authors have declared that no competing interests exist.

* Email: gks28@cam.ac.uk

⁹ These authors contributed equally to this work.

Introduction

The molecular and cellular mechanisms that facilitate learning and memory formation have been studied intensely for decades. In order to understand these complex cognitive processes, neuroscientists have developed 'simple' *in vitro* reductionist approaches that model the cellular basis of memory formation. Since the discovery by Bliss and Lømo [1] that high-frequency electrical stimulation (HFS) can lead to a long-lasting enhancement of synaptic transmission, it has been suggested that this experimentally-induced phenomenon, known as long-term potentiation (LTP), can recapitulate many of the molecular and cellular processes that facilitate memory formation [2–6]. Both LTP and memory formation have been shown to depend on new protein synthesis within stimulated cells [7–9]. Transcription factors such as cyclic AMP-responsive element binding protein (CREB) and nuclear factor-kappa B (NF-κB) are reported to play crucial roles in the gene transcription that drives enhanced synaptic transmission [10–18]. Upstream of gene transcription, however, are a multitude of intracellular signalling cascades involving several key protein kinases, including protein kinase A (PKA) and calcium calmodulin-dependent kinase II (CaMKII) [19]. Activation of these kinases is intimately linked to elevations in intracellular calcium concentration [20,21]. Therefore, calcium acts as a second messenger and initiates intracellular signalling that promotes transcription factor translocation to the nucleus and new protein synthesis required for LTP maintenance [22,23].

The role of calcium in LTP induction and maintenance is complex. Pre-synaptic glutamate release can activate post-synaptic AMPA receptors causing a depolarisation-induced unblocking of NMDA receptors which allows calcium influx to the post-synaptic cell [2,24]. Large increases in intracellular calcium concentration $[Ca^{2+}]_i$ can lead to the opening of voltage-dependent calcium channels (VDCC). Elevations in $[Ca^{2+}]_i$ can also promote calcium-induced calcium release (CICR) from intracellular stores [25]. Repeated activation of intracellular stores can produce sustained oscillations in $[Ca^{2+}]_i$ [26,27]. Because calcium is a ubiquitous second messenger and is involved in translating many extracellular stimuli into intracellular biochemical reactions, the precise dynamics of the calcium response may act as a coded message that allows the cell to decipher the initial stimulus. Therefore, the amount of extracellular calcium $[Ca^{2+}]_o$ that enters the cell and how fast this occurs could influence the intracellular signalling cascades that are activated. Similarly, the time it takes for elevated $[Ca^{2+}]_i$ to return to basal levels and whether intracellular calcium oscillations are initiated will influence the physiological response of the cell [28].

Theta-burst electrical stimulation mimics *in vivo* firing frequencies (3–12 Hz) in the CA1 region of the hippocampus of rats performing a spatial learning task [29–31]. Moreover, theta-burst stimulation (TBS) is arguably the most effective pattern of activity for LTP induction [31–33]. The TBS protocol used in this study has been shown to activate both NMDA receptors and VDCCs to produce a robust and long-lasting form of LTP [34–37]. To our knowledge, however, simultaneous calcium imaging of hundreds of individual cells in response to theta-burst stimulation has not yet been described in detail. There are many elegant studies that have concentrated on characterising the calcium response of individual synapses or small numbers of cells close to the stimulation site [38–43]. Therefore, not much is known about the network-level effects of TBS on $[Ca^{2+}]_i$ fluctuations at large distances from the site of electrical stimulation. Our aim, in this study, was to measure and characterise single-cell calcium responses to TBS in a large proportion of a hippocampal slice. We analysed the calcium dynamics of 6,536 cells located within 500 µm from the point of stimulation. TBS triggers an initial radially-propagating calcium wave that decays exponentially in intensity with respect to distance from the electrode. Moreover, this first wave induces multiple and regular calcium oscillations in the hippocampal cellular network.

It has been shown that protein kinase activation is sensitive to intracellular calcium oscillations [44,45] and CaMKII, for example, has been shown to activate the transcription factor, NF-κB, following glutamate-induced synaptic transmission [46]. Interestingly, it has also been reported that different $[Ca^{2+}]_i$ oscillation frequencies can preferentially activate different transcription factors, with low frequency $[Ca^{2+}]_i$ oscillations preferentially activating NF-κB over NF-AT and Oct/OAP transcription factor gene expression [47]. We, therefore, monitored changes in NF-κB activation 30 min after TBS in the three main neuronal populations of the hippocampus, i.e. dentate gyrus, CA3 and CA1. We report increased NF-κB activation in the CA1 region after TBS. More importantly, we also found the same temporal up-regulation in NF-κB activation in CA1 neurons in rats trained in the Morris water maze spatial learning task. These similar temporal and cell type-specific activations of NF-κB following both learning and TBS suggest that NF-κB is mobilised to a common goal in these two models of synaptic plasticity [48–50]. Moreover, the precise frequency of the sustained calcium oscillations in the hippocampal network, triggered by TBS, may be responsible for activating specific gene expression changes important to both LTP maintenance and to memory formation.

Materials and Methods

Organotypic hippocampal cultures

Organotypic hippocampal cultures were prepared according to Stoppini et al. [51]. Briefly, post-natal day 7 male Wistar rats were decapitated without anaesthetic and their brains quickly dissected out and placed into ice-cold Earle's balanced salt solution (EBSS) for 1 min. Both hippocampi were dissected and cut into 400 µm slices using a McIlwain tissue chopper. Slices were separated and arranged onto organotypic inserts (3 per insert, Millicell PICMORG50). The inserts were housed in standard 6-well cell culture plates which were kept in an incubator at 35°C and 5% CO_2. The slices were grown using an interface method with 1 ml organotypic medium supplying the undersurface of the slice. The organotypic medium consisted of 50% minimum essential medium (MEM, Gibco), 25% EBSS (Gibco), 25% heat-inactivated horse serum (Sigma) and supplemented with 2 mM glutamine, 28 mM D-glucose, 100 U/ml penicillin/streptomycin and 25 mM HEPES. The first medium change was conducted 24 h following slice preparation with subsequent medium changes occurring every 2 days. Slices were maintained for 21 days *in-vitro* (DIV) prior to experimentation.

Calcium imaging and theta-burst stimulation of organotypic hippocampal cultures

21 DIV organotypic hippocampal cultures were prepared for calcium imaging experiments by transferring inserts to room-temperature BSS (buffered salt solution) composed of 130 mM NaCl, 5.4 mM KCl, 1.8 mM $CaCl_2$, 2 mM $MgSO_4$, 5.5 mM D-glucose and 20 mM HEPES, pH 7.3. The insert membranes were cut using a scalpel and individual slices were transferred to 35 mm Petri dishes containing 2 ml of 3 µM fluo-4 AM calcium indicator (Molecular Probes) in BSS and allowed to incubate in the dark for 30 min. Following ester loading of the calcium dye, slices were transferred to a custom-built chamber containing fresh BSS to be imaged using the 10X/0.3W Ph1 water-immersion lens on a LSM 5 Pascal confocal microscope (Zeiss). All experiments were conducted at room temperature. A stimulating monopolar glass electrode was lowered onto the surface of the slice and positioned in the molecular layer of the dentate gyrus. The scanning laser on the microscope was programmed to capture 1 frame per second for 330 s allowing a baseline recording of 20 s before a theta-burst stimulus protocol of 10 volts in magnitude was delivered to the tissue (Figure 1). The electrode used was pulled from a borosilicate glass capillary (GC150F-10, Harvard Apparatus, USA) using a P-97 Brown-Flaming micropipette puller (Sutter Instruments Co.) and had a tip diameter of 4 µm and a resistance of approx. 1.5 MΩ for monopolar stimulation of organotypic slice cultures. The same stimulating electrode was used for each slice in order to minimise any inherent slice-to-slice variability in input/output relationships evoked by the stimulus voltage (Grass Instruments SIU5 stimulus isolation unit, 10 V output). Moreover, the magnitude, velocity and propagation distance of the TBS-induced calcium wave was similar in all slices tested. TBS consisted of 8 trains with an inter-burst interval of 2 s. Each train lasted 40 ms and consisted of 8 bursts at 200 Hz. Therefore, TBS was complete after 14.04 s (Figure 1A). The calcium response to TBS was visualized and recorded over a 5 min 10 s period. Slices were then transferred back into the incubator in 1 ml of fresh pre-equilibrated organotypic medium for 30 min post-TBS. Control slices received the exact same treatment minus theta-burst stimulation. A total of 15 slices were stimulated using this TBS protocol. Three control and three stimulated slices were chosen at random for immunofluorescent labelling of activated NF-κB.

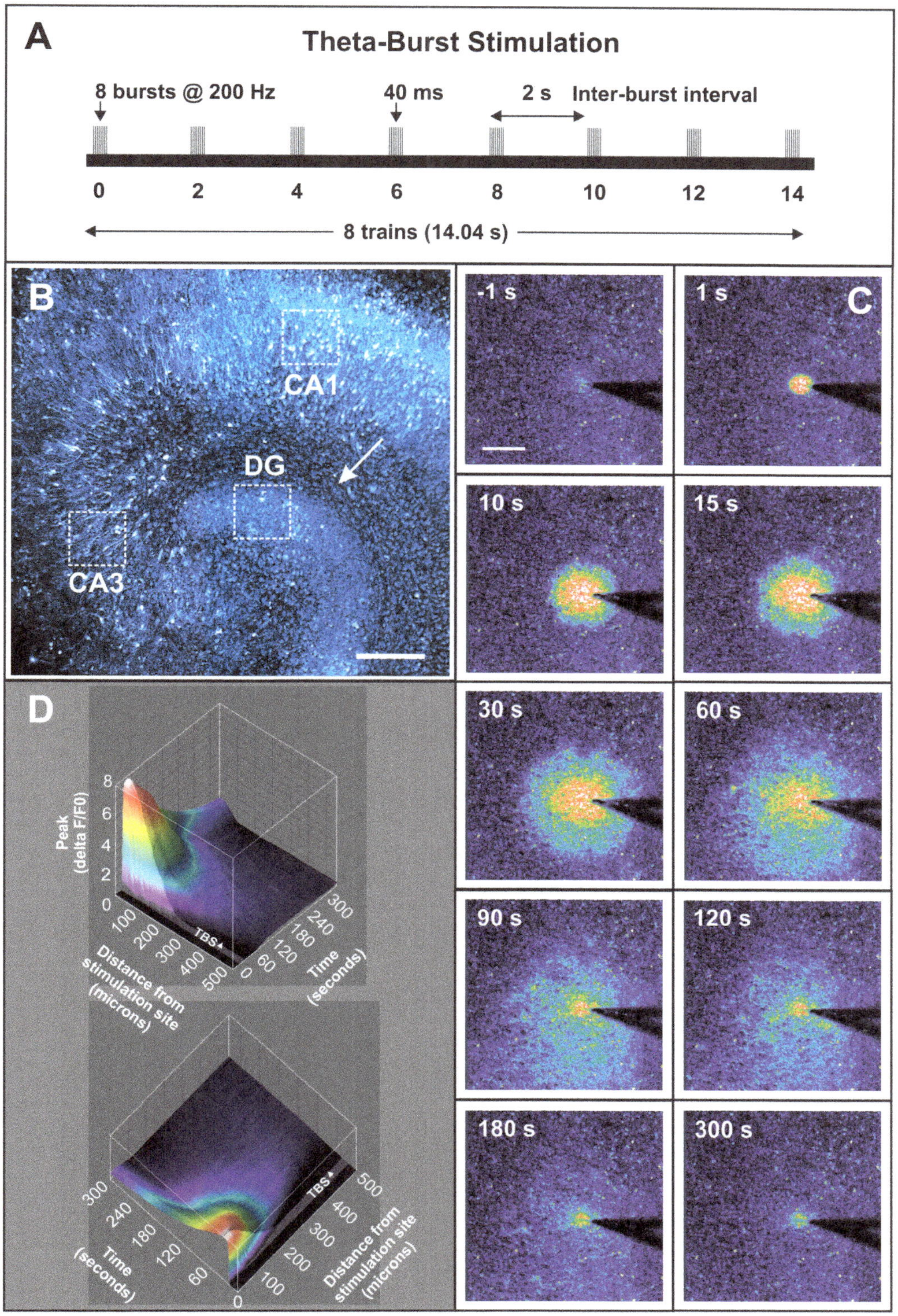

Figure 1. Theta-burst stimulation of hippocampal slice cultures. (A) Schematic representation of the theta-burst stimulation (TBS) protocol used. TBS consisted of 8 trains with 8 bursts in each train (i.e. 64 stimuli in total). The train duration was 40 ms making the burst frequency 200 Hz and the inter-burst interval was 2 s. Therefore, TBS took 14.04 s to complete. (B) 21 day *in vitro* (DIV) organotypic hippocampal culture loaded with Fluo-4 AM calcium indicator. A pseudo-colour fluorescence intensity palette (cyan → white) indicates levels of lowest to highest basal calcium concentration in the slice culture. The arrow indicates the point of electrical stimulation in the molecular layer of the dentate gyrus. The white boxes represent the areas imaged and analysed for changes in nuclear NF-κB activation. Scale bar = 200 μm. (C) Low-magnification (10X) images representing the calcium response at various time-points post theta-burst stimulation (TBS). A pseudo-colour rainbow palette (black/violet → red/white) is used to illustrate the changes in calcium levels more clearly, i.e. the 'hotter' the colour, the higher the relative intracellular calcium

concentration. The first image represents baseline calcium levels 1 s before TBS began. TBS lasts for 14.04 s but the calcium wave continues to propagate in a radial fashion after TBS has terminated. Scale bar = 200 μm. (D) A four-dimensional surface plot representing the changes in intracellular calcium levels in a 21 DIV organotypic hippocampal slice culture in response to TBS to the molecular layer of the dentate gyrus. The X-axis represents time, i.e. 20 s baseline followed by a 14.04 s shaded area representing the period of TBS, followed by a 4 min 56 s period (296 s) post-TBS. Graphed along the Y-axis is distance from the electrode tip, i.e. 0–500 μm. The Z-axis represents the peak calcium response (i.e. $\Delta F/F_0$). Also, mapped onto the surface plot is the 'time-to-peak' data which is represented by the rainbow palette, i.e. the 'hotter' the colour, the faster the cell achieved its peak calcium level in response to TBS.

Immunofluorescent staining of organotypic hippocampal cultures

Organotypic hippocampal cultures were prepared for immunofluorescence according to Gogolla et al. [52]. Briefly, slices were removed from the incubator and received two 30 s washes in phosphate buffered saline (PBS) before being fixed in an ice-cold solution of 4% formaldehyde for 5 min. Slices received another 1 min wash in PBS and were transferred to a solution of 20% methanol for 3 min. Slices were again washed in PBS for 5 min and transferred to a 0.5% solution of Triton X. The slices were permeabilized in this solution for 18 h at 4°C. They were then washed in PBS and transferred for 4 h into a blocking solution consisting of 20% BSA (bovine serum albumin) in PBS. Following this blocking step, slices were incubated with the primary antibody MAB3026 (Chemicon) for 18 h at 4°C in a solution containing 5% BSA. This antibody binds to an epitope overlapping the nuclear location signal on the p65 subunit of the NF-κB heterodimer. Thus, it selectively binds to the activated form of NF-κB. The slices were then washed and incubated with an anti-mouse secondary antibody labelled with Cy3 (Jackson ImmunoResearch) for 4 h at room temperature. Nuclei were counterstained using Hoechst 33258 (Molecular Probes). Slices were placed on microscope slides and mounted with coverslips using OCT (optimal cutting temperature compound, Agar Scientific) and sealed with clear nail varnish. Slides were stored in the dark at room temperature before being imaged.

Animal care and behavioural assessment

Postnatal day 80 male Wistar rats (330–380 g) were obtained from the Biomedical Facility at University College Dublin, Ireland. All experimental procedures were approved by the Animal Research Ethics Committee of the Biomedical Facility at UCD and were carried out by individuals who held the appropriate license issued by the Minister for Health and Children. Animals were socially housed in groups of 4 and given *ad libitum* access to food and water. The experimental room was kept on a 12 h light/dark cycle at 22±2°C. The animals' behaviour was assessed in an open field apparatus (620 mm long, 620 mm wide and 150 mm high) both 48 h and 24 h prior to commencement of training. All rats behaved normally in the open field apparatus. The base of the open field box was demarcated into an 8×8 grid. The rat was placed in the centre of the box and its locomotion was monitored by counting the number of squares crossed in a 5 min period. The number of times the rats reared on their hind legs was also noted. Behavioural assessment was conducted in a quiet room under low-level red light illumination. The rats displayed similar locomotion and rearing scores to one another and appeared to habituate to the open field arena by the second day of observation.

Morris water maze training in rats

On postnatal day 80, animals were trained in the Morris water maze spatial learning task. Briefly, the water maze apparatus consists of a large circular pool (150 cm diameter, 80 cm deep) and a hidden platform (11 cm diameter). Both are constructed from black polyvinyl plastic, offering no intra-maze visual cues that may help guide escape behaviour. The platform was submerged 1.5 cm below the water's surface (temperature 26±1°C) and positioned 30 cm from the edge of the maze wall. The platform remained in the same position throughout the training session. The experimental room contained several extra-maze visual cues. The rat was lowered into the water facing the wall of the maze (30 cm high) at one of three locations which were alternated with each trial. Trials lasted a maximum of 90 s and the length of time taken for the rat to find the hidden platform was recorded. Rats failing to find the platform within the 90 s were placed on it for 10 s and allowed orientate themselves. The training session consisted of 5 trials with an inter-trial interval of 300 s. Each trained animal was assigned a corresponding passive control partner that spent the same lengths of time swimming in the pool, minus the platform. The latencies to find the maze platform were recorded for each trained rat over the 5-trial session (n = 4 trained rats). Latency-to-platform times decreased significantly (two-way ANOVA, Bonferroni post-tests, $p<0.001$) over the 5 trials of the training session indicating that the animals learned the task. After training, the rats were dried-off and placed back into their home cages. This was designated 'Time 0 min' after training. They were then sacrificed 30 min later, without anaesthetic, by cervical dislocation (n = 4 trained and passive controls, i.e. 8 animals in total). Following decapitation, their brains were quickly dissected out, covered in OCT and snap frozen in CO_2-cooled n-hexane.

Cryosectioning and immunofluorescence of Morris water maze-trained rat brains

Whole brains were cryosectioned coronally at −3.3 mm with respect to Bregma in order to reveal the dorsal hippocampus [53]. 12 μm sections were adhered to glass slides coated with poly-L-lysine. Sections were permeabilized using a solution of 0.1% Triton X in PBS for 25 min. Following this, sections were fixed in 70% ethanol for 25 min. The sections were then incubated overnight (18 h) with the primary antibody MAB3026 (Chemicon), which binds to the activated form of NF-κB. Following two 10 min washes in PBS, sections were incubated for 3 h with an anti-mouse secondary antibody labelled with the fluorescent marker FITC (Sigma). The secondary antibody was then washed off and sections were incubated in a solution of propidium iodide (PI) in order to stain all nuclei. A drop of Citifluor glycerol PBS solution (Agar Scientific) was used to mount each section with a coverslip and the slides were stored in darkness at 4°C.

Confocal microscopy

All confocal images used for quantitative analysis of NF-κB activity (12-bit; 1024×1024 pixels) were captured using a 40X/0.8W water-immersion lens (Zeiss Achroplan). Images taken from Morris water maze-trained animals were captured from three defined regions of the hippocampus, i.e. CA1, CA3, and the apex of the dentate gyrus. The specific areas of the hippocampus that were imaged were kept consistent between sections. Confocal images of organotypic hippocampal cultures were captured from two distinct areas of the CA1, CA3 and dentate gyrus (i.e. 6 images

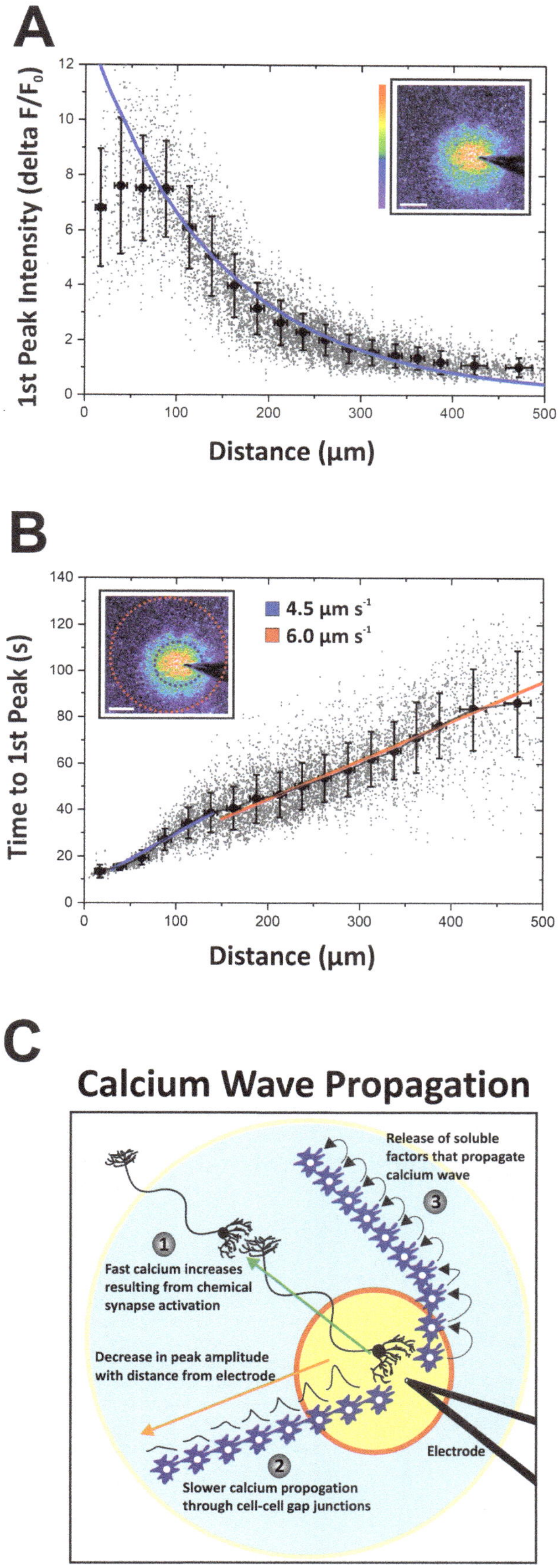

Figure 2. Calcium wave propagation in hippocampal slice cultures post-TBS. (A) Describes the relative increase in $[Ca^{2+}]_i$ concentration (i.e. 1st Peak Intensity) in every cell (n = 6,536) post-TBS, with respect to distance from the electrode (0–500 μm). Within the first 100 μm from the point of stimulation, the Ca^{2+} fluorescence intensity of the first peak displays a wide range of values. From 100–500 μm, however, the fluorescence intensity of the first peak follows an exponential decay rate. Inset: Relative increase in $[Ca^{2+}]_i$ fluorescence, depicted by a pseudo-colour rainbow palette, in hippocampal cells 15 s after TBS termination. (B) Graphed is the time it takes each cell to achieve its first peak in $[Ca^{2+}]_i$ versus the distance that cell is from the electrode. Cells located further from the electrode take a longer time to reach their first peak in $[Ca^{2+}]_i$; the calcium wave travels at an average velocity of 5.2 ± 1 μm s^{-1}. However, there appears to be a bi-phasic response in calcium wave propagation, illustrated by the blue and red linear fits of the data. The calcium wave travels slower 0–150 μm from the electrode, with an average speed of 4.5 μm s^{-1} (blue linear fit). Cells that lie 150–500 μm from the point of stimulation reach their first peak in $[Ca^{2+}]_i$ relatively faster (red linear fit) as the velocity of the calcium wave increases, reaching 6.0 μm s^{-1}. Inset: Illustrates how the velocity of calcium wave propagation increases >150 μm from the electrode. (C) Schematic diagram describing the mechanisms by which changes in $[Ca^{2+}]_i$ may propagate over long distances in hippocampal slice cultures. The first method (1) is through action potential-mediated release of excitatory neurotransmitter (e.g. glutamate) at synapses located large distances from TBS-stimulated dendrites and cell bodies. This may explain the relatively small number of cells in panel B that are 300–500 μm from the electrode tip but exhibit very fast increases in $[Ca^{2+}]_i$ and 'time-to-first peak' responses. Because the velocity of calcium wave propagation in hippocampal slice cultures appears to increase >150 μm from the point of stimulation, this may represent a transition from (2) gap junction-mediated $[Ca^{2+}]_i$ propagation to (3) release of soluble factors (such as ATP) that stimulate neighbouring cells and perpetuate the calcium wave over long distances through astrocyte networks.

per slice). Calcium imaging time-series frames (12-bit; 512×512 pixels) were captured using the 10X/0.3W Ph1 water-immersion lens (Zeiss Achroplan).

Image and data analysis

Image analysis was conducted using the software package EBImage (http://www.bioconductor.org/packages/2.12/bioc/html/EBImage.html) for R statistical programming environment. Briefly, taking the immunofluorescently-labelled sections from water maze-trained animals as an example, the red and green channels were first separated for each image. Every pixel (1024×1024) was assigned an intensity value between 0 and 1. Using the red channel as a reference, size and fluorescence intensity thresholds were set in order to select only propidium iodide-labelled nuclei. A distance map was then generated for the image which calculates the distance each pixel is from an edge pixel. The watershed segmentation algorithm is then employed which accurately separates clusters of nuclei that are very close together, or touching, into individual cells. Minimum distance between objects and minimum radius criteria are written into the analysis scripts which further refines object separation. NF-κB activation was measured in the nucleus of every cell and then the average nuclear fluorescence intensity for NF-κB was calculated for the CA1, CA3 and dentate gyrus.

Calcium imaging time-series data was analysed using EBImage and individual cells were detected using similar object detection criteria described above. Baseline calcium fluorescence (F_0) for each cell was taken as the average fluorescence intensity of that cell over the first 20 images, i.e. before TBS. The relative change in calcium fluorescence for every cell at increasing time points was then calculated using the equation $\Delta F/F_0$, where ΔF = [fluores-

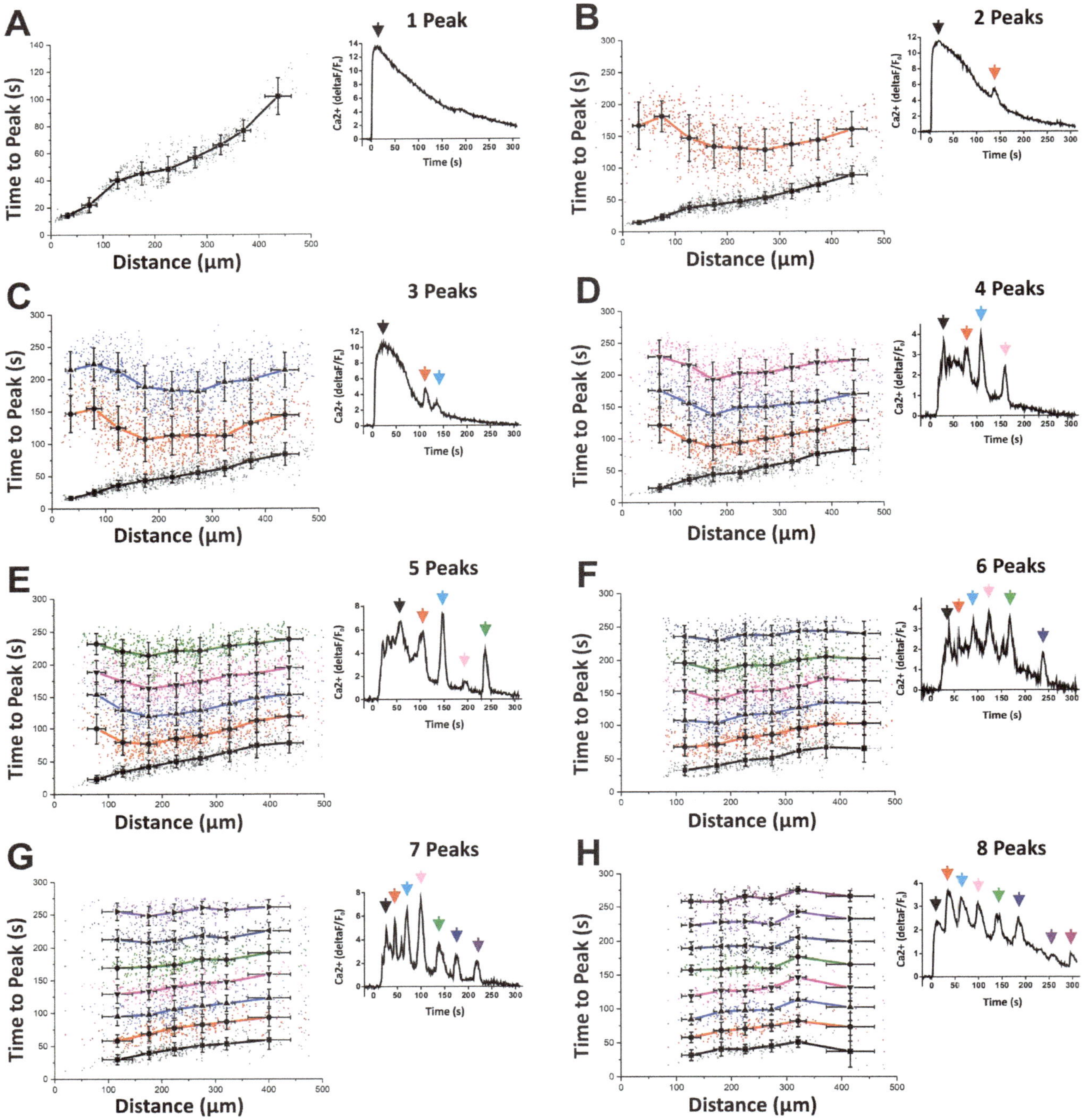

Figure 3. Time-to-peak for cells displaying multiple fluctuations in $[Ca^{2+}]_i$. (A) Time-to-peak versus distance from electrode for cells displaying one peak in $[Ca^{2+}]_i$. Inset: Relative changes in $[Ca^{2+}]_i$ over time for a single cell displaying one peak post-TBS. (B) Black line represents the 'time-to-first peak' in $[Ca^{2+}]_i$ for cells displaying two peaks. Red line represents the 'time-to-second peak'. Notice the long delay in the second peak in cells within 150 μm from the point of stimulation. Therefore, cells with large first peaks in $[Ca^{2+}]_i$ take a long time to display a second peak. Cells located >300 μm from the electrode, however, display shorter durations between peak one and two. Inset: Relative changes in $[Ca^{2+}]_i$ over time post-TBS for a single cell displaying two peaks. (C) Black line represents the 'time-to-first peak' in $[Ca^{2+}]_i$ for cells displaying three peaks. Red and blue lines represent the 'time-to-second and -third peaks', respectively. Notice again the relatively large time between peak one and two in cells located <150 μm from the electrode. The time between second and third peaks is shorter, however. (D) Cells displaying four peaks in $[Ca^{2+}]_i$ post-TBS. Notice the regular interval between peaks 2, 3 and 4 (red, blue and magenta lines, respectively). (E–H) Time-to-peak versus distance from electrode for cells displaying 5, 6, 7 and 8 peaks in $[Ca^{2+}]_i$.

cence at time X − baseline fluorescence (i.e. F_0)]. The XY coordinates of each cell were used to calculate their distances from the electrode tip. Calcium response curves were smoothed via MATLAB (The MathWorks Inc.) inbuilt functions. Briefly, a moving average filter spanning 9 data points was used to reduce noise in the fluorescence time-course data. Non-responsive cells were excluded from the analysis (5,414 'non-responders' in total). Non-responsive cells were defined as any cell that either achieved its peak calcium fluorescence prior to TBS, or any cell in which the difference between its maximum peak fluorescence signal and the mean of its signal was less than 0.25. To find the major peaks each calcium curve was processed by the MATLAB 'peak finder routines' (i.e. iPeak, developed by T. O'Haver: http://terpconnect.umd.edu/~toh/spectrum/PeakFindingandMeasurement.htm). Small local oscillations occurring near each major peak were neglected by selecting a time interval of 5 sec as the 'minimum peak width' and choosing an appropriate smoothing algorithm available in the options section of the 'iPeak' function. $[Ca^{2+}]_i$ oscillation frequency was calculated on a cell-by-cell basis by converting the 'distance between peaks' to millihertz (mHz).

Results

Theta-burst stimulation induces a radial-propagating calcium wave in the hippocampal network

We applied the theta-burst stimulation (TBS) protocol, described in figure 1A, to the molecular layer of the dentate gyrus of organotypic hippocampal slice cultures (figure 1B). The TBS electrical stimulus produced a slow-propagating calcium wave that spread radially from the electrode tip (figure 1C). We stimulated 15 slices in this way and, using automated image analysis, measured the average speed of calcium wave propagation to be 5.2±1 μm s^{-1}. Figure 1D shows the spatiotemporal evolution of the changes in $[Ca^{2+}]_i$ after TBS is applied to one hippocampal slice. An exponential decrease in the peak $[Ca^{2+}]_i$ with increasing distance from the point of stimulation was observed.

Next, we calculated the changes in calcium fluorescence over time for every cell positioned less than 500 μm from the electrode. Cells that did not exhibit significant calcium elevations were excluded from the analysis. As expected, cells located within 100 μm of the stimulation point displayed relatively large increases in $[Ca^{2+}]_i$ (figure 2A). Further than 150 μm from the electrode, however, the primary peak calcium signal was lower and decayed exponentially with increasing distance from the stimulation site (figure 2A). Cells located closer to the electrode, not surprisingly, achieved their first peak in $[Ca^{2+}]_i$ sooner than more distally-located cells. Interestingly, however, cells located within 150 μm of the electrode displayed a slower 'time-to-peak' $[Ca^{2+}]_i$ response after correcting for their absolute distance from the stimulation site. This is illustrated in figure 2B by the steeper slope of the blue linear fit (4.5 μm s^{-1}; 0–150 μm), compared to the shallower slope of red linear fit (6.0 μm s^{-1}; 150–500 μm), in the scatter plot. Cells located within 150 μm of the electrode achieved greater elevations in $[Ca^{2+}]_i$ post-TBS and, because of this, take slightly longer to achieve their peak calcium response. There were also notable differences in the 'return-to-baseline' kinetics of $[Ca^{2+}]_i$ at increasing distances from the electrode. The majority of cells exhibited semi-exponential decay rates after an initial peak in calcium, whereas a small proportion of cells (<1%) situated within 60 μm of the stimulation site, displayed linear decay constants (data not shown). This may indicate that different calcium-dependent signalling cascades are activated in a small number of cells very close to the TBS stimulus.

Cells displaying large primary peaks in $[Ca^{2+}]_i$ have a delayed 2nd peak

Almost all of the cells situated within 500 μm of the electrode achieved their primary peak in calcium within 120 s from the start of TBS (Figure 2B). Figure 3A graphs the 'time-to-peak' with respect to distance from the electrode for cells that possess only one peak. However, a large proportion of the total number of cells analysed (>85%) displayed multiple peaks in $[Ca^{2+}]_i$ following TBS. Therefore, we measured the 'time-to-second peak' (and also times to 3rd, 4th, 5th, 6th, 7th and 8th peaks) for all of these cells. Interestingly, the 'time-to-second peak', for cells displaying 2, 3 or 4 fluctuations in $[Ca^{2+}]_i$ and situated within 150 μm of the electrode, is delayed compared to more distal cells (figure 3B, C and D). This means that strongly stimulated cells close to the electrode display large first peaks in $[Ca^{2+}]_i$ and, therefore, require a longer latency period before a second spike in calcium can occur (figure 3B). In other words, the $[Ca^{2+}]_i$ has to drop to a certain level before a second peak can take place within the cell. This suggests that cells located further from the electrode, which display relatively modest primary peaks in $[Ca^{2+}]_i$, are more likely to begin oscillating sooner than cells located close to the electrode.

Theta-burst stimulation induces calcium oscillations in hippocampal cells

A striking result, clearly illustrated by figure 3, is that once a cell is stimulated with TBS and starts to display multiple oscillations in intracellular calcium, the time between subsequent peaks, i.e. peaks 2–3, peaks 3–4, peaks 4–5 etc., are remarkably regular. We analysed the frequencies of oscillations (i.e. 'time between peaks') in cells displaying up to 8 peaks in $[Ca^{2+}]_i$ (figure 3). Figure 4A summarises this analysis and charts the 'time between peaks' with respect to the number of peaks for each and every cell. Cells that exhibited 3 oscillations in $[Ca^{2+}]_i$ post-TBS did so at an average frequency of 17±8 mHz. For cells with 4 peaks, the frequency of $[Ca^{2+}]_i$ oscillations was 22±8 mHz. Cells displaying 5, 6, 7 or 8 peaks had corresponding frequencies of oscillation of 26±8 mHz, 29±8 mHz, 30±7 mHz or 33±7 mHz, respectively (figure 4A). Therefore, TBS induces large primary increases in $[Ca^{2+}]_i$ and also triggers calcium oscillations over a range of frequencies within stimulated cells. Moreover, our results indicate that the rhythm of oscillations, as determined by the 'time-between-peaks', was non-stochastic in nature and was strongly correlated with the cell's distance from the origin of electrical stimulation. This suggests that theta-burst stimulation induces a calcium wave that propagates large distances throughout the hippocampal neural network and may have far-reaching modulatory effects on synaptic plasticity.

Calcium oscillations are more likely to occur in cells located >100 μm from the point of stimulation

Next, we calculated the proportion of cells displaying 1–8 peaks with respect to their distance from the point of stimulation (figure 4B). Almost 50% of cells possessing just one peak lay within 50 μm of the electrode. Moreover, less than 5% of the cells within the first 50 μm exhibited 5 or more intracellular calcium oscillations. In fact, the further the cell was from the electrode, the more likely it was to display multiple calcium oscillations (figure 4B). The most common number of oscillations in intracellular calcium post-TBS was 3, with 1194 (18%) cells exhibiting 3 peaks (figure 4B, inset). Over 50% of cells exhibited 4 peaks or more in the 5 min post-tetanic period, highlighting the widespread prevalence of $[Ca^{2+}]_i$ oscillations following this form of repetitive synaptic stimulation. Having assessed the effects of TBS on calcium dynamics, our next aim was to investigate a possible

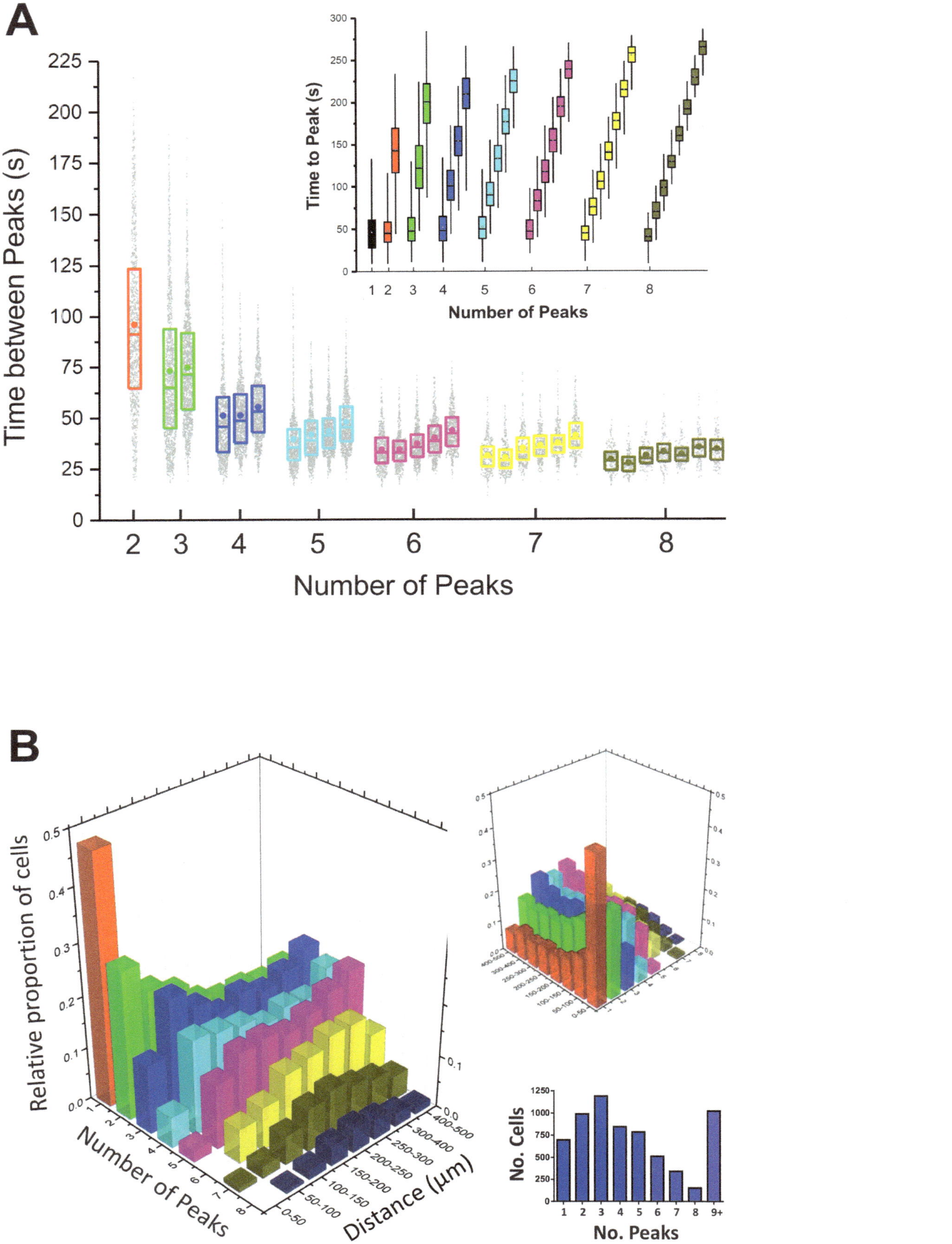
A
Time between Peaks (s)
Number of Peaks
Time to Peak (s)
Number of Peaks
B
Relative proportion of cells
Number of Peaks
Distance (µm)
No. Cells
No. Peaks

Figure 4. Calcium oscillation frequency with respect to distance from the point of TBS stimulation (A) Graphed is the 'time-between-peaks' for cells displaying between 2–8 fluctuations in $[Ca^{2+}]_i$. For cells containing either 2 or 3 peaks, there is large variability in the 'time-between-peaks'. Cells with 4 peaks or greater, however, show regular frequencies of oscillations in $[Ca^{2+}]_i$ between approx. 22–33 mHz. Inset: Graphed is the 'time-to-peak' for cells displaying between 1–8 peaks in $[Ca^{2+}]_i$. (B) 3D graph representing the frequency of $[Ca^{2+}]_i$ oscillations in cells post-TBS with respect to their distance from the stimulation site. Plotted on the X axis is the 'number of peaks' each cell displays. The Y axis represents the distance the cell is from the electrode. Graphed on the Z axis is the relative proportion of cells with 'n = 1–8 peaks' at a given distance from the electrode. The graph shows that almost 50% of cells with one peak in $[Ca^{2+}]_i$ lie within 50 µm from the electrode. The further a cell is from the point of stimulation, the more likely it is to display multiple peaks in $[Ca^{2+}]_i$. Inset: 1,194 cells displayed 3 peaks in $[Ca^{2+}]_i$ post-TBS, the most common number of peaks; whereas 153 cells displayed 8 peaks. The total number of cells analysed was 6,536 and of these, 5,512 exhibited 1–8 peaks in $[Ca^{2+}]_i$ with the rest exhibiting greater than 8.

functional consequence of the observed $[Ca^{2+}]_i$ oscillations post-TBS in terms of what is already known about the molecular underpinnings of LTP induction and maintenance in the hippocampus. Therefore, we measured changes in the glutamate-inducible and $[Ca^{2+}]_i$-responsive transcription factor, NF-κB, after theta-burst stimulation.

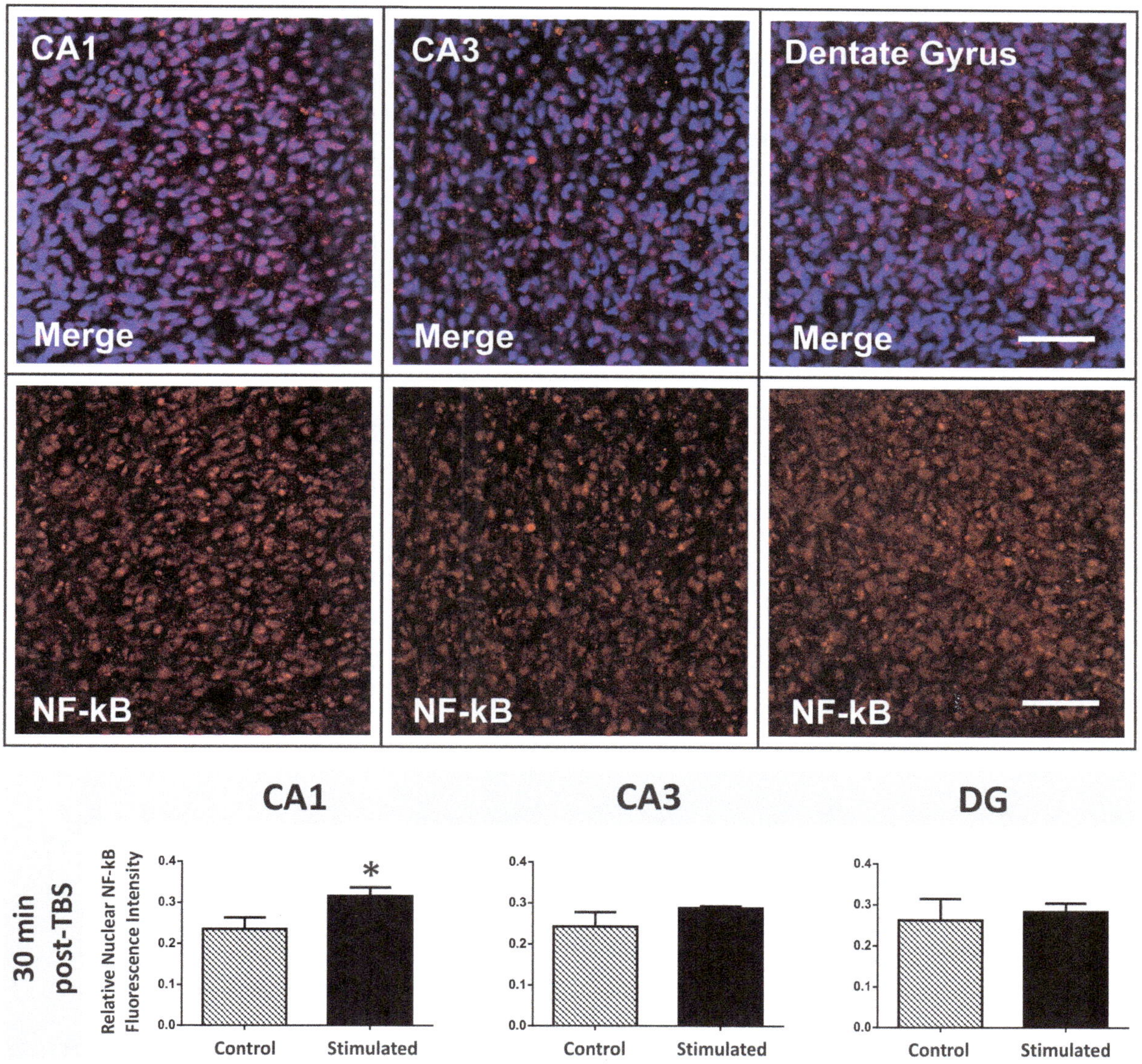

Figure 5. Changes in nuclear NF-κB levels 30 min post-TBS in the hippocampus. Top panel: NF-κB was immunofluorescently labelled in organotypic hippocampal slice cultures. The p65 subunit of activated NF-κB was stained red using a Cy3 secondary antibody and nuclei were counterstained blue using Hoechst 33258. High magnification confocal images (40X) of the CA1, CA3 and dentate gyrus neuronal cell populations were captured for each slice. Scale bar = 50 µm. Bottom graphs: Levels of activated nuclear NF-κB fluorescence were measured in organotypic hippocampal slices 30 min after theta-burst stimulation (TBS). CA1, CA3 and dentate gyrus cell populations were compared for control and stimulated slices. There is an up-regulation in activated nuclear NF-κB in the CA1 region (*two-tailed Student's t tests, p value $<$0.05).

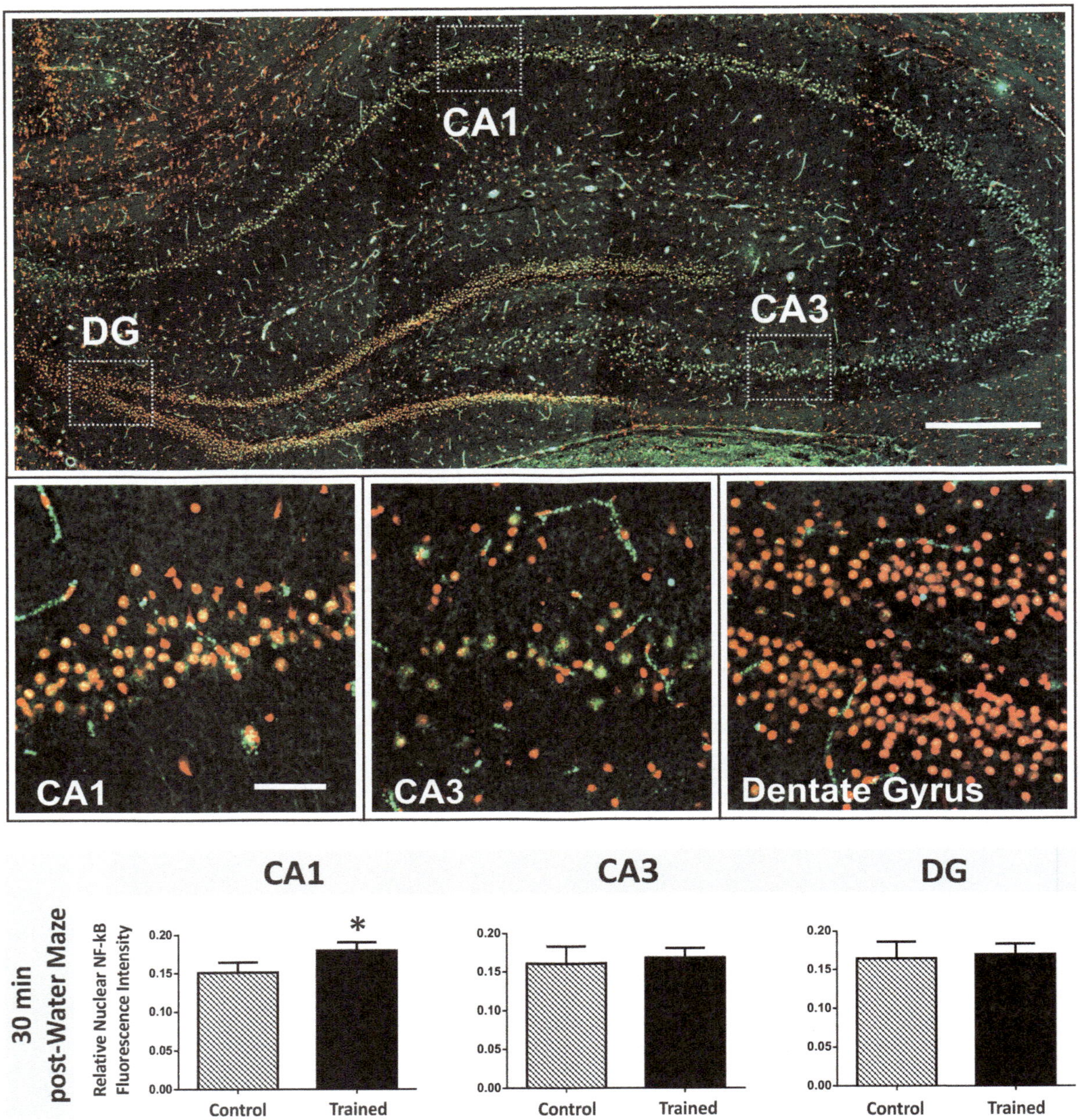

Figure 6. Changes in nuclear NF-κB levels 30 min post-spatial learning in the hippocampus. Top panel: Coronal section through the rat dorsal hippocampus (approx. −3.3 mm with respect to Bregma) immunofluorescently-labelled for the active form of the p65 subunit of NF-κB. Nuclei are stained red using propidium iodide and NF-κB labelled green using a FITC-conjugated secondary antibody. The white boxes represent the three regions of the hippocampal neuronal network that were analysed throughout this study. Scale bar = 400 μm. Middle panel: High-magnification images (40X) of the CA1, CA3 and DG illustrated by white boxes in the top montage. Scale bar = 50 μm. Bottom graphs: Levels of activated nuclear NF-κB fluorescence were measured in the rat hippocampus 30 min after water maze training ceased. CA1, CA3 and dentate gyrus cell populations were compared for passive control and trained rats. There is an up-regulation in activated nuclear NF-κB in the CA1 region (*two-tailed Student's t tests, p value<0.05).

TBS induces NF-κB activity in CA1 pyramidal cells of organotypic hippocampal cultures

Following theta-burst stimulation, organotypic hippocampal slices were fixed and stained for changes in the levels of activated nuclear NF-κB which could indicate the initiation of gene expression changes within stimulated cells. Changes in nuclear NF-κB levels were quantified in the CA1, CA3 and dentate gyrus 30 min post-TBS (figure 5). We found that NF-κB expression was significantly up-regulated in the CA1 region 30 min post-TBS. Nuclear NF-κB activation was unaltered in the CA3 and DG regions 30 min post-TBS, even though the stimulating electrode was positioned in the molecular layer of the DG. This suggests that theta-burst stimulation can activate transcription in cells located large distances from the stimulation site (CA1 >250 μm from electrode). This may, in part, be a consequence of the tri-synaptic feed-forward architecture of the hippocampal neuronal network.

Strongly stimulated cells in the DG could transfer this information to the CA3 and onto CA1 neurons through activity-driven synaptic communication. Moreover, the TBS-induced slow-propagating calcium wave may also contribute to these long-range effects on NF-κB activation. The increased frequency of calcium oscillations in stimulated cells at greater distances from the electrode may explain NF-κB activation in the CA1 hippocampal region, but not dentate gyrus [47,54]. Unfortunately, we were unable to retrospectively correlate TBS-induced calcium responses in individual cells with up-regulations in NF-κB activation specifically in the CA1 pyramidal cell layer.

Spatial learning induces NF-κB activation in the CA1 region of the rat hippocampus

We next investigated whether the activation of NF-κB measured in hippocampal slices following theta-burst stimulation is recapitulated *in vivo* in rats trained in the Morris water maze spatial learning task. Trained and passive control groups of rats were sacrificed 30 min post-training. Changes in nuclear NF-κB expression were quantified in the CA1, CA3 and dentate gyrus of the dorsal hippocampus; the area of the brain thought to be most important for spatial memory formation (figure 6). NF-κB activation was up-regulated specifically in the CA1 region 30 min post-water maze training. Therefore, similar cell type-specific changes in transcription factor activation in the hippocampus seem to underlie both *in vitro* theta-burst stimulation and spatial memory formation *in vivo*.

Discussion

Calcium signalling in hippocampal neurons is fundamental to many processes including synaptic plasticity, long-term potentiation (LTP) and memory formation [2,55–60]. Over the years, *in vitro* LTP studies in brain slices have reported a wide range of high-frequency stimulus (HFS) protocols used to model the cellular and molecular basis of learning and memory formation [61]. An important feature of the HFS protocol is the calcium response of directly stimulated, as well as interconnected, neurons and glial cells. In neuronal synapses, the magnitude of the calcium response is thought to determine whether the synapse will undergo a change in synaptic strength [62]. In astrocyte networks, the calcium response can influence the release of gliotransmitters which will have secondary modulatory effects on neuronal synapses in close proximity with glial cells [63]. In this study, we describe the propagating wave and oscillations in intracellular calcium $[Ca^{2+}]_i$ induced in a large proportion (>50%) of a transverse slice of the hippocampal network (an area of approx. 0.8 mm^2) when a theta-burst stimulus (TBS) is applied to the dentate gyrus (DG) dendritic field. We recorded the simultaneous calcium response of hundreds of cells to TBS which is crucial if we are to even begin to understand how functionally connected neuronal ensembles translate a given stimulus into activity-driven changes in plasticity, gene expression and behaviour [64].

TBS-induced $[Ca^{2+}]_i$ oscillations

Theta-burst stimulation mimics a physiologically-relevant frequency of neuronal activity exhibited in the hippocampus of behaving animals [29,65–67]. By monitoring the dynamics of calcium fluctuations in response to TBS in a large proportion of the hippocampus we have uncovered a novel post-tetanic phenomenon; network-wide rhythmic calcium oscillations that range between 17–33 mHz in periodicity. Multiple $[Ca^{2+}]_i$ oscillations are more common in cells positioned further from the stimulation source (>100 μm). Cells located close to the electrode (<100 μm) experience a larger rise in $[Ca^{2+}]_i$ and it takes longer for the intracellular calcium levels to drop sufficiently (and/or intracellular stores to refill) before a second spontaneous rise in $[Ca^{2+}]_i$ can occur. This explains the large delay between first and second peaks in cells located <100 μm from the electrode. After the spontaneous second peak in $[Ca^{2+}]_i$ occurs, however, most cells appear to enter a post-tetanic phase of rhythmic $[Ca^{2+}]_i$ oscillations. It is likely that the $[Ca^{2+}]_i$ oscillations are heavily-dependent on calcium-induced calcium release (CICR) from intracellular stores [26,27,68,69] and/or sustained extracellular calcium influx through store-operated calcium (SOC) channels that act to replenish calcium stores [70,71]. $[Ca^{2+}]_i$ oscillations may also be functionally important in the bi-directional communication between neurons and astrocytes that accompanies TBS-induced changes in hippocampal synaptic plasticity [72,73]. Since theta-burst stimulation mimics a physiologically-relevant frequency of neuronal activity in the hippocampus of behaving animals, we propose that these post-tetanic oscillations in $[Ca^{2+}]_i$ are functionally important for deciphering the information encoded in patterns of neuronal activation [72]. Moreover, the frequency of $[Ca^{2+}]_i$ oscillations triggered may be crucially important to the initial stimulus since the frequency increases with respect to distance from the stimulus origin. Cells situated within 100 μm of the electrode are likely to exhibit around 2 or 3 oscillations, whereas cells lying 400–500 μm from the stimulation point are more likely to display between 3–6 oscillations in $[Ca^{2+}]_i$. Therefore, the frequency of calcium oscillations in hippocampal cells post-TBS may be important in pattern separation, i.e. the ability of the hippocampus to process and code specific patterns of neuronal activity and to discriminate them from similar events. Therefore, since $[Ca^{2+}]_i$ oscillations exhibiting a frequency of 17–22 mHz are more likely to occur in cells located within 100 μm of the stimulation site and frequencies of 26–33 mHz are more common in cells situated 400–500 μm from the electrode, this information could facilitate the pattern separation needed for complex cognitive processes involving spatial learning and memory formation. Moreover, $[Ca^{2+}]_i$ oscillations of different frequencies are likely to activate distinct signalling cascades and changes in gene transcription within stimulated cells which could add a further layer of complexity to pattern separation and memory encoding in the hippocampus. In the present study, we report increased activation of the transcription factor, NF-κB, in the CA1 pyramidal cell layer of hippocampal slices 30 min after theta-burst stimulation to the dentate gyrus dendritic field. This cell-type specific translocation of activated NF-κB to the nucleus of CA1 cells may be functionally relevant for both LTP maintenance and memory formation since rats trained in the Morris water maze spatial learning task also displayed similar temporal and cell type-specific regulation of NF-κB activation.

NF-κB and memory-associated synaptic plasticity

Since LTP is dependent on the synthesis of new proteins to maintain enhanced synaptic transmission at stimulated synapses [74], NF-κB activation in the CA1 region of hippocampal slices stimulated with TBS may indicate the transcription of genes important for LTP expression. NF-κB is reportedly activated both *in vitro* and *in vivo* in the hippocampus by high-frequency stimulation [48,75] and is sensitive to both glutamate- and GABA-mediated synaptic transmission [76]. NF-κB is also present in synapses and can exhibit retrograde translocation to the nucleus upon activation [46,77,78]. Thus, as well as an activity-driven regulator of gene-expression, it is ubiquitously located within the cell and, therefore, ideally primed to act as a signalling molecule of glutamate-mediated calcium entry.

It is interesting that dentate granule cells display no alterations in NF-κB activation post-TBS. Either NF-κB up-regulation comes and goes within the first 30 min post-stimulation or dentate granule cells, being so close to the point of stimulation, are less likely to display multiple oscillations in $[Ca^{2+}]_i$ and, therefore, less NF-κB activation. Alternatively, NF-κB activation in the CA1 may not be a consequence of TBS-induced calcium oscillations. There are several studies, however, which do link $[Ca^{2+}]_i$ oscillations to NF-κB activity [79,80]. It has also been shown that CaMKII activity is sensitive to $[Ca^{2+}]_i$ oscillations and CaMKII has been shown to regulate NF-κB activation [28,44,46,81]. Consequently, if $[Ca^{2+}]_i$ oscillations are important for NF-κB activation, then DG cells, because of their close proximity to the electrode, may be less likely to exhibit up-regulations in NF-κB activation post-TBS. In addition to the propagating wave of calcium, the position of the electrode in the molecular layer of the dentate gyrus may directly stimulate some CA1 pyramidal neurons through axonal projections that synapse on dentate granule cells. The number of CA1 axons that synapse in the molecular layer of the dentate gyrus may also be exaggerated in organotypic slice cultures grown *in vitro* for 21 days since they tend to display more aberrant neuronal projections compared to acute hippocampal slices [82].

TBS-induced calcium wave propagation

As well as serving to potentiate synaptic transmission between neurons, TBS initiates a wave of calcium within the interconnected astrocyte networks of the hippocampus. There are at least three main methods by which calcium waves can travel in an *in vitro* hippocampal slice culture (figure 2C). The predominant method, at least in acute hippocampal slices, is reportedly through stimulation-induced release of ATP and subsequent paracrine activation of purinergic receptors which perpetuate the release of ATP from neighbouring cells, thus initiating a calcium wave through astrocyte networks [83,84]. Other signalling molecules, such as glutamate and nitric oxide, can also be released from astrocytes and contribute to calcium wave propagation [72,85,86]. The second is through cell-cell contacts and gap junctions which allow the movement of calcium ions and inositol 1,4,5-trisphosphate (IP3) into neighbouring cells, thus perpetuating the calcium wave over long distances [87,88]. As the calcium wave travels further from the point of stimulation, the amplitude of the $[Ca^{2+}]_i$ response decays exponentially with distance (illustrated in figure 2C). A third way in which calcium waves propagate through the hippocampal network is mediated by action potential generation in neurons close to the electrode which synapse on other neurons and glial cells located up to hundreds of microns away from the site of stimulation [89]. This can explain the small number of cells in figure 2B, located 300–500 μm from the point of stimulation, which display relatively fast 'time-to-first peak' kinetics. Because the velocity of calcium wave propagation in hippocampal slice cultures appears to increase >150 μm from the point of stimulation, this may represent a transition from gap junction-mediated $[Ca^{2+}]_i$ propagation to release of soluble factors (such as ATP) that stimulate neighbouring cells and perpetuate the calcium wave over long distances through astrocyte networks. ATP is also a well-known trigger of $[Ca^{2+}]_i$ oscillations which could explain the increased number of oscillations at further distances from the point of stimulation.

The importance of astrocytes and other glial cells in hippocampal synaptic plasticity is becoming more and more evident in recent years [90–92]. Astrocytes can release neuromodulatory chemicals that can serve to either enhance or dampen synaptic transmission [93–97]. The triggering of calcium oscillations in astrocyte networks in the hippocampus could activate the release of neuromodulators from glial cells. Therefore, astrocytes may contribute to the decoding of the initial theta-burst stimulus and likely serve a pertinent role in LTP and synaptic plasticity changes in the hippocampus post-TBS stimulation [89,98,99].

Conclusion

Here, we show that theta-burst stimulation, administered to the molecular layer of the dentate gyrus of hippocampal slices, induces similar temporal and cell-type specific activation of NF-κB to spatial learning in trained rats. This finding suggests that TBS in slice cultures may activate similar changes in gene expression that are important for memory formation in behaving animals. This confirms the validity and usefulness of this *in vitro* system to study the molecular basis of complex cognitive processes such as learning and memory formation. We have also uncovered a novel and interesting feature of theta-burst stimulation in the hippocampal network; the initiation of slow rhythmic $[Ca^{2+}]_i$ oscillations that may contribute to changes in synaptic plasticity and NF-κB-mediated changes in gene expression important for LTP maintenance. Moreover, changes in the frequency of $[Ca^{2+}]_i$ oscillations with increasing distance from the stimulation source may be important in pattern separation in the hippocampal network.

Author Contributions

Conceived and designed the experiments: GKS MP JJOC KJM. Performed the experiments: GKS MP. Analyzed the data: GKS EM. Contributed reagents/materials/analysis tools: JJOC KJM. Contributed to the writing of the manuscript: GKS.

References

1. Bliss TVP, Lømo T (1973) Long-lasting potentiation of synaptic transmission in the dentate area of the anaesthetized rabbit following stimulation of the perforant path. J Physiol 232: 331–356.
2. Bliss TVP, Collingridge GL (1993) A synaptic model of memory: long term potentiation and the hippocampus. Nature 361: 31–39.
3. Martin SJ, Grimwood PD, Morris RG (2000) Synaptic plasticity and memory: an evaluation of the hypothesis. A Rev Neurosci 23: 649–711.
4. Martin SJ, Morris RGM (2002) New life in an old idea: the synaptic plasticity and memory hypothesis revisited. Hippocampus 12: 609–636.
5. Malenka RC, Bear MF (2004) LTP and LTD: an embarrassment of riches. Neuron 44: 5–21.
6. Baez MV, Oberholzer MV, Cercato MC, Snitcofsky M, Aguirre AI, et al. (2013) NMDA receptor subunits in the adult rat hippocampus undergo similar changes after 5 minutes in an open field and after LTP induction. PLoS ONE 8(2): e55244.
7. Freeman FM, Rose SPR, Scholey AB (1995) Two time windows of anisomycin-induced amnesia for passive avoidance training in the day-old chick. Neurobiol Learn Mem 63: 291–295.
8. Meiri N, Rosenblum K (1998) Lateral ventricle injection of the protein synthesis inhibitor anisomycin impairs long-term memory in a spatial memory task. Brain Res 789: 48–55.
9. Igaz LM, Vianna MRM, Medina JH, Izquierdo I (2002) Two time periods of hippocampal mRNA synthesis are required for memory consolidation of fear-motivated learning. J Neurosci 22: 6781–6789.
10. Bailey CH, Bartsch D, Kandel ER (1996) Toward a molecular definition of long-term memory storage. Proc Natl Acad Sci USA 93: 13445–13452.
11. Kandel ER (2001) The molecular biology of memory storage: a dialogue between genes and synapses. Science 294: 1030–1038.
12. Cavallaro S, D'Agata V, Manickam P, Dufour F, Alkon DL (2002) Memory-specific temporal profiles of gene expression in the hippocampus. Proc Natl Acad Sci USA 99: 16279–16284.
13. Levenson JM, Choi S, Lee SY, Cao YA, Ahn HJ, et al. (2004) A bioinformatics analysis of memory consolidation reveals involvement of the transcription factor c-rel. J Neurosci 24: 3933–3943.
14. Kaltschmidt B, Ndiaye D, Korte M, Pothion S, Arbibe L, et al. (2006) NF-κB regulates spatial memory formation and synaptic plasticity through protein kinase A/CREB signalling. Mol Cell Biol 26: 2936–2946.

15. Romano A, Freudenthal R, Merlo E, Routtenberg A (2006) Evolutionarily-conserved role of the NF-kappaB transcription factor in neural plasticity and memory. Eur J Neurosci 24: 1507–1516.
16. O'Sullivan NC, McGettigan PA, Sheridan GK, Pickering M, Conboy L, et al. (2007) Temporal change in gene expression in the rat dentate gyrus following passive avoidance learning. J Neurochem 101: 1085–1098.
17. O'Sullivan NC, Sheridan GK, Murphy KJ (2012) Transcriptional profiling of hippocampal memory-associated synaptic plasticity: old friends and new faces. In: Transcription factors CREB and NF-kB: involvement in synaptic plasticity and memory formation. Sharjah, UAE: Bentham Science. pp. 43–65.
18. Ryan MM, Ryan B, Kyrke-Smith M, Logan B, Tate WP, et al. (2012) Temporal profiling of gene networks associated with the late phase of long-term potentiation in vivo. PLoS ONE 7(7): e40538.
19. Lisman J, Yasuda R, Raghavachari S (2012) Mechanisms of CaMKII action in long-term potentiation. Nat Rev Neurosci 13: 169–182.
20. Ashpole NM, Song W, Brustovetsky T, Engleman EA, Brustovetsky N, et al. (2012) Calcium/calmodulin-dependent protein kinase II (CaMKII) inhibition induces neurotoxicity via dysregulation of glutamate/calcium signaling and hyperexcitability. J Biol Chem 287: 8495–8506.
21. Gillespie JM, Hodge JJL (2013) CASK regulates CaMKII autophosphorylation in neuronal growth, calcium signaling, and learning. Front Mol Neurosci 6: 27.
22. Poser S, Storm DR (2001) Role of Ca^{2+}-stimulated adenylyl cyclases in LTP and memory formation. Int J Dev Neurosci 19: 387–394.
23. West AE, Chen WG, Dalva MB, Dolmetsch RE, Kornhauser JM, et al. (2001) Calcium regulation of neuronal gene expression. Proc Natl Acad Sci USA 98: 11024–11031.
24. MacDonald JF, Jackson MF, Beazely MA (2006) Hippocampal long-term synaptic plasticity and signal amplification of NMDA receptors. Crit Rev Neurobiol 18: 71–84.
25. Kato HK, Kassai H, Watabe AM, Aiba A, Manabe T (2012) Functional coupling of the metabotropic glutamate receptor, InsP3 receptor and L-type Ca2+ channel in mouse CA1 pyramidal cells. J Physiol 590: 3019–3034.
26. Dupont G, Goldbeter A (1993) One-pool model for Ca^{2+} oscillations involving Ca^{2+} and inositol 1,4,5-trisphosphate as co-agonists for Ca^{2+} release. Cell Calcium 14: 311–322.
27. Dupont G, Goldbeter A (1994) Properties of intracellular Ca^{2+} waves generated by a model based on $Ca^{(2+)}$-induced Ca^{2+} release. Biophys J 67: 2191–2204.
28. Li L, Stefan MI, Le Novere N (2012) Calcium input frequency, duration and amplitude differentially modulate the relative activation of calcineurin and CaMKII. PLoS One 7: e43810.
29. Ranck JB (1973) Studies on single neurons in dorsal hippocampal formation and septum in unrestrained rats. Part I. Behavioral correlates and firing repertoires. Exp Neurol 41: 461–555.
30. Hill AJ (1978) First occurrence of hippocampal spatial firing in a new environment. Exp Neurol 62: 282–297.
31. Otto T, Eichenbaum H, Wiener SI, Wible CG (1991) Learning-related patterns of CA1 spike trains parallel stimulation parameters optimal for inducing hippocampal long-term potentiation. Hippocampus 1: 181–192.
32. Larson J, Wong D, Lynch G (1986) Patterned stimulation at the theta frequency is optimal for the induction of hippocampal long-term potentiation. Brain Res 368: 347–350.
33. Staubli U, Lynch G (1987) Stable hippocampal long-term potentiation elicited by 'theta' pattern stimulation. Brain Res 435: 227–234.
34. Grover LM, Teyler TJ (1990) Two components of long-term potentiation induced by different patterns of afferent activation. Nature 347: 477–479.
35. Grover LM, Teyler TJ (1994) Activation of NMDA receptors in hippocampal area CA1 by low and high frequency orthodromic stimulation and their contribution to induction of long-term potentiation. Synapse 16: 66–75.
36. O'Connor JJ, Rowan MJ, Anwyl R (1994) Long-lasting enhancement of NMDA receptor-mediated synaptic transmission by metabotropic glutamate receptor activation. Nature 367: 557–559.
37. O'Leary DM, O'Connor JJ (1999) Potentiation of synaptic transmission by (S)-3,5-dihydroxy phenylglycine in the rat dentate gyrus in vitro: a role for voltage dependent calcium channels and protein kinase C. Prog Neuropsychopharmacol Biol Psychiatry 23: 133–147.
38. Emptage NJ, Reid CA, Fine A, Bliss TV (2003) Optical quantal analysis reveals a presynaptic component of LTP at hippocampal Schaffer-associational synapses. Neuron 38: 797–804.
39. Raymond CR, Redman SJ (2006) Spatial segregation of neuronal calcium signals encodes different forms of LTP in rat hippocampus. J Physiol 570: 97–111.
40. Ward B, McGuinness L, Akerman CJ, Fine A, Bliss TV, et al. (2006) State-dependent mechanisms of LTP expression revealed by optical quantal analysis. Neuron 52: 649–661.
41. Hamilton TJ, Wheatley BM, Sinclair DB, Bachmann M, Larkum ME, et al. (2010) Dopamine modulates synaptic plasticity in dendrites of rat and human dentate granule cells. Proc Natl Acad Sci USA 107: 18185–18190.
42. Piochon C, Levenes C, Ohtsuki G, Hansel C (2010) Purkinje cell NMDA receptors assume a key role in synaptic gain control in the mature cerebellum. J Neurosci 30: 15330–15335.
43. Kratzer S, Mattusch C, Kochs E, Eder M, Haseneder R, et al. (2012) Xenon attenuates hippocampal long-term potentiation by diminishing synaptic and extrasynaptic N-methyl-D-aspartate receptor currents. Anesthesiology 116: 673–682.
44. De Koninck P, Schulman H (1998) Sensitivity of CaM kinase II to the frequency of Ca2+ oscillations. Science 279: 227–230.
45. Dupont G, Houart G, De Koninck P (2003) Sensitivity of CaM kinase II to the frequency of Ca2+ oscillations: a simple model. Cell Calcium. 34: 485–497.
46. Meffert MK, Chang JM, Wiltgen BJ, Fanselow MS, Baltimore D (2003) NF-kappaB functions in synaptic signaling and behavior. Nat Neurosci 6: 1072–1078.
47. Dolmetsch RE, Xu K, Lewis RS (1998) Calcium oscillations increase the efficiency and specificity of gene expression. Nature 392: 933–936.
48. Freudenthal R, Romano A, Routtenberg A (2004) Transcription factor NF-kappaB activation after in vivo perforant path LTP in mouse hippocampus. Hippocampus: 14: 677–683.
49. Freudenthal R, Boccia MM, Acosta GB, Blake MG, Merlo E, et al. (2005) NF-kappaB transcription factor is required for inhibitory avoidance long-term memory in mice. Eur J Neurosci 21: 2845–2852.
50. O'Mahony A, Raber J, Montano M, Foehr E, Han V, et al. (2006) NF-κB/Rel regulates inhibitory and excitatory neuronal function and synaptic plasticity. Mol Cell Biol 26: 7283–7298.
51. Stoppini L, Buchs PA, Muller D (1991) A simple method for organotypic cultures of nervous tissue. J Neurosci Methods 37: 173–182.
52. Gogolla N, Galimberti I, DePaola V, Caroni P (2006) Staining protocol for organotypic hippocampal slice cultures. Nat Protoc 1: 2452–2456.
53. Paxinos G, Watson C (2005) The rat brain in stereotaxic coordinates, 5th ed. Elsevier Academic Press, San Diego, CA.
54. Li W, Llopis J, Whitney M, Zlokarnik G, Tsien RY (1998) Cell-permeant caged InsP3 ester shows that Ca^{2+} spike frequency can optimize gene expression. Nature 392: 936–941.
55. Guthrie PB, Segal M, Kater SB (1991) Independent regulation of calcium revealed by imaging dendritic spines. Nature 354: 76–80.
56. Müller W, Connor JA (1991) Dendritic spines as individual neuronal compartments for synaptic Ca^{2+} responses. Nature 354: 73–76.
57. Borroni AM, Fichtenholtz H, Woodside BL, Teyler TJ (2000) Role of voltage-dependent calcium channel long-term potentiation (LTP) and NMDA LTP in spatial memory. J Neurosci 20: 9272–9276.
58. Ismailov I, Kalikulov D, Inoue T, Friedlander MJ (2004) The kinetic profile of intracellular calcium predicts long-term potentiation and long-term depression. J Neurosci 24: 9847–9861.
59. Woodside BL, Borroni AM, Hammonds MD, Teyler TJ (2004) NMDA receptors and voltage-dependent calcium channels mediate different aspects of acquisition and retention of a spatial memory task. Neurobiol Learn Mem 81: 105–114.
60. Carter AG, Vogt KE, Foster KA, Regehr WG (2002) Assessing the role of calcium-induced calcium release in short-term presynaptic plasticity at excitatory central synapses. J Neurosci 22: 21–28.
61. Albensi BC, Oliver DR, Toupin J, Odero G (2007) Electrical stimulation protocols for hippocampal synaptic plasticity and neuronal hyper-excitability: are they effective or relevant? Exp Neurol 204: 1–13.
62. Graupner M, Brunel N (2012) Calcium-based plasticity model explains sensitivity of synaptic changes to spike pattern, rate, and dendritic location. Proc Natl Acad Sci USA 109: 3991–3996.
63. Rusakov DA, Zheng K, Henneberger C (2011) Astrocytes as regulators of synaptic function: a quest for the Ca^{2+} master key. Neuroscientist 17: 513–523.
64. Yuan Q, Isaacson JS, Scanziani M (2011) Linking neuronal ensembles by associative synaptic plasticity. PLoS ONE 6(6): e20486.
65. Kandel ER, WA Spencer (1961) Electrophysiology of hippocampal neurons. II. After-potentials and repetitive firing. J Neurophysiol 24: 243–259.
66. Hasselmo ME (2005) What is the function of hippocampal theta rhythm?—Linking behavioral data to phasic properties of field potential and unit recording data. Hippocampus 15: 936–949.
67. Bikbaev A, Neyman S, Ngomba RT, Conn PJ, Nicoletti F et al. (2008) MGluR5 mediates the interaction between late-LTP, network activity, and learning. PLoS ONE 3(5): e2155.
68. Aguado F, Espinosa-Parrilla JF, Carmona MA, Soriano E (2002) Neuronal activity regulates correlated network properties of spontaneous calcium transients in astrocytes in situ. J Neurosci 22: 9430–9444.
69. Nett WJ, Oloff SH, McCarthy KD (2002) Hippocampal astrocytes in situ exhibit calcium oscillations that occur independent of neuronal activity. J Neurophysiol 87: 528–537.
70. Pizzo P, Burgo A, Pozzan T, Fasolato C (2001) Role of capacitative calcium entry on glutamate-induced calcium influx in type-I rat cortical astrocytes. J Neurochem79: 98–109.
71. Sergeeva M, Strokin M, Wang H, Ubl JJ, Reiser G (2003) Arachidonic acid in astrocytes blocks Ca(2+) oscillations by inhibiting store-operated Ca(2+) entry, and causes delayed Ca(2+) influx. Cell Calcium 33: 283–292.
72. Pasti L, Volterra A, Pozzan T, Carmignoto G (1997) Intracellular calcium oscillations in astrocytes: a highly plastic, bidirectional form of communication between neurons and astrocytes in situ. J Neurosci. 17: 7817–7830.
73. Aguado F, Espinosa-Parrilla JF, Carmona MA, Soriano E (2002) Neuronal activity regulates correlated network properties of spontaneous calcium transients in astrocytes in situ. J Neurosci 22: 9430–9444.
74. Frey U, Krug M, Reymann K, Matthies H (1988) Anisomycin, an inhibitor of protein synthesis, blocks late phases of homo- and heterosynaptic long-term potentiation in the hippocampal CA1 region in vitro. Brain Res 452: 57–62.

75. Meberg PJ, Kinney WR, Valcourt EG, Routtenberg A (1996) Gene expression of the transcription factor NF-κB in hippocampus: regulation by synaptic activity. Mol Brain Res 38: 179–190.
76. Sheridan GK, Pickering M, Twomey C, Moynagh PN, O'Connor JJ et al. (2007) NF-κB activity in distinct neural subtypes of the rat hippocampus: Influence of time and GABA antagonism in acute slice preparations. Learn Mem 14: 525–532.
77. Wellmann H, Kaltschmidt B, Kaltschmidt C (2001) Retrograde transport of transcription factor NF-kappa B in living neurons. J Biol Chem 276: 11821–11829.
78. O'Riordan KJ, Huang IC, Pizzi M, Spano P, Boroni F, et al. (2006) Regulation of nuclear factor kappaB in the hippocampus by group I metabotropic glutamate receptors. J Neurosci 26: 4870–4879.
79. Hu Q, Deshpande S, Irani K, Ziegelstein RC (1999) $[Ca^{2+}]_i$ oscillation frequency regulates agonist-stimulated NF-kappaB transcriptional activity. J Biol Chem 274: 33995–33998.
80. Song S, Li J, Zhu L, Cai L, Xu Q, et al. (2012) Irregular Ca(2+) oscillations regulate transcription via cumulative spike duration and spike amplitude. J Biol Chem 287: 40246–40255.
81. Dupont G, Goldbeter A (1998) CaM kinase II as frequency decoder of Ca2+ oscillations. Bioessays 20: 607–610.
82. Caeser M, Aertsen A (1991) Morphological organization of rat hippocampal slice cultures. J Comp Neurol 307: 87–106.
83. Guthrie PB, Knappenberger J, Segal M, Bennett MV, Charles AC, et al. (1999) ATP released from astrocytes mediates glial calcium waves. J Neurosci 19: 520–528.
84. Schipke CG, Boucsein C, Ohlemeyer C, Kirchhoff F, Kettenmann H (2002) Astrocyte Ca2+ waves trigger responses in microglial cells in brain slices. FASEB J 16: 255–257.
85. Parpura V, Basarsky TA, Liu F, Jeftinija K, Jeftinija S, et al. (1994) Glutamate-mediated astrocyte-neuron signalling. Nature 369: 744–747.
86. Pasti L, Pozzan T, Carmignoto G (1995) Long-lasting changes of calcium oscillations in astrocytes. A new form of glutamate-mediated plasticity. J Biol Chem 270: 15203–15210.
87. Giaume C, Venance L (1998) Intercellular calcium signaling and gap junctional communication in astrocytes. Glia 24: 50–64.
88. Leybaert L, Sanderson MJ (2012) Intercellular Ca(2+) waves: mechanisms and function. Physiol Rev 92: 1359–1392.
89. Honsek SD, Walz C, Kafitz KW, Rose CR (2010) Astrocyte calcium signals at Schaffer collateral to CA1 pyramidal cell synapses correlate with the number of activated synapses but not with synaptic strength. Hippocampus 22: 29–42.
90. Huang YH, Sinha SR, Tanaka K, Rothstein JD, Bergles DE (2004) Astrocyte glutamate transporters regulate metabotropic glutamate receptor-mediated excitation of hippocampal interneurons. J Neurosci 24: 4551–4559.
91. Haydon PG, Carmignoto G (2006) Astrocyte control of synaptic transmission and neurovascular coupling. Physiol Rev 86: 1009–1031.
92. Pascual O, Ben Achour S, Rostaing P, Triller A, Bessis A (2012) Microglia activation triggers astrocyte-mediated modulation of excitatory neurotransmission. Proc Natl Acad Sci USA 109: E197–E205.
93. Bezzi P, Gundersen V, Galbete JL, Seifert G, Steinhauser C, et al. (2004) Astrocytes contain a vesicular compartment that is competent for regulated exocytosis of glutamate. Nat Neurosci 7: 613–620.
94. Domercq M, Brambilla L, Pilati E, Marchaland J, Volterra A, et al. (2006) P2Y1 receptor-evoked glutamate exocytosis from astrocytes: control by tumor necrosis factor-α and prostaglandins. J Biol Chem 281: 684–696.
95. Jourdain P, Bergersen LH, Bhaukaurally K, Bezzi P, Santello M, et al. 2007 Glutamate exocytosis from astrocytes controls synaptic strength. Nat Neurosci 10: 331–339.
96. Cali C, Marchaland J, Regazzi R, Bezzi P (2008) SDF 1-α (CXCL12) triggers glutamate exocytosis from astrocytes on a millisecond time scale: imaging analysis at the single-vesicle level with TIRF microscopy. J Neuroimmunol 198: 82–91.
97. Cali C, Bezzi P (2010) CXCR4-mediated glutamate exocytosis from astrocytes. J Neuroimmunol 224: 13–21.
98. Bernardinelli Y, Salmon C, Jones EV, Farmer WT, Stellwagen D, et al. (2011) Astrocytes display complex and localized calcium responses to single-neuron stimulation in the hippocampus. J Neurosci 31: 8905–8919.
99. Santello M, Bezzi P, Volterra A (2011) TNFα controls glutamatergic gliotransmission in the hippocampal dentate gyrus. Neuron 69: 988–1001.

15

Task-Specific and General Cognitive Effects in Chiari Malformation Type I

Philip A. Allen[1,2]*, James R. Houston[1], Joshua W. Pollock[1,2], Christopher Buzzelli[1], Xuan Li[1], A. Katherine Harrington[1], Bryn A. Martin[2,3], Francis Loth[2,3], Mei-Ching Lien[4], Jahangir Maleki[5], Mark G. Luciano[6]

1 Department of Psychology, University of Akron, Akron, Ohio, United States of America, **2** Conquer Chiari Research Center, University of Akron, Akron, Ohio, United States of America, **3** Department of Mechanical Engineering, University of Akron, Akron, Ohio, United States of America, **4** School of Psychological Science, Oregon State University, Corvallis, Oregon, United States of America, **5** Neurological Center for Pain, Cleveland Clinic Foundation, Cleveland, Ohio, United States of America, **6** Department of Neurological Surgery, Cleveland Clinic Foundation, Cleveland, Ohio, United States of America

Abstract

Objective: Our objective was to use episodic memory and executive function tests to determine whether or not Chiari Malformation Type I (CM) patients experience cognitive dysfunction.

Background: CM is a neurological syndrome in which the cerebellum descends into the cervical spine causing neural compression, severe headaches, neck pain, and number of other physical symptoms. While primarily a disorder of the cervico-medullary junction, both clinicians and researchers have suspected deficits in higher-level cognitive function.

Design and Methods: We tested 24 CM patients who had undergone decompression neurosurgery and 24 age- and education-matched controls on measures of immediate and delayed episodic memory, as well as three measures of executive function.

Results: The CM group showed performance decrements relative to the controls in response inhibition (Stroop interference), working memory computational speed (Ospan), and processing speed (automated digit symbol substitution task), but group differences in recall did not reach statistical significance. After statistical control for depression and anxiety scores, the group effects for working memory and processing speed were eliminated, but not for response inhibition. This response inhibition difference was not due to overall general slowing for the CM group, either, because when controls' data were transformed using the linear function fit to all of the reaction time tasks, the interaction with group remained statistically significant. Furthermore, there was a multivariate group effect for all of the response time measures and immediate and delayed recall after statistical control of depression and anxiety scores.

Conclusion: These results suggest that CM patients with decompression surgery exhibit cognitive dysfunction compared to age- and education-matched controls. While some of these results may be related to anxiety and depression (likely proxies for chronic pain), response inhibition effects, in particular, as well as a general cognitive deficit persisted even after control for anxiety and decompression.

Editor: Robert Sutherland, University of Lethbridge, Canada

Funding: The Conquer Chiari Foundation supported portions of this work. The funders had no role in study design, data collection and analysis, decision to publish, or preparation of the manuscript.

* E-mail: paallen@uakron.edu

Introduction

Chiari Malformation Type I (CM), affecting approximately 300,000 individuals in the USA, is approximately as common as multiple sclerosis (MS).[1,2] CM is a clinical syndrome in which the cerebellar tonsils are displaced/descend by 5 mm or greater caudal to the foramen magnum[3,4] (Figure 1). Even though neuroimaging technologies have led to the improvement of anatomical diagnoses, little is known about the incidence of cognitive symptoms, if any, associated with this syndrome.

While headache and neck pain are the most common symptoms in CM [5], CM patients also may show motoric and cognitive symptoms [3,6], although studies using precise tests of these potential cognitive deficits are uncommon. Cognitive deficits in CM may result from direct injury of cerebellar [7–12] or brainstem [13] systems, or from less direct effects based on anxiety and depression which are commonly seen in CM patients with chronic pain [14–19]. In the present study, anxiety and depression were also measured and used as covariates. Note that this argument does require certain assumptions. For example, general pain as an illness is more prevalent than anxiety and

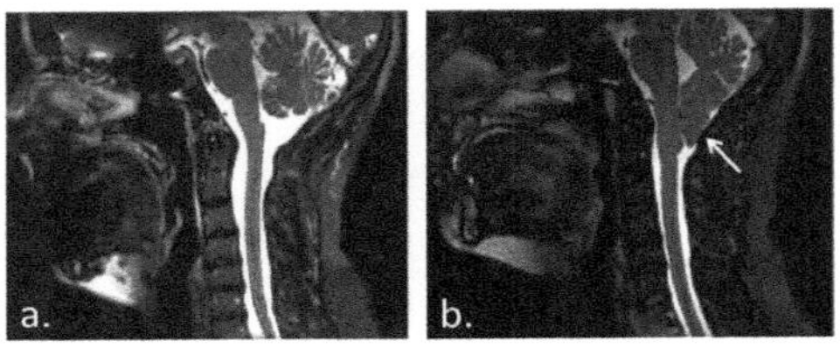

Figure 1. T2-weighted mid-sagittal MRI scan of (a) a healthy subject (b) and Chiari Type I malformation patient with arrow indicating location of tonsillar herniation through the foramen magnum and an asterisk indicating the medullary (brainstem) compression.

depression taken together, although some, but not all, patients with pain end up developing anxiety/depression. However, if we can show that anxiety and depression are significantly correlated with pain in CM patients, then it seems reasonable to use this as a starting place for separating pain-related and other predictors of potential cognitive deficits in CM. However, if group differences (CM vs. controls) in cognition persist after depression and anxiety are covaried out, then other causes of observed cognitive deficit(s) will need to be considered.

We hypothesize that CM patients will show executive dysfunction and episodic memory deficits relative to age- and education-matched controls. However, because both fiber-tract damage and chronic pain models of cognitive dysfunction involve similar brain areas (the cerebellum and the prefrontal cortex), it is difficult to separate fiber-tract damage in CM from chronic pain effects.

Evidence for Cognitive Deficits in Chiari Malformation

Our present hypothesis is that the downward herniation of the cerebellar tonsils (and/or their cardiac-cycle-based compression of the medulla) result either in direct pressure-related structural damage to the regional neural circuitry and/or cause dysfunction by generating chronic disorders such as pain. We further hypothesize that such damage to the cerebellum and its afferent/efferent circuits can result in cognitive deficits in executive function and episodic memory [12–20]. However, published evidence for cognitive deficits resulting from CM is surprisingly limited even though such deficits are hinted at in Yassari and Frim [6].

Kumar et al. [3] reported a neuroimaging study using diffusion tensor imaging (DTI) and intelligence testing on 10 CM patients and 10 controls. Kumar et al. observed that CM patients exhibited decreased fractional anisotropy (or FA) in the genu, splenium, fornix, and cingulum (areas of the brain that connect the limbic system to the medial temporal lobes). Given this location of decreased white-matter integrity, one might expect a CM-related deficit in episodic memory. Kumar et al. also observed cognitive deficits on the picture connection test, digit symbol, block design, picture arrangement, and 5-object assembly test (Wechsler Adult Intelligence Scale, or WAIS), as well as the Trail-Making B test, but no tests of episodic memory were administered. Kumar et al. also did not assess depression and anxiety, and as noted earlier, these variables are correlated with chronic pain that is a key symptom of CM patients. Thus, the present study was conducted to extend the Kumar et al. study to a new set of cognitive tasks to further test for cognitive dysfunction in CM.

Issues in the Diagnosis of Chiari Malformation Type I

Additionally, it is not clear whether the Kumar et al. [3] CM patients had undergone decompression surgery or were candidates for such a procedure. Because there have been no previous "comprehensive" tests of cognitive dysfunction in Chiari I Malformation that included measures of episodic memory and response inhibition, we felt that it was important in the present study that we obtain a conclusive diagnosis on CM. This is because diagnosis of CM is still somewhat ambiguous—even though it typically requires a 5 mm decension of the cerebellar tonsils into the cervical spinal canal, many neurologists and neurosurgeons also require observable symptoms, such as headache, and that there also be MRI evidence of CSF blockage and medulary compression.

One of the most direct methods to optimize the likelihood that an individual really does have conclusive CM is to select participants who have undergone posterior cranial fossa decompression surgery. CM can first present during childhood or adulthood, although pediatric-onset CM may show differences from adult-onset CM, both age groups frequently receive the same surgical intervention called craniospinal decompression surgery [21]. This surgery entails bone removal in the posterior cranial fossa, to varying degrees, along with the upper arch of the C1, and sometimes the C2, vertebrae. The objective is to restore space at the craniospinal junction in order to relieve the direct pressure on the brain stem and cerebellum. However, one consequence of this method is that the surgical procedure itself (rather than CM) could potentially result in cognitive dysfunction. However, most neurosurgeons feel that this procedure tends to alleviate symptoms associated with CM (e.g., headache), so it is likely that our present approach is a more conservative test of cognitive dysfunction in CM than using pre-decompression-surgery participants. An added benefit to the present approach is that if we were to use candidates for decompression surgery (who have not yet had surgery), patients' anxiety and/or depression might have been elevated due to the uncertainty of imminent neurosurgery. Thus, we decided that the optimal method for a comprehensive test of cognitive dysfunction in CM should use individuals who have already undergone decompresion surgery (at least six months prior to cognitive testing).

The Present Study

The present study examined the cognitive performances of CM patients who had undergone decompression surgery in addition to a sample of age- and education-matched, healthy controls. A secondary goal of this study was to use statistical control methods to distinguish between measures of anxiety and depression (likely related to chronic pain), and fiber-tract damage accounts of cognitive symptoms. To assess cognitive performance, we used a variation of the Rey Auditory Verbal Learning Test (RAVLT; a test of immediate and delayed episodic memory) using non-timed written responses and three computerized measures of executive function: an automated digit symbol substitution task [22] (a measure of processing speed with some memory load), a Stroop interference task [23] (a measure of response inhibition), and the Operation Span task (or Ospan, a measure of working memory) [24] using timed, button-press responses from a computer keyboard. To assess anxiety, depression, and stress levels in all participants, we used the 21-item, self-report Depression Anxiety and Stress Scale (DASS21) [25]. To directly assess self-reported head and neck pain in CM patients, we used the self-report Neck Pain Disability Index Questionnaire [26].

Methods

Ethics Statement

The present study was approved by the University of Akron Institutional Review Board (Akron, Ohio) and all participants (or their guardians) provided written informed consent.

Participants

Twenty-four CM patients (22 females, 2 males) who had undergone decompression surgery (age range: 15–59 years, mean age = 38.6 years, mean education = 14.6 years) and 24 age- and education-matched controls (15 females, 9 males; age range: 15–56 years, mean age = 39.2 years, mean education = 15.1 years) participated in the present study. There were no group differences in either age, $F(1, 46) = .03$, $p = .86$, or in years of education, $F(1, 46) = .50$, $p = .48$.

We selected post-decompression CM patients in order to assess potential cognitive deficits in more severe cases. All of these CM participants had considerable MRI evidence of cerebellar herniation below the foramen magnum in addition to being symptomatic with headache, dizziness and/or balance issues. In order to make sure that postoperative recovery was not contributing to the present results, we required at least a six-month interval between decompression surgery and participation in the present study. Approximately 80% of pre-decompression surgery CM patients experience severe headaches [5–6], and many of these patients are given opiate-based analgesics (e.g., Vicodin). However, because such analgesics can have an effect on cognition and/or contribute to ongoing headache in the long run, we limited participation in the present study of post-decompression participants to individuals who used just anti-inflammatories (NSAIDs) and acetaminophen (no opiate-based analgesics). In selecting post-decompression CM patients, though, we understand that we may have underestimated some CM cognitive deficits secondary to recovery.

Tasks and Procedure

Participants were tested individually on a computer and completed all of the tasks in one session. Each session began with immediate recall, followed by the digit symbol, Stroop, and working memory tasks assessing executive function. Finally, participants then completed the delayed recall task, followed by the depression, anxiety, and stress paper-and-pencil assessments. In addition, the CM patients but not the controls completed a pain and disability survey after the other tasks. The total testing time was approximately one hour.

RAVLT. To assess performance on episodic memory recall [27], we used a modified version of the Rey Auditory Verbal Learning Test [28]. Participants were presented orally the 15 words individually (approximately one second per word) and were asked to recall the words immediately after the first presentation of all of the words (the immediate recall) and also to recall the words 40 minutes later (the delayed recall) after the participants had completed the three executive function tasks. Participants wrote down their responses for both the immediate and delayed recall tasks, so the dependent variable was the number of written correct responses.

Stroop Test. Performance on the Stroop task has commonly been used as one indicator of frontal-lobe function measuring inhibitory control [29,30]. Specifically, it is important to note that the Stroop task is a measure of prepotent response inhibition [31]. The present Stroop test [32] involved the presentation of a single color word on a computer monitor (either "RED," "BLUE," "GREEN," or "PURPLE"). Words could be printed either in a color that matched the word (congruent trial) or in a different color than the word (incongruent trial). Participants were asked to identify the word or identify the color in which the word was printed. Responses for the four response alternatives were collected through the use of computer keys (the "1," "2," "3," and "4" keys). Reaction and accuracy served as the dependent variables. There were 20 practice trials and 96 experimental trials (48 "word meaning" trials and 48 "color" trials: 24 congruent and 24 incongruent of each).

Ospan Test. Working memory is the cognitive system that allows individuals to temporarily hold information in memory and to manipulate this information [33]. The Ospan test [24] is one of the most widely used measures of working memory capacity that includes both short-term memory maintenance (remembering sequences of letter string from 3–7 letters in length) as well as manipulation of math problems. However, it should be noted that the Ospan task has also been commonly used to measure fluid intelligence, which has been found to be correlated with the Raven's Progressive Matrices and mentally rotated blocks [24]. However, as noted in Unsworth et al. (2005, Figure 2) [24], fluid intelligence and working memory capacity (as measured by the Ospan task) form separate latent factors in structural equation models, implying that working memory capacity forms a separate construct from fluid intelligence. Thus, it is reasonable to assume that the Ospan task is a separate measure of working memory capacity independent of fluid intelligence.

There were 75 letters and 75 math problems in the presently used automated Ospan task based on Unsworth et al [24]. In the present study we report absolute Ospan scores and a measure of mean RT for the mental arithmetic solution time (the "working" portion of working memory), as well as accuracy of math computations.

Digit Symbol Substitution Task. We used a computer-administered version of the digit symbol substitution task [22]. Across the top of the computer screen, nine digits (from 0–9) were presented in a key along with nine symbols. Each digit was associated with a given symbol. In each trial, a single digit-symbol pair was presented directly below the middle of the key. Participants were instructed to respond whether the present pair was correct or incorrect. There were a total of 72 experimental trials.

We used SAS (Version 9.3) and SPSS (IBM SPSS Version 20) software to analyze the present results.

Results

For the RAVLT analysis, we had a 2 (group: CM vs. controls)×2 (retention interval: immediate vs. delayed recall) mixed design in which group was measured across participants and retention interval was measured within participants. The main effect of group approached significance, $F(1, 46) = 3.46$, $p = .07$, $\eta_P^2 = .07$ (words recalled: CM group = 6.00, Control group = 7.04, and there was a main effect of retention interval, $F(1, 46) = 67.26$, $p < .0001$, $\eta_P^2 = .60$ (immediate recall = 7.44 words, delayed recall = 5.60 words), but group did not interact with retention interval ($p = .71$) (see Figure 2).

For the digit symbol substitution task [22], a measure of processing speed, we compared means across group for response time (RT, in milliseconds) and accuracy (in mean percent error). There was a main effect of group for RT, $F(1, 46) = 4.95$, $p = .03$, $\eta_P^2 = .097$, (CM = 1767 ms, controls = 1544 ms) (Figure 3), but there was no main effect for accuracy ($p = .80$).

The Ospan task [24] is a set of measures of working memory capacity. There was a main effect of group for math computation RT, $F(1, 46) = 13.05$, $p < .001$, $\eta_P^2 = .18$, indicating that the CM

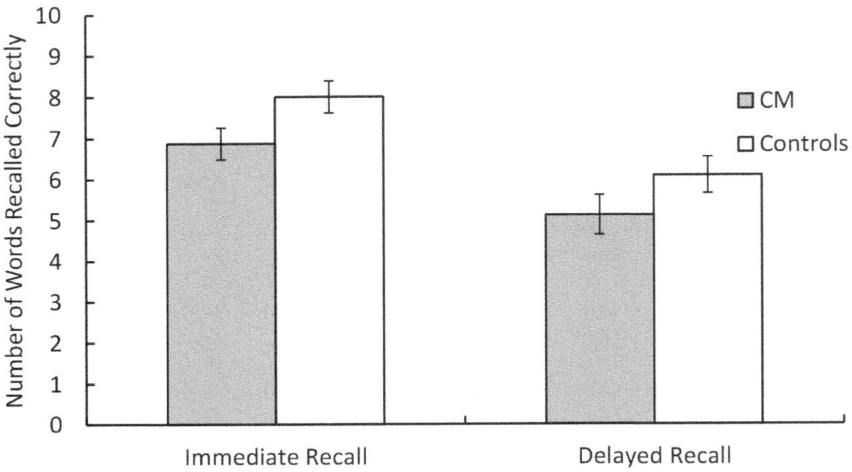

Figure 2. The mean total number of words correctly recalled in the immediate and delayed recall conditions for the Chiari Patients (CM) and Controls. Error bars represent the standard errors of the means.

Panel A:

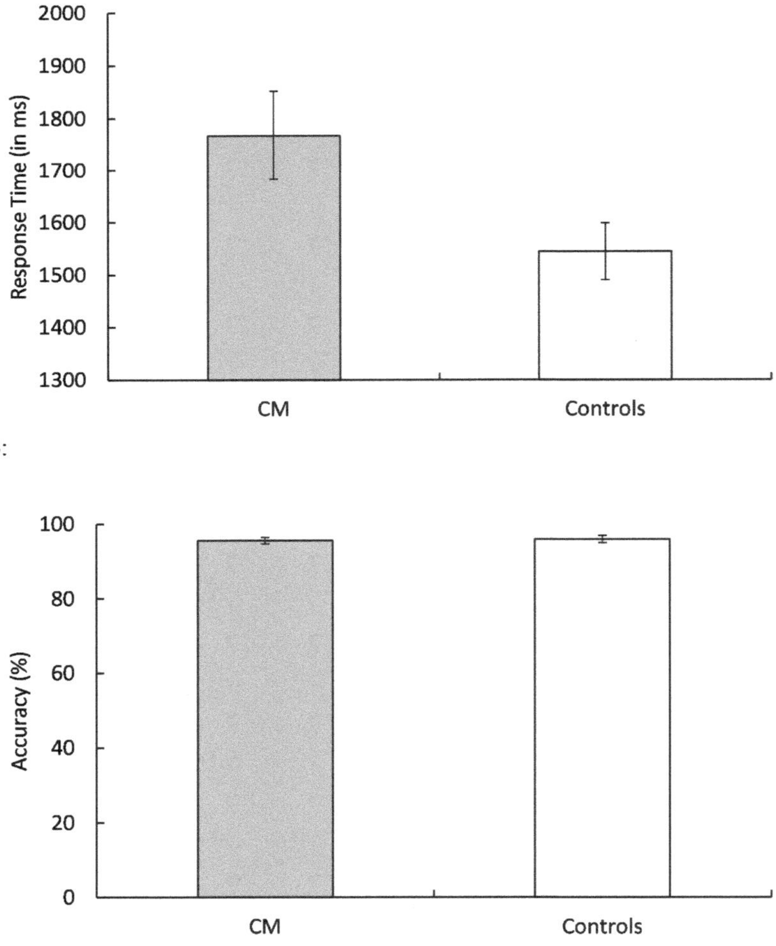

Figure 3. The mean response time (Panel A) and accuracy (Panel B) in digit symbol substitution task for the Chiari Patients (CM) and Controls. Error bars represent the standard errors of the means.

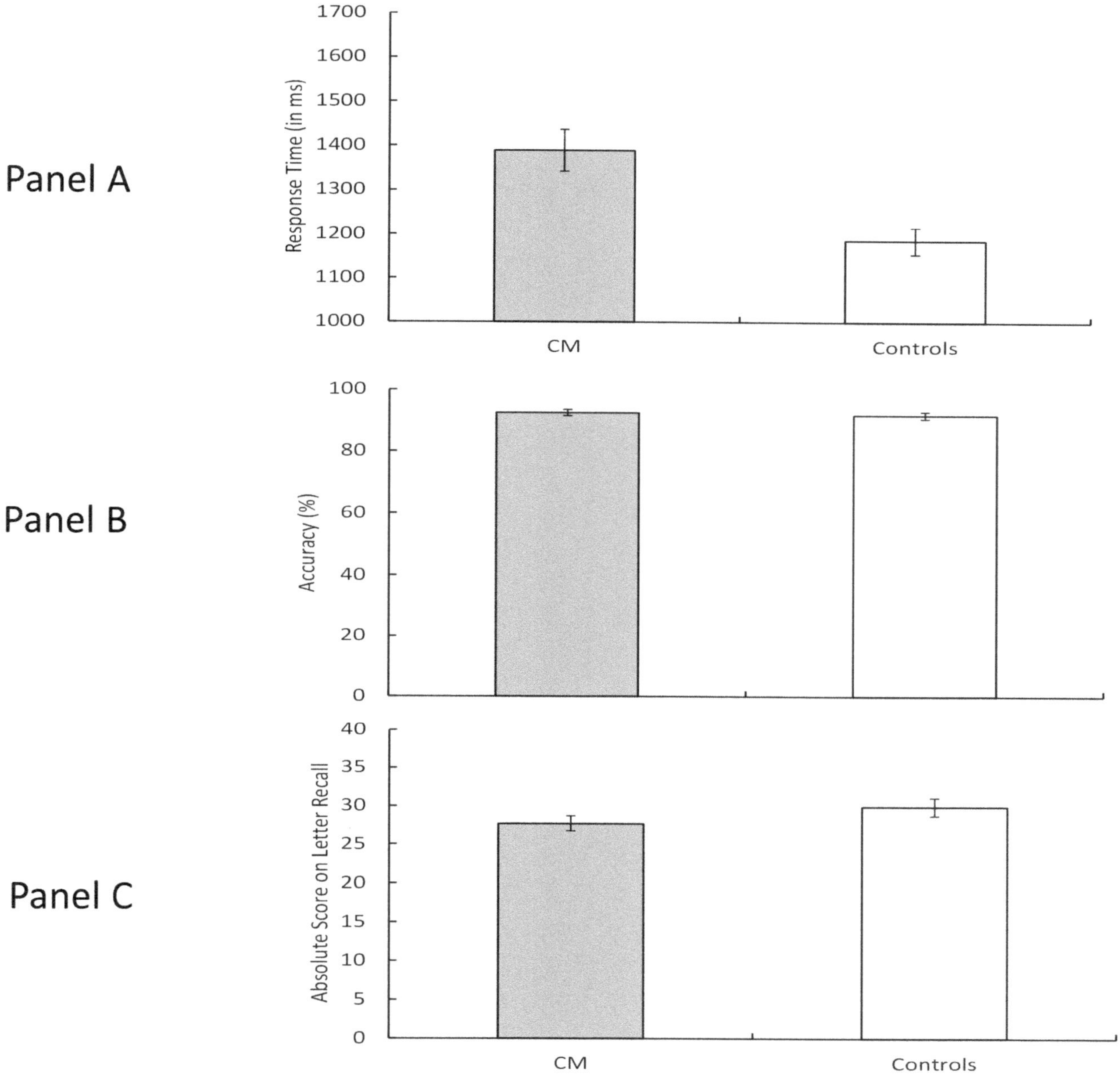

Figure 4. The mean response time (Panel A) and accuracy (Panel B) in Automated Operation Span (Ospan) computation time and accuracy as well as the total number of letters correctly recalled (Ospan Absolute Score; Panel C) for the Chiari Patients (CM) and Controls. Error bars represent the standard errors of the means.

group was significantly slower in computing the answers to math problems than were the controls (CM group = 1389 ms, controls = 1186 ms) (Figure 4). There was no effect of group for computational accuracy ($p = .69$). Also, there was no group effect for the total number of correctly recalled letter sequences ($p = .68$).

The Stroop task is a measure of response inhibition [23,31]. A 2 (group; a between-subject variable) ×2 (task type: color vs. word; a within-subject variable) ×2 (congruency: congruent vs. incongruent; a within-subject variable) mixed analysis of variance (ANOVA) was used to analyze the Stroop data. For RT, there were main effects for group, $F(1, 46) = 11.58$, $p < .01$, $\eta_P^2 = .25$ (CM = 1685 ms, controls = 1293 ms), task type, $F(1, 46) = 28.21$, $p < .0001$, $\eta_P^2 = .06$ (color = 1646 ms, word = 1332 ms), and congruency, $F(1, 46) = 46.22$, $p < .0001$, $\eta_P^2 = .50$ (congruent = 1406 ms, incongruent = 1572 ms). The key finding was a Group x Task Type x Congruency interaction, $F(1, 46) = 5.65$, $p < .05$, $\eta_P^2 = .11$, that occurred because the CM group showed a relatively larger congruency effect for the color condition (376 ms) versus the word condition (71 ms), relative to the control group for the color condition (162 ms) versus the word condition (54 ms) (Figure 5). To confirm this interpretation, we ran separate analyses for the Group x Congruency simple effects by task type. The Group x Congruency interaction was significant for color type, $F(1, 46) = 12.17$, $p = .001$; but this interaction was not significant for word type, $F < 1.0$.

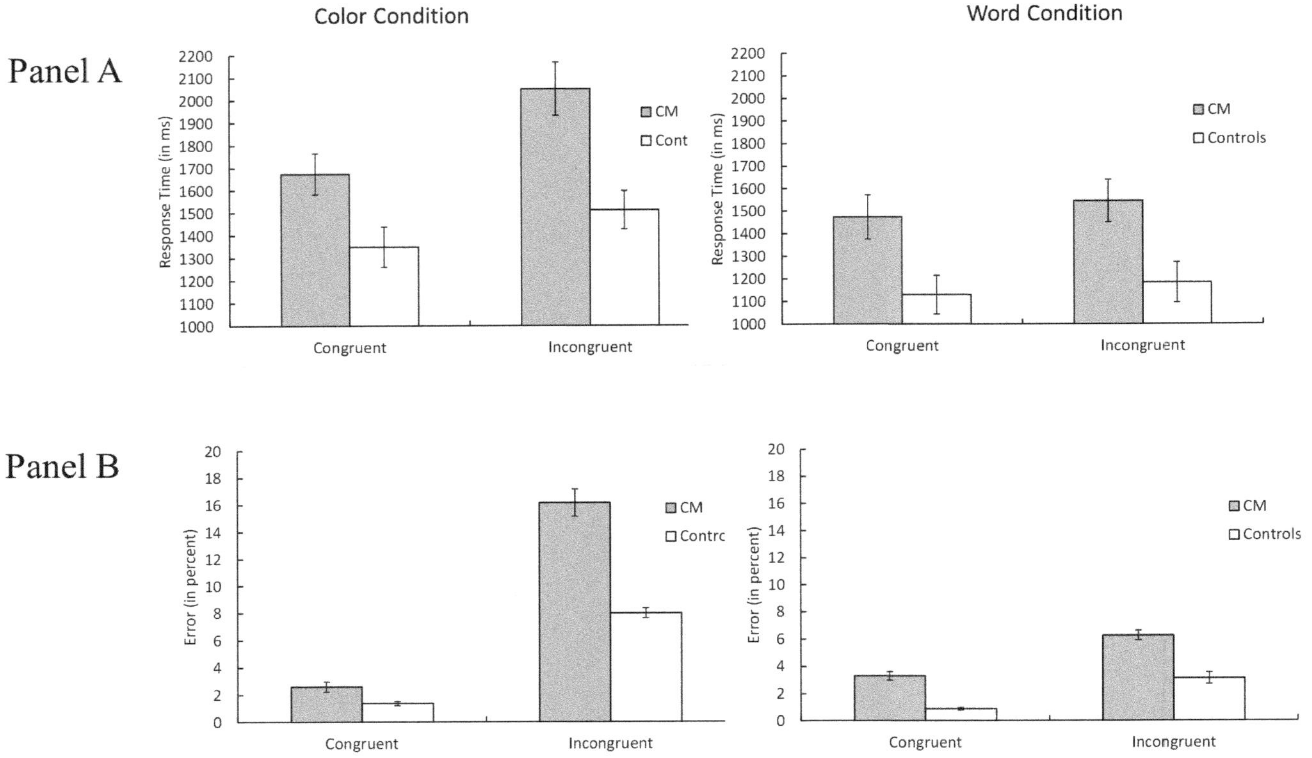

Figure 5. The mean response time (Panel A) and percent error (Panel B) in Stroop task (Color vs. Word) as a function of congruency between color and word (congruent vs. incongruent) for the Chiari Patients (CM) and Controls. Error bars represent the standard errors of the means.

No effects in the accuracy analysis for the Stroop data reached significance (all p's>.05).

Generalized Slowing Analyses for the Stroop Task

The observed slower responses for the CM group compared to the control group could be due to generalized slowing, such as psychomotor speed, rather than to task-specific slowing [34]. Madden, Pierce and Allen (1992) [35] reported a method that can be used to examine this possibility. First, one needs to find the best-fitting linear equation for $RT_{CM} = mRT_{controls} + b$ (reaction time, or RT, for CM patients should be a linear combination of controls' RT). Because we collected RT data from three different tasks (Stroop, Ospan, and Digit Symbol), in order to consider true general slowing rather than task-specific slowing, we needed to compute the linear slowing function for all three tasks. For the present tasks, this best fitting linear slowing function was $RT_{CM} = (1.16)RT_{controls} + 120$ ms, $R^2 = .76$. The next step was to transform the controls' RT data from the Stroop task using this linear function. This procedure will eliminate the main effect for group [35], and if task-related slowing is generalized, then the Group x Color Type x Task Type interaction for the Stroop task will also be eliminated [35]. However, if the task-specific slowing for the Stroop task goes beyond that predicted by general slowing, then this three-way interaction should remain statistically significant even after the controls' data are transformed into "generalized" replicas of CM patients' data [35]. When we transformed the controls' RT data for the Stroop task using the aforementioned generalized slowing equation and then added the non-transformed CM patients' data, the main effect for group was no longer significant, $F(1, 46) = .28$. $p = .60$. However, the Group x Color Type x Task Type interaction remained statistically significant, $F(1, 46) = 4.31$, $p = .0435$. Using the same logic as Madden et al. [35], we can conclude that the present Stroop response inhibition results for Chiari patients relative to controls cannot be accounted for by generalized slowing. Instead, it appears that these results are primarily due to task-specific slowing.

Depression, Anxiety, and Pain Analyses

Chiari patients, even after decompression surgery, still frequently experience severe headaches. To assess neck pain disability (including headache), we tested just the CM group on the Neck Pain Disability Index Questionnaire [26] (because individuals in the control group would typically score zero). Using the scoring criteria proposed by Fairbanks et al. [26], the present Chiari sample had a percent disability score of 47% (substantial disability due to neck and head pain). Next, we correlated the CM group's pain score with the DASS21 [25] scores (see Table 1 for correlation matrix). Pain and depression ($r = .51$, $p = .01$, $r^2 = .26$), as well as pain and anxiety ($r = .56$, $p = .006$, $r^2 = .31$) were significantly correlated, but pain and stress were not ($r = .32$, $p = .12$, $r^2 = .10$). This indicates that pain, depression, and anxiety (but not stress) scores were significantly related in CM patients.

The next step was to correlate depression, anxiety, and pain scores for CM patients with immediate recall, digit symbol RT (DSRT), Ospan computation RT, and Stroop congruency effects for the color condition (i.e., the four cognitive variables that showed statistically significant group differences). The correlation matrix for these analyses is presented in Table 1. Depression, anxiety, and pain all showed significant correlations with DSRT and Ospan computational RT, but not with Stroop congruency

Table 1. Correlation Matrix (Pearson's r) for Just Chiari Malformation Patients (N = 24) for Depression, Anxiety, Stress, Pain, Digit Symbol RT, Ospan RT, the Stroop Congruity Effect for Color, and Immediate Recall.

	Depression	Anxiety	Stress	Pain	DSRT	OspanRT	StroopRT
Depression							
Anxiety	.67*						
Stress	.52*	.49*					
Pain	.51*	.56*	.32				
DSRT	.66*	.52*	.04	.56*			
OspanRT	.46*	.48*	.08	.46*	.66*		
StroopRT	.10	.11	.08	.34	.58*	.55*	
Immediate Recall	−.09	−.01	−.17	−.37	.006	.201	.04

* $p<.05$

effects for the color condition or immediate recall. These results suggest that pain scores, depression, and anxiety in the CM group were significantly related to DSRT and working memory computational RT performance, but not with response inhibition (Stroop) or immediate recall performance.

We also compared depression, anxiety, and stress levels across groups (i.e., all 48 participants—not just the 24 CM patients' data) using the DASS21 scale data. The CM group showed significantly higher scores in depression (CM group = 6.5, controls = 2.6), $F(1, 46) = 8.48$, $p<01$, $\eta_P^2 = .16$, anxiety (CM group = 8.6, controls = 1.8), $F(1, 46) = 31.79$, $p<.0001$, $\eta_P^2 = .41$, and stress (CM group = 9.2, controls = 5.3), $F(1, 46) = 8.35$, $p<.01$, $\eta_P^2 = .15$. The present results showing that CM patients show symptoms of depression and anxiety are consistent with the findings of Mueller and Oro [36] who screened a much larger sample of CM patients for symptoms and observed that CM patients showed increases in depression and anxiety.

Because neck and head pain were correlated with cognitive performance in CM patients, and with depression ($r = .51$) and anxiety ($r = .56$), we conducted an analysis of covariance (ANCOVA) on the four measures showing significant effects for groups (or interactions with group) in the earlier ANOVAs (see Table 2). For the digit symbol substitution task, $F(1, 44) = .086$, $p = .77$, $\eta_P^2 = .002$, the Ospan RT task, $F(1, 44) = 2.46$, $p = .12$, $\eta_P^2 = .05$, and the immediate recall task, $F(1, 44) = 1.83$, $p = .18$, $\eta_P^2 = .087$, the main effects of group were no longer significant when depression and anxiety were entered as covariates. However, the Group x Task Type x Congruency interaction for the Stroop analysis remained significant, $F(1, 44) = 6.69$, $p<.02$, $\eta_P^2 = 13$, even after depression and anxiety were entered as covariates. These results suggest that variables correlated with chronic pain (i.e., anxiety and depression) accounted for all cognitive deficits in CM except for response inhibition (Stroop) effects.

Multivariate Analyses

Because we have reported results from four different tasks (Stroop, Ospan, Digit Symbol, and episodic memory: immediate and delayed recall), an important issue to consider is whether Chiari patients showed an "overall" cognitive deficit relative to age- and education-matched controls. One way to test for this possibility is to use latency scores from the Stroop, Ospan (math computational speed), and Digit Symbol tasks, and recall data from the memory tasks as dependent variables, and to use group as the independent variable and conduct a multivariate analysis of variance, or MANOVA. When we conducted this MANOVA, the multivariate effect of group was significant, Wilks' Lambda = .58, $p = .004$. In the univariate "step-down" analyses, all of the dependent variables were statistically significant except for delayed recall. These results indicate that the composite cognitive dependent variable in the present study varied across group. That is, Chiari patients performed significantly more poorly than controls did on global cognitive function. However, in the present study, we also need to consider the effects of anxiety and depression. In particular, was there a multivariate effect of group even after the effects of anxiety and depression are covaried out? The answer to this question is "yes." Namely, the multivariate analysis of covariance, or MANCOVA showed a statistically significant multivariate effect of group even when anxiety and depression were entered as covariates, Wilks' Lambda = .654, $p = .031$.

Table 2. Correlation Matrix (Pearson's r) for Chiari Malformation Patients and Controls (N = 48) for Depression, Anxiety, Stress, Digit Symbol RT, Ospan RT, the Stroop Congruity Effect for Color, and Immediate Recall.

	Depression	Anxiety	Stress	Processing Speed	Working Memory	Inhibitory Control
Depression						
Anxiety	.73*					
Stress	.62*	.57*				
Processing Speed	.56*	.49*	.23			
Working Memory	.39*	.50*	.17	.56*		
Stroop RT	.21	.34*	.17	.43*	.47*	
Immediate Recall	−.17	−.22	−.03	−.08	−.24	−.02

*$p<.05$.

Discussion

We assessed cognitive performance in CM patients with a firm diagnosis of CM who had undergone decompression surgery (minimum six months prior to testing in the present study). Little is known about the cognitive consequences of CM except for one study by Kumar et al. [3]. In an attempt to gain a more thorough understanding of the cognitive consequences of CM, we measured group differences between CM patients and age- and education-matched controls in response inhibition (Stroop), working memory (Ospan computational speed), processing speed (Digit/Symbol task), and episodic memory performance (modified RAVLT). The present results provide evidence that CM patients showed deficits in response inhibition, working memory speed, and processing speed relative to age- and education-matched controls. Also, CM patients showed deficits in episodic recall that approached statistical significance.

Cognitive Deficits in CM

With regard to working memory, CM patients did show significantly slower computational responses (Ospan RT) than controls, but group differences for this variable were eliminated when we statistically controlled for depression and anxiety scores as covariates—suggesting that group differences in working memory speed may be accounted for by chronic pain. Processing speed showed similar results—CM patients showed significantly slower digit symbol RT (DSRT) than did controls, but, again, group differences in processing speed were eliminated when we statistically controlled for anxiety and depression effects. On the other hand, response inhibition deficits (as measured by Stroop interference effects) in the CM group persisted even after statistical control of anxiety and depression effects. Furthermore, this color congruency effect was not significantly correlated with pain, depression, or anxiety in the CM group (see Table 1). This appears to be a response inhibition deficit [31].

Response inhibition, a type of attentional guidance [37], is related to selective attention. Human observers focus on information relevant to a task (in the Stroop task, "which response do I select?"), but must filter out (inhibit) non-relevant response information. Thus, a strong emphasis is placed on inhibitory control so that individuals can operate efficiently within this limited-capacity attentional system. Inhibitory control processing is typically associated with the dorsolateral prefrontal cortex and the anterior cingulate cortex [23] as well as areas of the parietal cortex—the frontoparietal attentional pathway [38]. However, it is known that CM is most commonly associated with damage to the cerebellum and brainstem [5], so it seems to suggest that performance deficits associated with the prefrontal cortex would be present. Could it be, then, that the response inhibition component of the Stroop task [31] is actually related to the cerebellar and/or brainstem damage in CM? We cannot conclusively answer this question in the present study because it did not include neuroimaging analyses (e.g., DTI-based tractography or fMRI-based functional connectivity) that would allow an examination of the integrity of fiber tracts connecting the cerebellum and/or brainstem to the front-parietal attentional pathway. However, Hesselmann, Flandin, and Dehaene (2011) [38] did report an fMRI/Event-Related Potential (ERP) study on a task known to have a response selection locus—the psychological refractory period (or PRP) paradigm. When they subtracted single-task from dual-task performance, they found significant activation for just the dual-task (PRP) component in the left middle and superior frontal gyrus areas—essentially Brodmann's area 46—part of the dorsolateral prefrontal cortex. Furthermore, when the fMRI subtracted data (i.e., the task component known to be related to response selection—of which a critical component is response inhibition) were synchronized with the ERP (P3) data, Broadmann's area 46 and areas in the parietal cortex were activated. These results showing that a task known to have a response selection/inhibition locus (the PRP effect) activated the fronto-parietal (or dorsal) attentional pathway suggest that response inhibition shares the same attentional pathway known to affect stimulus selection. This provides inductive evidence that the present response inhibition (Stroop) deficit observed in individuals diagnosed with CM might be associated with a prefrontal cortex deficit, although additional neuroimaging support for this CM assertion is needed to confirm the present hypothesis because there is evidence that the relationship between individual neuropsychological test data and specific brain regions is not necessarily specific [39].

What is not clear from the present study, though, is why CM patients showed specific deficits in response inhibition (Stroop interference), even when the effects of anxiety and depression were statistically controlled for, but not in working memory or processing speed—two other measures of executive function. Perhaps the most parsimonious interpretation is that response inhibition is more closely related to motoric processing known to be associated with cerebellar function (although response inhibition is an attentional process rather than a motoric process, per se) or reflexive processing known to be associated with medullary function. On the other hand, working memory and processing speed do not appear to be as closely associated with cerebellar and/or brainstem function as is response inhibition [8]. A more direct test of this issue would be to assess CM patients on both response inhibition and distractor interference tasks (e.g., an Eriksen flanker task) [31]. If CM patients showed performance decrements on both tasks, then this would provide evidence of a more general executive function deficit. On the other hand, if CM patients showed a deficit on the response inhibition task, but not on the distractor interference task, then this would provide evidence of a more specific deficit perhaps more localized at the cerebellar and/or brainstem level. Thus, while there is good reason to believe that response selection/inhibition, at least as measured by the psychological refractory period effect, shows a clear prefrontal attentional effect [38], it could be that response inhibition is also closely linked to cerebellar and/or medullary processing.

Another issue germane to the seemingly larger Stroop effects for CM patients than for controls is whether this effect was the result of generalized slowing in CM patients. To test for this possibility, we transformed the controls' data using the slowing function taken from the CM patients' data [34], which were then analyzed with the untransformed data from the CM patients. In this analysis, we still observed the Groups x Color Type x Task Type interaction. According to Madden et al. [35], these results suggest that the group-related differences are specific to a given task—not the result of generalized slowing across all tasks (in this case, Stroop, Ospan working memory, and automated digit/symbol). Thus, the presently observed larger response inhibition effects for CM patients relative to controls are the result of task-specific effects.

Episodic Memory Effects in CM?

Episodic memory is defined as contextual memory (events associated with time-, space-, or emotion-based contexts [27,40]. We observed marginally poorer episodic recall in individuals diagnosed with CM than in controls in a modified version of the RAVLT [28]. However, the group effect for recall was eliminated after statistical control for anxiety and depression effects. This suggests that the marginally significant group effects in recall were associated with a variable related to anxiety and depression—likely chronic pain.

Multivariate Effects

Given that all of the cognitive deficits other than the Stroop (response inhibition) effect were eliminated, an important issue to address is whether there was an "overall" cognitive deficit—especially after the effects of anxiety and depression (thought to index chronic pain effects in CM) were controlled. We addressed this issue using MANOVA and MANCOVA analyses. When all of the reaction time and memory recall data were included as dependent variables, and group (CM vs. controls) was included as an independent variable, the resulting MANOVA showed that the main effect of group was significant. However, this multivariate effect for group (i.e., that CM patients showed an overall cognitive performance deficit relative to age- and education-matched controls) could have been the result of anxiety and depression effects. To test for this possibility, we also conducted a multivariate analysis on group while including anxiety and depression as covariates. The resulting MANCOVA showed that the main effect of group remained statistically significant even after we controlled for anxiety and depression. Consequently, an overall cognitive deficit in CM patients was observed that cannot be explained by increased anxiety and depression levels in CM patients.

Locus of the Cognitive Effects

As illustrated in Figure 6, there are several possible causes of the presently observed cognitive dysfunction in the CM group relative to the controls. The two broad categories are: compression injury (e.g., chronic compression from CM or acute decompression from surgery-based injury) and non-specific (e.g., chronic pain). Also, the cognitive deficits observed for the CM group in the present study may have been the result of cerebellar tonsillar injury. However, most of the observable cerebellar damage in CM is done to the floculonodular lobe of the cerebellum (i.e., the caudal portion), and altered CSF pressure (cardiac-induced and/or through coughing or Valsalva maneuvers) may also damage other portions of the cerebellum that have known connections with the prefrontal cortex [7–12], however this is speculative. Another likely possibility of fiber-tract damage affecting prefrontal cortex (the area associated with executive function) is the medulla. As illustrated in Figure 1 (in the CM MRI), the cerebellum descends and impacts the brainstem (i.e., the medulla is compressed) in CM. Thus, it could be that brainstem damage rather than cerebellar damage is the culprit of potential fiber tract damage to other portions of the brain—such as the prefrontal cortex—resulting in executive dysfunction, or more diffuse cognitive deficits that indirectly affect executive function. There is evidence of fiber-tract connections between the brainstem and prefrontal cortex [13]. Also, it is known that there are medullary projections to the reticular activating system, the limbic system, and ultimately to the prefrontal cortex [41]. Thus, whether it is based on a cerebellar or a brainstem origin (or both), there are known fiber-tract pathways that link these areas to the prefrontal cortex (associated with executive function).

Limitations

We choose to test decompressed CM patients knowing that this might result in an underestimate of cognitive deficits due to recovery. Alternatively, there may also be a small chance of surgically induced trauma to the already Chiari-compressed area. As a result, some of the deficits seen may have occurred from surgical cerebellar injury rather than CM-based cerebellar compression (see Figure 6). In this event, it remains true that injury to the Chiari cerebellum would be responsible for the higher-level cognitive effects. In addition, a decompressed sample of CM patients was used to lessen pre-operative anxiety effects and to better insure a conclusive CM diagnosis. Previous studies [42] have demonstrated intraoperative sensorimotor (auditory evoked potentials) improvement within CM patients. This observation supports the idea that the use of post-decompression CM patients is a reasonable strategy because improved, rather than poorer information processing resulted from the decompression procedure.

This study employed statistical control to partial out the effects of anxiety and depression rather than using experimental control. While experimental control is always preferred, it is impractical if not impossible for this patient population. In addition, adult-diagnosed CM patients are largely female, but our CM patient group may have a relatively greater number of female participants than male (22 vs. 2) than is typical of adult CM (probably at least 70% female). We did have more males in the control group (9) than in in the CM group (2), but this was because we used a "yoked" control group when possible. That is, we used spouses or other relatives when possible as controls.

Conclusion

We provided evidence in this study that CM patients showed poorer cognitive performance on reaction time tasks (working memory, inhibitory control, and processing speed) compared to age- and education-matched controls, but that there were no group differences observed in episodic memory. These results are

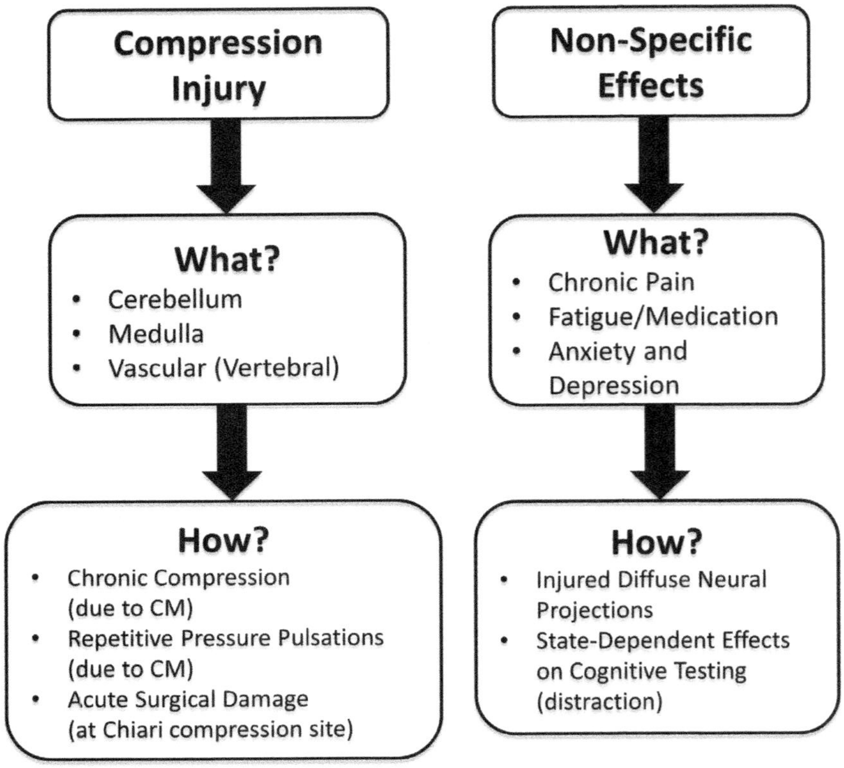

Figure 6. A flow diagram of Chiari I Malformation compression injury and non-specific effects is presented. Under "What," the anatomical areas or types of non-specific effects are presented. Under "How," the type of injury or state-dependent effect is presented.

consistent with both a general cognitive deficit and a specific deficit associated with response (Stroop) inhibition in CM. The locus of the observed response inhibition effect has frequently been associated with prefrontal, executive function [29,30]. However, the present finding that this response inhibition effect remained statistically significant even after statistical control of anxiety and depression effects, as well as general slowing, whereas other known executive function tasks such as working memory and processing speed were not, provides another potential explanation. For example, it suggests that the observed response inhibition deficit may be more influenced by known areas of damage in CM—namely the brainstem and cerebellum. It is important to note, though, that brain-imaging evidence for localized brain damage in CM for areas other than the cerebellum or brainstem (e.g., the prefrontal cortex) is needed to confirm this speculation. So far, Kumar et al. [3] have provided the only evidence of white-matter integrity losses (based on DTI data) in CM with a relatively small sample size, so more evidence is needed to confirm this possibility.

Finally, while there were task-specific group differences observed for response inhibition, we also observed a multivariate effect of group for all the reaction time tasks and the two episodic memory tasks, and this effect remained significant after statistical control of anxiety and depression. These MANOVA and MANCOVA results suggest that there is also a "global" cognitive deficit in CM.

Acknowledgments

We gratefully acknowledge support from the Conquer Chiari Foundation for recruitment of CM patients.

Author Contributions

Conceived and designed the experiments: PAA BAM FL JM MGL JRH JWP. Performed the experiments: JRH JWP CB XL AKH PAA. Analyzed the data: PAA BAM FL JRH. Contributed reagents/materials/analysis tools: PAA ML JM. Wrote the paper: PAA BAM FL MGL JM ML JRH CB JWP. XL AKH.

References

1. Anderson DW, Ellenberg JH, Leventhal CM, Rheingold SC, Rodriguez M, et al. (1992) Revised estimate of the prevalence of multiple sclerosis in The United States. Ann Neurol: 31, 333–336.
2. Speer MC, Enterline DS, Mehltretter L, Hammock P, Joseph J, et al. (2003) Chiari Type I Malformation with or without syringomyelia: Prevealence and genetics. J Gen Counsel: 12, 297–311.
3. Kumar M, Rathore RKS, Srivastava A, Yadav SK, Behari S, et al. (2011) Correlation of diffusion tensor imaging metrics with neurocognitive function in Chiari I malformation. World Neurosurg: 76, 189–194.
4. Shaffer N, Martin B, Loth F (2011) "Cerebrospinal fluid hydrodynamics in type I Chiari malformation." Neurol Res: 33(3), 247–260.
5. Milhorat TH, Chou MW, Trinidad EM, Kula RW, Mandell M, et al. (1999) Chiari I malformation redefined: clinical and radiographic findings for 364 symptomatic patients. Neurosurg: 44(5), 1005–1017.
6. Yessari R, Frim D (2004) Evaluation and management of the Chiari malformation type 1 for the primary care physician. Pediatr Clin N Am: 51, 477–490.
7. Schmahmann JD, Sherman JC (1998) The cerebellar cognitive affective syndrome. *Brain*, 121: 561–579.
8. O'Halloran CJ, Kinsella GJ, Storey E (2012) The cerebellum and neuropsychological functioning: A critical review. J Clin Exp Neuropsyc: 34, 35–56.

9. Riva D, Usilla A, Saletti V, Esposito S, Bulgheroni S (2011) Can Chiari malformation negatively affect higher mental functioning in developmental age? Neurol Sci: 32, S307–S309.
10. Riva D, Giorgi C (2000) The cerebellum contributes to higher functions during development. Brain: 123, 1051–1061.
11. Wakana S, Jlang H, Nagae-Poetscher LM, van Zijl PCM, Mori S (2004) Fiber tract-based atlas of human white matter anatomy, Radiology: 78, 77–87.
12. Krienen FM, Buckner RL (2009) Segregated fronto-cerebellar circuits revealed by intrinsic functional connectivity. Cereb Cortex: 19, 2485–2497.
13. Selemon LD, Goldman-Rakic PS (1988) Common Cortical and Subcortical Targets of the Dorsolateral Prefrontal and Posterior Parietal Cortices in the Rhesus Monkey: Evidence for a Distributed Neural Network Subserving Spatially Guided Behavior. J Neurosci: 8, 4049–4068.
14. Moriarty O, McGuire BE, Finn DP (2003) The effect of pain on cognitive function: A review of clinical and preclinical research. *Prog Neurobiol*, 93: 385–404.
15. Karp JF, Reynolds CF, Butters MA, Dew MA, Mazumdar S, et al. (2006) The relationship between pain and mental flexibility in older adult pain clinic patients. *Pain Med*, 7: 444–452.
16. Bosma FK, Kessels RP (2002) Cognitive impairments, psychological dysfunction, and coping styles in patients with chronic whiplash syndrome. *Neuropsychiatry: Neuropsychol. Behav. Neurol.* 15: 56–65.
17. Apkarian AV, Sosa Y, Sonty S, Levy RM, Harden RN, et al. (2004) Chronic back pain is associated with decreased prefrontal and thalamic gray matter density. J Neurosci: 24, 10410–10415.
18. Linton SJ, Bergbom S (2011) Understanding the link between depression and pain. Scand J Pain: 2, 47–54.
19. Chung S-D, Lin H-C (2013) Association between chronic prostatitis/chronic pelvic pain syndrome and anxiety disorder: A population-based study. PLoS ONE: 8, e64630.
20. Rogers TD, Dickson PE, Heck DH, Goldowitz D, Mittleman G, et al. (2011) Connecting the Dots of the Cerebro-Cerebellar Role in Cognitive Function: Neuronal Pathways for cerebellar Modulation of Dopamine Release in the Prefrontal Cortex, Synapse: 65, 1204–1212.
21. Luciano M (2011) Chiari malformation: Are children little adults? Neurol Res: 33, 272–277.
22. Salthouse TA (1996) A processing-speed theory of adult age differences in cognition. Psychol Rev: 103, 403–428.
23. Baena E, Allen PA, Kaut KP, Hall RJ (2010) On age differences in prefrontal function: The importance of emotional/cognitive integration. Neuropsychologia: 48, 319–333.
24. Unsworth N, Heitz RP, Schrock JC, Engle RW (2005). An automated version of the operation span task. Behav Res Methods: 37, 498–505.
25. Henry JD, Crawford JR (2005) The short-form version of the Depression Anxiety Stress Scales (DASS21): Construct validity and normative data in a large non-clinical sample. Brit J Clin Psychol: 44, 227–239.
26. Fairbanks CT, Couper C, Davies JB, O'Brien JP (1980) The Oswestry low back-pain disability questionannaire, Physiol Ther: 66, 271–273.
27. Allen PA, Kaut KP, Baena E, Lien M-C, Ruthruff E (2011) Individual differences in positive affect moderate age-related declines in episodic long-term memory. J of Cognitive Psychol: 23, 768–779.
28. Schmidt M (1996) *Rey auditory and verbal learning test: A handbook.* Los Angeles, CA: Western Psychological Services.
29. Schroeter ML, Zysset S, Wahl M, von Cramon DY (2004) Prefrontal activation due to Stroop interference increases during development—An event-related fNIRS study. NeuroImage: 23, 1317–1325.
30. Lezak M D, Howieson DB, Loring DW (2004) *Neuropsychological assessment* (4th ed.). New York, NY: Oxford University Press.
31. Friedman NP, Miyake A (2004) The relations among inhibition and interference control functions: A latent-variable analysis. J Exp Psychol Gen: 133, 101–135.
32. Stroop JR (1935) Studies of interference in serial verbal reactions. J Exper Psychol: 18, 643–662.
33. Rypma B, D'Esposito M (1999) The roles of the prefrontal brain regions in the components of working memory: Effects of memory load and individual differences. P Natl Acad Sci USA: 96, 6558–6563.
34. Cerella J (1991) Age effects may be global, not local: Comment of Fisk and Rogers (1991). J Exp Psychol Gen: 120, 215–223.
35. Madden DJ, Pierce TW, Allen PA (1992) Adult age differences in attentional allocation during memory search. Psychol Aging: ,7 594–601.
36. Mueller ND, Oro JJ (2004) Prospective analysis of presenting symptoms among 265 patients with radiographic evidence of Chiari Malformation Type I with or without Syringomyelia. J Am Acad Nurse Prac: 16, 134–138.
37. Madden DJ (2007) Aging and visual attention. Cur Dir Psychol Sci: 16, 70–74.
38. Hesselmann G, Flandin G, Dehaene S (2011) Probing the cortical network underlying the psychological refractory period: A combined EEG-fMRI study. NeuroImage: 56, 1608–1621.
39. Salthouse TA, Fristoe N, Rhee SH (1996) How localized are age-related effects on neuropsychological measures? Neuropsychology: 10, 272–285.
40. Allen PA, Kaut KP, Lord RG, Hall RJ, Bowie T, et al. (2005) An emotional mediation theory of differential age effects in episodic and semantic memory. Exp Aging Res: 31, 355–391.
41. Grafman J (2002) The structured event complex and the human prefrontal cortex. In D. T. Stuss, & R. T. Knight (Eds.), *Frontal lobe function* (pp. 292–310). New York: Oxford.
42. Chen JA, Coutin-Churchman CE, Nuwer MR, Lazareff JA (2012) Suboccipital craniotomy for Chiari I results in evoked potential conduction changes. Surg Neurol Int: 3, 165. doi: 10.4103/2152-7806.105277.

16

Time and Frequency-Dependent Modulation of Local Field Potential Synchronization by Deep Brain Stimulation

Clinton B. McCracken, Zelma H. T. Kiss*

Department of Clinical Neurosciences and Hotchkiss Brain Institute, University of Calgary, Calgary, Alberta, Canada

Abstract

High-frequency electrical stimulation of specific brain structures, known as deep brain stimulation (DBS), is an effective treatment for movement disorders, but mechanisms of action remain unclear. We examined the time-dependent effects of DBS applied to the entopeduncular nucleus (EP), the rat homolog of the internal globus pallidus, a target used for treatment of both dystonia and Parkinson's disease (PD). We performed simultaneous multi-site local field potential (LFP) recordings in urethane-anesthetized rats to assess the effects of high-frequency (HF, 130 Hz; clinically effective), low-frequency (LF, 15 Hz; ineffective) and sham DBS delivered to EP. LFP activity was recorded from dorsal striatum (STR), ventroanterior thalamus (VA), primary motor cortex (M1), and the stimulation site in EP. Spontaneous and acute stimulation-induced LFP oscillation power and functional connectivity were assessed at baseline, and after 30, 60, and 90 minutes of stimulation. HF EP DBS produced widespread alterations in spontaneous and stimulus-induced LFP oscillations, with some effects similar across regions and others occurring in a region- and frequency band-specific manner. Many of these changes evolved over time. HF EP DBS produced an initial transient reduction in power in the low beta band in M1 and STR; however, phase synchronization between these regions in the low beta band was markedly suppressed at all time points. DBS also enhanced low gamma synchronization throughout the circuit. With sustained stimulation, there were significant reductions in low beta synchronization between M1-VA and STR-VA, and increases in power within regions in the faster frequency bands. HF DBS also suppressed the ability of acute EP stimulation to induce beta oscillations in all regions along the circuit. This dynamic pattern of synchronizing and desynchronizing effects of EP DBS suggests a complex modulation of activity along cortico-BG-thalamic circuits underlying the therapeutic effects of GPi DBS for conditions such as PD and dystonia.

Editor: Adriano B. L. Tort, Federal University of Rio Grande do Norte, Brazil

Funding: This work was supported by a grant from the Canadian Institutes of Health Research. Dr. Kiss is a Clinical Scholar of the Alberta Heritage Foundation for Medical Research. Dr. McCracken received fellowship support from Parkinson Society Canada and Hotchkiss Brain Institute. The funders had no role in study design, data collection and analysis, decision to publish, or preparation of the manuscript.

Competing Interests: The authors have declared that no competing interests exist.

* Email: zkiss@ucalgary.ca

Introduction

High-frequency electrical stimulation of specific brain regions, known as deep brain stimulation (DBS), is an effective treatment strategy for a number of refractory neurological conditions. DBS of the globus pallidus internus (GPi) provides significant symptom relief for both Parkinson's disease (PD) and dystonia [1,2], however, despite widespread clinical use, consensus regarding the therapeutic mechanisms of action is lacking.

Initial clinical reports that the effects of DBS appeared to be qualitatively similar to those produced by a lesion of the same region [3,4] led to the idea that DBS exerted its effects by creating a reversible "functional lesion" of the stimulated nucleus. A variety of animal studies demonstrated that DBS inhibited activity in the stimulated region, through either depolarization blockade, neurotransmitter depletion, or enhanced local GABAergic transmission [5–9]. However, recent evidence suggests that other mechanisms may also be important. Electrical brain stimulation at clinically effective intensities preferentially excites axons as opposed to cell bodies [10], such that activation of afferent and efferent axons can modulate neuronal activity in sites distal to the stimulated nucleus [11–15]. Thus, GPi DBS can both inhibit local firing [5,16,17] as well as activate efferent GPi axons projecting to thalamus [18–20].

Both dystonia and PD show evidence of pathological hypersynchrony in local field potential (LFP) oscillations in the basal ganglia (BG) and cortex (Brown et al. 2001; Chen et al. 2006b; Weinberger et al. 2012), and reduction of these oscillations has been suggested as a potential mechanism of DBS [21]. How DBS affects LFP oscillations in intact animals with no obvious pathology is not known, and assessing the effects of DBS in normal animals is critical for informing the interpretation of the effects produced in disease states (Chiken and Nambu, 2003). This is particularly true when considering that PD and dystonia, both effectively treated by GPi DBS, are hypo- and hyper-kinetic movement disorders, respectively, with different pathophysiologic features [22,23]. Mechanistic studies have typically examined the effects of GPi DBS acutely over seconds [9,24–26]; however, how the immediate effects of stimulation relate to clinical improvement is not clear. Although the therapeutic effects of GPi DBS on PD symptoms occur very rapidly [27], maximum clinical benefit for dystonia can take much longer, i.e., weeks to years [28–32]. Accordingly, clarifying how the effects of DBS evolve over time is a high priority. Furthermore, many studies have not controlled for non-specific effects of stimulation by comparing the effects of low-frequency (LF) to therapeutic, high frequency (HF) stimulation. LF DBS generally does not produce beneficial effects and in some cases may be deleterious [33–38]; it is therefore important to identify changes in neural activity that are specific to high-frequency (i.e., therapeutic) stimulation.

Given the evidence for circuit-wide effects of DBS, we examined how DBS delivered to the entopeduncular nucleus (EP; the rat homolog of the primate GPi) affected spontaneous and evoked synchronous LFP activity both within and between a number of regions comprising the primary motor circuit. We recorded LFP activity simultaneously from the dorsal striatum (STR), primary motor cortex, (M1), and ventroanterior thalamus (VA), while DBS was applied to EP for 90 minutes, with short breaks after 30 and 60 minutes to assess activity induced by acute EP stimulation. Given the hypersynchrony associated with PD and dystonia, and the beneficial effects produced by GPi DBS, our working hypothesis was that the EP DBS would be globally desynchronizing. Although we saw widespread reduction in low beta synchronization both within and between regions, we identified more complex and time-dependent changes in both power within and functional connectivity between regions.

Methods

All procedures were performed in accordance with Canadian Council for Animal Care guidelines, and were approved by the Institutional Animal Care and Use Committee of the University of Calgary.

Animals and surgery

Male Sprague-Dawley rats (275–400 g) were anesthetized with urethane (1.5 g/kg, i.p.) and placed in a stereotaxic frame. Body temperature was maintained at 37°C with a temperature-controlled heating pad. In all surgical preparations the scalp was exposed and burr holes were drilled in the skull overlying M1, dorsocentral striatum, VA, and over the contralateral cerebellum to allow for insertion of the stimulating electrode into EP at a 30 degree angle to avoid potential damage to EP-VA connections. A concentric bipolar stimulating electrodes (SNEX-100; Kopf, Tujunga, CA) was placed in EP - anteroposterior (AP) −3.0 mm (from bregma), mediolateral (ML) +2.6 mm, dorsoventral (DV) −8.0 mm (vertical from skull); epoxy-insulated tungsten recording electrodes (0.125 mm shank diameter, 0.8–2 MΩ impedance at 1000 Hz, FHC, Bowdoin, ME) were slowly lowered into M1 (AP: +2.2 mm, ML: +2.8 mm, DV: −2.2 mm), striatum (AP: +1.2 mm, ML: +2.8 mm, DV: −5.0 mm) and VA (AP: −1.8 mm, ML: +1.8 mm, DV: −6.0 mm). Following implantation, electrodes were allowed to settle for at least 20 minutes before recording commenced.

Recording

LFP signals from the recording electrodes were amplified (gain: 1000), analog filtered (0.1–1000 Hz) by a multichannel amplifier (A-M Systems) and displayed on an oscilloscope (Tektronics, Wilsonville, OR). The data were digitized at 10 kHz using an Axon Digidata 1440 (Molecular Devices, Sunnyvale, CA), acquired using Clampex 10.2 (Molecular Devices), and stored for off-line analysis. LFP signals were referenced to a skull screw over the contralateral cerebellum. DBS was applied to separate groups of rats at 130 Hz (HF) or 15 Hz (LF) using parameters (80 µA, 0.2 ms pulse duration) that preliminary experiments indicated was below the threshold for evoking a motor response. Given the electrode surface area, the selected current intensity generates a charge density (20 $\mu C/cm^2$/phase) that approximates that which is clinically effective in humans [39], and shows effects in various rat behavioral studies [40,41] while remaining below the recommended clinical safety limit of 30 $\mu C/cm^2$/phase [42]. To control for the effects of electrode implantation and surgery, another group had the DBS implanted but did not receive stimulation (SHAM). DBS was applied for three 30 minute sessions for a total of 90 minutes; sessions were separated by 6 minute intervals where spontaneous and evoked LFP data were sampled with DBS off. Figure 1 shows electrode placements, and a schematic of the recording procedure.

We analyzed both spontaneous LFP oscillations and those induced by single-pulse stimulation of EP to address separate dimensions of neural activity. Spontaneous recordings assess the state of the system at rest, whereas evoked/induced activity provides an index of how the system responds to activation (analogous to an organism reacting to a stimulus). For spontaneous recordings, LFPs were recorded for 3 minutes at a number of different time points with DBS on or off (Fig. 1). We recorded baseline (BL) LFPs, LFPs with DBS ON during the first 5 and 25 minutes of DBS (referred to as On5 and On25), and then with stimulation OFF after 30 minutes of DBS had been applied (Off30). This protocol was repeated twice to examine changes over longer time periods, giving the additional time points of On35, On55, Off60, On85 and Off90. During OFF periods, spontaneous LFP data were recorded, followed immediately by evoked data, after which DBS was turned ON again. For induced LFP responses, EP stimulation was delivered at 0.4 Hz (600 µA, 0.2 ms pulse duration, 20 stimulation sweeps). This stimulus intensity was chosen based on preliminary experiments, with this intensity being the lowest that consistently resulted in an oscillatory response. LFP data were recorded for 1 s pre- and post-stimulus. Induced activity was reassessed following 30, 60 and 90 minutes of DBS.

Histology

At the end of each experiment, small lesions were made at the tip of the electrodes (250 µA, 10 sec current pulse) and visualized by adding potassium ferrocyanide during post-fixation. Animals were euthanized with an overdose of urethane and decapitated. The brain was removed and fixed for at least 48 h in 8% w/v paraformaldehyde (in PBS) and cryoprotected in 25% w/v sucrose (in PBS). Brains were then sectioned (50 µm coronal sections), placed on gelatin-chromalum-coated slides, and stained with cresyl violet for histochemical verification of the recording/stimulation electrode placements (Fig. 1C). Only animals with the cathode located in EP were included for analysis. This pole was also used to record LFP activity from EP when DBS was off.

Analysis

The spectral power of LFP oscillations in each region was analyzed using routines from the Chronux software package (www.chronux.org) for Matlab (MathWorks, Natick, MA) as previously described [43]. As certain measures of functional connectivity (e.g., coherence) are impacted by volume conduction, we used the debiased weighted phase lag index (WPLI) which is both insensitive to volume conduction effects and more sensitive to true phase synchronization [44] using the FieldTrip software toolbox for Matlab [45]. Before analysis of power and WPLI, signals were processed to remove stimulus artifacts using an offline algorithm (Fig. S1). The algorithm detects stimulus artifacts by thresholding the first derivative of the signal and deleting a defined period surrounding each artifact. The missing values in the signal

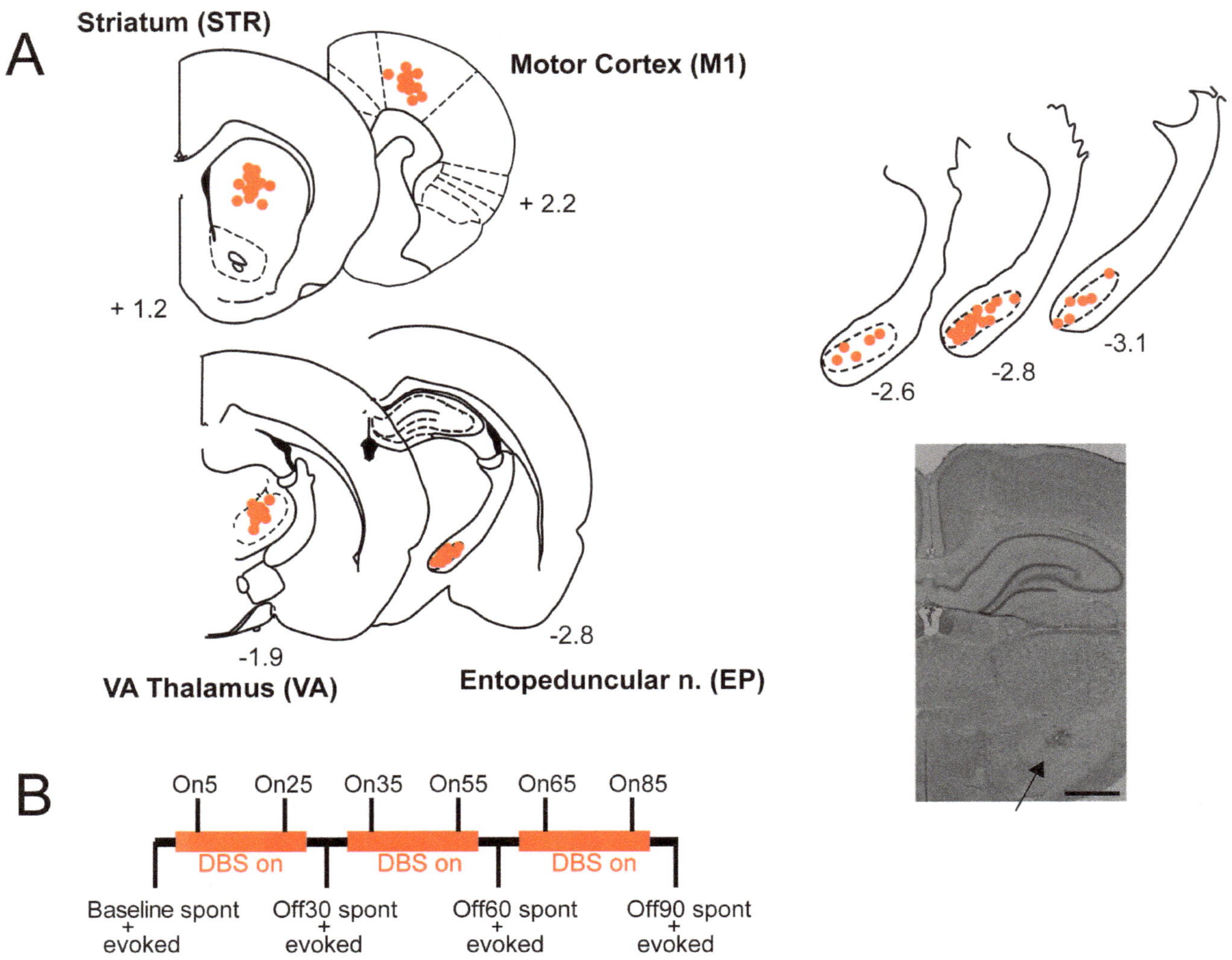

Figure 1. Electrode placements and experimental design. A: Left: Dots show recording electrode placements in striatum (STR), primary motor cortex (M1), and ventroanterior thalamus (VA) and DBS electrode placements in entopeduncular nucleus (EP), and; numbers represent antero-posterior distance from bregma. Overlapping placements have been omitted for clarity, and placements have been collapsed into the same plane and may be slightly anterior or posterior (±~200 μm) to the indicated distance from bregma. Right: Enlarged sections showing placements in EP and photomicrograph showing marked electrode location in EP. Scale bar = 1 mm. **B:** Outline of stimulation and recording protocol.

are then reconstructed using cubic spline interpolation. To ensure this procedure did not introduce any spurious effects or artifacts due to processing, simulated artifacts were added to non-stimulated LFPs (OFF periods and SHAM animals) and then removed using the same algorithm. Furthermore, spontaneous LFP recordings were downsampled to 500 Hz, and segmented (10 s window). Each segment was detrended to remove any slow DC components and padded with zeros to increase frequency resolution.

Multitaper spectral power and WPLI were calculated for each segment in the following frequency bands: slow/delta (0.5–4 Hz); theta (4–12 Hz); low beta (12–20 Hz), high beta (20–30 Hz), low gamma (30–59 Hz) and high gamma (61–90 Hz). The traditional beta and gamma bands were subdivided as reports have suggested differences in generation and function in the low and high beta bands [46–48], as well as low and high gamma bands [49–52]. Data for each frequency band were then averaged over segments. To compare across different groups and over time, power and WPLI values for each animal in a group were normalized to the mean baseline values for that group. For induced LFP oscillations, power values from the 1 s post-stimulus were normalized to pre-stimulus baseline (1 s) and averaged across stimulation sweeps for each time point. To compare across different groups, the values for each animal in a group were normalized to the mean baseline values for that group.

Statistics

Changes in spontaneous and evoked power in each region and WPLI between regions due to time and DBS frequency were analyzed using 3-way ANOVA with "stimulation frequency" as a between subjects factor; time and "frequency band" were within subject measures, followed by Bonferroni's post-hoc test, corrected for multiple comparisons. If the assumption of sphericity was violated according to Mauchley's test, the Greenhouse-Geisser correction was applied and corrected F values are reported. Significance was set at $p<0.05$.

Results

While multisite LFP data were recorded from a total of 36 animals (n = 12/group), all animals with incorrectly placed EP stimulating electrodes were excluded. In the remaining animals, exclusions were made due to incorrectly placed recording electrodes on a region-by-region basis, leaving final group sizes of 6–8 animals/group. In the LF group, DBS stimulation produced acute voltage deflections lasting tens to hundreds of milliseconds (see Figure S1) that corrupted the analysis of oscillations even after removal of the stimulus artifact itself. This did not occur in the HF group, likely due to the short latency between pulses. Accordingly, analysis of the LF group was restricted to acute-stimulus evoked responses in the OFF periods.

Spontaneous Oscillatory Activity

Power. Analysis of the effects of EP DBS on LFP power in M1 (Fig. 2) revealed that HF DBS significantly reduced low beta power in the first five minutes of stimulation (On5) compared to SHAM DBS at that time point, as well as compared to within-subject baseline (BL) [significant main effect of time ($F_{3.57, 42.84} = 12.35$, $p<0.001$) and frequency band ($F_{2.06, 24.68} = 6.70$, $p = 0.004$) and a significant time × stimulation frequency interaction ($F_{3.57, 42.84} = 2.98$, $p = 0.036$); no effects of stimulation frequency, and no other interactions ($F<1.47$, NS)]. Of note, this effect was not evident in any other frequency band, including high beta, and was transient – these group differences were not present at the next time point (On25). Although this reduction in low beta power was only significant at On5, when data are pooled according to relative time point (i.e., "OFF" = BL, On30, Off60; "ON+ 5" = On5, On35, On55; and "ON+25" – On25, On55, On85) the effect remains (Fig. 2D) – low beta power is significantly reduced in the "ON+5" period in the HF group compared to "OFF" and "ON+25", and compared to SHAM [(main effect of time, $F_{2,80} = 5.451$, $p = 0.006$; no effect of stimulation frequency and no interactions ($F<1.04$, NS)]. In addition, high gamma power was elevated significantly in the HF group compared to baseline at selected later time points (i.e., Off30, Off60, On85 and Off90). There were no significant within-subject differences in the SHAM group at any time point in any frequency band.

The effects on LFP activity produced by EP DBS in STR were qualitatively similar to those observed in M1 (Fig. 2A, B), with low beta power significantly reduced in the HF group at ON5 compared to BL, and compared to SHAM at On5 [significant main effect of time ($F_{3.54, 42.50} = 11.97$, $p<0.001$) and frequency band ($F_{1.97, 23.66} = 5.07$, $p = 0.015$), and a significant time × stimulation frequency interaction ($F_{3.54, 42.50} = 3.54$, $p = 0.020$); no effect of stimulation frequency and no other interactions ($F<1.75$, NS)]. As with M1, this effect was transient and frequency band-specific, and no other significant differences were present between HF and SHAM groups. Furthermore, pooled data showed similar effects as in M1; low beta power was significantly reduced in the HF group compared to SHAM at "ON+5", and also compared to BL [main effects of time ($F_{2,80} = 12.158$, $p<0.001$) and a time×stimulation frequency interaction ($F_{2,80} = 8.017$, $p<0.001$); no effect of stimulation frequency ($F<0.91$, NS)]. However, unlike in M1, theta power in STR was significantly increased in the HF group at Off60 and Off90 compared to BL. There were no other significant within-subject effects in the HF group, and no within-subjects differences in the SHAM group.

By contrast with M1 and STR, analysis of the effects of EP DBS in LFP power in VA (Fig. 2A, B) indicated no significant differences between HF and SHAM groups in any frequency band at any time point [significant effect of time ($F_{2.67, 31.99} = 13.56$, $p<0.001$) and frequency band ($F_{1.10, 28.09} = 4.43$, $p = 0.017$); no effect of stimulation frequency and no interactions ($F<1.86$, NS)]. However, in the HF group, theta power was significantly enhanced at Off60 compared to BL. Furthermore, low beta power was significantly elevated compared to BL at Off30, On85, Off90, whereas high beta power was significantly elevated compared to BL at Off30 and Off90. There were no significant within-subject differences in the SHAM group at any time point in any frequency band.

Due to the size of EP, it was only possible to record EP LFP activity through one pole of the stimulating electrode during OFF periods. During the OFF periods, there were no significant effects on EP oscillation power in any region or band (data not shown).

Thus, HF DBS produced an early and transient reduction in low beta power compared to SHAM in M1 and STR, but not VA. Furthermore, HF DBS produced time-dependent enhancements in fast oscillation power that were region- and frequency-band specific and not present in the SHAM group.

Functional connectivity. EP DBS also produced widespread changes in functional connectivity along the circuit, as assessed using WPLI (Fig. 3). M1-STR WPLI was significantly increased in the HF group compared to SHAM in the delta (at On5, On25, and Off60) and low gamma bands (at On5, On25, and On35); and significantly decreased in the theta (at ON5), low beta (all time points) and high beta (at Off30, On35, Off60, and Off90) [significant frequency band × stimulation frequency interaction ($F_{2.84, 34.08} = 7.803$, $p = 0.001$); no other main effects or interactions ($F<2.09$, NS)]. There were no within-subject effects in either group.

EP DBS also produced effects on M1-VA connectivity (Fig. 3A, B). Low beta band WPLI was significantly decreased in the HF group compared to SHAM at Off30, Off60, On65, On85, and Off90 [significant frequency band × stimulation frequency interaction ($F_{2.53, 30.38} = 2.75$, $p = 0.042$); no other main effects or interactions ($F<1.96$, NS)]. In addition, WPLI in the low gamma band was significantly higher in the HF group than the SHAM group at On5, On25, On35, and On65. In SHAM animals, there was a general enhancement of synchronization in the low beta band relative to baseline and other frequency bands, but this effect did not reach significance; there were no within-subject effects in either group.

Analysis of the effects of EP DBS on STR-VA connectivity (Fig. 3A, B) indicated that HF DBS produced significant increases in WPLI in the high beta (at On5 and On65), low gamma (at On5, On25, On35, On65, and Off85) and high gamma (at On5, On85) bands, and a significant decrease in low beta synchronization at Off60. [significant frequency band × stimulation frequency × time interaction ($F_{5.64, 67.69} = 2.46$, $p = 0.025$); no effects of time or frequency band, and no other interactions ($F<1.30$, NS)]. There were no within-subject effects in either group.

As mentioned above, it was only possible to record EP LFP activity (and WPLI between EP and the other regions) during OFF periods. In the HF group, EP-M1 WPLI was significantly reduced compared to SHAM in the delta band (at Off30, Off60, and Off90) as well as the low beta band at Off60 and Off90 [significant main effect of stimulation frequency ($F_{1.22, 14.65} = 4.386$, $p = 0.048$)], and a significant time × frequency band interaction ($F_{3.89, 46.73} = 2.101$, $p = 0.025$); no effect of time, frequency band, and no other interactions ($F<1.32$, NS)]. There were no within-subject effects in either group.

EP-STR coherence was also affected by EP DBS [significant band × stimulation frequency ($F_{1.41, 16.96} = 1.922$, $p = 0.039$) interaction, no other significant main effect or other interactions ($F<1.29$, NS)]. Post-hoc analysis showed a significant reduction in

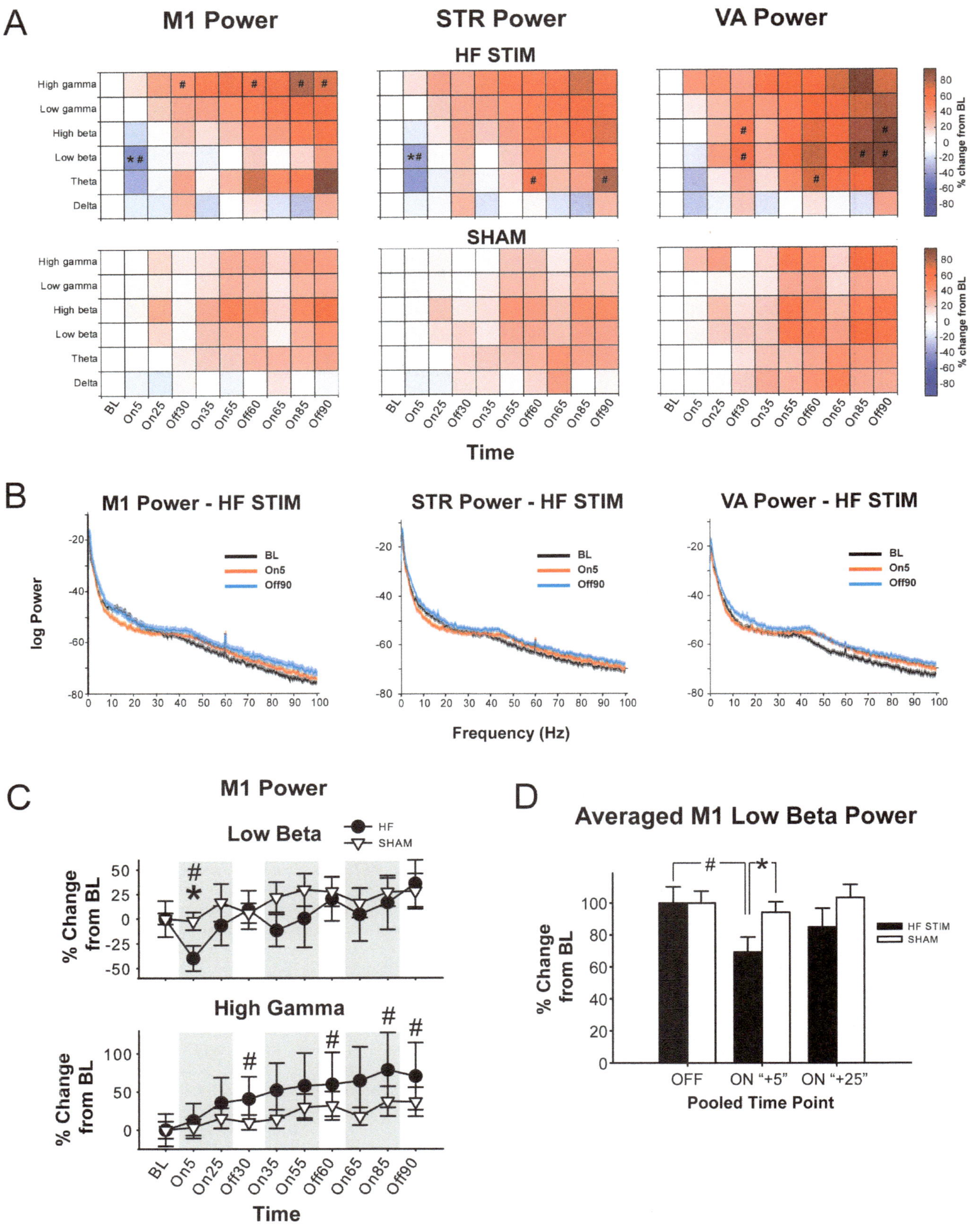
A
M1 Power
STR Power
VA Power
HF STIM
SHAM
High gamma
Low gamma
High beta
Low beta
Theta
Delta
BL
On5
On25
Off30
On35
On55
Off60
On65
On85
Off90
Time
% change from BL
B
M1 Power - HF STIM
STR Power - HF STIM
VA Power - HF STIM
log Power
Frequency (Hz)
C
M1 Power
Low Beta
High Gamma
HF
SHAM
% Change from BL
D
Averaged M1 Low Beta Power
HF STIM
SHAM
OFF
ON "+5"
ON "+25"
Pooled Time Point

Figure 2. High-frequency (HF) EP DBS produces frequency band-specific and time-dependent increases and decreases in LFP oscillation power in primary motor cortex (M1), striatum (STR) and ventroanterior thalamus (VA). A. Color plots showing effects of high-frequency (HF; top) or SHAM (bottom) EP DBS on normalized LFP power in M1, STR, and VA according to frequency band and time point. * = significantly different from SHAM; # significantly different from within-group BL ($p<0.05$). * = significantly different from SHAM; # significantly different from within-group BL ($p<0.05$). **B.** Representative power spectra from a rat receiving HF EP DBS at BL, in the first five minutes of stimulation (On5), and after 90 minutes of stimulation (Off90). Shaded area represents 95% confidence interval generated using "leave one out" jackknife statistics. **C.** Effects of HF and SHAM EP DBS on normalized M1 low beta (top) and high gamma (bottom) power over time. Error bars represent S.E.M. **D.** Effects of EP DBS on M1 low beta power, pooled according to relative stimulation time point. OFF = pooled average of BL, Off30, Off60; "ON+5" = pooled average of On5, On35, On 65; "ON+25" = average of On25, On55, On85. * = significantly different from SHAM; # = significantly different from within-group BL ($p<0.05$).

WPLI in the HF group compared to SHAM in the theta (at Off30) and low beta (at Off60) bands. There were no within-subject effects in either group.

With respect to EP-VA connectivity, there was a significant stimulation frequency × time × frequency band interaction ($F_{5.81, 46.73} = 2.170$, $p = 0.029$); WPLI was significantly reduced in the HF group compared to SHAM in both the delta and low beta bands (at Off 30 and Off 90).

Thus, the predominant effect of HF EP-DBS on functional connectivity was desynchronization in the low beta band, initially only between M1 and STR, but between all other regions with sustained stimulation, and enhanced synchronization in the low gamma band that was most prominent between VA and other regions along the circuit. Interestingly, enhanced gamma connectivity was only observed when stimulation was on; beta desynchronization persisted into OFF periods.

Stimulus-induced Oscillations

Acute EP stimulation often resulted in induced oscillations (i.e., not time-locked to the stimulus; see Fig. 4A) at all recording sites. Changes in induced oscillations as a function of time and stimulation frequency were quantified by examining the spectral power within regions and coherence between regions in the 1 s following stimulation, normalized to activity in the 1 s prior to stimulation during the four OFF periods.

Induced Power. In M1, EP DBS had a number of effects on induced LFP power (Fig. 4). Induced low and high beta power were both significantly reduced in the HF group compared to both SHAM and LF groups at all three OFF time points (Off30, Off60, Off90) [significant main effects of stimulation frequency ($F_{2, 19} = 3.633$, $p = 0.046$), time ($F_{1.96, 37.28} = 3.559$, $p = 0.039$), and frequency band ($F_{2.09, 39.76} = 3.466$, $p = 0.039$), as well as a significant stimulation frequency × frequency band interaction ($F_{4.19, 39.76} = 8.040$, $p<0.001$); but no other interactions ($F<2.01$, NS)]. There were no significant between-group differences in any other frequency bands at any other time points. In addition, induced power in the low and high beta bands was significantly reduced in the HF group at all time points compared to BL. No significant within-subject effects were observed in the other groups at any time point.

The effects of EP DBS on induced oscillatory activity in STR were largely similar to those observed in M1 (Fig. 4). Induced theta power was significantly reduced in the HF group compared to both SHAM and LF at Off90, whereas induced low and high beta were both significantly reduced compared to SHAM (but not LF) at Off30 and Off60, and significantly reduced compared to both LF and SHAM at Off90 [significant main effect of time ($F_{2.08, 39.48} = 6.44$, $p = 0.003$), and a significant stimulation intensity × frequency band interaction ($F_{4.47, 42.43} = 4.196$, $p = 0.005$); no effect of stimulation frequency or frequency band, and no other interactions ($F<2.39$, NS)]. In the HF group, compared to BL there was significant reduction in low beta power at Off30 and Off90, a significant reduction in high beta power at all 3 time points, and a significant reduction in low gamma power at Off90. No within subject effects were observed in the LF and SHAM groups.

Analysis of the effects of EP DBS on induced LFP activity in VA (Fig. 4) revealed that induced low beta power was significantly attenuated compared to LF and SHAM at OFF60 and OFF90 [significant main effects of time ($F_{3, 57} = 7.651$, $p<0.001$), and frequency band ($F_{2.23, 42.28} = 3.855$, $p = 0.025$); no effect of stimulation frequency and no interactions ($F<2.23$, NS)]. Furthermore, induced high beta power was reduced compared to SHAM but not LF at Off60. With respect to within-subject effects, in the HF group there was a significant decrease in both induced low and high beta at all time points compared to BL. In the LF group, there was a significant reduction in induced high beta at Off90 compared to BL, and in induced high gamma at Off30 compared to BL. There were no significant within-subject effects in the SHAM group.

Thus, compared to SHAM and LF, HF EP DBS produced a robust decrease in evoked oscillatory activity that was predominantly confined to the beta band (both low and high). While small differences were apparent, these effects were for the most part similar in all recorded areas. LF stimulation produced effects that were either similar in direction as the changes produced by HF stimulation (i.e., in VA) or not different from SHAM or LF BL (i.e, in M1 and STR).

Discussion

EP DBS delivered for 90 minutes generated widespread alterations in spontaneous and stimulus-induced LFP oscillations along a motor cortical-basal ganglia-thalamic circuit known to exhibit pathological activity in PD and dystonia (summarized in Table 1). The most prominent effect was a reduction in beta synchronization and enhancement of gamma synchronization; however, although some effects appeared similar across regions, others occurred in a region- and frequency band-specific manner, and importantly, many evolved over time. We also observed a dissociation of the effects of DBS on power within a region and functional connectivity between regions. Although EP DBS produced an initial transient reduction in power in the low beta band in M1 and STR, synchronization between these two regions in this band was dramatically reduced at all time points, and EP DBS markedly suppressed the ability of acute EP stimulation to induce beta oscillations in all regions along the circuit. These stimulus-induced effects were specific to HF DBS and were not present with LF (i.e. non-therapeutic) DBS. Gamma synchronization between regions along the circuit was enhanced when DBS was on, and with time, sustained DBS enhanced power in the faster frequency bands.

Neural circuitry

The aim of this study was to assess the effects of EP DBS simultaneously in a number of regions that comprise a primary

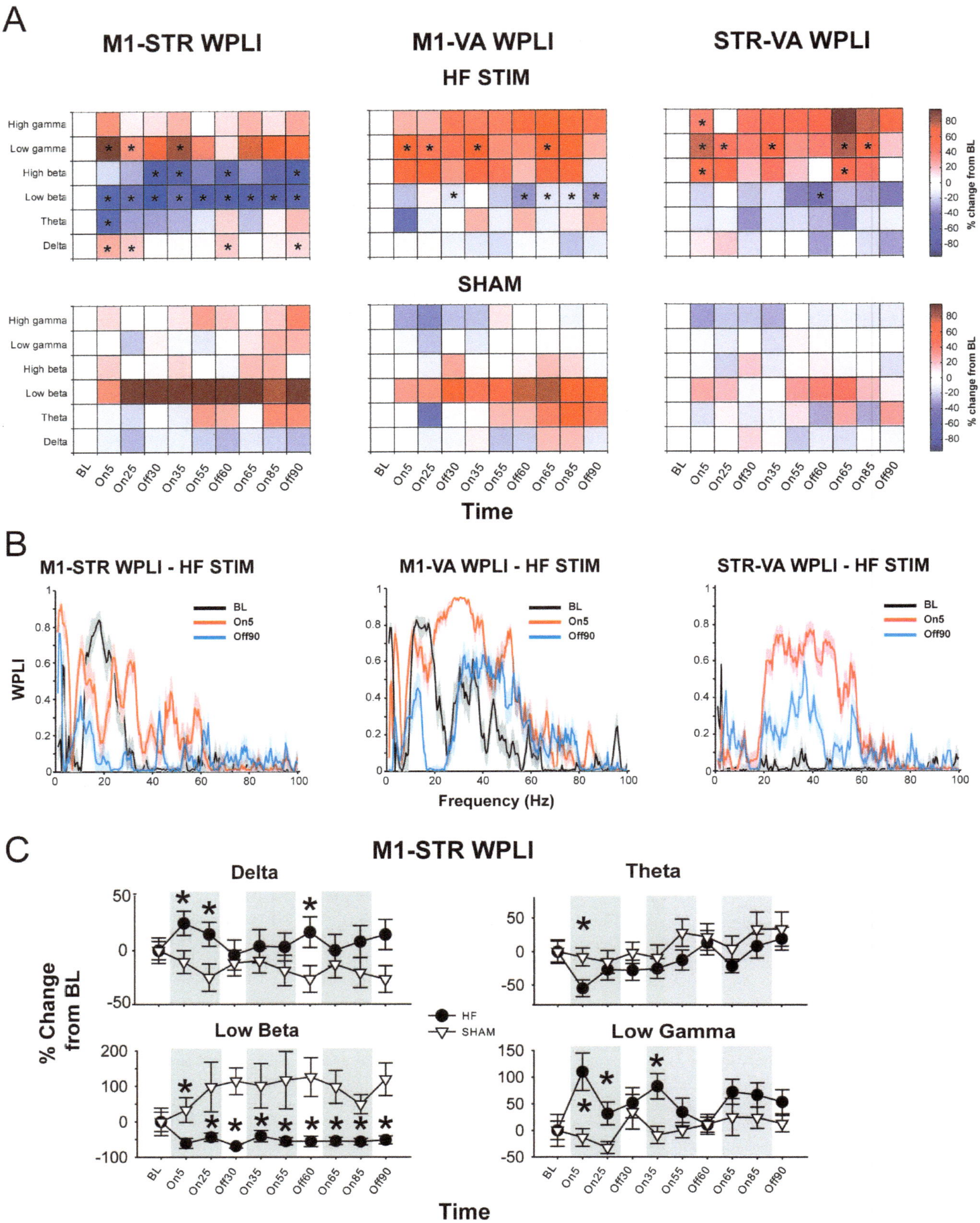

Figure 3. High-frequency (HF) EP DBS produces region- and frequency band-specific effects on functional connectivity. A. Color plots showing effects of high-frequency (top) or SHAM (bottom) EP DBS on debiased weighted phase lag index (WPLI) between regions according to frequency band and time point. * = significantly different from SHAM ($p<0.05$). **B.** Representative WPLI plots from a rat receiving HF stimulation at

baseline (BL), in the first five minutes of stimulation (On5), and after 90 minutes of stimulation (Off90). Shaded area represents 95% confidence interval generated using jackknife statistics. **C.** Effects of HF and SHAM EP DBS on M1-STR WPLI over time. Error bars represent S.E.M. * = significantly different from SHAM ($p<0.05$).

motor circuit. The direct efferent pathway from the striatum projects directly to the entopeduncular nucleus [53,54], which in turn projects to the VA/VL thalamus [55,56]. Thalamocortical projections to primary motor cortex have been well-studied (Jones, 2005) as have projections from M1 to the striatum [57,58]. Together, these regions are proposed to create a functional segregated motor processing loop [59]. In rats and pigs, respectively, EP DBS produced changes in immediate early gene expression [60] and BOLD imaging [61] in all regions along this circuit; GPi DBS in primates has been shown to produce effects consistent with activation of GPi axons [19,20], and modulates neuronal firing in M1 [62]. The present work allowed us to examine how circuit-wide changes in neural activity evolve over time and allowed comparison to human DBS studies that report changes in LFP oscillations.

LFP oscillations, movement disorders and DBS

Accumulating evidence suggests that DBS may exert beneficial effects by reducing pathological beta synchronization. Thus,

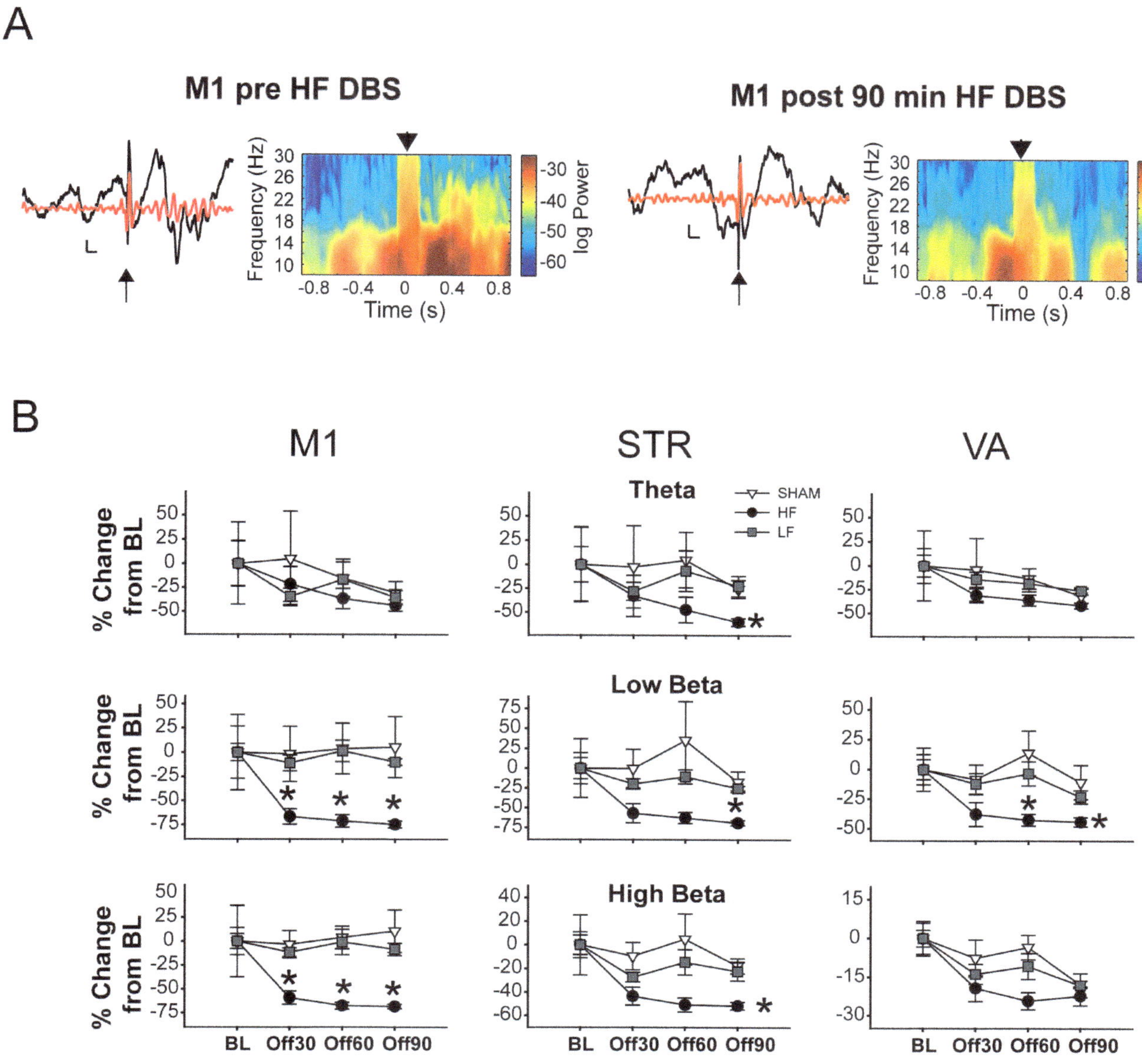

Figure 4. High-frequency (HF) EP DBS suppresses acute EP-induced beta oscillations in all recorded regions. A. Representative raw (black) and filtered (6–30 Hz; red) voltage traces from M1 (calibration: 200 ms, 0.2 mV) and time-frequency spectrograms showing effects of acute EP stimulation before (left) and after (right) 90 minutes of high-frequency (HF) EP DBS. **B.** Changes in induced oscillation power according to region and time point. Low-frequency (LF) EP DBS does not suppressed induced oscillations as HF DBS does. Error bars represent S.E.M. * = significantly different from SHAM and LF ($p<0.05$).

Table 1. Summary of major effects.

	M1			STR			VA		
	Spont	Evoked		Spont	Evoked		Spont	Evoked	
POWER	HF	HF	LF	HF	HF	LF	HF	HF	LF
Slow/delta	–	–	–	–	–	–	–	–	–
Theta	–	–	–	↑	–	–	↑	–	–
Beta	**↓**	**↓** ↓	–	**↓**	↓	–	↑	↓	–
Gamma	↑	–	–	–	–	–	–	–	–

	M1-VA	M1-STR	STR-VA
WPLI	Spont HF	Spont HF	Spont HF
Slow/delta	**↑** ↑	–	–
Theta	**↓**	–	–
Beta	**↓** ↓	↓	↓
Gamma	**↑**	**↑** ↑	**↑** ↑

Arrows signify significant increases or decreases ($p<0.05$) in oscillation power or functional connectivity (assessed using debiased weighted phase lag index; WPLI). Bold arrows represent early effects and thin arrows represent late effects, which are more widespread.

prominent oscillatory activity in the beta band throughout the basal ganglia and motor cortex is reported in PD patients off dopaminergic medications [63–66], as well as animal models of PD that involve destruction of dopamine neurons [67–70]. Moreover, L-DOPA administration reduces beta oscillation power concomitantly with movement facilitation [46,63,71], and beta desynchronization is associated with movement initiation [72–74]. While beta oscillations are associated with akinesia/bradykinesia, gamma oscillations are generally associated with movement, with movement-related gamma synchronization found in a number of regions [75–77]. Furthermore, in PD patients the prokinetic effects of levopoda are accompanied by increases in gamma power [63,64,78,79].

The relationship between synchronization in BG and dystonia is less clear. LFPs recorded from the BG of dystonia patients display oscillation peaks at a lower frequency than PD patients, typically at 4–10 Hz [80–84]. In dystonia there is also less coherence between LFP oscillation and single neuron firing than in PD patients [85]. These oscillations are coherent with [86] and thought to drive [87] EMG oscillation in the affected muscle groups; using a sensory trick to alleviate dystonic contractions is associated with desynchronization in this frequency band [83].

DBS of the subthalamic nucleus (STN) has been shown to reduce BG beta oscillations in PD patients either during stimulation or in the period immediately following stimulation, while therapeutic effects persist [88–94]. Although the effects of GPi DBS on oscillatory activity are not well studied, GPi DBS suppresses oscillatory activity in the beta range in MPTP-treated macaques [95].

EP DBS and LFP oscillations

Based on this literature, we hypothesized that EP DBS would promote desynchronization, particularly in the lower frequency bands. While this was indeed the case, the effects we observed were more complex, including enhancements in gamma synchronization, and dissociations between changes in power within a region and synchronization between regions. While DBS produced an initial reduction in low beta power in both M1 and STR, this effect was transient and did not persist over sustained stimulation. However, synchronization in this band between these two regions was profoundly suppressed at all time points. DBS also enhanced low gamma synchronization between regions throughout the circuit, particularly between VA and other regions, and with longer stimulation, DBS enhanced oscillation power in the faster frequency bands within both M1 and VA. The SHAM group displayed a gradual non-significant enhanced broadband power over time. This effect may be due to changes in network activity stemming tissue damage during electrode insertion, or is a side effect of urethane anesthesia. We believe the latter is more probable, as urethane has a variety of effects on neural activity that could contribute to the observed power changes, including effects on catecholamine levels and ion channel function [96,97] (Maggi and Mello, 1986; Hara and Harris, 2002). The reduction in low beta power and functional connectivity that we observed is consistent with the ability of therapeutic DBS to reduce pathological beta oscillations in PD patients. The fact that significant changes occurred in the low beta band only is also consistent with specific reduction in this band following L-DOPA administration and associated with movement facilitation [46–48]. Spontaneous measures represent the general activity state of the system; stimulated responses provide an index of how the system responds to activation. We saw a pronounced effect of HF DBS but not LF DBS on the ability of acute stimulation of the EP to induce beta oscillation in all recorded regions. This effect is consistent with the desynchronization of spontaneous beta oscillations and connectivity seen with DBS.

LF stimulation of the STN is reported to worsen movement performance on a variety of tasks [33–35]. We expected LF EP DBS to produce effects opposite in direction to those produced by HF EP DBS, however, LF stimulation either produced no significant effects, or in the same direction as HF DBS but reduced in magnitude. This may have occurred because we applied the same amplitude of DBS for both LF and HF, resulting in overall lower current injection into the tissue with LF [98].

Time-dependent effects of EP DBS

Our most notable finding is the differential time course of the observed changes in LFP activity (i.e., early vs. late). To our knowledge, virtually all studies examining the effects of DBS on neuronal firing or LFP oscillations have focused on the short-term effects of stimulation, on a time scale ranging from seconds to a few minutes. While understanding the initial effects of stimulation is essential, DBS is applied chronically over years, and the effects of DBS may evolve over time. For example, in PD patients, although therapeutic effects are seen within minutes of DBS application [27], not all symptoms respond equally quickly to DBS [1] and DBS for dystonia can take months to years to achieve maximum benefit [28–30]. The early low beta desynchronization in (and between) M1 and STR we report here ma-y be similar to changes seen immediately in PD patients and together with enhanced gamma connectivity may be sufficient for facilitating voluntary movement. The more slowly developing beta desynchronization between the other regions and enhancement of faster oscillation power along the circuit may represent the early stages of the plastic reorganization that relate to the therapeutic effects of GPi DBS in dystonia [32]. The enhanced fast oscillatory synchronization we observed throughout this motor circuit may act as a stabilizing influence, promoting coordinated physiological information flow throughout the circuit, and dampening the effects of pathological synchronization in lower frequency bands.

There are several limitations to this study. One is that our "extended" stimulation remains considerably less than days or weeks; however, the time-dependent changes observed here may represent the initial stages of a plastic or compensatory response to the hyperacute effects of DBS. Two other limitations are the use anesthesia and normal intact animals. Even with anesthetics like urethane that are thought to preserve many aspects physiological responses, neuronal activity and the synchronization thereof are likely to be differently regulated in the awake and anesthetized states (Hara and Harris, 2002). Several studies support the relevance of our data. Dopamine-depleted rats show prominent spontaneous cortical and subcortical beta oscillations in both awake and anesthetized states (Mallet et al., 2008a, Mallet et al., 2008b). Furthermore, Ahrens and Freeman (2001) reported similar profiles of electrically-evoked entorhinal cortex LFP activity in awake and anesthetized rats. In normal animals it can be different to ensure the stimulation applied is in the appropriate therapeutic range. Preliminary work showed that the stimulation parameters used caused no motor side effects in normal animals, produce a charge density approximating what is clinically effective in humans (Fakhar et al., 2013), and produced effects in various rat behavioral studies (Creed et al., 2011, Creed et al., 2012a), suggesting our parameters are consistent with those used in the preclinical and clinical literature. The question remains as to whether the effects on synchronization that we observe in normal animals are relevant and generalizable to disease states. Given that the effects of EP/GPi DBS on oscillatory activity have not been characterized in intact animals, and that GPi DBS is clinically effective for both dystonia and PD, diseases with unique pathological profiles, the findings reported here will help identify how responses to DBS may vary under different physiological and pathological conditions. Furthermore, the reduction and enhancement beta and gamma synchronization, respectively, is consistent with what is observed in the clinic with DBS for PD (Wingeier et al., 2006, Kuhn et al., 2008, Bronte-Stewart et al., 2009, Eusebio et al., 2011, Giannicola et al., 2012).

Implications

The effects of DBS on LFP activity are not static, but rather reflect an evolving pattern of effects that vary by time, frequency band, and region. In addition, the widespread and specific alterations in oscillatory activity provide further evidence that DBS can modulate neural activity distant to the stimulated nucleus; indeed, our results point to a constellation of changes across the entire cortico-BG-thalamic circuit. The time-dependent effects DBS are likely to be most relevant for conditions that show a more gradual response to stimulation, and suggest that studies of therapeutic mechanisms should examine the effects of both short-duration and more extended stimulation.

Supporting Information

Figure S1 Representative voltage traces and power spectrum during HF (left) and LF (right) DBS, before (top) and after (bottom) stimulus artifact removal. Note the acute responses to stimulation in the LF trace that contaminate the power spectrum even after artifact removal.

Author Contributions

Conceived and designed the experiments: CM ZK. Performed the experiments: CM. Analyzed the data: CM. Wrote the paper: CM ZK.

References

1. Rodriguez-Oroz MC, Obeso JA, Lang AE, Houeto JL, Pollak P, et al. (2005) Bilateral deep brain stimulation in Parkinson's disease: a multicentre study with 4 years follow-up. Brain 128: 2240–2249.
2. Kupsch A, Benecke R, Muller J, Trottenberg T, Schneider GH, et al. (2006) Pallidal deep-brain stimulation in primary generalized or segmental dystonia. N Engl J Med 355: 1978–1990.
3. Benabid AL, Pollak P, Louveau A, Henry S, de Rougemont J (1987) Combined (thalamotomy and stimulation) stereotactic surgery of the VIM thalamic nucleus for bilateral Parkinson disease. Appl Neurophysiol 50: 344–346.
4. Limousin P, Pollak P, Benazzouz A, Hoffmann D, Le Bas JF, et al. (1995) Effect of parkinsonian signs and symptoms of bilateral subthalamic nucleus stimulation. Lancet 345: 91–95.
5. Boraud T, Bezard E, Bioulac B, Gross C (1996) High frequency stimulation of the internal Globus Pallidus (GPi) simultaneously improves parkinsonian symptoms and reduces the firing frequency of GPi neurons in the MPTP-treated monkey. Neurosci Lett 215: 17–20.
6. Benazzouz A, Gao DM, Ni ZG, Piallat B, Bouali-Benazzouz R, et al. (2000) Effect of high-frequency stimulation of the subthalamic nucleus on the neuronal activities of the substantia nigra pars reticulata and ventrolateral nucleus of the thalamus in the rat. Neuroscience 99: 289–295.
7. Beurrier C, Bioulac B, Audin J, Hammond C (2001) High-frequency stimulation produces a transient blockade of voltage-gated currents in subthalamic neurons. J Neurophysiol 85: 1351–1356.
8. Anderson TR, Hu B, Iremonger K, Kiss ZH (2006) Selective attenuation of afferent synaptic transmission as a mechanism of thalamic deep brain stimulation-induced tremor arrest. J Neurosci 26: 841–850.
9. Chiken S, Nambu A (2013) High-frequency pallidal stimulation disrupts information flow through the pallidum by GABAergic inhibition. J Neurosci 33: 2268–2280.
10. Nowak LG, Bullier J (1998) Axons, but not cell bodies, are activated by electrical stimulation in cortical gray matter. I. Evidence from chronaxie measurements. Exp Brain Res 118: 477–488.
11. Vitek JL (2002) Mechanisms of deep brain stimulation: excitation or inhibition. Mov Disord 17 Suppl 3: S69–72.
12. McIntyre CC, Savasta M, Kerkerian-Le Goff L, Vitek JL (2004) Uncovering the mechanism(s) of action of deep brain stimulation: activation, inhibition, or both. Clin Neurophysiol 115: 1239–1248.
13. McCracken CB, Grace AA (2007) High-frequency deep brain stimulation of the nucleus accumbens region suppresses neuronal activity and selectively modulates afferent drive in rat orbitofrontal cortex in vivo. J Neurosci 27: 12601–12610.
14. Li S, Arbuthnott GW, Jutras MJ, Goldberg JA, Jaeger D (2007) Resonant antidromic cortical circuit activation as a consequence of high-frequency subthalamic deep-brain stimulation. J Neurophysiol 98: 3525–3537.
15. Li Q, Ke Y, Chan DC, Qian ZM, Yung KK, et al. (2012) Therapeutic deep brain stimulation in Parkinsonian rats directly influences motor cortex. Neuron 76: 1030–1041.
16. Dostrovsky JO, Levy R, Wu JP, Hutchison WD, Tasker RR, et al. (2000) Microstimulation-induced inhibition of neuronal firing in human globus pallidus. J Neurophysiol 84: 570–574.
17. Wu YR, Levy R, Ashby P, Tasker RR, Dostrovsky JO (2001) Does stimulation of the GPi control dyskinesia by activating inhibitory axons? Mov Disord 16: 208–216.
18. Montgomery EB, Jr. (2006) Effects of GPi stimulation on human thalamic neuronal activity. Clin Neurophysiol 117: 2691–2702.
19. Bar-Gad I, Elias S, Vaadia E, Bergman H (2004) Complex locking rather than complete cessation of neuronal activity in the globus pallidus of a 1-methyl-4-phenyl-1,2,3,6-tetrahydropyridine-treated primate in response to pallidal microstimulation. J Neurosci 24: 7410–7419.
20. Anderson ME, Postupna N, Ruffo M (2003) Effects of high-frequency stimulation in the internal globus pallidus on the activity of thalamic neurons in the awake monkey. J Neurophysiol 89: 1150–1160.
21. Eusebio A, Cagnan H, Brown P (2012) Does suppression of oscillatory synchronisation mediate some of the therapeutic effects of DBS in patients with Parkinson's disease? Front Integr Neurosci 6: 47.
22. Tang JK, Moro E, Mahant N, Hutchison WD, Lang AE, et al. (2007) Neuronal firing rates and patterns in the globus pallidus internus of patients with cervical dystonia differ from those with Parkinson's disease. J Neurophysiol 98: 720–729.
23. Sani S, Ostrem JL, Shimamoto S, Levesque N, Starr PA (2009) Single unit "pauser" characteristics of the globus pallidus pars externa distinguish primary dystonia from secondary dystonia and Parkinson's disease. Exp Neurol 216: 295–299.
24. Shin DS, Samoilova M, Cotic M, Zhang L, Brotchie JM, et al. (2007) High frequency stimulation or elevated K+ depresses neuronal activity in the rat entopeduncular nucleus. Neuroscience 149: 68–86.
25. McCairn KW, Iriki A, Isoda M (2012) High-frequency pallidal stimulation eliminates tic-related neuronal activity in a nonhuman primate model of Tourette syndrome. Neuroreport 23: 206–210.
26. Cleary DR, Raslan AM, Rubin JE, Bahgat D, Viswanathan A, et al. (2013) Deep brain stimulation entrains local neuronal firing in human globus pallidus internus. J Neurophysiol 109: 978–987.
27. Hristova A, Lyons K, Troster AI, Pahwa R, Wilkinson SB, et al. (2000) Effect and time course of deep brain stimulation of the globus pallidus and subthalamus on motor features of Parkinson's disease. Clin Neuropharmacol 23: 208–211.
28. Coubes P, Cif L, El Fertit H, Hemm S, Vayssiere N, et al. (2004) Electrical stimulation of the globus pallidus internus in patients with primary generalized dystonia: long-term results. J Neurosurg 101: 189–194.
29. Bittar RG, Yianni J, Wang S, Liu X, Nandi D, et al. (2005) Deep brain stimulation for generalised dystonia and spasmodic torticollis. J Clin Neurosci 12: 12–16.
30. Magarinos-Ascone CM, Regidor I, Gomez-Galan M, Cabanes-Martinez L, Figueiras-Mendez R (2008) Deep brain stimulation in the globus pallidus to treat dystonia: electrophysiological characteristics and 2 years' follow-up in 10 patients. Neuroscience 152: 558–571.
31. Kiss ZH, Doig-Beyaert K, Eliasziw M, Tsui J, Haffenden A, et al. (2007) The Canadian multicentre study of deep brain stimulation for cervical dystonia. Brain 130: 2879–2886.
32. Ruge D, Tisch S, Hariz MI, Zrinzo L, Bhatia KP, et al. (2011) Deep brain stimulation effects in dystonia: time course of electrophysiological changes in early treatment. Mov Disord 26: 1913–1921.
33. Timmermann L, Wojtecki L, Gross J, Lehrke R, Voges J, et al. (2004) Ten-Hertz stimulation of subthalamic nucleus deteriorates motor symptoms in Parkinson's disease. Mov Disord 19: 1328–1333.
34. Chen CC, Litvak V, Gilbertson T, Kuhn A, Lu CS, et al. (2007) Excessive synchronization of basal ganglia neurons at 20 Hz slows movement in Parkinson's disease. Exp Neurol 205: 214–221.
35. Chen CC, Lin WY, Chan HL, Hsu YT, Tu PH, et al. (2011) Stimulation of the subthalamic region at 20 Hz slows the development of grip force in Parkinson's disease. Exp Neurol 231: 91–96.
36. Moro E, Esselink RJ, Xie J, Hommel M, Benabid AL, et al. (2002) The impact on Parkinson's disease of electrical parameter settings in STN stimulation. Neurology 59: 706–713.
37. Kupsch A, Klaffke S, Kuhn AA, Meissner W, Arnold G, et al. (2003) The effects of frequency in pallidal deep brain stimulation for primary dystonia. J Neurol 250: 1201–1205.

38. Florin E, Reck C, Burghaus L, Lehrke R, Gross J, et al. (2008) Ten Hertz thalamus stimulation increases tremor activity in the subthalamic nucleus in a patient with Parkinson's disease. Clin Neurophysiol 119: 2098–2103.
39. Fakhar K, Hastings E, Butson CR, Foote KD, Zeilman P, et al. (2013) Management of deep brain stimulator battery failure: battery estimators, charge density, and importance of clinical symptoms. PLoS One 8: e58665.
40. Creed M, Hamani C, Nobrega JN (2011) Deep brain stimulation of the subthalamic or entopeduncular nucleus attenuates vacuous chewing movements in a rodent model of tardive dyskinesia. Eur Neuropsychopharmacol 21: 393–400.
41. Creed MC, Hamani C, Bridgman A, Fletcher PJ, Nobrega JN (2012) Contribution of decreased serotonin release to the antidyskinetic effects of deep brain stimulation in a rodent model of tardive dyskinesia: comparison of the subthalamic and entopeduncular nuclei. J Neurosci 32: 9574–9581.
42. Kuncel AM, Grill WM (2004) Selection of stimulus parameters for deep brain stimulation. Clin Neurophysiol 115: 2431–2441.
43. McCracken CB, Grace AA (2009) Nucleus accumbens deep brain stimulation produces region-specific alterations in local field potential oscillations and evoked responses in vivo. J Neurosci 29: 5354–5363.
44. Vinck M, Oostenveld R, van Wingerden M, Battaglia F, Pennartz CM (2011) An improved index of phase-synchronization for electrophysiological data in the presence of volume-conduction, noise and sample-size bias. Neuroimage 55: 1548–1565.
45. Oostenveld R, Fries P, Maris E, Schoffelen JM (2011) FieldTrip: Open source software for advanced analysis of MEG, EEG, and invasive electrophysiological data. Comput Intell Neurosci 2011: 156869.
46. Marceglia S, Foffani G, Bianchi AM, Baselli G, Tamma F, et al. (2006) Dopamine-dependent non-linear correlation between subthalamic rhythms in Parkinson's disease. J Physiol 571: 579–591.
47. Priori A, Foffani G, Pesenti A, Tamma F, Bianchi AM, et al. (2004) Rhythm-specific pharmacological modulation of subthalamic activity in Parkinson's disease. Exp Neurol 189: 369–379.
48. Lopez-Azcarate J, Tainta M, Rodriguez-Oroz MC, Valencia M, Gonzalez R, et al. (2010) Coupling between beta and high-frequency activity in the human subthalamic nucleus may be a pathophysiological mechanism in Parkinson's disease. J Neurosci 30: 6667–6677.
49. Crone NE, Miglioretti DL, Gordon B, Lesser RP (1998) Functional mapping of human sensorimotor cortex with electrocorticographic spectral analysis. II. Event-related synchronization in the gamma band. Brain 121 (Pt 12): 2301–2315.
50. Edwards E, Soltani M, Deouell LY, Berger MS, Knight RT (2005) High gamma activity in response to deviant auditory stimuli recorded directly from human cortex. J Neurophysiol 94: 4269–4280.
51. van der Meer MA, Kalenscher T, Lansink CS, Pennartz CM, Berke JD, et al. (2010) Integrating early results on ventral striatal gamma oscillations in the rat. Front Neurosci 4: 300.
52. Pogosyan A, Kuhn AA, Trottenberg T, Schneider GH, Kupsch A, et al. (2006) Elevations in local gamma activity are accompanied by changes in the firing rate and information coding capacity of neurons in the region of the subthalamic nucleus in Parkinson's disease. Exp Neurol 202: 271–279.
53. Kita H (2001) Neostriatal and globus pallidus stimulation induced inhibitory postsynaptic potentials in entopeduncular neurons in rat brain slice preparations. Neuroscience 105: 871–879.
54. Nagy JI, Carter DA, Fibiger HC (1978) Anterior striatal projections to the globus pallidus, entopeduncular nucleus and substantia nigra in the rat: the GABA connection. Brain Res 158: 15–29.
55. Kha HT, Finkelstein DI, Pow DV, Lawrence AJ, Horne MK (2000) Study of projections from the entopeduncular nucleus to the thalamus of the rat. J Comp Neurol 426: 366–377.
56. Carter DA, Fibiger HC (1978) The projections of the entopeduncular nucleus and globus pallidus in rat as demonstrated by autoradiography and horseradish peroxidase histochemistry. J Comp Neurol 177: 113–123.
57. Wilson CJ (1986) Postsynaptic potentials evoked in spiny neostriatal projection neurons by stimulation of ipsilateral and contralateral neocortex. Brain Res 367: 201–213.
58. Hoffer ZS, Alloway KD (2001) Organization of corticostriatal projections from the vibrissal representations in the primary motor and somatosensory cortical areas of rodents. J Comp Neurol 439: 87–103.
59. Alexander GE, Crutcher MD, DeLong MR (1990) Basal ganglia-thalamocortical circuits: parallel substrates for motor, oculomotor, "prefrontal" and "limbic" functions. Prog Brain Res 85: 119–146.
60. Creed MC, Hamani C, Nobrega JN (2012) Early gene mapping after deep brain stimulation in a rat model of tardive dyskinesia: comparison with transient local inactivation. Eur Neuropsychopharmacol 22: 506–517.
61. Min HK, Hwang SC, Marsh MP, Kim I, Knight E, et al. (2012) Deep brain stimulation induces BOLD activation in motor and non-motor networks: An fMRI comparison study of STN and EN/GPi DBS in large animals. Neuroimage 63: 1408–1420.
62. Johnson MD, Vitek JL, McIntyre CC (2009) Pallidal stimulation that improves parkinsonian motor symptoms also modulates neuronal firing patterns in primary motor cortex in the MPTP-treated monkey. Exp Neurol 219: 359–362.
63. Brown P, Oliviero A, Mazzone P, Insola A, Tonali P, et al. (2001) Dopamine dependency of oscillations between subthalamic nucleus and pallidum in Parkinson's disease. J Neurosci 21: 1033–1038.
64. Williams D, Tijssen M, Van Bruggen G, Bosch A, Insola A, et al. (2002) Dopamine-dependent changes in the functional connectivity between basal ganglia and cerebral cortex in humans. Brain 125: 1558–1569.
65. Kuhn AA, Kupsch A, Schneider GH, Brown P (2006) Reduction in subthalamic 8–35 Hz oscillatory activity correlates with clinical improvement in Parkinson's disease. Eur J Neurosci 23: 1956–1960.
66. Weinberger M, Hutchison WD, Dostrovsky JO (2009) Pathological subthalamic nucleus oscillations in PD: can they be the cause of bradykinesia and akinesia? Exp Neurol 219: 58–61.
67. Sharott A, Magill PJ, Harnack D, Kupsch A, Meissner W, et al. (2005) Dopamine depletion increases the power and coherence of beta-oscillations in the cerebral cortex and subthalamic nucleus of the awake rat. Eur J Neurosci 21: 1413–1422.
68. Mallet N, Pogosyan A, Marton LF, Bolam JP, Brown P, et al. (2008) Parkinsonian beta oscillations in the external globus pallidus and their relationship with subthalamic nucleus activity. J Neurosci 28: 14245–14258.
69. Mallet N, Pogosyan A, Sharott A, Csicsvari J, Bolam JP, et al. (2008) Disrupted dopamine transmission and the emergence of exaggerated beta oscillations in subthalamic nucleus and cerebral cortex. J Neurosci 28: 4795–4806.
70. Leblois A, Meissner W, Bioulac B, Gross CE, Hansel D, et al. (2007) Late emergence of synchronized oscillatory activity in the pallidum during progressive Parkinsonism. Eur J Neurosci 26: 1701–1713.
71. Levy R, Ashby P, Hutchison WD, Lang AE, Lozano AM, et al. (2002) Dependence of subthalamic nucleus oscillations on movement and dopamine in Parkinson's disease. Brain 125: 1196–1209.
72. Courtemanche R, Fujii N, Graybiel AM (2003) Synchronous, focally modulated beta-band oscillations characterize local field potential activity in the striatum of awake behaving monkeys. J Neurosci 23: 11741–11752.
73. Crowell AL, Ryapolova-Webb ES, Ostrem JL, Galifianakis NB, Shimamoto S, et al. (2012) Oscillations in sensorimotor cortex in movement disorders: an electrocorticography study. Brain 135: 615–630.
74. Miller KJ, Leuthardt EC, Schalk G, Rao RP, Anderson NR, et al. (2007) Spectral changes in cortical surface potentials during motor movement. J Neurosci 27: 2424–2432.
75. Brucke C, Huebl J, Schonecker T, Neumann WJ, Yarrow K, et al. (2012) Scaling of movement is related to pallidal gamma oscillations in patients with dystonia. J Neurosci 32: 1008–1019.
76. Kempf F, Brucke C, Salih F, Trottenberg T, Kupsch A, et al. (2009) Gamma activity and reactivity in human thalamic local field potentials. Eur J Neurosci 29: 943–953.
77. Kempf F, Kuhn AA, Kupsch A, Brucke C, Weise L, et al. (2007) Premovement activities in the subthalamic area of patients with Parkinson's disease and their dependence on task. Eur J Neurosci 25: 3137–3145.
78. Cassidy M, Mazzone P, Oliviero A, Insola A, Tonali P, et al. (2002) Movement-related changes in synchronization in the human basal ganglia. Brain 125: 1235–1246.
79. Foffani G, Bianchi AM, Baselli G, Priori A (2005) Movement-related frequency modulation of beta oscillatory activity in the human subthalamic nucleus. J Physiol 568: 699–711.
80. Silberstein P, Kuhn AA, Kupsch A, Trottenberg T, Krauss JK, et al. (2003) Patterning of globus pallidus local field potentials differs between Parkinson's disease and dystonia. Brain 126: 2597–2608.
81. Liu X, Griffin IC, Parkin SG, Miall RC, Rowe JG, et al. (2002) Involvement of the medial pallidum in focal myoclonic dystonia: A clinical and neurophysiological case study. Mov Disord 17: 346–353.
82. Liu X, Wang S, Yianni J, Nandi D, Bain PG, et al. (2008) The sensory and motor representation of synchronized oscillations in the globus pallidus in patients with primary dystonia. Brain 131: 1562–1573.
83. Tang JK, Mahant N, Cunic D, Chen R, Moro E, et al. (2007) Changes in cortical and pallidal oscillatory activity during the execution of a sensory trick in patients with cervical dystonia. Exp Neurol 204: 845–848.
84. Chen CC, Kuhn AA, Trottenberg T, Kupsch A, Schneider GH, et al. (2006) Neuronal activity in globus pallidus interna can be synchronized to local field potential activity over 3–12 Hz in patients with dystonia. Exp Neurol 202: 480–486.
85. Weinberger M, Hutchison WD, Alavi M, Hodaie M, Lozano AM, et al. (2012) Oscillatory activity in the globus pallidus internus: comparison between Parkinson's disease and dystonia. Clin Neurophysiol 123: 358–368.
86. Chen CC, Kuhn AA, Hoffmann KT, Kupsch A, Schneider GH, et al. (2006) Oscillatory pallidal local field potential activity correlates with involuntary EMG in dystonia. Neurology 66: 418–420.
87. Sharott A, Grosse P, Kuhn AA, Salih F, Engel AK, et al. (2008) Is the synchronization between pallidal and muscle activity in primary dystonia due to peripheral afferance or a motor drive? Brain 131: 473–484.
88. Eusebio A, Thevathasan W, Doyle Gaynor L, Pogosyan A, Bye E, et al. (2011) Deep brain stimulation can suppress pathological synchronisation in parkinsonian patients. J Neurol Neurosurg Psychiatry 82: 569–573.
89. Meissner W, Leblois A, Hansel D, Bioulac B, Gross CE, et al. (2005) Subthalamic high frequency stimulation resets subthalamic firing and reduces abnormal oscillations. Brain 128: 2372–2382.
90. Kuhn AA, Kempf F, Brucke C, Gaynor Doyle L, Martinez-Torres I, et al. (2008) High-frequency stimulation of the subthalamic nucleus suppresses oscillatory beta activity in patients with Parkinson's disease in parallel with improvement in motor performance. J Neurosci 28: 6165–6173.

91. Silberstein P, Pogosyan A, Kuhn AA, Hotton G, Tisch S, et al. (2005) Cortico-cortical coupling in Parkinson's disease and its modulation by therapy. Brain 128: 1277–1291.
92. Brown P, Mazzone P, Oliviero A, Altibrandi MG, Pilato F, et al. (2004) Effects of stimulation of the subthalamic area on oscillatory pallidal activity in Parkinson's disease. Exp Neurol 188: 480–490.
93. Bronte-Stewart H, Barberini C, Koop MM, Hill BC, Henderson JM, et al. (2009) The STN beta-band profile in Parkinson's disease is stationary and shows prolonged attenuation after deep brain stimulation. Exp Neurol 215: 20–28.
94. Wingeier B, Tcheng T, Koop MM, Hill BC, Heit G, et al. (2006) Intra-operative STN DBS attenuates the prominent beta rhythm in the STN in Parkinson's disease. Exp Neurol 197: 244–251.
95. McCairn KW, Turner RS (2009) Deep brain stimulation of the globus pallidus internus in the parkinsonian primate: local entrainment and suppression of low-frequency oscillations. J Neurophysiol 101: 1941–1960.
96. Hara K, Harris RA (2002) The anesthetic mechanism of urethane: the effects on neurotransmitter-gated ion channels. Anesth Analg 94: 313–318, table of contents.
97. Maggi CA, Meli A (1986) Suitability of urethane anesthesia for physiopharmacological investigations in various systems. Part 1: General considerations. Experientia 42: 109–114.
98. Lai HY, Younce JR, Albaugh DL, Kao YC, Shih YY (2014) Functional MRI reveals frequency-dependent responses during deep brain stimulation at the subthalamic nucleus or internal globus pallidus. Neuroimage 84: 11–18.

17

Deep Brain Stimulation of the Antero-Medial Globus Pallidus Interna for Tourette Syndrome

Perminder S. Sachdev[1,2]*, Adith Mohan[1,2], Elisabeth Cannon[1], John D. Crawford[2], Paul Silberstein[3], Raymond Cook[3], Terrence Coyne[4,5], Peter A. Silburn[4,5]

1 Neuropsychiatric Institute, Prince of Wales Hospital, Randwick, NSW, Australia, **2** Centre for Healthy Brain Ageing, School of Psychiatry, The University of New South Wales, Sydney, Australia, **3** North Shore Private Hospital, St. Leonards, Sydney, NSW, Australia, **4** Centre for Clinical Research, University of Queensland, Herston, QLD, Australia, **5** St. Andrew's War Memorial Hospital, Spring Hill, QLD, Australia

Abstract

Background: We have previously reported the results of Deep Brain Stimulation (DBS) of the antero-medial globus pallidus interna (GPi) for severe Tourette Syndrome (TS) in 11 patients. We extend this case series to 17 patients and a longer follow-up to a maximum of 46 months.

Methods: 17 patients (14 male; mean age 29.1 years, range 17–51 years) with severe and medically intractable TS were implanted with Medtronic quadripolar electrodes bilaterally in the antero-medial GPi. The primary outcome measure was the Yale Global Tic Severity Scale (YGTSS). Secondary outcome measures included the Yale-Brown Obsessive Compulsive Scale, Hamilton Depression Rating Scale, Gilles de la Tourette Quality of Life Scale and Global Assessment of Functioning. Follow up was at one month, three months and finally at a mean 24.1 months (range 8–46 months) following surgery.

Results: Overall, there was a 48.3% reduction in motor tics and a 41.3% reduction in phonic tics at one month, and this improvement was maintained at final follow-up. 12 out of 17 (70.6%) patients had a>50% reduction in YGTSS score at final follow up. Only 8 patients required ongoing pharmacotherapy for tics post-surgery. Patients improved significantly on all secondary measures. Adverse consequences included lead breakage in 4 patients, infection (1), transient anxiety (2), dizziness (1), poor balance (1) and worsening of stuttering (1).

Conclusions: This case series provides further support that antero-medial GPi DBS is an effective and well tolerated treatment for a subgroup of severe TS, with benefits sustained up to 4 years.

Editor: Krystof Bankiewicz, University of California at San Francisco, United States of America

Funding: Employment: PSS and AM – University of New South Wales (UNSW) Australia & Prince of Wales Hospital; EC – Prince of Wales Hospital; JDC – UNSW Australia; PS and RC – North Shore Private Hospital; TC and PAS – University of Queensland and St. Andrew's War Memorial Hospital. Grants: PSS and AM – National Health and Medical Research Council of Australia Program Grant (no. 401162); EC – NSW Institute of Psychiatry Training Fellowship. The funders had no role in study design, data collection and analysis, decision to publish, or preparation of the manuscript.

Competing Interests: The authors have declared that no competing interests exist.

* Email: p.sachdev@unsw.edu.au

Introduction

The last decade has seen an increasing number of reports of deep brain stimulation (DBS) for the treatment of medically-intractable Tourette Syndrome (TS), with nearly 100 cases having been reported in the published literature [1–4]. Although nine different brain targets have been reported [5], the most commonly used targets have been the centromedian-parafascicular and ventralis oralis complex of the thalamus [6], and the globus pallidus interna (GPi) [7].

We recently reported an open case series of 11 TS patients who were treated with DBS of the antero-medial GPi and were followed up for a mean 14 months, with the longest follow-up periods being 30 months [8]. The study showed that the acute benefit of DBS was maintained over this follow-up period, and adverse effects were encountered in only a few patients. Since TS is a chronic disorder, the long-term outcome over many years is important to determine. In the longest follow-up reported so far in the literature, 15 patients with thalamic stimulation were followed up for 5–6 years and three patients for 3–4 years. While the overall improvement was maintained, some notable findings were that four patients had a worsening of their obsessive compulsive symptoms and two requested device removal more than 5 years after implantation. Issues with non-compliance and repeated infections were also noted, highlighting the importance of longer-term follow-up in these cases.

We report the results of an extended series of TS patients with a longer follow-up to complement our previous report. The 17 patients being reported are inclusive of the 11 reported previously.

Methods

Ethics statement: All information collected was entered into a dedicated, purpose designed data registry. The data registry is regarded as an audit activity that does not require patient consent. The Uniting Care Health Human Research Ethics Committee

(Ref. 0813) deemed that a formal ethical review was not required. This follow-up study was undertaken at St Andrew's War Memorial Hospital, Spring Hill, QLD 4000, and at the North Shore Private Hospital, St Leonards, NSW 2065, Australia.

Patients with severe, disabling and medically resistant TS were recruited from the Movement Disorders Clinic of St Andrew's War Memorial Hospital, Brisbane (n = 15) and Neuropsychiatric Institute, Sydney (n = 2). Criteria for selection for DBS have been described previously (5). A summary of individual patient characteristics is shown in Table 1.

Prior to surgery, each patient completed a series of questionnaires, including the Yale Global Tic Severity Scale (YGTSS) [9] which was the primary outcome measure. Secondary outcome measures included the Yale-Brown obsessive-compulsive Scale (Y-BOCS) [10], Hamilton Depression Rating Scale (HDRS) [11], Gilles de la Tourette Quality of Life Scale (GTS-QOL) [12] and the Global Assessment of Functioning (GAF) scale [13].

Surgeries were performed by a team comprising a psychiatrist, a neurologist and neurosurgeon, and were performed solely on the basis of clinical indication. The assessments for this paper were performed by psychiatrists who were independent of the decision to perform the surgery. Consent was obtained by the surgeon for the surgical procedure. For the rating scales and the assessment, written consent was obtained from the patient. In the case of two patients who were <18 years at the time of surgery, the consent was obtained in the presence of the mother in each case.

A Medtronic multi-programmable quadripolar deep brain stimulation system was implanted under general anesthetic using a stereotaxic procedure as described previously [5]. Each patient received either the Soletra system (Model 7426) which has a separate battery for each side, or the Activa PC/RC device (Model 37601/37612) (Medtronic, Inc, Minneapolis MN, USA) which has a single battery for both sides. Medtronic leads 3389 in cases 1–15, and 3387 in cases 16 and 17, were placed with active contacts spanning the GPi/GPe, the choice of leads reflecting the surgeon's preference.

The anatomical target was a modification of the posteroventral pallidal (PVP) target popularized by Laitinen [14]. We have described this target previously [15].

In reference to the anterior commissure/posterior commissure (AC/PC) line, the PVP target was 2 mm anterior to the midpoint of the AC/PC line, between 18–21 mm lateral to the midline and 3–5 mm below the AC/PC plane. The antero-medial pallidal target used in this series was approximately 6 mm anterior to the AC/PC midpoint and 14–17 mm lateral to the midline at the same depth as the PVP target 3–5 mmm below the AC/PC plane. With reference to the PVP target, it is approximately 4 mm anterior and 4 mm medial to this target. Indirect calculations based on the AC/PC plane or line are however only a guide as the use of 3T MRI/CT fusion is standard practice owing to the inherent variability in brain dimensions, and the real anatomical target is seen in Figure 1 as the red marker in relation to the internal pallidum and surrounding structures. Once the target is defined anatomically, microelectrode techniques are used mainly to define the inferior pallidal border. The inferior electrode (0) is placed 2 mm above the pallidal base with the remaining 3 electrodes spaced and angled 50–70 degrees in the sagittal plane with the plane of the base ring (CRW)/arc parallel to the AC/PC plane. The coronal angle is wide, varying 15–25 degrees from the midpoint of the arc. This allows for a DBS electrode trajectory from the above-defined target passing through the internal and external GPi, the GPe/GPi raphe into the external pallidum.

The Medtronic impulse generator was placed in the subclavicular region. A post-operative brain CT scan was undertaken and fused to the pre-operative MRI image to confirm correct lead positioning.

DBS stimulation was commenced in the immediate post-operative period when the patient had recovered from the propofol anesthetic and all patients were closely monitored. Initial stimulation parameters were bilateral 1.0 V, pulse width 90 μs and frequency 130 Hz with unipolar activation of the contacts most commonly 0, 1 or 2 and rarely 3. Stimulation parameters were adjusted at follow up visits depending on residual tic severity and presence of side effects. The most commonly used increments were 0.5 V every second day. The mean stimulation parameters at final follow up were amplitude 4.14 V (SD 0.63), pulse width 95.2 μs (SD 21.8) and frequency 139.4 Hz (SD 19.5). The final stimulation parameters for each of the patients are documented in Table S1 in File S1.

Patients were followed up weekly for 1 month, monthly for 3 months and then 3 monthly. Stimulation parameters were adjusted as required over the course of follow up. Rating scales were repeated at one month after surgery and at final follow up (mean: 23.4 months, range: 8–46 months). At these time points, information was obtained on any adverse effects. Assessments were performed by three authors (PSS, EC and AM) independently of the surgical teams (PSilburn, TC, PSilberstein, RC).

Data were analyzed using IBM SPSS Statistics 21 (SPSS, IBM Corp, Armonk NY, USA). The non-parametric Friedman test was used to test for the statistical significance of variation of measures across the 4 time points. Paired comparisons between measures at the pre-DBS and 3 post-DBS time points were performed using the Wilcoxon Signed-Ranks Tests. Relationships between treatment response, as evaluated by changes in the primary outcome measures derived from the YGTSS, and a number of potential predictors were evaluated. Spearman's rank-order correlations were used for continuous predictors and the Mann-Whitney U test for binary predictors. Due to multiple tests, an alpha of 0.01 was considered statistically significant.

Results

Treatment response

Out of 17, 16 (94%) patients reported having a positive response to DBS, with self-perceived reduction in tic number, severity and frequency. Defining response as >50% reduction in the Total TYGTSS score, 12 out of 17 (70.6%) patients responded to DBS, although three others also had a meaningful improvement at final follow up, as evidenced by changes in GTS-QOL and GAF scores (Table S3 in File S1).

Significant improvements were noted in all four components of the YGTSS scores, as was the case with secondary outcome measures. At final follow up 47.8% reduction in motor tics and 51.5% reduction in phonic tics were noted. In the 12 patients considered 'responders', there was greater than 50% reduction in both motor (72.5%) and phonic (60.4%) tics at final follow up. Overall, there was a reduction in the mean TYGTSS score from 81.18 before surgery to 37.12 at final follow-up representing a 54.3% reduction in total tic severity ($Z = 3.52$, $p \leq 0.001$) (see Table 2 and Tables S2 and S3 in File S1). The mean TYGTSS scores, and those for individual patients at each of the four assessment occasions, are presented in Figure 2.

Compared with changes from baseline, variation in mean scores for the four YGTSS measures across the last three occasions was much smaller, with none of the differences between the post DBS occasions being statistically significant. The decrease in the phonic tic scale at 1 month to final assessment ($Z = 1.99$, $p = 0.049$; see

Table 1. Summary of individual patient characteristics.

No.	Age	Sex	Consent	Electrode location	Follow up (mths)	Severity of illness	No. drugs tried before DBS	OCD	MD	Attentional Problems
1	27	M	Y	Bilat Gpi	28	Severe	4	Y	Y	N
2	19	F	Y	Bilat Gpi + Nac	46	very severe	6	Y	Y	Y
3	35	F	Y	Bilat Gpi	30	severe	4	Y	Y	N
4	26	F	Y	Bilat Gpi	36	severe	5	Y	N	N
5	34	M	Y	Bilat Gpi + Nac	41	Severe	4[1]	Y	Y	N
6	28	M	Y	Bilat Gpi	22	Severe	6	Y	Y	Y
7	23	M	Y	Bilat Gpi	30	Severe	3	N	N	N
8	31	M	Y	Bilat Gpi	22	Severe	4	N	N	N
9	28	M	Y	Bilat Gpi	35	Severe	4	Y	Y	N
10	39	M	Y	Bilat Gpi	20	Severe	6	Y	N	N
11	51	M	Y	Bilat Gpi	23	Severe	3	N	N	N
12	42	M	Y	Bilat Gpi	12	Severe	>3	N	N	N
13	17	M	Y	Bilat Gpi	16	very severe	6	N	Y	Y
14	19	M	Y	Bilat Gpi	9	Severe	>3	Y	N	N
15	18	M	Y	Bilat Gpi	8	Severe	>3	Y	Y	N
16	17	M	Y	Bilat Gpi	18	very severe	6	Y	N	Y
17	30	M	Y	Bilat Gpi	13	Severe	6	Y	N	N

[1]including botulinum toxin.

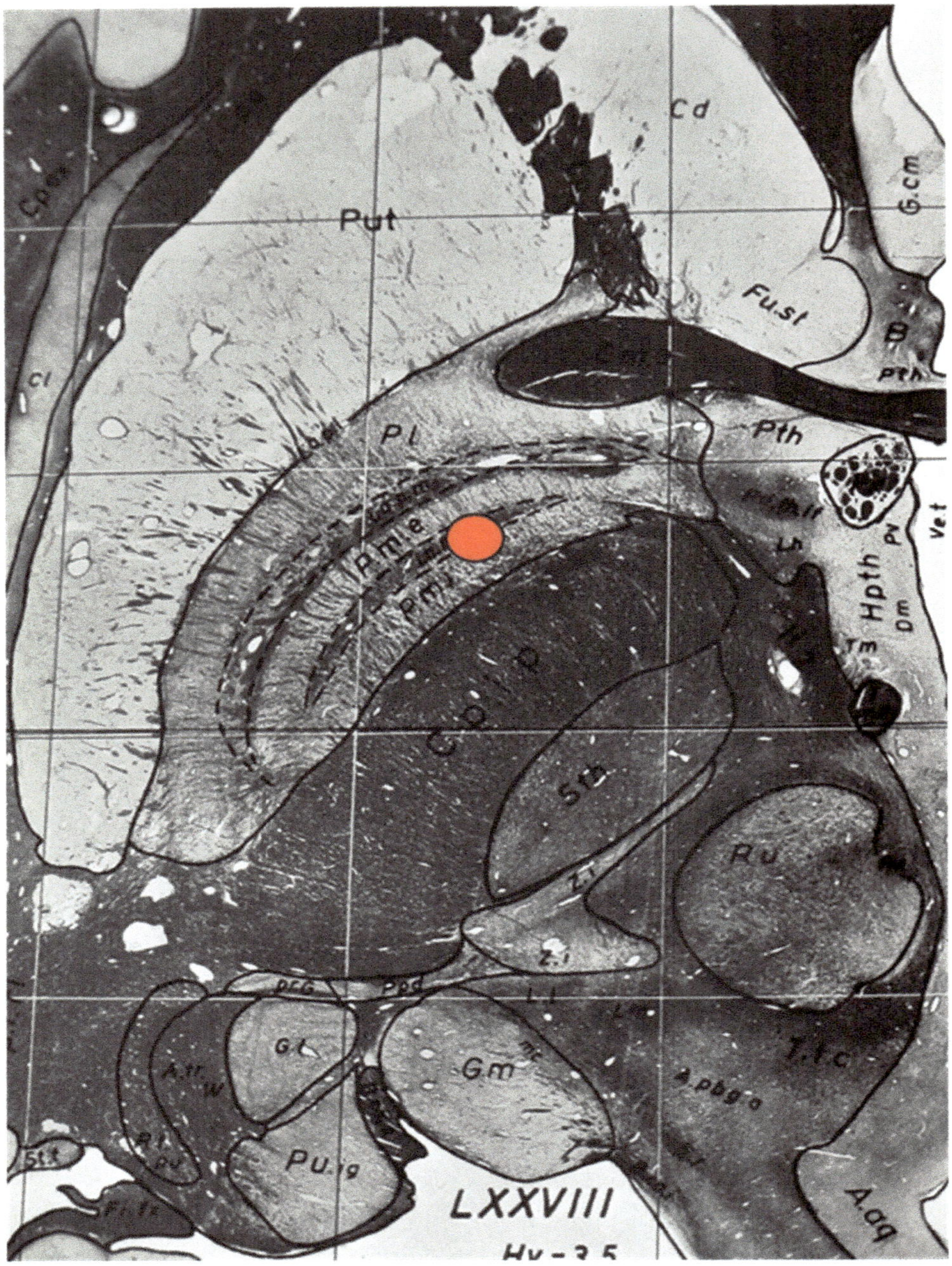

Figure 1. An image from the "Atlas for Stereotaxy of the Human Brain": Schaltenbrand and Wahren, Plate 54 [25] showing a the stimulation target as red marker overlying the anteromedial pallidum on an axial brain slice at 3.5 mm below the AC/PC line.

Table 2) was not statistically significant after correction for multiple testing ($\alpha = 0.01$).

Of the 17 patients in the study, 11 (64.7%) patients reported clinically significant obsessive compulsive symptoms prior to DBS on the Y-BOCS, which decreased from a mean score of 13.88 at pretest to 5.29 at the final assessment ($Z = 2.94$, $p = 0.001$). There was also a reduction in mean HDRS scores from 15.35 at pretest to 8.00 at the final assessment ($Z = 3.03$, $p = 0.001$). There were significant improvements between pretest and final scores in the GTS-QOL, from 40.88 to 66.47 ($Z = -3.53$, $p < 0.001$), and in GAF scale, from 50.0 to 72.12 ($Z = 3.45$, $p < 0.001$).

As with the YGTSS measures, variation across the three post-DBS occasions for the secondary measures were much smaller than between these and the pretest scores. The HDRS score increased slightly from the 3 months value of 5.07 to the final assessment score of 8.00 ($Z = 2.58$, $p = 0.007$), although the final value was still well below the pre-DBS score of 15.35. There was also a relatively small decline in the Quality of Life score from the 3 months value of 76.43 to the final assessment mean score of 66.43 ($Z = 2.51$, $p = 0.014$), although, again, the final value was still well below the pre-DBS score of 40.88.

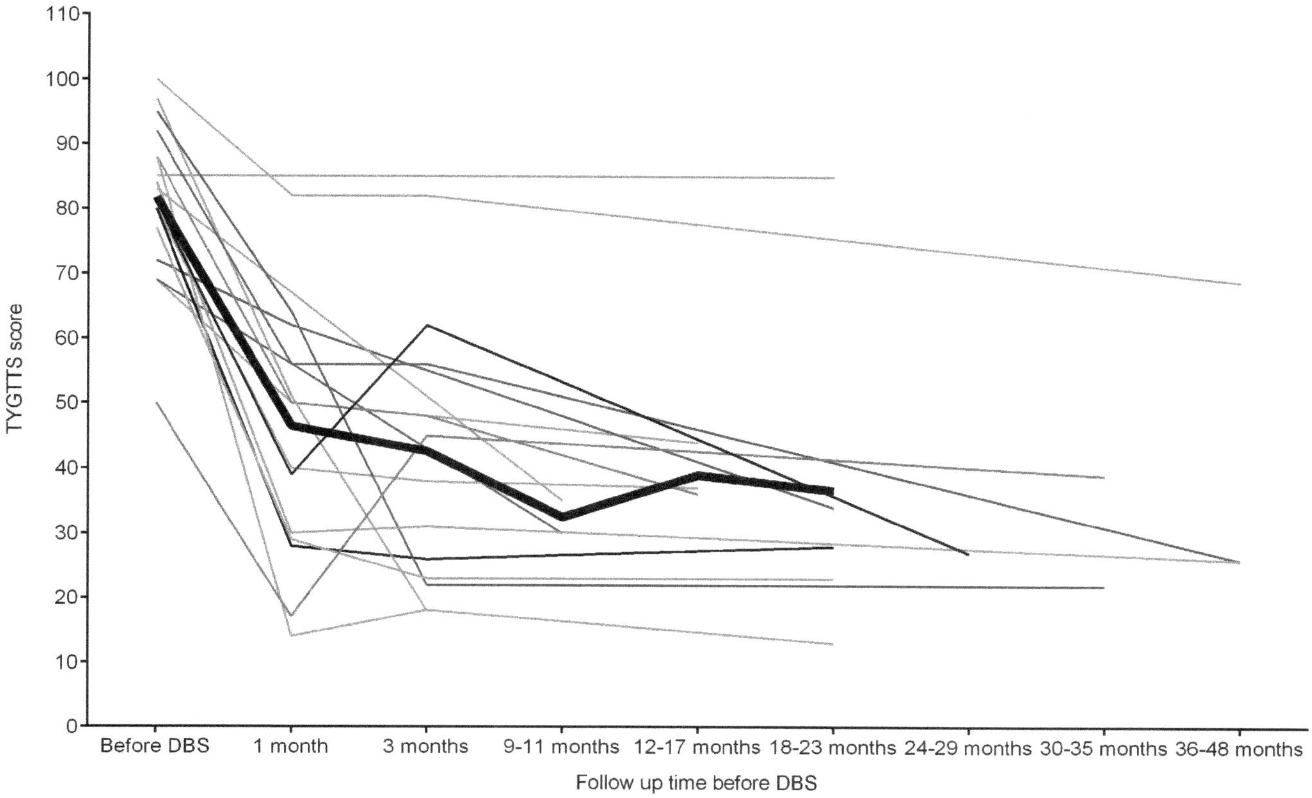

Figure 2. Change in Total Yale Global Tic Severity Score (TYGTTS) at different time points pre and post-DBS. Bold line indicates the mean of the scores. Mean scores were only displayed when more than 3 data points were present. There was a downward trend or no change in the mean scores after 23 months.

Outlying patients

Only two patients failed to gain clinically significant benefit from DBS stimulation (Patients 9 and 11). The first of these, patient 9, was in fact a treatment responder at the end of the first wave follow up period, but had a device battery failure associated with severe tic recurrence and a relapse of pre-DBS pattern of substance abuse. The consequent family discord culminated in an acute psychiatric admission. This patient had his device explanted in the aftermath of these events.

The second patient (no. 11), reported previously [5], suffered a worsening of his tics and somatic symptoms with the stimulation and elected to have it switched off at 3 months. At 51 years of age, he was the oldest patient in the cohort, and had a chronically severe condition.

Predictors of treatment response

No significant relationships were found between treatment response, as measured by change in TYGTSS score, and a number of potential predictors, which included patient characteristics shown in Table 1, and pre-DBS scores on YBOCS, HDRS, GAF and GTS_QOL. Whether the tics were primarily motor or phonic was also not a predictor of response. This was true even when using the liberal type-one error rate of 0.10.

Adverse effects

No procedure related complications were noted. The main device related adverse effect was cable breakage in 4 patients, due to a motor vehicle accident in one, an inadvertent self-inflicted blow to the chest as a complex motor tic in another, a self-injurious tic in the third, and no obvious cause in the fourth. One patient developed an infection around the leads in the neck 3 months after surgery and required bilateral lead replacement. In 3 patients, hardware malfunction resulted in interruption to stimulation during which time worsening in tic severity was the main adverse effect, with subsequent improvement once stimulation was re-established. Relapse of substance abuse and subsequent device explantation in patient 9 have been previously noted. The psychological distress experienced by patients upon cessation of stimulation following a therapeutic response, has been documented by other investigators [12].

Side effects related to stimulation itself were mostly temporary, and attenuated with adjustment of stimulation parameters. These included transient anxiety (2 patients), agitation upon stimulation of most caudal contacts (2 patients), dizziness (1 patient), poor balance (1 patient) and worsening of pre-existing stuttering (1 patient). The phenomenology of the stuttering in this last patient was of significance in that it he appeared to suffer intermittent speech arrest, manifesting as a stutter that improved to pre-operative levels with stimulation reduction. Speech dysfluency has been previously been reported as a stimulation related consequence of both pallidal [17] and subthalamic nucleus DBS [18]. Patient 11 reported worsening in tic severity with stimulation and eventually elected to have his stimulator switched off.

Table 2. Rating scale scores for 17 patients with Tourette syndrome with deep brain stimulation of the globus pallidus interna.

	BL (N = 17)	1 month (N = 15)	3 months (N = 14)	Final (N = 17)	Friedman test for overall effect of time (N = 14)	Wilcoxon Signed Ranks tests for paired comparisons, Z (p)		
	Mean (SD)	Mean (SD)	Mean (SD)	Mean (SD)	Chi Squared (d.f. = 3) (p)	1 month versus BL	3 months versus BL	Final versus BL
M	21.53 (2.58)	11.13 (6.41)	10.50 (6.54)	11.24 (5.98)	25.8 (.000)	3.30 (.000)	3.18 (.000)	3.52 (.000)
V	17.59 (4.87)	10.33^a (5.86)	8.00 (6.19)	8.53^a (5.77)	26.5 (.000)	3.24 (.000)	3.19 (.000)	3.52 (.000)
TTSS	39.12 (6.99)	21.47 (10.52)	18.43 (11.24)	19.76 (10.65)	27.2 (.000)	3.30 (.000)	3.19 (.000)	3.52 (.000)
TYGTSS	81.18 (12.32)	45.80 (20.16)	41.29 (20.92)	37.12 (19.53)	28.7 (.000)	3.30 (.000)	3.18 (.000)	3.52 (.000)
YBOCS	13.88 (11.73)	6.80 (9.14)	5.29 (8.52)	5.29 (7.07)	14.6 (.001)	2.55 (.008)	2.55 (.008)	2.94 (.001)
HDRS	15.35 (7.57)	6.60 (4.55)	5.07^b (4.20)	8.00^b (5.60)	15.8 (.001)	2.96 (.002)	2.96 (.002)	3.03 (.001)
GAF	50.00 (14.14)	76.00 (14.04)	75.71 (12.84)	72.12 (14.60)	27.7 (.000)	3.29 (.000)	3.20 (.000)	3.45 (.000)
GTS_QOL	40.88 (20.48)	72.67 (15.57)	76.43^a (16.81)	66.47^a (17.03)	32.5 (.000)	3.45 (.000)	3.32 (.000)	3.53 (.000)

M = motor tics; V = vocal/phonic tics; TTSS = Total Tic Severity Scale; TYGTSS = Total Yale Global Tic Severity Scale; YBOCS = Yale-Brown Obsessive-Compulsive Scale; HDRS = Hamilton Depression Rating Scale; GAF = Global Assessment of Functioning; GTS-QOL = Gilles de la Tourette Syndrome Quality of Life Scale.

Discussion

We present extended follow up data from a case series of patients who underwent DBS for intractable TS. In addition to the 11 patients described previously [8], we have described data on 6 more patients, making this amongst the largest series of TS patients treated with DBS of the antero-medial globus pallidus interna (GPi) from one centre. The extended duration of follow up makes it possible to comment on the time course of symptom remission in these patients and the long-term outcome of DBS.

Using a>50% reduction in the TYGTSS score as the criterion for treatment response, 12 out of 17 (70.6%) patients responded to DBS of the antero medial GPi. This was a cohort of severely to very severely affected patients with Tourette syndrome, all of whom had failed treatment with at least 3 or more pharmacological therapies. In considering the patients reported in our previous paper first [8], of the 6 patients classed as responders at a mean of 14 months after surgery (range = 4–30 months), 5 remained responders, with TYGTSS scores at second wave follow up closely resembling their earlier final follow up scores. All 5 had attained responder status between 1 and 3 months follow up. 1 patient classed as non responder in the first report (patient 1) had in fact achieved treatment responsiveness at 1 month, but had a subsequent worsening, although remaining clinically much improved relative to baseline. This patient had re-attained responder status by the time of second wave follow up as reported in this paper.

Only 1 new responder was added to this data set from the initial cohort of 11 patients (patient 5), reaching >50% TYGTSS reduction between 26 and 41 months. It is possible that this represents a propensity to delayed treatment response in a minority of these patients, though this is difficult to extrapolate from just one patient.

On the whole, our data would suggest that the time to respond to antero medial GPi DBS in this cohort is short, being between 1–3 months, and that symptomatic gains, once achieved, remain stable over time. The percentage reductions in tics were remarkably similar in both first and second waves of follow up, for both motor (48% and 47.8%) as well as phonic (54.5% and 51.5%) tics respectively. The time difference between the mean follow up durations for these two waves was about 10 months. This stability of effect on tic reduction in TS with DBS has been noted by another group as well [19], with patients continuing to show significant reduction in tic severity, and consistently requiring less medication or treatment of their TS as well as associated comorbidities over 6 years of follow up. Similarly, in long term follow up data at 3–6 years reported on by Kennedy and colleagues [20] for DBS in depression, short and long term response, and remission rates remained stable over time. Holtzheimer and colleagues made the important observation that none of their depressed patients who remitted on being treated with DBS of the subcallosal cingulate, suffered a spontaneous relapse over 2 years of follow up [16]. In a review of DBS in OCD undertaken across four centers in the United States and Europe [21], symptomatic improvements were noted to occur by 3 months on average, and to remain stable over 3 to 36 months of follow. Taken together, converging evidence appears to indicate that in DBS for refractory neuropsychiatric disorders, relatively early treatment response is to be expected in most, and in those that do respond, treatment benefit is maintained over several years.

Most importantly, stable symptom improvement in our cohort was translated in the majority of patients into substantial improvements in vocational functioning, as well as in the patient's relationships with family and friends. The wide ranging impact of

TS on sufferers is well known, and although almost all our patients continued to display clinically relevant symptomatology, it is notable that the degree of improvement noted with DBS in these patients leads to significant gains in their day to day lives. Modest gains noted on symptom rating scores, often translate into greater functional gains, reflective of the high pretreatment severity of illness in such DBS cohorts. This is reflected more accurately in the improvements noted in the quality of life, and functional status ratings of this cohort (GTS-QOL and GAF respectively) for responders and the majority of non responders alike. All but the two patients described as outliers in the results, elected to continue with stimulation in light of these improvements.

It is worthwhile noting that all 6 patients recruited into our study between the first and current time points were responders. Better outcomes with patients enrolled later in DBS trials have been conceptualized as being a 'learning effect'. This has been attributed to refinements in targeting, advances in surgical technique and better patient management including programming protocols, with similar improvements noted with patients [22] recruited over time in DBS for other movement disorders as well. Even though our surgical target remained the antero medial GPi, given inter-individual neuroanatomical variability, and small target size in TS, relative to more conventional targets in DBS for movement disorders such as PD, future work focusing on more detailed comparisons of responders and non responders in terms of final lead location within GPi, and computer modeling to predict the field of stimulation would be instructive.

The importance of long term follow data in this patient population is beginning to become increasingly apparent. In a recent report, follow up data were reported on for 15 patients at 5–6 years and 3 patients at 3–4 years who underwent thalamic DBS for refractory TS [19]. In this, the authors make note of the emergence of a number of issues over time, chief amongst these being infections, treatment discontinuation, and a concerning lack of consensus between clinician's and patient's perspectives on the extent of improvement. In our long term data by contrast, we noted consistency across clinician and patient ratings over time, and lower rates of treatment discontinuation. The adverse effect profile has differed in DBS for TS depending on the target chosen [23], which in turn affect patient compliance. The antero medial GPi in this context, appears to be a relatively safe, with comparable efficacy to thalamic targets for TS DBS.

Limitations

We, along with others [24], have previously commented on the limitations of an open study without placebo control and with non-blinded assessments. However, the long-term follow-up data further support the argument against this being a placebo response. This case series is still limited by the lack of a comparison site of stimulation, making it difficult to argue that this is indeed the optimal implantation site. Moreover, more refined analysis in terms of simulation of the anatomical region actually stimulated, and neuroimaging to understand likely mechanisms of response have not been possible in this study and will serve as objectives for future work.

Supporting Information

File S1 Table S1) Stimulation parameters for the patients at time of final assessment. **Table S2)** Individual patient Total Yale Global Tic Severity Scale scores before DBS and at final follow up. **Table S3)** Individual patient Yale-Brown Obsessive Compulsive Scale (YBOCS), Hamilton Depression Rating Scale (HDRS), and Gilles de la Tourette Quality of Life Scale (GTS-QOL) scores before DBS and at final follow up.

Acknowledgments

We thank Karen O'Maley and Lyndsey Jones for their assistance in patient management and Sophia Dean for help with manuscript preparation.

Author Contributions

Conceived and designed the experiments: PSS AM PS RC TC PAS. Performed the experiments: PSS AM EC PS RC TC PAS. Analyzed the data: PSS AM JDC. Wrote the paper: PSS AM EC.

References

1. Müller-Vahl KR (2013) Surgical treatment of Tourette syndrome. Neurosci Biobehav Rev 37: 1178–1185. doi: 10.1016/j.neubiorev.2012.09.012.
2. Massano J, Sousa C, Foltynie T, Zrinzo L, Hariz M, et al. (2013) Successful pallidal deep brain stimulation in 15-year-old with Tourette syndrome: 2-year follow-up. J Neurol 260: 2417–2419. doi: 10.1007/s00415-013-7049-1.
3. Martínez-Fernández R, Zrinzo L, Aviles-Olmos I, Hariz M, Martinez-Torres I, et al. (2011) Deep brain stimulation for Gilles de la Tourette syndrome: a case series targeting subregions of the globus pallidus internus. Mov Disord 26: 1922–1930. doi: 10.1002/mds.23734.
4. Motlagh MG, Smith ME, Landeros-Weisenberger A, Kobets AJ, King RA, et al. (2013) Lessons Learned from Open-label Deep Brain Stimulation for Tourette Syndrome: Eight Cases over 7 Years. Tremor Other Hyperkinet Mov (N Y) Nov 1;3. pii: tre-03-170-4428-1.
5. Hariz MI, Robertson M (2010) Gilles de la Tourette syndrome and deep brain stimulation. Eur J Neurosci 32: 1128–1134. doi: 10.1111/j.1460-9568.2010.07415.x.
6. Servello D, Sassi M, Brambilla A, Defendi S, Porta M (2009) Long-term, post-deep brain stimulation management of a series of 36 patients affected with refractory Gilles de al Tourette Syndrome. Neuromodulation 10: 187–194. doi: 10.1111/j.1525-1403.2009.00253.x.
7. Welter ML, Mallet L, Houeto JL, Karachi C, Czernecki V, et al. (2008) Internal pallidal and thalamic stimulation in patients with Tourette syndrome. Arch Neurol 65: 952–957. doi: 10.1001/archneur.65.7.952.
8. Cannon E, Silburn P, Coyne T, O'Maley K, Crawford JD, et al. (2012) Deep brain stimulation of anteromedial globus pallidus interna for severe Tourette syndrome. Am J Psychiatry 169: 860–866. doi: 10.1176/appi.ajp.2012.11101583.
9. Leckman J, Riddle M, Hardin M, Ort S, Swartz B, et al. (1989) The Yale Global Tic Severity Scale: Initial Testing of a Clinician-Rated Scale of Tic Severity. J Am Acad Child Adolesc Psychiatry 28: 566–573.
10. Goodman W, Price L, Rasmussen S, Mazure C, Fleischmann RL, et al. (1989) The Yale-Brown Obsessive Compulsive Scale. Arch Gen Psychiatry; 46: 1006–1011.
11. Hamilton M (1960) A rating scale for depression. J Neurol Neurosurg Psychiatry 23: 56–62.
12. Cavanna AE, Schrag A, Morley D, Orth M, Robertson MM, et al. (2008) The Gilles de la Tourette syndrome-quality of life scale (GTS-QOL): development and validation. Neurology 71: 1410–1416. doi: 10.1212/01.wnl.0000327890.02893.61.
13. Jones H, Thornicroft G, Goffey M, Dunn G (1995) A brief mental health outcome scale - reliability and validity of the Global Assessment of Functioning (GAF). Br J Psychiatry 166: 654–659.
14. Laitinen LV, Bergenheim AT, Hariz MI (1992) Ventroposterolateral pallidotomy can abolish all parkinsonian symptoms. Stereotact Func Neurosurg 58(1–4): 14–21.
15. Cook RJ, Fracchia G, Hoban P, Joffe R, O'Sullivan D (1998) Evolution of a surgical technique for posteroventral pallidotomy using CT/MR fusion and intraoperative macrostimulation. J Clin Neurosci 5: 20–27.
16. Holtzheimer PE, Kelley ME, Gross RE, Filkowski MM, Garlow SJ, et al. (2012) Subcallosal cingulate deep brain stimulation for treatment-resistant unipolar and bipolar depression. Arch Gen Psychiatry 69: 150–158. doi: 10.1001/archgenpsychiatry.2011.1456.
17. Nebel A, Reese R, Deuschl G, Mehdorn HM, Volkmann J (2009) Acquired stuttering after pallidal deep brain stimulation for dystonia. J Neural Transm 116: 167–169. doi: 10.1007/s00702-008-0173-x.
18. Toft M, Dietrichs E (2011) Aggravated stuttering following subthalamic deep brain stimulation in Parkinson's disease - two cases. BMC Neurology 11: 44. doi: 10.1186/1471-2377-11-44.
19. Porta M, Servello D, Zanaboni C, Anasetti F, Menghetti C, et al. (2012) Deep brain stimulation for treatment of refractory Tourette syndrome: long-term

follow-up. Acta Neurochir (Wien) 154: 2029–2041. doi: 10.1007/s00701-012-1497-8.
20. Kennedy M, Giacobbe P, Rizvi S, Placenza F, Nishikawa Y, et al. (2011) Deep brain stimulation for treatment-resistant depression: follow-up after 3 to 6 years. Am J Psychiatry 168: 502–510. doi: 10.1176/appi.ajp.2010.10081187.
21. Greenberg BD, Gabriels LA, Malone DA Jr, Rezai AR, Friehs GM, et al. (2010). Deep brain stimulation of the ventral internal capsule/ventral striatum for obsessive-compulsive disorder: worldwide experience. Mol Psychiatry 15: 64–79. doi: 10.1038/mp.2008.55.
22. Starr PA, Christine CW, Theodosopoulos PV, Lindsey N, Byrd D, et al. (2002) Implantation of deep brain stimulators into the subthalamic nucleus: technical approach and magnetic resonance imaging-verified lead locations. J Neurosurg 97: 370–387.
23. Ackermans L, Duits A, van der Linden C, Tijssen M, Schruers K, et al. (2011) Double-blind clinical trial of thalamic stimulation in patients with Tourette syndrome. Brain 134: 832–844. doi: 10.1093/brain/awq380.
24. Denys D, Mantione M, Figee M, van den Munckhof P, Koerselman F, et al. (2010) Deep brain stimulation of the nucleus accumbens for treatment-refractory obsessive-compulsive disorder. Arch Gen Psychiatry 67: 1061–1068. doi: 10.1001/archgenpsychiatry.2010.122.
25. Schaltenbrand G, Wahren W (1977) Atlas for stereotaxy of the human brain. Stuttgart: Thieme.

18

Interdisciplinary Approaches of Transcranial Magnetic Stimulation Applied to a Respiratory Neuronal Circuitry Model

Stéphane Vinit[1], Emilie Keomani[1], Thérèse B. Deramaudt[1,2], Victoria M. Spruance[3], Tatiana Bezdudnaya[3], Michael A. Lane[3], Marcel Bonay[1,2,4]ᘒ, Michel Petitjean[1,4]*ᘒ

1 Université de Versailles Saint-Quentin-en-Yvelines, Unité End:icap, UFR des Sciences de la Santé – Simone Veil, Montigny-le-Bretonneux, France, **2** LIA-BAHN (Laboratoire International Associé – Biologie Appliquée Handicap Neuromusculaire), CSM (Centre Scientifique de Monaco), Monaco, Monaco, **3** Drexel University College of Medicine, Department of Neurobiology and Anatomy, Philadelphia, Pennsylvania, United States of America, **4** Service de Physiologie-Explorations Fonctionnelles, Hôpital Ambroise Paré, Assistance Publique-Hôpitaux de Paris (AP-HP), Groupe Hospitalier Paris Ile-de-France Ouest, Boulogne-Billancourt, France

Abstract

Respiratory related diseases associated with the neuronal control of breathing represent life-threatening issues and to date, no effective therapeutics are available to enhance the impaired function. The aim of this study was to determine whether a preclinical respiratory model could be used for further studies to develop a non-invasive therapeutic tool applied to rat diaphragmatic neuronal circuitry. Transcranial magnetic stimulation (TMS) was performed on adult male Sprague-Dawley rats using a human figure-of-eight coil. The largest diaphragmatic motor evoked potentials (MEPdia) were recorded when the center of the coil was positioned 6 mm caudal from Bregma, involving a stimulation of respiratory supraspinal pathways. Magnetic shielding of the coil with mu metal reduced magnetic field intensities and improved focality with increased motor threshold and lower amplitude recruitment curve. Moreover, transynaptic neuroanatomical tracing with pseudorabies virus (applied to the diaphragm) suggest that connections exist between the motor cortex, the periaqueductal grey cell regions, several brainstem neurons and spinal phrenic motoneurons (distributed in the C3-4 spinal cord). These results reveal the anatomical substrate through which supraspinal stimulation can convey descending action potential volleys to the spinal motoneurons (directly or indirectly). We conclude that MEPdia following a single pulse of TMS can be successfully recorded in the rat and may be used in the assessment of respiratory supraspinal plasticity. Supraspinal non-invasive stimulations aimed to neuromodulate respiratory circuitry will enable new avenues of research into neuroplasticity and the development of therapies for respiratory dysfunction associated with neural injury and disease (e.g. spinal cord injury, amyotrophic lateral sclerosis).

Editor: Alexander Rabchevsky, University of Kentucky, United States of America

Funding: This work was supported by funding from the European Union Seventh framework Programme (FP7/2007-2013) under grant agreement No. 246556 (European project RBUCE-UP), HandiMedEx allocated by the French Public Investment Board, the Chancellerie des Universités de Paris (Legs Poix), the « Centre d'Assistance Respiratoire à Domicile d'Ile de France (CARDIF) », the « Fonds de Dotation de Recherche en Santé Respiratoire » and LVL Medical. Financial support for neuroanatomical studies was provided through internal funds awarded to Michael Lane at Drexel University – College of Medicine, Department of Neurobiology & Anatomy. The funders had no role in study design, data collection and analysis, decision to publish, or preparation of the manuscript.

Competing Interests: The financial support received from LVL Medical to the authors' laboratory is financial support for basic research without any profit. The funders had no role in our study design, data collection and analysis, decision to publish, or preparation of the manuscript.

* Email: michel.petitjean134@gmail.com

ᘒ These authors contributed equally to this work.

Introduction

There is a wide spread appreciation for developing new and powerful non-invasive strategies, particularly enhancing neural activity and neuroplasticity with the therapeutic potential of transcranial magnetic stimulation. While numerous studies have reported various effects of repetitive transcranial magnetic stimulation (rTMS) on different rat cortical and brainstem structures by increasing neuroplasticity involved molecules [1,2], the effect of rTMS on respiratory function and respiratory neuroplasticity remains unknown. Interdisciplinary synergies (neuroanatomy and electrophysiology principally) have been the first crucial step to address this gap in knowledge.

Cortical influence over respiratory neuronal control has been demonstrated in several animal preparations [3] and clinically in humans [4–6], by electrically stimulating primary motor cortex and recording motor evoked responses with diaphragmatic electromyograms. Although the precise anatomical and functional relationship between cortical and bulbar neurons remains unclear, there is some physiological evidence for a descending corticospinal pathway innervating the phrenic motoneuron pool in cat [7] and rat [8]. Transcranial magnetic stimulation (TMS) in humans has proven to be effective in the study of diaphragmatic motor evoked potential (MEP) [9–13]. This provides an easy, non-invasive and painless clinical tool for studying respiratory supraspinal pathway excitability and plasticity in response to neuromodulation techniques in humans and animals [14,15]. Recent clinical studies in healthy patients [16–18] have demonstrated that repetitive transcranial magnetic stimulation (rTMS) and transcranial direct current stimulation (tDCS) could increase or decrease diaphragmatic MEP amplitude respectively in response to a TMS single pulse. In case of respiratory neuronal disordered breathing patients such as partial tetraplegia or amyotrophic lateral sclerosis, the ability of supraspinal neuromodulation techniques, such as rTMS, to potentiate diaphragmatic output could lead to respiratory functional recovery. However, clinical studies in respiratory deficiency patients are extremely limited and having a viable, reliable and quantifiable preclinical respiratory model is dramatically needed to further understand the consequences of supraspinal neuromodulation as therapeutics. Based on the results from these human studies, the aim of the present work was 1) to demonstrate the suitability of these stimulation techniques to the supraspinal respiratory pathways of adult rats and 2) to determine whether TMS represents a therapeutic strategy for enhancing diaphragmatic motor activity and neuroplasticity in preclinical models aimed to mimic various human respiratory insufficiencies.

Materials and Methods

Ethics statement

All experiments reported in this manuscript conformed to policies laid out by the National Institutes of Health (USA) in the Guide for the Care and Use of Laboratory Animals. The majority of these experiments were performed on 2 month-old male Sprague–Dawley rats (Janvier, France). The animals were dual-housed in individually ventilated cages in a state-of-the-art animal care facility (2CARE animal facility, accreditation A78-322-3, France), with access to food and water *ad libitum* with a 12 h light/dark cycle. These experiments were approved by the Ethics committee of the RBUCE-UP chair of Excellence (University of Paris-Sud, grant agreement No. 246556) and the University of Versailles Saint-Quentin-en-Yvelines. Neuroanatomical tracing was performed at Drexel University, College of Medicine (Philadelphia, USA) using male and female adult Sprague-Dawley rats (purchased from Harlan Laboratories). Tracing studies were also conducted with Institutional Animal Care and Use Committee (Drexel University) approval. This manuscript has been prepared in accordance with ARRIVE guidelines.

Transcranial magnetic stimulation (TMS)

TMS was performed using a magnetic stimulator MAGPRO X100 (Magventure, Farum, Denmark) connected to a figure-of-eight coil (CB60; dimensions: 165×85×20 mm) delivering a unique biphasic pulse (380 µs in duration) with an intensity of the stimulus expressed as a percentage of maximum output of the stimulator (% MO), from 60 to 100% MO in this study. Magnetic shielding was established by inserting a 2 mm thick plate of Mu-METAL (Magnetic Shield Corp, Bensenville, IL, USA) designed by MecaMagnetic (Amilly, France) (85 mm×165 mm), with a 30×30 mm centered open window, between the coil and the animals scalp (group labeled "Shielded" in the figure). MuMETAL is an alloy patented and distributed worldwide by Magnetic Shield Corp (Bensenville, IL, USA). MuMETAL is made with Nickel (80%), Iron (15%) and Molybdene (5%) (MECAMAGNETIC, Amilly, France). The total size corresponds to the coil dimensions. The "Unshielded" group throughout the manuscript refers to the use of the coil without magnetic shielding.

Magnetic field quantification

Mapping of the magnetic field intensities was done to evaluate the influence of magnetic field shape over the coil relative to the rat central nervous system structures, and the effect of a magnetic shielding with a centered open window. Single magnetic pulses were recorded using a solenoid (Magprobe, Magventure, Farum, Denmark). The solenoid is a 2.5 cm diameter copper coil converting a magnetic field into a measurable electrical current (in Volts). The solenoid was placed as close as possible to the CB60 coil (570 different points of recording, 30×19 matrix) in all three dimensional directions of the magnetic field (x, y and z axes). The induced electrical current for each direction (x, y and z) was recorded by using the Powerlab device and the LabChart 7 Pro software (AD Instrument). The whole magnetic field recorded with the solenoid was calculated using the following formula: $\sqrt{(x^2+y^2+z^2)}$. Each dimension of the electrical field induced in the solenoid was reconstructed in 3D with a 2D Z-axis projection (Sigmaplot 12.5 software).

Electrophysiological recordings

A total of 20 animals were used for terminal electrophysiological assessment, randomly divided into those that received a single pulse of TMS with magnetic shielding on the stimulating coil ("Shielded, n = 9) and those that have no shield on it ("Unshielded", n = 11). Each animal received about 100 TMS single pulses throughout the different experimental conditions. Interpulse duration was always above 10 s to avoid low frequency repetitive TMS like effects known to induce neuroplasticity and dramatically reduce motor excitability [14,15]. As described previously [19], anesthesia was induced using isoflurane (100% O_2 balanced). A 25 G catheter was placed in the tail vein, then the rats were tracheotomized and pump ventilated (Rodent Ventilator, model 683; Harvard Apparatus, South Natick, MA, USA). The ventilation rate was adjusted to maintain the animal below its central apneic threshold throughout the experiment. $EtCO_2$ was monitored using an infrared capnograph (Viamed, VM-2500-M). Anesthesia was maintained using isoflurane (3.5% in 21% O_2, continuously monitored by an oxygen sensor (Viamed, AX300). Animals were placed on a heating pad to maintain a constant body temperature and rectal temperature was monitored throughout the experiment. A catheter was inserted in the right femoral artery to measure arterial pressure. Arterial and tracheal pressures were monitored continuously with transducers connected to a bridge amplifier (AD Instruments). Isoflurane anesthesia was then slowly converted to urethane anesthesia (1.8 g/kg, i.v.; Sigma-Aldrich). A single dose of urethane is sufficient to keep the animal deeply anesthetized throughout the experiment. The depth of anesthesia was confirmed by the absence of any response to toe pinch. A laparotomy was performed, and the liver was gently moved caudally to access the diaphragm. Gauze soaked with warm buffered saline was placed on the liver to prevent dehydration.

A custom-made silver bipolar electrode was placed on the right mid-costal part of the diaphragm. Diaphragm EMG and motor evoked potential induced by a single pulse of TMS (MEPdia) were amplified (gain, 1 k; A-M Systems, Everett, WA, USA) and band pass-filtered (100 Hz to 10 kHz). The signal was digitized with an 8-channel Powerlab data acquisition device (Acquisition rate: 100 k/s; AD Instruments) connected to a computer. The data was recorded and analyzed using LabChart 7 Pro software (AD Instruments). The head of the animal was placed on a non-magnetic custom-made stereotaxic apparatus which allowed moving the head of the animal from the center of the figure-of-eight coil along rostro-caudal axis and rotational positions in line with previous publications [9,20–24]. At the end of the study, a bilateral vagotomy followed by a paralytic agent (gallamine trietiodide, 1 mg, Sigma, n = 8, 4 from each group) or a complete transection of the spinal cord at the C2 level (n = 8, 4 from each group) were performed on all animals. At the end of the experiment (around 3 hours of anesthesia), the animal is euthanized with an i.v. overdose of urethane.

Neuroanatomical Tracing

A total of 8 adult Sprague Dawley rats (n = 4 female; n = 4 male) were used for transneuronal retrograde tracing studies to determine the distribution of neurons throughout the brain and brainstem that are associated with the phrenic circuitry. While female rats have been used for previous similar transneuronal tracing studies [25,26], the present study used males also to be consistent with those animals used for TMS and ensure there were no gender-specific differences in underlying circuitry. As previously described [25], animals were surgical anesthetized and received a laparotomy to expose the peritoneal surface of the diaphragm. The transneuronal tracer pseudorabies virus (PRV614, 2.0×10^8 pfu) was topically applied to the entire surface of the left hemi-diaphragm. Musculature and skin were then sutured and closed with wound clips, respectively. Animals were given lactated Ringer's solution (5 ml subcutaneous) to prevent dehydration, Yohimbine (1.2 mg/kg subcutaneous) as a xylazine reversal agent, and buprenorphine (0.05 mg/kg subcutaneous) for pain relief.

Histology and Microscopy

Seventy two hours following PRV-delivery, animals used for neuroanatomical tracing were euthanized with either Beuthanasia (n = 4; 9:1, sodium pentobarbitone to phenytoin solution; 0.45 ml i.p.) or Euthasol (n = 4; 0.5 ml i.p.). Tissues were then intracardially perfuse-fixed with paraformaldehyde (4% w/v in 0.1 M phosphate buffered saline (PBS), pH ~7.4). Spinal cord and brain tissue was dissected and post-fixed by immersion in paraformaldehyde (4%). Brain, brainstem and cervical spinal cord tissues were cryoprotected (sucrose, 30% w/v in 0.1 M PBS) and frozen. Transverse sections (Cryostat, 40 micron thick) were made throughout the entire brain, brainstem and upper cervical spinal cord. Every section was immunolabeled with primary antibodies for PRV (Rabbit anti-PRV (Rb134) - raised against whole, purified PRV particles that were acetone inactivated; provided by Dr. Lynn Enquist, Princeton University, as a service of the National Center for Experimental Neuroanatomy with Neurotropic Viruses: NCRR P40 RRO118604). Prior to immunohistochemical methods, floating sections were washed in PBS (0.1 M (pH = 7.4), 3×5 min), blocked against endogenous peroxidase activity (30% methanol, 0.6% hydrogen peroxide in 0.1 M PBS, incubated for 1 h), re-washed in PBS and blocked against non-specific protein labeling (10% serum in 0.1 M PBS with 0.03% Triton-X, incubated for 1 h). Tissue was then incubated in Rb134 at 4°C overnight. The following day, sections were washed (3×PBS), incubated in secondary antibodies (biotinylated donkey anti-rabbit, Jackson Immunocytochemicals; 1:200) for 2 hours at room temperature, and washed again (3×PBS). Finally, sections were incubated in a Vectastain ABC solution (2 hours at room temperature), washed (3×PBS) and processed for DAB reactivity. Labeled sections were washed, slide mounted, counterstained with cresyl violet and coverslipped. Sections were examined using a Zeiss AxioImager M2 with motorized stage and images captured using an AxioCam HRc (high resolution, color digital camera) and Zen Pro 2012 software on a PC computer. For images taken with a 40x objective, Z-stacks were created (10–13 images, ~1.0 micrometer apart) and processed for extended depth of focus images.

Data processing

A minimal average of 5 MEPdia for each condition was calculated with LabChart Pro software (AD Instruments). The peak-to-peak amplitude of the first negative wave (N1) of each averaged MEPdia were measured. MEP latency was defined as the first electrical (positive or negative) deviation following the magnetic pulse artefact. Given that MEP onset latency can be difficult to determine, the first negative peak latency was also used (as has been described previously in rodent TMS studies [27]).

Normality of data distribution was assessed using a Kolmogorov-Smirnoff test and log transformation was performed if necessary. Two way ANOVA with Bonferonni correction for multiple comparisons were performed between animal's groups followed by post-hoc Student t-test. A Student paired t-test was performed to demonstrate the effect of magnetic shielding. All the data are presented as mean ± one SEM. A test was considered significant if $p<0.05$.

Results

Effect of magnetic shield on the magnetic field generated by the TMS coil

The entire recorded magnetic field is located in the center of the coil without the magnetic shield, with two hot spots located in the middle of the two holes of the figure-of-eight (represented in red, Figure 1A). The magnetic field is statistically reduced by 32% with shielding (average "Unshielded" = 5.76±0.1 V, average "Shielded" = 3.89±0.06 V, $p<0.001$, paired t-test; Figure 1A and 1B) and focused in the center of the 30×30 mm window (Figure 1B). All the 3 dimensional x, y and z of the magnetic field are statistically reduced in presence of the magnetic shield (average "Unshielded" in x = 3±0.09 V, average "Shielded" in x = 2.03±0.06 V, reduction of 32%, $p<0.001$, paired t-test; average "Unshielded" in y = 2.74±0.07 V, average "Shielded" in y = 1.78±0.04 V, reduction of 35%, $p<0.001$, paired t-test; average "Unshielded" in z = 2.75±0.11 V, average "Shielded" in z = 2.07±0.07 V, reduction of 24%, $p<0.001$, paired t-test).

Physiological effect of a single magnetic pulse on the diaphragmatic motor evoked response (MEPdia)

No statistical differences were observed in physiological parameters (body weight, body temperature, $EtCO_2$, blood pressure) between treatment groups ("Unshielded" vs. "Shielded"; Table 1). A single pulse of magnetic stimulation at different locations of the brain and spinal cord (Figure 2A) induced different MEPdia depending on the origin of the stimulus. A stimulation (100% MO for the "Shielded" group; 85% MO for the "Unshielded" group, representing 140% of resting motor threshold (MT) value in each condition) applied at the C1 spinal cord, 12 and 6 mm caudal to Bregma (−12 and −6), at Bregma, and 6 mm rostral to Bregma (+6) locations, induced an observable MEPdia whereas a stimulation of the snout did not induce a detectable MEPdia in either group (Figure 2B and 2C).

The magnetic shield does not affect the presence/absence of the MEPdia. However, it statistically reduced the amplitude of MEPdia for the stimulation at −12 mm caudal to Bregma ("Unshielded": 2.49±0.48 μV compared to "Shielded": 1.11±0.26 μV, p = 0.04; Figure 2D) and for the stimulation of the upper cervical spinal cord (C1; "Unshielded": 5.95±1.34 μV compared to "Shielded": 2.15±0.51 μV, p = 0.045; Figure 2D). No statistical differences were observed on the MEPdia amplitude

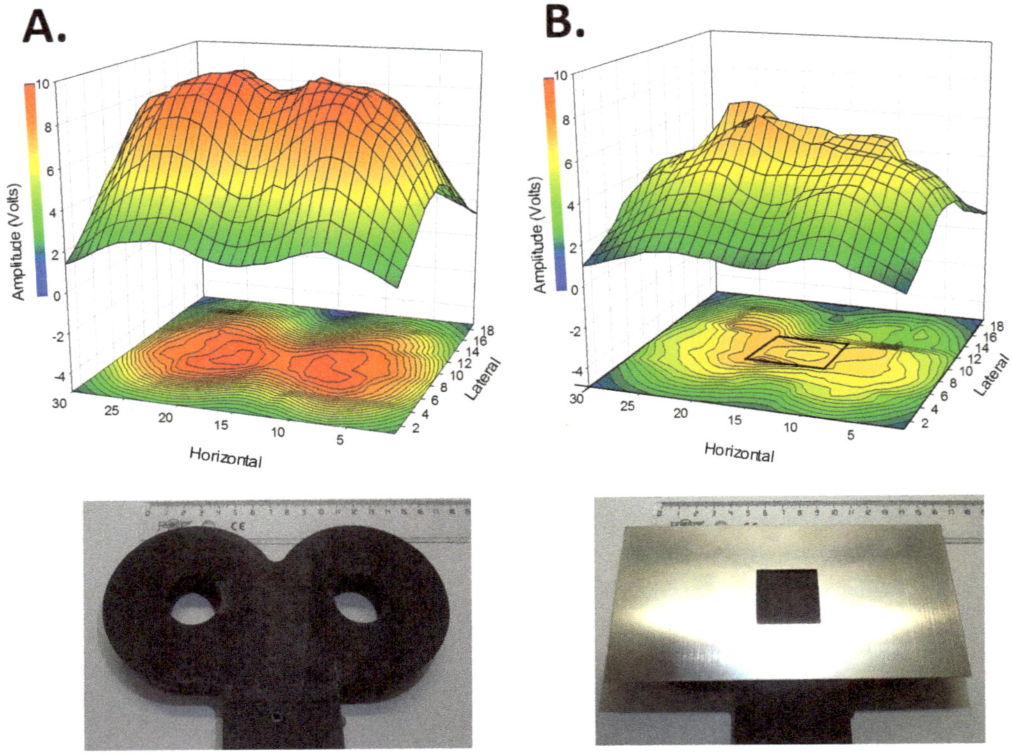

Figure 1. Effect of magnetic shield on the induced magnetic field intensity from the TMS coil. A) 3D representation and its 2D projection (bottom of the graph) of the whole magnetic field intensity (represented as intensity colors) recorded in volts with the solenoid from the "Unshielded" TMS coil. Picture at the bottom represents the coil. B) 3D representation and its 2D projection (bottom of the graph) of the whole magnetic field intensity (represented as intensity colors) recorded with the shield on the TMS coil (Noted as "Shielded"). Picture at the bottom represents the coil with the shield on it with the 30×30 mm window. Note that black square in the 2D projection representing the 3×3 cm window. The intensity is statistically reduced by 32% ($p<0.001$) compared to the one obtained in the "Unshielded" coil, and better concentrated where the rat head will be placed on (Middle of the window). Horizontal and Lateral scale represent the side of the coil, which each measured point represents half centimeter.

for the stimulation at −6 mm from Bregma ("Unshielded": 1.23±0.36 µV compared to "Shielded": 0.62±0.06 µV, $p=0.751$; Figure 2D), at Bregma ("Unshielded": 0.67±0.19 µV compared to "Shielded": 0.74±0.24 µV, $p=0.597$; Figure 2D) and +6 mm rostral to Bregma ("Unshielded": 0.27±0.05 µV compared to "Shielded": 0.47±0.09 µV, $p=0.102$; Figure 2D).

The magnetic shield significantly increased the latency of the recorded MEPdia for the stimulation at C1 location ("Unshielded": 7.84±0.98 ms compared to "Shielded": 11.07±0.86 ms, $p=0.009$; Figure 2E), −12 mm to Bregma ("Unshielded": 7.71±0.81 ms compared to "Shielded": 10.58±0.77 ms, $p=0.031$; Figure 2E) and +6 mm to Bregma ("Unshielded": 6.36±0.39 ms compared to "Shielded": 9.59±0.82 ms, $p=0.003$; Figure 2E). No significant differences in the latency of the MEPdia are observed for the stimulation at Bregma location ("Unshielded": 7.71±0.79 ms compared to "Shielded": 9.42±1.14 ms, $p=0.161$; Figure 2E) and −6 mm to Bregma ("Unshielded": 9±0.77 ms compared to "Shielded": 10.41±0.83 ms, $p=0.252$; Figure 2E). However, no difference in MEPdia latency was observed between groups "Unshielded" and "Shielded" at the different locations of the stimuli ($p>0.05$; Figure 2E).

The amplitude of the MEPdia was dependent on the stimulus intensity of the magnetic stimulator (expressed as % of maximum output (MO)). The MEPdia starts to be recorded at a resting motor threshold (MT), namely the stimulus intensity of around 70% MO in both groups ("Unshielded" Figure 3A; "Shielded" Figure 3B) at −6 mm from Bregma's stimulation site. The amplitude of the observed MEPdia increases with the stimulus intensity in both "Unshielded" and "Shielded" groups (Figure 3A and 3B respectively). Quantitatively, the MEPdia amplitudes for the "Unshielded" group (Figure 3C, black circles) follow a S-shape curve, with a plateau at a stimulus intensity of 85% MO, whereas, for the "Shielded" group (black x), a plateau is not yet reached at the stimulus of 100% MO (MEPdia amplitude at 95% MO = 4.9±0.2 µV compared to 100% MO = 8.1±1.0 µV, $p<0.05$). A statistical difference in MEPdia amplitudes was observed between groups, starting from 80% MO up to 100% MO ($p<0.05$). The stimulus intensities do not have any statistical effects ($p>0.05$) on the MEPdia latency in each group or between groups (Figure 3D) at −6 mm from Bregma.

Moreover, the orientation of the coil also plays a role in the amplitude, shape and latency of the MEPdia recordings after occipital cortex stimulation (Figure 4). When the coil is at 0°, the figure-of-eight is perpendicular to the rostrocaudal axis of the animals head (See figure 4). The amplitude of the MEPdia in the "Unshielded" group varies with the coil orientation, with a maximum amplitude at +90° and −90° (Figure 4A, the figure-of-eight is in-line with the rostrocaudal axis). This correlates with the shape of the magnetic field (Figure 1A) where the maximal field intensity (in red) is represented in both holes of the eight-shape

Table 1. Physiological parameters.

Treatment Group	Body weight (g)		Temperature (°C)		$EtCO_2$ (mmHg)		MAP Start (mmHg)		MAP End (mmHg)	
	Mean	SEM	Mean	SEM	Mean	SEM	Mean	SEM	Mean	SEM
No permalloy	339	16	37.3	0.2	38.8	0.8	108	4	111	5
3×3 cm permalloy	327	21	36.9	0.1	38	1.8	90	5	93	5

coil. A similar tendency is also observed in the "Shielded" group with an evident reduction in MEPdia amplitude (Figure 4B).

Distribution of neurons associated with the phrenic circuitry in the rat model

Transynaptic PRV tracing of spinal and supraspinal neurons associated with the diaphragm on one side provided an insight into those cells that can be stimulated by TMS. The number of labelled cells were not quantified in these tracing experiments as they were intended only to provide a map of the distribution of labelled cells.

PRV-positive interneurons in the upper cervical (C1) spinal cord were primarily detected bilaterally in laminae 7 and 10, with fewer cells seen also seen in laminae 1, 5 and 8 (see Figure 5). Within the brainstem (Figure 5D, 5H), PRV-labeled neurons were observed in the following regions: serotonergic nuclei (raphe obscuris (ROb); raphe pallidus (RPa); group B5 serotonergic cells), reticular nuclei (gigantocellular (Gi); ventral gigantocellular (GiV); lateral paragigantocellular (LPGi); rostroventrolateral (RVL), the epifascicular nucleus (EF), nucleus of the solitary tract (or nucleus tractus solitarius (NTS) which forms the 'dorsal respiratory group'), and the ventral respiratory column (VRC; comprised of the rostral and caudal ventral respiratory groups, the pre-Bötzinger and Bötzinger complexes, the retrotrapezoid nucleus and the parafacial respiratory group). Examining tissue more rostrally (~9 mm caudal of Bregma) also revealed labelling in the periaqueductal grey matter (lateral (LPAG), ventrolateral and dorsomedial, tegmental nuclei, the dorsal aspect of the subcoeruleus and the Kölliker-Fuse nucleus. Around 6 mm caudal of Bregma (Figure 5C, 5G), PRV-positive neurons were seen within the periaqueductal grey matter, the rubral and pararubral nuclei (or Red nuclei, PaR and R) and the Edinger-Westphal nucleus. Another millimetre more rostrally labeled neurons were seen in the lateral hypothalamic area (LH), the reticular aspect of the substantia nigra (SNR), pre-commissural nucleus (PrC) and the ventral part of zona incerta (ZIV). At approximately the level of Bregma, PRV-labeled neurons were seen in the periventricular and paraventricular and hypothalamic nuclei, and the primary (M1) and secondary (M2) motor cortex (Figure 5B). No PRV-positive neurons were detected rostral to those seen in the motor cortex (~1.5 to 0.0 mm rostral of Bregma).

Early neuronal PRV infection is usually indicated by PRV within the nucleus and cytoplasm, with limited dendritic labelling (Figure 5, inset in G). During later stages of infection PRV is detectable through neuronal dendrites and may be seen in surrounding glia that take up viral particles at synapses (Figure 5, inset in F and H). Final stages of PRV-infection are marked by neuronal pathology associated with cell death, as the cell is compromised by long-term infection (Figure 5, inset in H).

Specificity of the recorded diaphragmatic motor evoked potential

A single magnetic stimulation at −6 mm from the Bregma induced an observable MEPdia before vagotomy in both groups (Figure 6A "Unshielded" and 6B "Shielded"). A bilateral vagotomy did not affect the amplitude of the recorded MEPdia in either the "Unshielded" (before vagotomy: 7.4±1.7 μV, after vagotomy: 8.4±2.4 μV, $p = 0.25$; Figure 6C) or "Shielded" groups (before vagotomy: 5.9±1.2 μV, after vagotomy: 4.5±0.4 μV, $p = 0.36$; Figure 6C). No difference in latency was observed (data not shown). However, an injection of a paralytic agent (gallamine trietiodide) abolished the MEPdia in both "Unshielded" (after vagotomy: 8.4±2.4 μV, after muscular paralysis: 0.3±0.08 μV, $p = 0.018$) and "Shielded" (after vagotomy: 4.5±0.4 μV, after

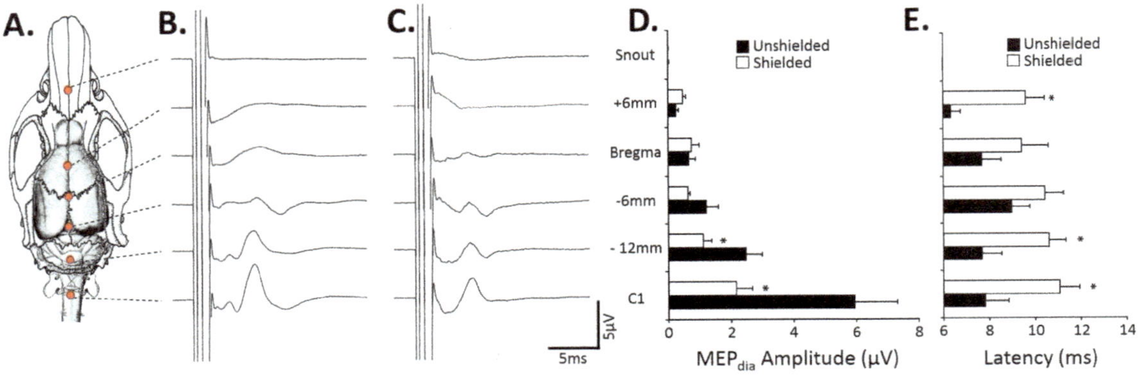

Figure 2. Antero-posterior stimulation with a single TMS pulse on the amplitude and latency of the observed MEPdia. A) Representation of the different stimulated sites on a rat brain skull with a schematic representation of the rat brain and upper spinal cord. B) Representative MEPdia induced with a single stimulation using the "Unshielded" coil from different rostro-caudal stimulation sites. C) Representative MEPdia induced with a single stimulation using the "Shielded" coil from different rostro-caudal stimulation sites. D) Histogram of the MEPdia amplitudes (in μV) from the different rostro-caudal stimulated position with "Shielded" (white) and "Unshielded" (black) coil in all animals. E) Histogram of the MEPdia latencies (in ms) from the different rostro-caudal stimulated positions with "Shielded" (white) and "Unshielded" (black) coil in all animals. *: $p<0.05$.

muscular paralysis: 0.03±0.1 μV, p = 0.001) groups (Figure 6C). Magnetic stimulations at −6 mm from Bregma (100% MO) and the C1 spinal cord evoked a MEPdia in the "Unshielded" group (Figure 7A). However, a complete transection of the cervical spinal cord at the C2 level abolished the observable MEPdia after stimulation at −6 mm from Bregma. In contrast, the observable MEPdia is enhanced following a C1 spinal cord magnetic stimulation (Figure 7B). Similar results for all the animals are observed in the "Shielded" group (data not shown).

Discussion

This study represents the first demonstration of diaphragmatic motor response to TMS in adult rat and provides a rationale for the use of TMS in animal studies of respiratory neuroplasticity. While preliminary in nature, these results support the feasibility of using TMS to study respiratory dysfunction associated with neurological injury and disease. In addition, we predict that these experiments will enable new avenues of research into the development of therapeutic strategies to treat respiratory dysfunction.

Previous studies in rat have demonstrated that limb muscle MEPs could be induced by figure-of-eight coil and suggested that pyramidal tract cells were recruited [27–30]. Although fore-and hind-limb muscle MEP have been described in awake animals [29], most studies were carried out in anesthetized rats. Most anesthetics are known to reduce or abolish MEP, although propofol [27,28], ketamine [31], pentobarbital [30] and anesthetics cocktail with urethane [31] have been successfully used in some rat strains (Wistar, Long-Evans). In the present study, urethane anesthesia in Sprague-Dawley rats did not abolish MEPdia evoked by TMS. Moreover, vital physiological signs (e.g. Table 1) were constant all through the experiments and blood pressure was similar to that previously published [19,32]. Nevertheless, several technical and physiological features have to be discussed regarding i) the use of a magnetic stimulator connected to a large figure-of-eight coil usually used in humans and ii) the specificity those pathways that are stimulated.

Besides testing the feasibility of evoking a diaphragmatic MEP in rat with a conventional magnetic stimulator, we also tested the influence of magnetic shielding designed to focalize or improve the efficiency of the magnetic field over specific brain regions to more selectively depolarize supraspinal cells associated with the phrenic system. The use of magnetic shield has been reported previously in cats [33], suggesting that the focality and the efficiency of the magnetic field was significantly improved while using it, with lower resting motor threshold values and increased MEP amplitude in the flexor carpi radialis. In contrast, the results from the present work using rats with a much smaller brain relative to the coil size show an increase in resting motor threshold with shielding. Physical measurements demonstrate that the focality of magnetic field density is slightly improved by the shield in the middle of the coil surface whereas the intensity is then globally reduced. These results may partly explain why the "Shielded" recruitment curve in figure 4 looks very different from that seen in the "Unshielded" group. Moreover, a recent paper have been shown that it is possible to lateralize the MEP responses in the rat forelimb [30], suggesting that the magnetic field is concentrated enough to stimulate primary motor cortex individually from the two hemispheres.

It is worth noting that the diaphragmatic resting motor threshold values obtained in our experiments are almost in the same range as the ones observed in rat limb muscles [27,31] as well as in humans in more recent published studies [17,34]. Moreover, there is an increase of about 10% of resting motor threshold value by adding the magnetic shield, as was reported with the same size shield in cats [33]. By increasing stimulation intensities, there is an obvious recruitment effect, implying that the magnetic field at the center of the coil is high enough to recruit the most excitable supraspinal cells, which are then able to depolarize phrenic motoneurons. However, shielding seems to limit the effect of ectopic stimulation of extra-cortical cell populations as the recruitment curve in animals with shielded TMS displayed a continuous increase up to a plateau of MEPdia, whereas the "Unshielded" recruitment curve exhibits an upward shift as stimulation intensity reaches a threshold value of 80% MO. In addition, stimulation above 80% MO resulted in an increase in SEM amplitude values, suggesting that a first recruitment mode has changed. With this in mind, given the relatively small region of the rat primary motor cortex area devoted to respiration (compared to the muscles of the extremities [35]) shielded TMS

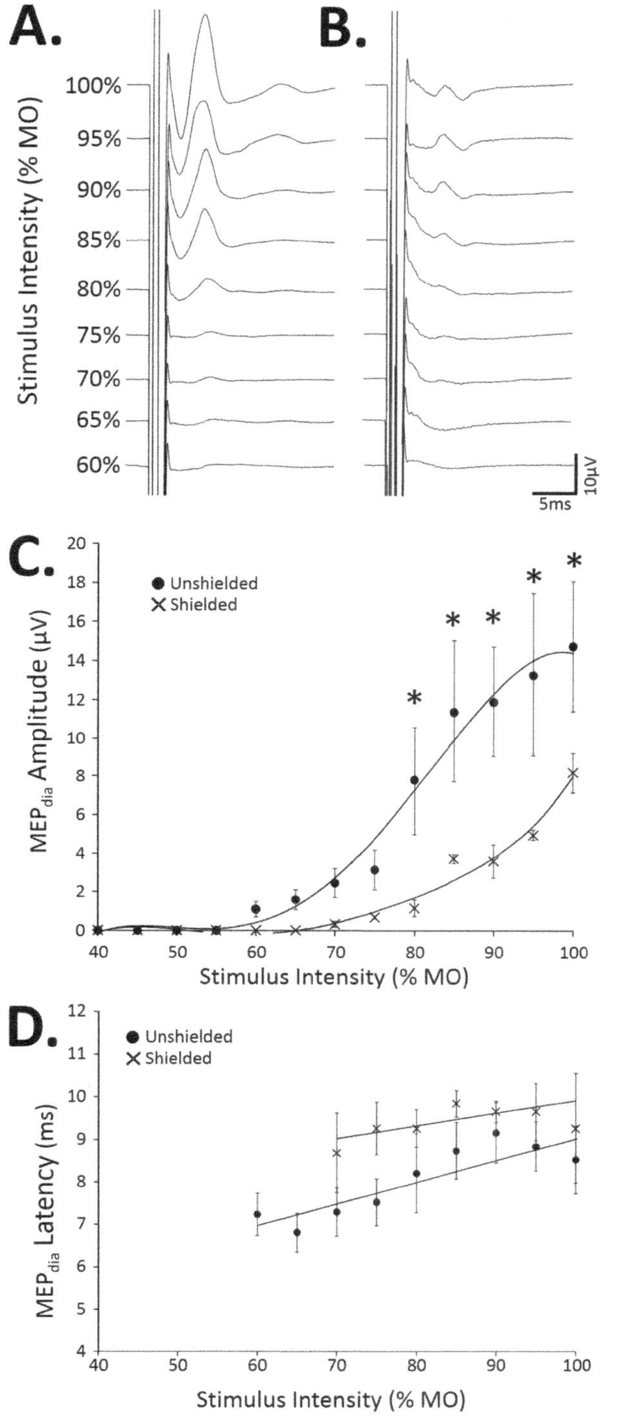

Figure 3. Effect of the stimulus intensity on the MEPdia following a single TMS at −6 mm from Bregma. A) Representative MEPdia obtained with different stimulus intensities (60 to 100% MO) using the "Unshielded" coil. B) Representative MEPdia obtained with different stimulus intensities (60 to 100% MO) using the "Shielded" coil. C) Correlation between MEPdia amplitude (in μV) and stimulus intensity (% MO) for the animals stimulated in "Unshielded" (black circles) or "Shielded" (black x) coil. D) Correlation between MEPdia latency (in ms) and stimulus intensity (% MO) for the animals stimulated with the "Unshielded" (black circles) or "Shielded" (black x) coil. MO: Maximal output; *: $p<0.05$.

is necessary to limit stimulation at the peripheral regions of the coil and the recruitment of extra cortical excitable cells.

Even with shielded TMS, the possibility that neurons ventral to the cortical layers are stimulated cannot be ruled out. For instance, it is likely that neurons within the periaqueducal grey matter (PAG) which are also shown to be associated with phrenic circuitry (transynaptically labelled with PRV), were stimulated in the present study when the coil was positioned over the occipital cortex (~6 mm caudal to Bregma). For this reason, it was essential to map the distribution of cells throughout the brain and brainstem that are in some way associated with spinal phrenic neurons. Transynaptic tracing was employed to address this for the preliminary needs of the present study, but further work is needed to quantify the number of labelled neurons within each anatomical region, elucidate the connectivity between each nucleus of cells and assess whether cells within each region have excitatory or inhibitory functions. The distribution of cells outlined in the present work is consistent with previous reports of supraspinal neurons involved with phrenic circuitry [36].

Based on the labelling of neurons within the PAG, it is worth noting electrical stimulation of the neurons within this region in rat has been reported to increase breathing frequency and increase the amplitude of respiratory muscle contraction [37]. Consistent with these previous findings, the results from the present work show that TMS in the region of the PAG can alter respiratory output. This therefore supports the rationale for future studies to investigate whether directly stimulating PAG neurons can modulate respiratory function and plasticity, and whether TMS of deep brain stimulation of the PAG could serve as a therapeutic tool to enhance respiratory activity.

The present work also revealed interactions between "Shielded" and "Unshielded" stimulation conditions, and rostro-caudal position of the coil. Without shielding, no MEP was recordable with the coil positioned over the snout even for the highest stimulation intensities. In contrast, stimulation revealed greater recordable MEP at stereotaxic locations more caudally, where PRV-positive neurons were observed within the respiratory motor cortex and periaqueducal grey matter areas. These results are consistent with a previous report describing an excitable region at Bregma (electrically or magnetically evoked MEP [31]). However, a bigger electrical response was recorded when the coil was located over the cerebellum/brainstem regions and the cervical spinal cord. This is to be expected given the density brainstem neurons associated with respiratory control (e.g. the dorsal and ventral respiratory columns), and the transynaptically labelled cells shown in the present tracing studies and reported previously [26,36,38]. It should also be noted that cervical neuroforamina root stimulation at high stimulation intensities (almost around 80–90% MO) is possible in animal models [39], and is known to spread out stimulation sites of peripheral motor fibres [40].

Effects of an acute C2 spinal cord transection

When an acute cervical cord total C2 transection was performed (figure 7), MEPdia could no longer be obtained with a single pulse of TMS at −6 mm from Bregma, confirming that the signal had been relayed to spinal neurons. Nevertheless, following a spinal cord complete transection and magnetic stimulation performed over cervicomedullary region (−12 mm from Bregma), an increased MEPdia amplitude and reduced latency are observed. This increased MEPdia could be due to the removal of inhibitory connections and/or hyperexcitability of the spinal stub due to the release of glutamate following complete injury. Thus C1 stimulation in both unshielded and shielded groups must result in activation of neurons caudal to the C2

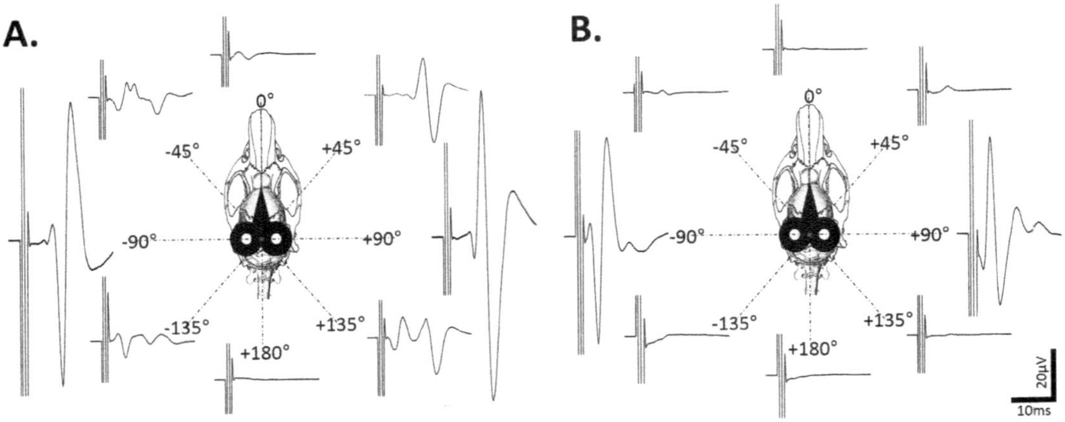

Figure 4. Effect of the coil rotation on the MEPdia. A) Representative MEPdia recorded after a single TMS pulse with the "Unshielded" coil at different orientation degrees (from 0° to 360°, 45° steps) of the coil (black coil represented on the top at −6 mm from Bregma in black). B) Representative MEPdia recorded after a single TMS pulse with "Shielded" coil at different orientation degrees (from 0° to 360°, 45° steps).

transection. These results as well as those from antero-posterior stimulation site shifting indicated the specificity of cortical excitability without any contamination from spinal cord excitable cells when a MEPdia is recorded.

Results concerning the MEP amplitude were confirmed with MEP latency analyses. Data from figure 2, examining the effect of antero-posterior position of the coil, do not show significant change in MEPdia first negative wave (N1) peak latency mean values for the most posterior sites – over cerebellum (−12 mm from Bregma) and cervicomedullary sites (positioned over the C1 spinal cord) – suggesting that closer to the diaphragm, different cell populations could be depolarized and emit action potential volleys with lower propagation velocity. In addition, an antidromic volley could inhibit output from upper respiratory pathways, resulting in the same latency. Thus, it is important to consider the stereotaxic location of stimulation and whether it has the potential to attenuate evoked responses and affect latency related to magnetic shielding. While not significantly different, MEPdia latency mean values were always shorter in unshielded than in shielded conditions. This suggests that shielding would definitively induce a small delay due to the fact that magnetic stimulation would be more effective at motor cortex than supraspinal level. In addition, latency mean values are in the same range as those reported for limb muscles taken either the onset latency [28,29,31] or the MEP first negative wave latency (N1) [27] suggesting that evoked potentials originate in the same central nervous system structure rather than at spinal or phrenic nerve locations.

Definitively, our data suggest that the position of the coil over the cortex or deeper brain structures is crucial to record specific diaphragmatic MEP in a rat model, as has been described in humans [9,11]. MEP amplitude showed a higher response when the coil is centred over specific motor cortex area.

Consistent with previous work [9], the present study also revealed that rotating the orientation of the coil (see Figure 4) resulted in robust differences in MEP. MEP amplitude was increased for −90° as well as +90° positions, which is likely due to the geometry of the magnetic field under the coil, with or without shielding. These two positions correspond to the alignment of the greater axis of the coil and rostro-caudal (antero-posterior) axis of the central nervous system. This also extends the magnetic field over the cervical spinal cord increasing the likelihood of depolarizing phrenic motoneuron axons at neuroforamina portions of the cervical roots. This is not shield dependant, and it is likely that the reduction in the magnetic field is less at the widest part of the coil than in the center. Moreover, the fact that almost no signal was recorded for +180° gives some insight into the influence of magnetic field direction.

Human TMS studies [9,22] have revealed that the motor cortex is sensitive to magnetic field direction and preferentially recruited for 45° position. This had been interpreted as the orientation of the magnetic field, being perpendicular to primary motor cortex cell orientation in the frontal sulcus [9,23]. However, the rat cortex is much less complex than human cortex (lissencephalic vs gyrencephalic). Given that stimulation of the rat motor cortex may be affected by coil orientation in a similar manner to that seen in humans, there may be a closer correlation between magnetic field geometry and motor cell intrinsic excitable properties, than with brain surface architecture (as has been suggested in humans).

The major goal of this paper was to demonstrate that recorded MEPdia reflects a response to direct activation of supraspinal respiratory pathways following stimulation of cortical neurons or deeper brain structure stimulation in order to modulate the activity of these pathways to induce a respiratory neuroplasticity. As previously discussed, the correlation between the MEPdia latency and amplitude with the magnitude of the magnetic stimulation output, suggests that the recorded MEP is initiated at the cortical level [41]. However, we cannot rule out that MEPs might be contaminated by stimulation of neurons within other brain and peripheral structures. For example, the size and wideness of the magnetic field induced by a single stimulation could activate respiratory related nerves, such as the vagus nerve, by which one pass through some diaphragmatic afferents. However, despite the fact that the magnetic field is large and powerful enough to depolarize antidromically vagus nerve fibres and could induce an ectopic activation of some diaphragmatic motor units, no changes in MEPdia following a bilateral vagotomy was observed. This confirms the specificity of the magnetic stimulation.

In addition, no MEPdia were recorded following a magnetic stimulation if the animal was pre-treated with a cholinergic blocker (gallamine trietiodide)to induce muscular paralysis. This result reinforces that diaphragmatic motor unit recruitment recorded as a MEPdia is induced by TMS activating supraspinal neurons, and not directly or by local electrical currents induced by the magnetic

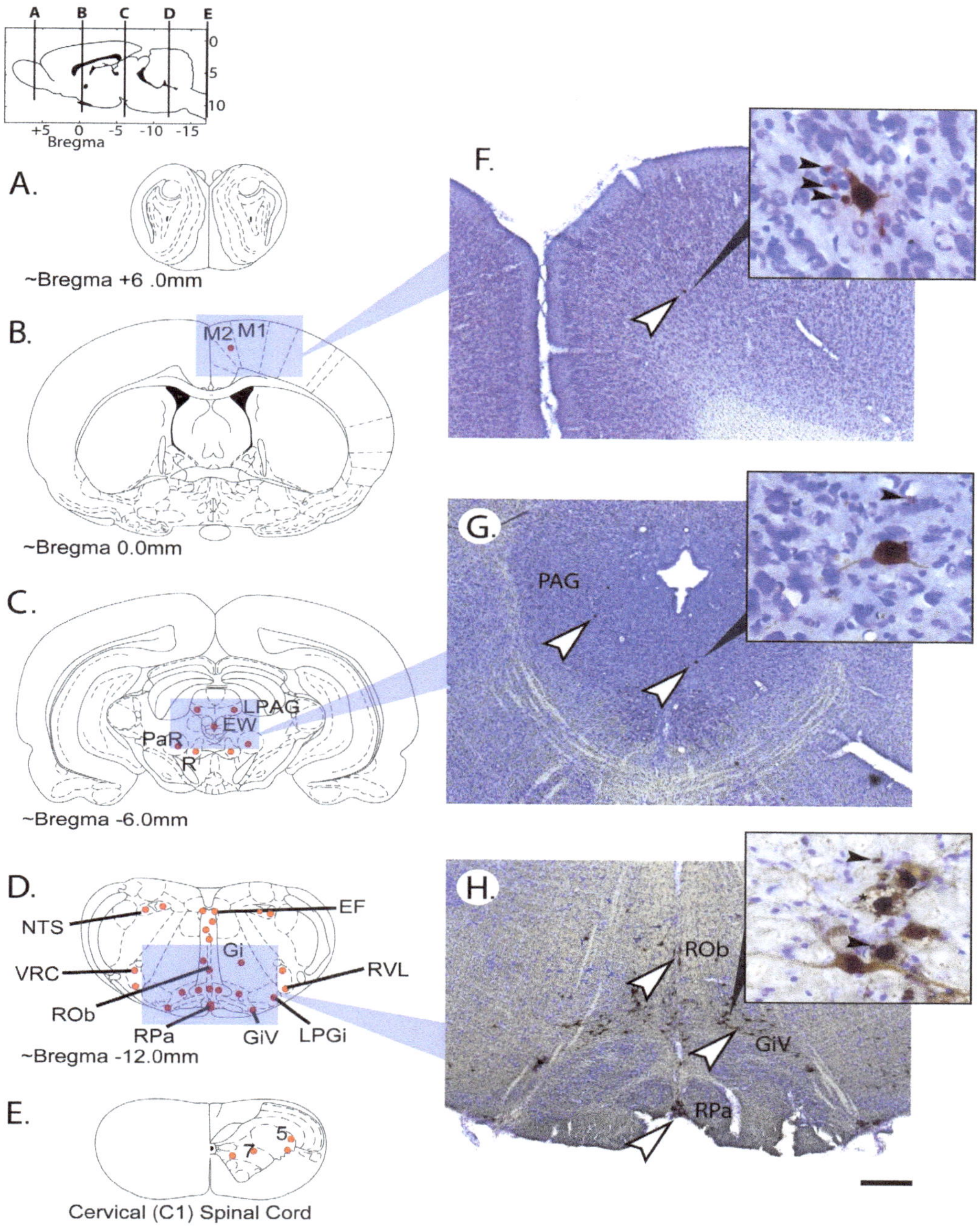

Figure 5. Schematic diagrams (modified from [43]) representing cross sections of the brain (A–C), brainstem (D) and spinal cord (E), and corresponding images of tissue that has been immunolabeled for the presence of PRV (brown; white arrowheads) and counterstained with cresyl violet (F–G). Inset show examples of PRV-labeled neurons at higher magnification. Schematic diagrams are representative of the stereotaxic positions that the TMS coil was used in the present work. Each of these positions relative to Bregma is also indicated on the sagittal diagram above. The qualitative distribution of PRV labelled neurons is indicated by red dots. PRV-positive neurons were detected in the cortex, the midbrain, the medulla, and spinal cord 72 hours following delivery of PRV to the diaphragm. Only few PRV-positive neurons were detected within the motor cortex at this post-PRV time point (primary (M1) and secondary (M2) motor cortex). Approximately 6 mm caudal to bregma, several PRV-positive cells were seen within midbrain in the periaqueductal grey (PAG) and Edinger-Westphal nucleus (EW), and some also in the Red (R) and pararubral nucleus (PaR) nuclei. Several PRV-positive neurons were seen throughout the brainstem 12 mm caudal to Bregma, predominantly in the Raphe (including raphe obscuris (ROb), pallidus (RPa)) and reticular nuclei (gigantocellular (Gi), ventral gigantocellular (GiV), lateral paragigantocellular (LPGi) and rostroventrolateral reticular nucleus (RVL)). Labelling was also seen in two key respiratory centers: the ventral respiratory column (VRC) and the solitary nucleus (nucleus tractus solitarius; NTS) (which comprises the 'dorsal respiratory group'). Finally some labelling was seen within the epifascicular nucleus. PRV labelled spinal interneurons were observed bilaterally in the C1, primarily in the intermediate grey matter (laminae 7 and 10), but fewer neurons seen in laminae 1, 5, and 8. Note the differences in morphology of PRV-labeled neurons shown in the insets (e.g. late-stage neuronal infection results in cell death (*), additional description in the text) and the presence of some smaller PRV-positive cells (black arrowheads; likely glia). Scale bar is 200 (F–H) and 40 micrometres (insets).

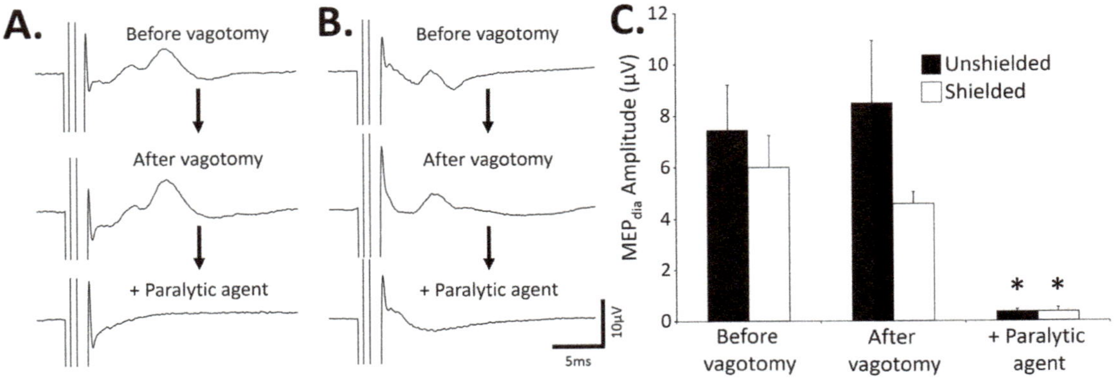

Figure 6. Effect of vagotomy and muscular paralysis on the MEPdia induced by a single TMS pulse at −6 mm from Bregma. A) Representative MEPdia before vagotomy, after vagotomy and injection of a paralytic agent (gallamine trietiodide) obtained with the "Unshielded" coil. B) Representative MEPdia before vagotomy, after vagotomy and injection of a paralytic agent (gallamine trietiodide) obtained with the "Shielded" coil. Note that the vagotomy does not affect the MEPdia, and the paralytic agent abolish the MEPdia in both conditions in A and B. C) Histogram of the MEPdia amplitude before vagotomy, after vagotomy and following the injection of paralytic agent in the "Unshielded" (black histogram) and "Shielded" (White histogram) on the TMS coil. *: $p<0.001$.

field depolarized phrenic motor axons [42]. The recorded MEPdia is therefore the consequence of a single TMS pulse which induces an action potential volley from stimulated supraspinal neurons (cortical or deeper brain structures) to phrenic motoneurons innervating the diaphragm. Future studies should employ direct stimulation of brain structures to further elucidate which regions have the greatest influence over respiratory activity and plasticity. Knowledge of these structures could identify targets for developing and testing the potential therapeutic benefits of TMS in order to enhance respiratory corticospinal excitability and/or activate and strengthen pre-existing pathways.

The present work suggests that TMS may be a safe, non-invasive and readily usable strategy for neuromodulation and treatment of respiratory function. The therapeutic effects of TMS can be easily investigated further with either molecular or functional techniques. While these experiments are preliminary and the extent to which TMS applied repeatedly (rTMS) can be used therapeutically needs to be more extensively characterized, there are a wide range of potential therapeutic applications for TMS that can now be explored. Future experiments should investigate whether rTMS could be used to treat respiratory deficits associated with neurological injury and disease.

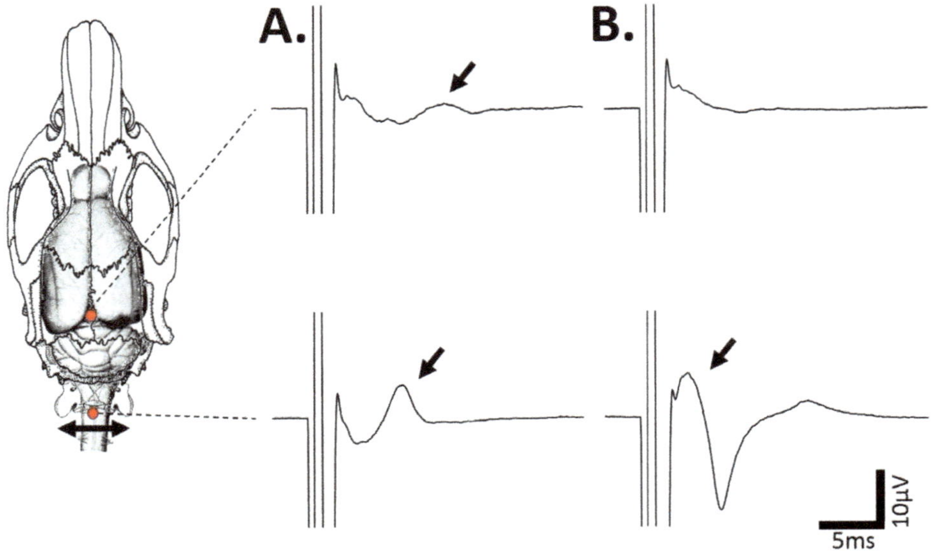

Figure 7. Effect of a total transection of the spinal cord at the C2 level on the MEPdia upon stimulation at −6 mm from Bregma and at the C1 spinal cord. A) Representatives MEPdia (black arrows) obtained after a single TMS pulse at −6 mm from Bregma (top trace) and at C1 spinal cord site (bottom trace) in the "Unshielded" coil group before complete C2 spinal cord transection. B) Representatives MEPdia (black arrows) obtained after a single TMS pulse at −6 mm from Bregma (top trace) and at C1 spinal cord site (bottom trace) in the "Unshielded" coil group after the complete C2 spinal cord transection. Note the absence of MEPdia when the stimulation is applied at −6 mm from Bregma, and the presence of an enhanced MEPdia when the C1 spinal cord is stimulated.

Acknowledgments

This work was supported by funding from the European Union Seventh framework Programme (FP7/2007–2013) under grant agreement No. 246556 (European project RBUCE-UP), HandiMedEx allocated by the French Public Investment Board, the Chancellerie des Universités de Paris (Legs Poix), the « Centre d'Assistance Respiratoire à Domicile d'Ile de France (CARDIF) », the « Fonds de Dotation de Recherche en Santé Respiratoire » and LVL Medical. Financial support for neuroanatomical studies was provided through internal funds awarded to Michael Lane at Drexel University – College of Medicine, Department of Neurobiology & Anatomy. We would like to thanks Marie Baubrand and Christian Pichault for their technical assistance and Vitaliy Marchenko for his comments on the manuscript. Primary antibodies to pseudorabies virus were provided by Lynn W. Enquist, Princeton University, as a service of the National Center for Experimental Neuroanatomy with Neurotropic Viruses: NCRR P40 RRO118604. PRV614 was produced by David Bloom, University of Florida (original viral stocks donated by Bruce Banfield, University of Colorado).

Author Contributions

Conceived and designed the experiments: SV MAL MB MP. Performed the experiments: SV EK TBD VMS TB MP. Analyzed the data: SV EK VMS TB MAL MP. Contributed reagents/materials/analysis tools: SV MAL MP. Contributed to the writing of the manuscript: SV TBD VMS TB MAL MB MP.

References

1. Gersner R, Kravetz E, Feil J, Pell G, Zangen A (2011) Long-term effects of repetitive transcranial magnetic stimulation on markers for neuroplasticity: differential outcomes in anesthetized and awake animals. J Neurosci 31: 7521–7526.
2. Wang HY, Crupi D, Liu J, Stucky A, Cruciata G, et al. (2011) Repetitive transcranial magnetic stimulation enhances BDNF-TrkB signaling in both brain and lymphocyte. J Neurosci 31: 11044–11054.
3. Planche D (1972) [Effects of cerebral cortex stimulation on the activity of the phrenic nerve]. J Physiol (Paris) 64: 31–56.
4. Gandevia SC, Rothwell JC (1987) Activation of the human diaphragm from the motor cortex. J Physiol 384: 109–118.
5. Macefield G, Gandevia SC (1991) The cortical drive to human respiratory muscles in the awake state assessed by premotor cerebral potentials. J Physiol 439: 545–558.
6. Zifko U, Remtulla H, Power K, Harker L, Bolton CF (1996) Transcortical and cervical magnetic stimulation with recording of the diaphragm. Muscle Nerve 19: 614–620.
7. Lipski J, Bektas A, Porter R (1986) Short latency inputs to phrenic motoneurones from the sensorimotor cortex in the cat. Exp Brain Res 61: 280–290.
8. Alexandrov VG, Ivanova TG, Alexandrova NP (2007) Prefrontal control of respiration. J Physiol Pharmacol 58 Suppl 5: 17–23.
9. Maskill D, Murphy K, Mier A, Owen M, Guz A (1991) Motor cortical representation of the diaphragm in man. J Physiol 443: 105–121.
10. Lissens MA (1994) Motor evoked potentials of the human diaphragm elicited through magnetic transcranial brain stimulation. J Neurol Sci 124: 204–207.
11. Khedr EM, Trakhan MN (2001) Localization of diaphragm motor cortical representation and determination of corticodiaphragmatic latencies by using magnetic stimulation in normal adult human subjects. Eur J Appl Physiol 85: 560–566.
12. Sharshar T, Ross E, Hopkinson NS, Dayer M, Nickol A, et al. (2003) Effect of voluntary facilitation on the diaphragmatic response to transcranial magnetic stimulation. J Appl Physiol 95: 26–34.
13. Davey NJ, Murphy K, Maskill DW, Guz A, Ellaway PH (1996) Site of facilitation of diaphragm EMG to corticospinal stimulation during inspiration. Respir Physiol 106: 127–135.
14. Hunanyan AS, Petrosyan HA, Alessi V, Arvanian VL (2012) Repetitive spinal electromagnetic stimulation opens a window of synaptic plasticity in damaged spinal cord: role of NMDA receptors. J Neurophysiol 107: 3027–3039.
15. Muller PA, Dhamne SC, Vahabzadeh-Hagh AM, Pascual-Leone A, Jensen FE, et al. (2014) Suppression of motor cortical excitability in anesthetized rats by low frequency repetitive transcranial magnetic stimulation. PLoS One 9: e91065.
16. Raux M, Xie H, Similowski T, Koski L (2010) Facilitatory conditioning of the supplementary motor area in humans enhances the corticophrenic responsiveness to transcranial magnetic stimulation. J Appl Physiol (1985) 108: 39–46.
17. Azabou E, Roche N, Sharshar T, Bussel B, Lofaso F, et al. (2013) Transcranial direct-current stimulation reduced the excitability of diaphragmatic corticospinal pathways whatever the polarity used. Respir Physiol Neurobiol 189: 183–187.
18. Laviolette L, Nierat MC, Hudson AL, Raux M, Allard E, et al. (2013) The supplementary motor area exerts a tonic excitatory influence on corticospinal projections to phrenic motoneurons in awake humans. PLoS One 8: e62258.
19. Vinit S, Windelborn JA, Mitchell GS (2011) Lipopolysaccharide attenuates phrenic long-term facilitation following acute intermittent hypoxia. Respir Physiol Neurobiol 176: 130–135.
20. Brasil-Neto JP, Cohen LG, Panizza M, Nilsson J, Roth BJ, et al. (1992) Optimal focal transcranial magnetic activation of the human motor cortex: effects of coil orientation, shape of the induced current pulse, and stimulus intensity. J Clin Neurophysiol 9: 132–136.
21. Mills KR, Boniface SJ, Schubert M (1992) Magnetic brain stimulation with a double coil: the importance of coil orientation. Electroencephalogr Clin Neurophysiol 85: 17–21.
22. Niehaus L, Meyer BU, Weyh T (2000) Influence of pulse configuration and direction of coil current on excitatory effects of magnetic motor cortex and nerve stimulation. Clin Neurophysiol 111: 75–80.
23. Dubach P, Guggisberg AG, Rosler KM, Hess CW, Mathis J (2004) Significance of coil orientation for motor evoked potentials from nasalis muscle elicited by transcranial magnetic stimulation. Clin Neurophysiol 115: 862–870.
24. Ni Z, Charab S, Gunraj C, Nelson AJ, Udupa K, et al. (2011) Transcranial magnetic stimulation in different current directions activates separate cortical circuits. J Neurophysiol 105: 749–756.
25. Lane MA, White TE, Coutts MA, Jones AL, Sandhu MS, et al. (2008) Cervical prephrenic interneurons in the normal and lesioned spinal cord of the adult rat. J Comp Neurol 511: 692–709.
26. Lane MA, Lee KZ, Fuller DD, Reier PJ (2009) Spinal circuitry and respiratory recovery following spinal cord injury. Respir Physiol Neurobiol 169: 123–132.
27. Luft AR, Kaelin-Lang A, Hauser TK, Cohen LG, Thakor NV, et al. (2001) Transcranial magnetic stimulation in the rat. Exp Brain Res 140: 112–121.
28. Fishback AS, Shields CB, Linden RD, Zhang YP, Burke D (1995) The effects of propofol on rat transcranial magnetic motor evoked potentials. Neurosurgery 37: 969–974.
29. Linden RD, Zhang YP, Burke DA, Hunt MA, Harpring JE, et al. (1999) Magnetic motor evoked potential monitoring in the rat. J Neurosurg 91: 205–210.
30. Rotenberg A, Muller PA, Vahabzadeh-Hagh AM, Navarro X, Lopez-Vales R, et al. (2010) Lateralization of forelimb motor evoked potentials by transcranial magnetic stimulation in rats. Clin Neurophysiol 121: 104–108.
31. Kamida T, Fujiki M, Hori S, Isono M (1998) Conduction pathways of motor evoked potentials following transcranial magnetic stimulation: a rodent study using a "figure-8" coil. Muscle Nerve 21: 722–731.
32. Huxtable AG, Vinit S, Windelborn JA, Crader SM, Guenther CH, et al. (2011) Systemic inflammation impairs respiratory chemoreflexes and plasticity. Respir Physiol Neurobiol 178: 482–489.
33. Nakatoh S, Kitagawa H, Kawaguchi Y, Nakamura H, Takano H, et al. (1998) Effects of coil orientation and magnetic field shield on transcranial magnetic stimulation in cats. Muscle Nerve 21: 1172–1180.
34. Sharshar T, Desmarais G, Louis B, Macadou G, Porcher R, et al. (2003) Transdiaphragmatic pressure control of airway pressure support in healthy subjects. Am J Respir Crit Care Med 168: 760–769.
35. Kolb B, Tees RC (1990) The Cerebral Cortex of the Rat.; Press M, editor. Cambridge, MA: A Bradford Book.
36. Dobbins EG, Feldman JL (1994) Brainstem network controlling descending drive to phrenic motoneurons in rat. J Comp Neurol 347: 64–86.
37. Subramanian HH, Holstege G (2013) Stimulation of the midbrain periaqueductal gray modulates preinspiratory neurons in the ventrolateral medulla in the rat in vivo. J Comp Neurol 521: 3083–3098.
38. Lane MA, Fuller DD, White TE, Reier PJ (2008) Respiratory neuroplasticity and cervical spinal cord injury: translational perspectives. Trends Neurosci 31: 538–547.
39. Bader SR, Fischer A, Emrich D, Juetting U, Weyh T, et al. (2011) Evaluation of lumbosacral nerve root conduction in chickens by electrophysiological testing including high-resolution spinal magnetic stimulation. J Neurosci Methods 194: 342–349.
40. Cros D, Day TJ, Shahani BT (1990) Spatial dispersion of magnetic stimulation in peripheral nerves. Muscle Nerve 13: 1076–1082.
41. Devanne H, Lavoie BA, Capaday C (1997) Input-output properties and gain changes in the human corticospinal pathway. Exp Brain Res 114: 329–338.
42. Maccabee PJ, Nagarajan SS, Amassian VE, Durand DM, Szabo AZ, et al. (1998) Influence of pulse sequence, polarity and amplitude on magnetic stimulation of human and porcine peripheral nerve. J Physiol 513 (Pt 2): 571–585.
43. Paxinos G, Watson C (1997) The rat brain in stereotaxic coordinates.; Ed. Cr, editor. San Diego: Academic Press.

VGF Changes during the Estrous Cycle: A Novel Endocrine Role for TLQP Peptides?

Barbara Noli, Carla Brancia, Filomena D'Amato, Gian-Luca Ferri*, Cristina Cocco*

Department of Biomedical Sciences, University of Cagliari, Monserrato (Cagliari), Italy

Abstract

Although the VGF derived peptide TLQP-21 stimulates gonadotropin-releasing hormone (GnRH) and gonadotropin secretion, available data on VGF peptides and reproduction are limited. We used antibodies specific for the two ends of the VGF precursor, and for two VGF derived peptides namely TLQP and PGH, to be used in immunohistochemistry and enzyme-linked immunosorbent assay complemented with gel chromatography. In cycling female rats, VGF C-/N-terminus and PGH peptide antibodies selectively labelled neurones containing either GnRH, or kisspeptin (VGF N-terminus only), pituitary gonadotrophs and lactotrophs, or oocytes (PGH peptides only). Conversely, TLQP peptides were restricted to somatostatin neurones, gonadotrophs, and ovarian granulosa, interstitial and theca cells. TLQP levels were highest, especially in plasma and ovary, with several molecular forms shown in chromatography including one compatible with TLQP-21. Among the cycle phases, TLQP levels were higher during metestrus-diestrus in median eminence and pituitary, while increased in the ovary and decreased in plasma during proestrus. VGF N- and C-terminus peptides also showed modulations over the estrous cycle, in median eminence, pituitary and plasma, while PGH peptides did not. In ovariectomised rats, plasmatic TLQP peptide levels showed distinct reduction suggestive of a major origin from the ovary, while the estrogen-progesterone treatment modulated VGF C-terminus and TLQP peptides in the hypothalamus-pituitary complex. In *in vitro* hypothalamus, TLQP-21 stimulated release of growth hormone releasing hormone but not of somatostatin. In conclusion, various VGF peptides may regulate the hypothalamus-pituitary complex *via* specific neuroendocrine mechanisms while TLQP peptides may act at further, multiple levels *via* endocrine mechanisms involving the ovary.

Editor: Hubert Vaudry, University of Rouen, France, France

Funding: This study was sponsored by the ARS (Autonomous Region of Sardinia) through the 'Sardinia PO FSE 2007-1013' funds (the L.R. 7/2007 for the 'Promotion of the Scientific Research and of the Technological Innovation in Sardinia'). The funders had no role in study design, data collection and analysis, decision to publish, or preparation of the manuscript.

Competing Interests: The authors have declared that no competing interests exist.

* Email: cristina.cocco@unica.it (CC); ferri@unica.it (GLF)

Introduction

The VGF gene product, and/or its derived peptides, appear to be involved in reproduction since *vgf* null mice were sexually immature and almost completely infertile [1]. The 66 kDa VGF precursor [1–6] is composed of 617 or 615 amino acid residues (in rat or human, respectively), and gives rise to several low molecular weight VGF peptides which are abundant in multiple brain regions, peripheral neurones, and certain endocrine and neuroendocrine cell populations [7–13]. Despite their abundance and wide distribution, limited data are available on their role and function/s. Among the VGF peptides with proven biological activity are included TLQP-21 [14], TLQP-62 [15] and the peptides called NERPs [16]. TLQP-21 was shown to act on various mechanisms, including the regulation of energy balance [14], inflammatory and neuropathic pain [17,18], chronic stress [19], and gastric motility and emptying [20]. With respect to reproduction, induction of VGF mRNA was reported in the pituitary immediately after the estrus, in parallel with a clear-cut decrease in certain VGF peptides, as well as changes in their localisation in gonadotrophs and lactotrophs [21]. A distinct seasonal modulation in cell-type-specific processing of the VGF precursor was revealed in the anterior pituitary of female sheep [22], while significant upregulation of VGF mRNA was found related to reproductive maturation in baboon ovary [23]. More recently, TLQP-21 was shown to exert a number of actions on the rat reproductive axis [24,25]. Central administration of TLQP-21 in pubertal and adult male rats induced gonadotrophin secretion *via* release of gonadotropin-releasing hormone (GnRH), and stimulated testosterone secretion *in vitro* in pre-pubertal animals [24]. In female pre-pubertal rats, TLQP-21 induced *in vitro* secretion of luteinising hormone (LH) and follicle-stimulating hormone (FSH) from the pituitary, with no detectable effect on GnRH release from the hypothalamus [25]. On the same rats, upon *i.p.* injection of the same peptide at high doses, serum LH showed a moderate increase, while after central administration of TLQP-21 in adults animals, the LH response was dependent on the stage of the reproductive cycle [25]. On the whole, TLQP-21 would so far appear to affect female reproduction by stimulating pituitary LH release. We produced antisera selective for the C-and N-terminal portions of the VGF precursor, and for two cleaved peptides "TLQP" and "PGH" (named from the corresponding four N-terminal, and three C-terminal amino-acids, respectively, immediately adjacent to their respective sites of cleavage from the

VGF precursor), to be used for immunohistochemistry (IHC) and enzyme-linked immunosorbent assay (ELISA), complemented with gel chromatography. We addressed the localisation and changes of VGF peptides in the female rat reproductive axis in connection with the estrous cycle, as well as after ovariectomy. Their presence and modulation in plasma was outlined in parallel, as a clue to their possible endocrine significance. In addition, in view of its selective distribution in the hypothalamus, the ability of the TLQP-21 peptide to release somatostatin or growth-hormone-releasing hormone (GHRH) was tested *in vitro*.

Materials and Methods

Animals and tissue samples

Sprague Dawley adult female rats (from Charles River, Italy, 200–250 g body weight) were kept at 22°C (12:12-h light/dark cycle, lights on 7 am–7 pm), 3 to 4 rats *per* cage, with food and water *ad libitum*. All animals were killed at the same time of day (approximately 10 am), with a diethyl ether overdose. Group 1 ("cycling rats") included females showing regular 4 days estrous cycles (vaginal smears were taken daily at 8.30–9.30 during about 2 consecutive cycles, on average). Rats were killed at the age of 12–14 weeks, at proestrus, estrus, diestrus, or metestrus (n = 12 *per* each cycle phase). Group 2 rats ("ovariectomy + estrogen/progesterone treatment", n = 8) were bilaterally ovariectomised at 3–4 weeks' age, hence received intraperitoneal beta-estradiol (200 ug/200 ul, 2 days before sacrifice) and progesterone (500 ug/200 ul, on the day of sacrifice). Group 3 rats ("ovariectomy controls", n = 7) were as for group 2, but received the corresponding solvent only (seed oil). Rats from groups 2 and 3 were sacrificed in parallel, 4 hours after the progesterone/oil injection. All experimental protocols were approved by the Ethical Committee at the University of Cagliari, and were performed in accordance with the guidelines for the care and use of animals approved by the American Physiological Society, the EEC Council Directive of 24 November 1986 (86/609) and the relevant Italian legislation. For ELISA experiments, the brain, hypophysis and ovaries were extracted from each rat as follows: group 1, n = 8 *per* phase; group 2, n = 5; group 3, n = 4. For group 1, the median eminence was dissected (under a stereomicroscope) from the remainder of the hypothalamus, and the two were separately extracted. The whole hypothalamus, inclusive of the median eminence, was taken from rats of groups 2 and 3. Blood (approximately 5 ml) was drawn at sacrifice (hence for cycling rats at the morning of each cycle phase as above mentioned) from the left heart of every animal, collected in an EDTA (1.78 mg/ml) containing tube, and rapidly centrifuged (3,000× *g*, 10–15 minutes), hence plasma was stored frozen. Tissues were extracted in ice-cold phosphate buffered saline (PBS, 0.01 mol/l PO_4, pH 7.2–7.4, 0.15 mol/l NaCl: 10 ml/g tissue) containing protease inhibitor cocktail (P8340, Sigma-Aldrich, Schnelldorf, Germany), homogenized for 3 minutes using an ultra Turrax (Ika-Werke, Staufen, Germany), hence tubes were heated in a vigorously boiling water bath for 10 minutes, and centrifuged (3,000×*g*, 10 minutes). Supernatants were stored frozen until use (−20°C or lower). For IHC, rats (group 1, n = 4; groups 2 and 3, n = 3 each) were transcardially perfused with 4% paraformaldehyde (in 0.2 mol/l PO_4 buffer, pH = 7.2), hence brain, pituitary and ovary were dissected out, and rinsed overnight in PBS containing 7% sucrose. Samples were oriented in aluminum foil moulds with cryoembedding media [26], snap-frozen and stored in a liquid nitrogen tank (vapour phase). Sections (5–7 um) were obtained using a cold-blade cryomicrotome [27] (Microm HM-560, Walldof, Germany), and collected on poly-L-lysine treated slides.

Antibodies

The antibodies used are summarized in Table 1. VGF peptides used for immunizations (Fig. 1) encompassed: (i) the rat VGF C-terminal nonapeptide; (ii) the N-terminal decapeptide of the rat VGF precursor (VGF24-33, upon cleavage of the rat VGF1-23 signal peptide); (iii) the N-terminal decapeptide of rat TLQP peptides (rat VGF556-565), and: (iv) the C-terminal nonapeptide of PGH peptides (rat VGF422-430). These were conjugated with bovine thyroglobulin or keyhole limpet haemocyanin, via either an additional N-terminal D-tyrosine residue (for VGF C-terminus and PGH), or an additional C-terminal cysteine (for VGF N-terminus and TLQP), as previously described (Tables 1–2). Hormone and hypothalamic factor antibodies (Table 1) showed negligible (<0.5%) cross reactivity with other pituitary hormones [21,22].

Characterization of VGF antibodies

Specificity was addressed in parallel *via* immunohistochemistry and ELISA. In the former, labeling with each VGF antibody was prevented by pre-absorbed with the relevant peptide (up to 50 nmol/ml). At the C-terminus of VGF, the rat sequence shows a single amino acid difference *versus* human VGF (Table 2). Both the human nonapeptide and other peptide missing the last three C-terminal amino acids (HVLL) showed negligible reactivity in ELISA (Table 2), while in IHC the rat VGF C-terminus antibody showed: (i) low reactivity on human tissues; (ii) clear-cut no-colocalisation of VGF C-terminus and HVLL immunostaining [28]. On such basis, the latter antibody is considered to recognise a short intact sequence at the extreme C-terminus of rat VGF. Species differences are shown in the VGF N-terminal decapeptide (Table 2), with very low reactivity of mouse and human forms in ELISA. Hence, antibody reactivity would depend on a comparatively long portion of the immunogen sequence. Cleaved peptides with an exposed TLQP or PGH sequence (i.e. with such sequence present at their N-terminus, and C-terminus, respectively) can be formed via proteolysis at the adjacent cleavage sequence: Arg_{553}-Pro_{554}-Arg_{555}, for TLQP peptides [12], and: Arg_{431}-Arg_{432}, for PGH peptides. Synthetic peptides similar to immunogens, with the addition of one extra Arginine in the location of their respective cleavage sequence ("Arginine-extended", see Table 2), were used to gain insight into the potential cross-reactivity of antibodies with native extended peptides (these may include the whole VGF precursor, or any peptides cleaved from VGF and including the TLQP or PGH sequence internally). In ELISA, the coating of specific peptide antigen onto the wells, together with high antibody dilutions, results in selection of the antibodies taking part in the reaction, hence in a major increase in specificity for cleaved peptides. Furthermore, most native peptides will be extended by many more than the one (Arginine) residue we tested, thus favouring low cross-reactivity.

Immunostaining

Sections were incubated overnight in a humid chamber, with antibodies diluted in PBS containing 30 ml/l of normal donkey serum, 30 ml/l of normal rat serum, and 0.02 g/l NaN_3. Double and triple immunofluorescence experiments were carried out mixing a VGF antibody with one hormone or hypothalamic factor antibody (Table 1) obtained in a different donor species. The relevant species-specific secondary antibody/ies (all from donkey, affinity purified IgG preparations absorbed with serum proteins from multiple species, conjugated with either Cy_3, Cy_2 or AMCA: Jackson Immunoresearch Laboratories, West Grove, PA) were used to reveal the sites of primary antibody binding. Slides were coverslipped with PBS-glycerol, observed and photographed using

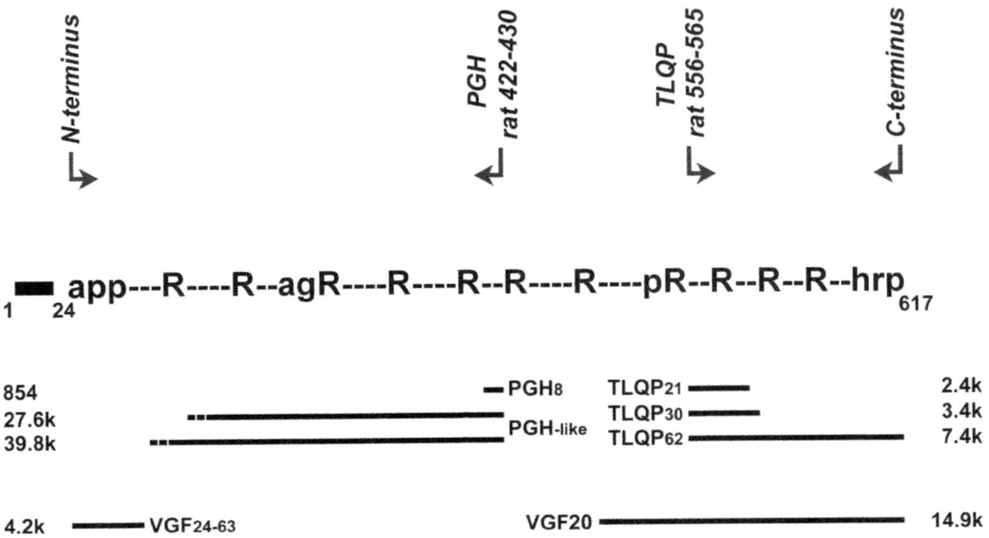

Figure 1. The VGF precursor, amino acid stretches used to raise antibodies, and known/putative VGF peptides. Top panel: arrows are aligned with 9 or 10 amino acid stretches used to raise antibodies, directed towards the site of conjugation with carrier protein. Middle panel: along the primary sequence of VGF (not drawn to scale) are shown: dibasic cleavage sites (R, or: pR) and a cleavage-amidation site (agR), the N- and C-terminal ends of the VGF precursor ("app-" and "-hrp", respectively: single letter notation of the corresponding amino acids), and the signal peptide (1–24 black box). Antibodies raised against VGF C-or N-terminus peptides are expected to react with any peptide cleaved from VGF, which includes the corresponding sequence. Antibodies to PGH and TLQP are expected to react well with any peptide extended on the "conjugation" side (N-terminal side of PGH, and C-terminal side of TLQP, respectively). Bottom panel: several known VGF peptides (relevant to the present study) together with their MW are aligned with the precursor. "PGH-like" peptides are intended to outline two putative peptides, running from: the PGH sequence, to: the N-terminal VGF_{24-36} peptide for the 39.8 kDa form, or to: a cleavage site (rat $VGF_{178-179}$) implicated in the biosynthesis of NERP-3 for the 27.6 kDa peptide. Their hypothetical N-terminal extreme is pointed out (dotted bar).

BX41 and BX51 fluorescence microscopes (Olympus, Milan, Italy) equipped with Fuji S2 and S3 Pro digital cameras (Fujifilm, Milan, Italy). Further to absorption controls (see above), routine controls included substitution of each antibody, in turn, with PBS, the use of pre-immune or non-immune sera, and the testing of each secondary antibody with their respective non-relevant primary antibodies.

Table 1. Antisera and antibodies used in the study.

	Antigen	Specie	Ref.	Dilutions	use
VGF peptides	C-t.	Rabbit	Ferri *et al.* 1995	1:250 K/1:3 K	E/I
			Cocco *et al.* 2007		
	TLQP	G. Pig	Brancia *et al.* 2005	1:60 K/1:1000	E/I
			D'Amato *et al.* 2008		
	PGH	Rabbit	D'Amato *et al.* 2008	1:60 K/1:1000	E/I
	N-t.	G. Pig	Cocco *et al.* 2010	1:400 K/1:800	E/I
Hormones	FSH	Mouse	Berger *et al.* 1990	1:500	I
	GH	Monkey	AF Parlow	1:600	I
	LH	Sheep	Biomol/Enzo	1:600	I
	PRL	Mouse	Berger *et al.* 1990	1:600	I
	GHRH	Rabbit	Phoenix	1:16000	E
	GHRH	GHRH Rabbit	Phoenix	1:6000	E
h. factors	GnRH	Mouse	Sternb	1:2000	I
	SRIF	Rabbit	Abcam	1:20 K/ 1:600	E/I
	Kissp	Rabbit	Millipore	1:800	I

C-term: VGF C-terminus; N-term: VGF N-terminus; FSH: follicle-stimulating hormone; GH: growth hormone; LH: luteinising hormone; PRL: prolactin; h. factor: hypothalamic factor, GHRH: growth hormone-releasing hormone; GnRH: gonadotrophin-releasing hormone; SRIF: somatostatin, Kissp: kisspeptin; Ref: references; E: ELISA; I: immunohistochemistry.

Table 2. ELISA characterization.

	Peptide	Sequence	IC_{50}	CV1	CV2	% cross- reactivity
	$rVGF_{609-617}$[2]	**--dY-IEHV LLHRP**				100
C-t	$hVGF_{607-615}$	**IEHV LLRRP**	0.02	2–3	4	<0.01
	$hVGF_{603-612}$	**LEN YIEHV LL**				<0.01
	$rVGF_{556-565}$[2]	**TLQPP ASSRR-C--**				
	$rVGF_{556-564}$	**TLQPP ASSRR**				100
TLQP	$rVGF_{556-567}$	**TLQPP ASSRR R**	1.1	3–5	6	122
	$rVGF_{556-576}$	**TLQPP ASSRR RHFHH ALPPA R**				183
	$rVGF_{556-564}$-R^3	**R-TLQPP ASSR**				3.5
	$rVGF_{422-430}$[2]	**-dY-RSQEE APGH**				100
PGH	$hVGF_{422-431}$-R^4	**RSQEE APGH-R**	0.3	4–6	6–8	<0.015
	$hVGF_{419-427}$	**RSQEE TPGH**				3.5
	$hVGF_{419-428}$-R^4	**RSQEE TPGH-R**				<0.015
	$rVGF_{24-31}$[2]	**APPGR SDVYP-C--**				100
N-t	$rVGF_{23-30}$	**APPGR PEAQP**	10	3–7	5–8	<0.001
	$mVGF_{24-31}$	**APPGR PDVFP**				<0.001

Sequence differences versus rat VGF are underlined; IC50: dose producing 50% inhibition (pmol per well); CV1 and CV2: intra and inter assay variation, respectively, C-t and N-t: VGF C-terminus and N-terminus, respectively; [2] "immunogen": peptide used for conjugation to carrier protein and immunizations; used for plate coating and assay standards; R^3: Arg-extended: with addition of Arginine residue at the peptide N- or C-terminus, respectively; R^4 additional Arginine residue from adjacent cleavage site; "dY" and "C": additional d-Tyrosine, or Cysteine residue used for conjugation; r: rat, h: human, m: mouse.

ELISA

VGF assays were carried out as described previously [28–29]. Briefly, multiwell plates were coated with either the relevant VGF peptide (Table 2), or synthetic GHRH (Bachem, Bubendorf, Switzerland, 120 pmol/ml), as appropriate, and blocked with PBS containing 9% normal donkey serum and 0.05% NaN_3 (2 h). Primary incubations were carried out with a mixture of the relevant primary antibody (in PBS containing 9% normal donkey serum, 20 nmol/L aprotinin, 1 mg/ml EDTA and 0.05% NaN_3), and either samples (diluted 1:5 to 1:40), or serial dilutions of the relevant standard peptide, or the relevant peptides to be tested for characterization purposes (Table 2). Detection was carried out with the relevant secondary antibody (affinity purified donkey IgG, absorbed with serum proteins from multiple species, biotin conjugated: 1 h, from: Jackson), streptavidin-peroxidase conjugate (Biospa, Milan, Italy: 30 min), and tetramethylbenzidine substrate (TMB X-tra, Kem-En-Tec Diagnostics, Taastrup, Denmark). Optical density was measured at 450 nm using a multilabel plate reader (Chameleon, Hidex, Turku, Finland). For the somatostatin assay, plates were coated with donkey anti-rabbit IgG (as above, 1:3000), blocked as above, and incubated with a mixture of somatostatin antibody (diluted in the above medium), biotin-conjugated somatostatin (Bachem, 100 pmol/ml), and either samples of heat-treated culture medium (diluted 1:10), or serial dilutions of unconjugated somatostatin (Bachem). Detection was carried out with streptavidin-peroxidase, as above. VGF assay characterization is summarised in Table 2. GHRH and somatostatin assays showed low intra- and inter-assay variation (CV% < 10%).

Chromatography

Extracts (2 ml) were individually loaded onto a Sephadex G-50S column (Sigma; 2 $cm^2 \times 1$ m), equilibrated with 50 mM ammonium bicarbonate and eluted with the same buffer. A molecular weight (MW) marker kit (MWGF70: Sigma) was used for column calibration. Fractions (3 ml) were reduced in volume with a Vacufuge Concentrator (Eppendorf, Milan, Italy) and assessed by ELISA. For all VGF peptides studied, overall recovery of loaded immunoreactivity ranged between 80% and 100%.

In vitro experiments

In view of the specific localisation of TLQP peptides in median eminence somatostatin-containing terminals, we hypothesized a possible action onto secretion of somatostatin and its GHRH neurone targets. Adult male rats (Sprague Dowley, 300–350 g body weight, n = 12) were killed by decapitation, and their brain was rapidly dissected out. Each hypothalamus (from optic chiasm to mammilary bodies, about 2 mm wide) was incubated in Dulbecco's modified Eagle's medium (DMEM, with 4.5 g/L glucose, without glutamine) in a 95% O_2 and 5% CO_2 atmosphere, at 37°C, as previously described [24]. After 30 min, the medium was removed and substituted with fresh medium with/without TLQP-21 (10^{-6} mol/L; n = 6 and 6 hypothalami). After a further 45 minutes incubation, culture media were collected, heat treated in a boiling water bath for 30 min, and stored frozen pending somatostatin and GHRH assays.

Statistical analysis

Data were expressed as mean ± SEM throughout. Statistical analyses were carried out by one-way ANOVA, followed by *t*-test as appropriate (StatistiXL software, www.statistixl.com), and a $P< 0.05$ was considered statistically significant.

Results

VGF peptide immunolocalisation

Immunoreactive VGF peptides were revealed in multiple areas of the reproductive axis as hypothalamus, including the preoptic area (POA) and median eminence, as well as in hypophyseal and ovarian cells (Fig. 2 and 3). Experiments focussed on the POA showed PGH peptide immunoreactivity in the majority of GnRH axons and terminals (Fig. 2, A and B), with weak labeling of some GnRH containing perikarya (not shown). The same applied to VGF C-and N-terminus antibodies, with the latter additionally labeling almost all kisspeptin containing fibres (Fig. 2C and D). In the median eminence, TLQP peptides were brightly immunostained (Fig. 2, E), confined to somatostatin containing axons and terminals (Fig. 2, F). VGF C-and N-terminus peptides were far more widely distributed throughout the external and internal median eminence, including axons and terminals containing GnRH (Fig. 2, G and H), or kisspeptin (VGF N-terminus only, not shown). PGH peptides showed a discrete localisation, in the lateral portion of the median eminence, virtually completely colocalised with GnRH (Fig. 2, I and J). The above distribution profiles of VGF peptides in the POA and median eminence remained broadly similar over the estrous cycle (not shown). In the anterior pituitary (Fig. 2, K–Q), all VGF antisera labelled large numbers of endocrine cells. The majority (80–90%) proved to be LH containing gonadotrophes (Fig. 2, K–N and O, P: TLQP and PGH peptides, respectively). A small proportion (about 10–20%) of VGF C- or N-terminus, or PGH immunoreactive cells (Fig. 2, O, Q) were prolactin containing lactotropes. In the morning following estrus, immunostaining of gonadotropes (especially with VGF C-and N-terminus and TLQP antibodies) was reduced, with an increase of visible labeling in a fraction of lactotropes, as shown previously [21] (Fig. 2, K, L *versus* M, N: diestrus *versus* estrus, respectively).

In the ovary (Fig. 3), TLQP peptide immunoreactivity was revealed in the granulosa (Fig. 3A) as well as in the theca and interstitial cells (Fig. 3B). Conversely, PGH peptide/s were restricted to oocytes (Fig. 3, C), and VGF C- and N- terminus peptide labeling was scanty. In ovariectomised rats, most hypertrophic pituitary gonadotropes showed VGF peptide immunoreactivity, with intense to moderate labeling intensity, as reported previously [21].

Changes in cycling females

As with any other quantitative method based on the use of antibodies, the numerical values of peptide concentrations measured in ELISA ought to be considered with caution, pending sequencing of the relevant native peptide/s, hence use of proper standards.

Nonetheless, TLQP peptides appeared to be most abundant in all areas we studied, as well as in plasma (Fig. 4), with lowest levels for VGF C-and N-terminus peptides in ovary and plasma. Along the estrous cycle, TLQP levels were higher during metestrus in median eminence and during metestrus and diestrus in pituitary. The same peptides were more abundant in ovary and lower in plasma during proestrus, compared to the other phases. VGF C- and N-terminus peptides, too, increased during metestrus and/or diestrus in median eminence and pituitary, as well as in plasma. PGH peptides failed to show significant modulation.

Ovariectomy and hormonal treatment

In the absence of hormonal treatment, upon ovariectomy TLQP peptides were greatly reduced in plasma (roughly 20% of average levels in cycling females: Figs. 4, 5). The other VGF peptides studied were also decreased, to very low levels. As measured in the "whole hypothalamus", post-ovariectomy TLQP and PGH peptides were roughly comparable to cycling females, while VGF N- and C-terminus peptides were reduced (Figs. 4, 5). In the pituitary, most VGF peptides studied were distinctly increased, except for VGF C-terminus containing ones. Upon estrogen-progesterone treatment, a differential response was shown for TLQP and VGF C-terminus peptides, both further increasing in the pituitary, while in hypothalamus TLQP increased, and VGF C-terminus peptides were reduced (Fig. 5). In plasma, all VGF peptides studied showed a tendency to increase after hormonal treatment, with significant differences for VGF N-terminus peptides only.

Molecular heterogeneity

To resolve small to medium MW peptides we resorted to gel chromatography, with detection by ELISA in view of its enhanced selectivity for internally cleaved peptides (see above). Three major peaks were shown for TLQP peptides (Fig. 6, left: a, b, c), closely matching the elution positions shown previously for TLQP-62, TLQP-30 and TLQP-21 [30]. Such forms were found in all tissues studied and in plasma, with a lower TLQP-21 peak in the ovary. Higher MW forms were seen, at approximately 10–12 kDa and in the void volume, or in the region overlapping the void volume in plasma (Fig. 6, left). VGF C-terminus immunoreactivity was revealed in the void volume (Fig. 6, mid-left: d), compatible with VGF precursor, and in a major broad peak in the approximately 10–15 kDa range (ibidem: e), possibly representing previously described VGF18 or VGF20 [11,12]. A lower peak (ibidem: f) appeared to relate to the TLQP "a" peak described above. The same peptides were mostly seen as low MW fragments in the ovary, while migrating as large forms in plasma (Fig. 6, mid-left). The VGF N-terminus assay also showed abundant reactivity in the large MW fractions from plasma (Fig. 6, mid-right: refer "g" to bottom panel), with lower levels at varied MW in tissue extracts. In the hypothalamus, the N-terminal VGF24–63 peptide [31] may take part in the lower MW portion (Fig. 6, mid-right: h) of a broad, approximately 3–10 kDa interval of immunoreactive fractions. PGH peptides were revealed as different MW forms, especially in the hypothalamus (Fig. 6, right). The largest MW forms eluting in the void volume were low in tissues and abundant in plasma (ibidem: i). Interestingly, an intermediate MW peak (ibidem: m, roughly 30–50 kDa) might correspond to PGH peptide/s encompassing the whole portion between the PGH sequence and either of the known cleaved rat peptides: $VGF_{180-209}$, or VGF_{24-36} [31;32], see (Fig. 1). The low MW peak shown (ibidem: n) fits well with the reported PGH8 peptide [33], running between the PGH sequence and the immediately preceding cleavage site (rat VGF: Lys_{421}-Arg_{422}).

In vitro experiments

A single dose of TLQP-21 was tested, comparable to the one shown to induce release of GnRH from male rat hypothalami [24]. Upon addition of TLQP-21 to the culture medium, somatostatin release into the medium showed a non-significant tendency to decrease (Fig. 7, left panel). Conversely, GHRH release was significantly enhanced (approximately 50%, Fig. 7, right panel).

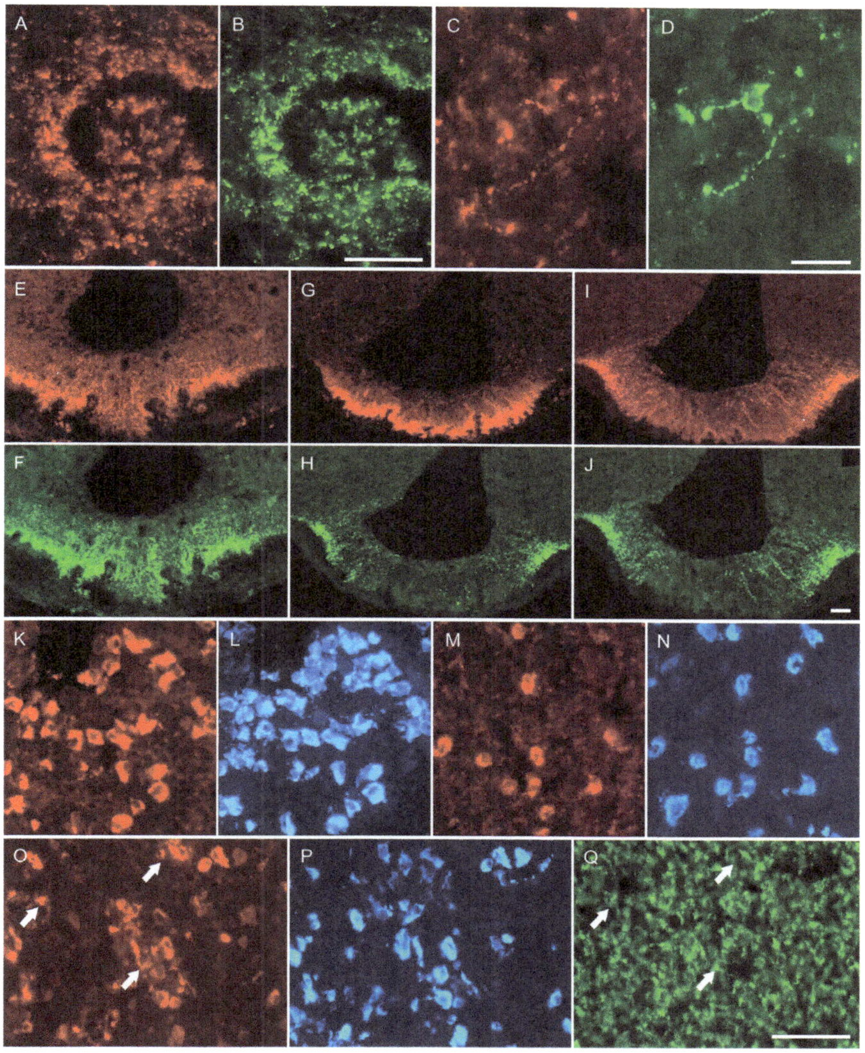

Figure 2. VGF peptide localisation in hypothalamus and pituitary. In the preoptic area (A–D), PGH peptides (A) were immunostained within almost all neuronal terminals containing GnRH (B) conversely, VGF N-terminus peptides (C) were also revealed in most kisspeptin neuronal terminals (D): A, C: Cy3 red labeling; B, D: Cy_2 green labeling. In the median eminence (E–J), TLQP peptides (E) were selectively found in almost all somatostatin neuronal terminals and axons (F). Conversely, VGF C-terminus (G) and PGH (I) antibodies labeled GnRH neurone terminals (H and J, respectively): E, G, I: Cy3 red labeling; F, H, J: Cy_2 green labeling. In the pituitary (K–Q), the number of cells positive with both TLQP (K, M) and LH (L, N) antibodies was higher in diestrous (K, L) than in estrous phase (M, N). Conversely, the PGH peptides (O) were found in a large number of LH cells (P) and in a few PRL cells (Q, colocalised cells are identified by the arrows). Scale bars: A–B, E–Q: 100 um, C–D: 50 um.

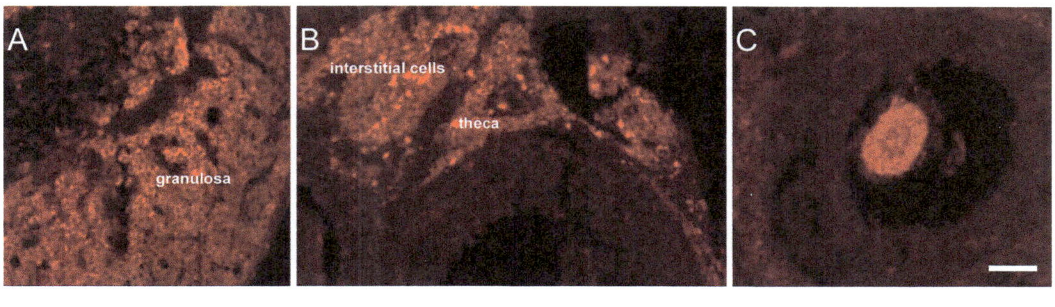

Figure 3. VGF peptide localisation in Ovary. TLQP peptide immunoreactivity was found in the granulosa (A) as well as in the theca and interstitial cells (B), while PGH peptides were restricted to the oocyte (C). All VGF staining: Cy_3 red labeling. Scale bar: 50 um.

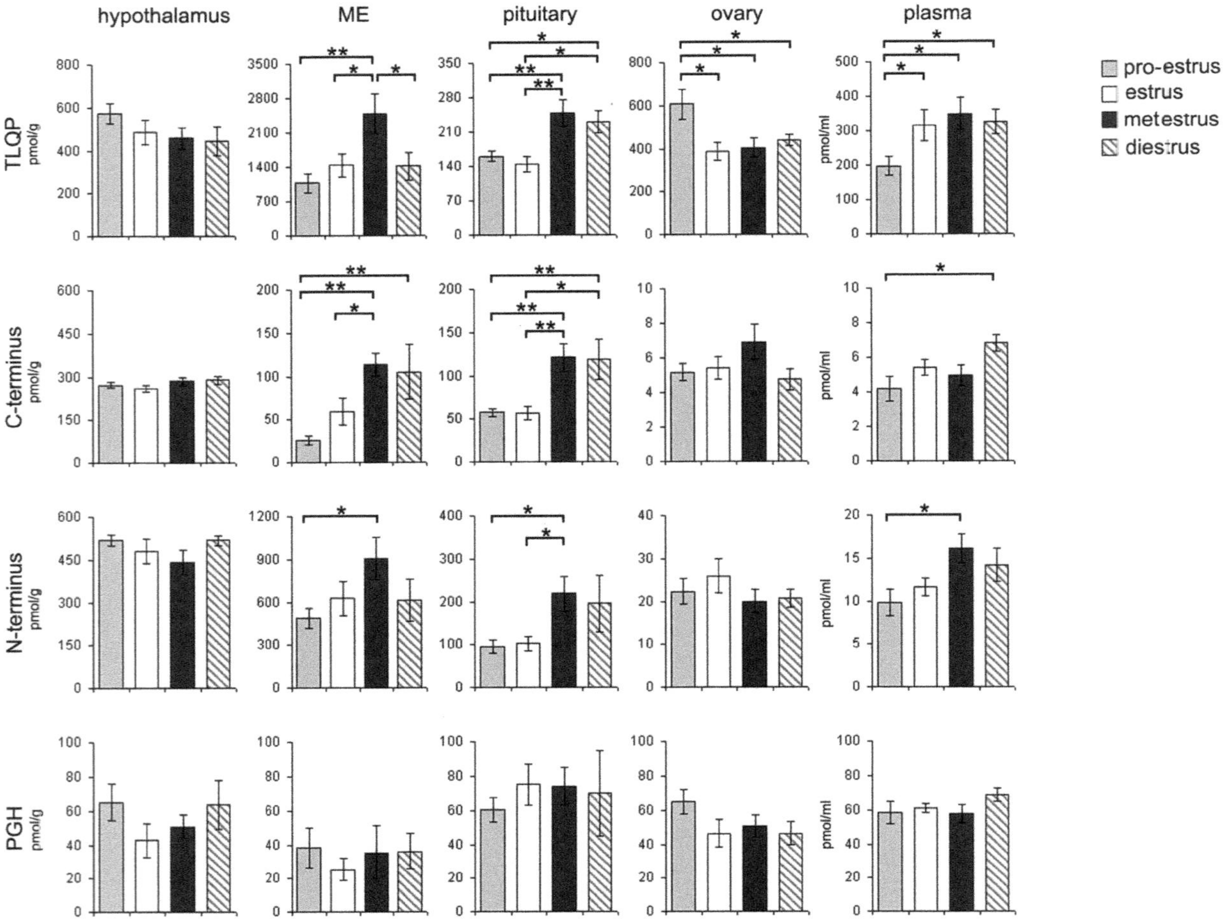

Figure 4. VGF peptide levels in cycling females. Levels of TLQP, C-/N- terminus and PGH peptides were measured in hypothalamus, median eminence (M.E), pituitary, ovary and plasma in each phase of the estrous cycle. During metestrus and/or diestrus, enhancement was revealed for TLQP and the C-/N-terminal peptides in M.E, pituitary and also in plasma. In the pro-estrous phase, exclusively TLQP peptides were found to be increased in ovary and decreased in plasma. PGH peptides did not show any change. Pmol/g: picomoles per grams; pmol/ml: picomoles per millilitres; *p<0.05, **p<0.005.

Discussion

Our study demonstrated the presence of several peptides derived from the VGF precursor, with selective differential profiles at all levels of the hypothalamic-pituitary-ovarian axis. A striking modulation in peptide tissue levels including plasma was shown across the estrous cycle, implicating VGF peptides in events and mechanisms relevant to reproduction.

In view of the proposed role of VGF as multifunctional precursor of bioactive peptides our study was focused on end products of the VGF precursor, rather than on the primary VGF gene product itself. The primary sequence of VGF shows at least ten putative cleavage sites, in the form of two or more basic amino acid residues, highly conserved across species. Recently, further fragments including bioactive VGF peptides have been shown to derive from cleavage at single basic amino acids [16,34,35]. In view of the lower proteomic complexity of the cerebro-spinal fluid (CSF), the precise chemical nature of VGF derived end products has so far been mostly studied in such body fluid [36] with the addition of neuro-endocrine cells lines [33]. An array of VGF peptides and fragments have been revealed, with striking changes in neurodegenerative and other disease conditions [37–40]. Certain VGF peptides proved to be released *in vivo* in the brain upon neuronal depolarization [31] while an interactomic investigation revealed selective domains of VGF, including the TLQP-21 region, as likely binding partners for the amyloid precursor protein [41]. Similarly, two peptides derived from non-overlapping regions of the VGF precursor were reported in the protein-bound and unbound fractions, respectively, from CSF [42]. In the present study, TLQP-antibodies showed several chromatography peaks fitting well with known VGF peptides, such as TLQP-21, -30 and -62 [30]. Products derived from the C-terminal domain of VGF have been studied in some detail [11,12] and the major molecular form/s we found in hypothalamus and pituitary may represent so-called VGF18 and 20 (such denomination refers to migration in western blot, not to MW). In connection with the TLQP-62 peak shown here with the relevant N-terminal antibody ("TLQP rat 556–565" antibody), a lower amount of reactivity was revealed in chromatography with the corresponding C-terminus antibody. The very high selectivity of such antibody that we found for the unmodified C-terminal sequence suggests that TLQP-62 peptide/s may partly undergo limited processing at their C-terminal end. Other peptides derived from the C-terminal domain of the VGF precursor may have gone undetected in our study, due to a degree of processing or change at their C-terminus. At the other extreme

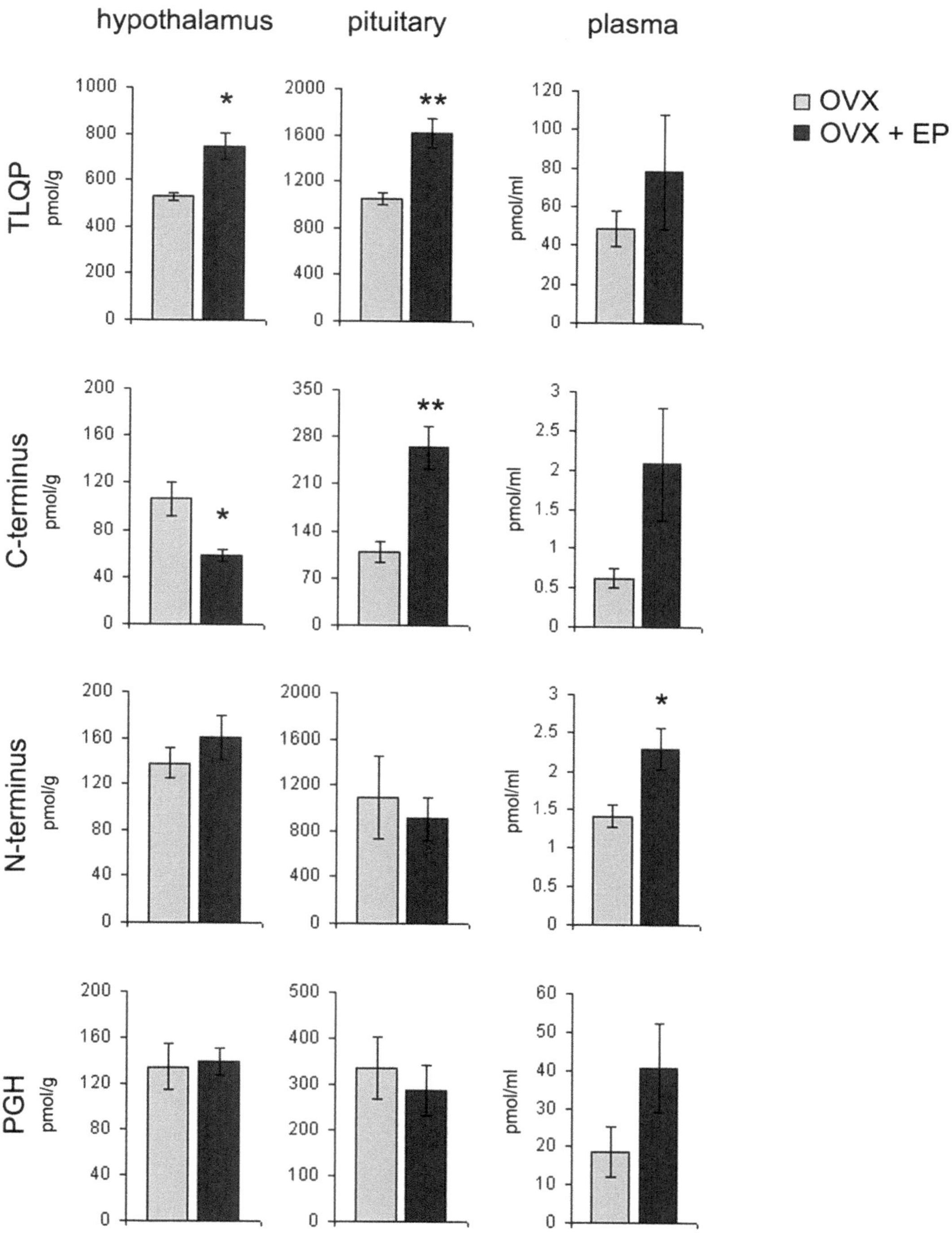

Figure 5. VGF peptide levels in ovariectomised (OVX) rats. Levels of TLQP, C-/N-terminus and PGH peptides were measured in the hypothalamus (including median eminence), pituitary, and plasma of OVX rats with and without oestradiol-progesterone (EP) treatment: OVX+EP and OVX, respectively. OVX+EP rats revealed an increase for TLQP peptides in hypothalamus and pituitary as well as changes for C-terminal peptides. In plasma, after EP treatment an increase was revealed for N-terminal peptides only. The PGH peptides did not reveal any change. Pmol/g: picomoles *per* grams; pmol/ml: picomoles per millilitres; $*p<0.05$, $**p<0.005$.

of VGF, a fully N-terminal 40 amino acid peptide has been proved to be released upon neuronal depolarization [31]. Such peptide may take part in a broad region of immunoreactivity we found in the hypothalamus and probably elsewhere. A small PGH peptide ("PGH8"), corresponding to a sequence running from the C-terminal peptide sequence we used to raise antibodies ("PGH rat$_{422-430}$" antibody), to the immediately preceding putative cleavage site (Lys-Arg, rat VGF$_{421-422}$, "R" preceding the "PGH rat 422–430") was demonstrated in mouse neuroblastoma cells [33]. While several intermediate MW PGH peptides are difficult to interpret, one may speculate that the broad immuno-reactive peak close to the void volume that we found in gel

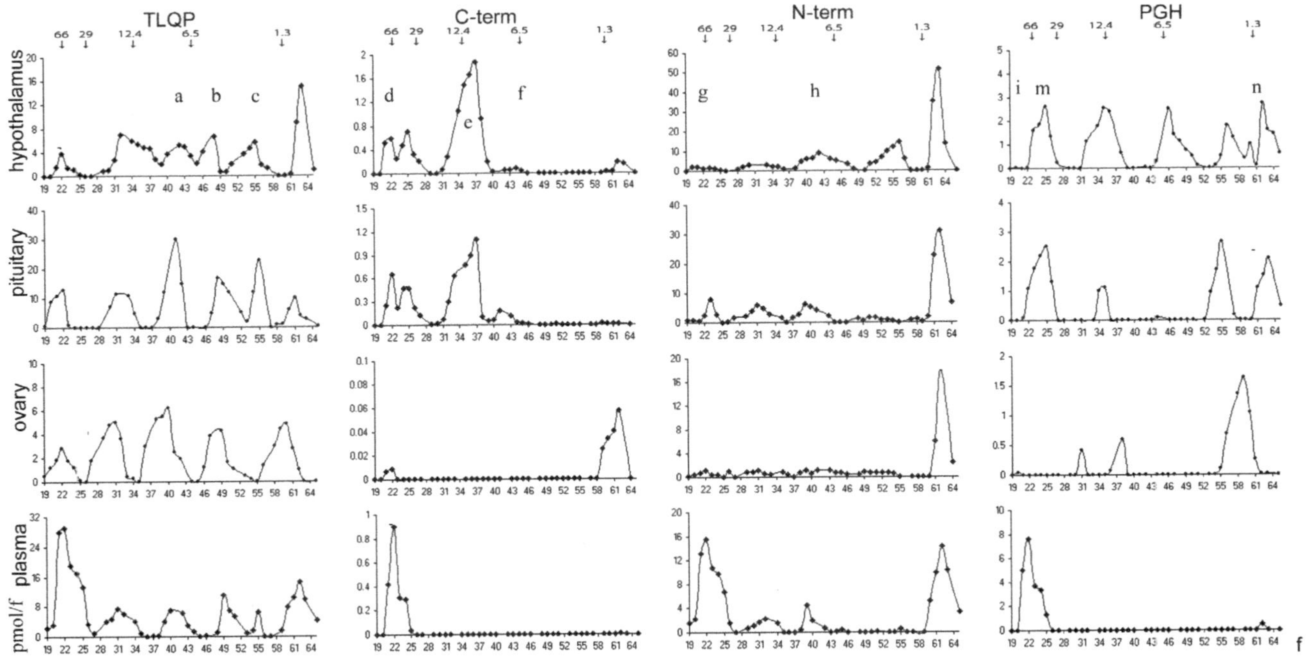

Figure 6. Sephadex chromatography. Three major peaks were shown for TLQP peptides (left: a, b, c), corresponding to TLQP-62, TLQP-30 and TLQP-21 and found in all tissue extracts. Higher MW forms were seen, at approximately 10–12 kDa and in the void volume, or in the region overlapping the void volume in plasma. VGF C-terminus immunoreactivity was revealed in the void volume (mid-left: d), compatible with VGF precursor, and in a major broad peak in the approximately 10–15 kDa range (ibidem: e), while a lower peak (ibidem: f) appeared related to the TLQP "a" peak described above. The same peptides were mostly seen as low MW fragments in the ovary, while migrating as large forms in plasma (mid-left). The VGF N-terminus assay revealed abundant reactivity in the large MW fractions from plasma (mid-right: refer "g" to bottom panel), with lower levels at varied MW in the other tissue extracts. PGH peptides were revealed as different MW forms, especially in the hypothalamus while the largest MW forms eluting in the void volume were abundant in plasma (ibidem: i). Molecular weight markers are shown with the corresponding arrows. Pmol/f:picomoles/fraction; f:fraction.

chromatography could include putative, large VGF fragments running from the PGH sequence to a region close to the N-terminus of VGF. In plasma, we revealed certain VGF peptides possibly including TLQP-21, TLQP-30 and TLQP-62, however, in general, a large MW peak was prominent with all VGF assays. This may indicate that one or more VGF peptides travel in the circulation bound to plasma proteins. In fact, many polypeptides are known to bind to major plasma proteins, and/or to their selective transporter/s. Concerning to our study, one ought to notice that tissue extracts underwent at least some treatment steps (e.g. heat tratment) which would reduce molecular interactions of VGF peptides with other molecules, while plasma samples was

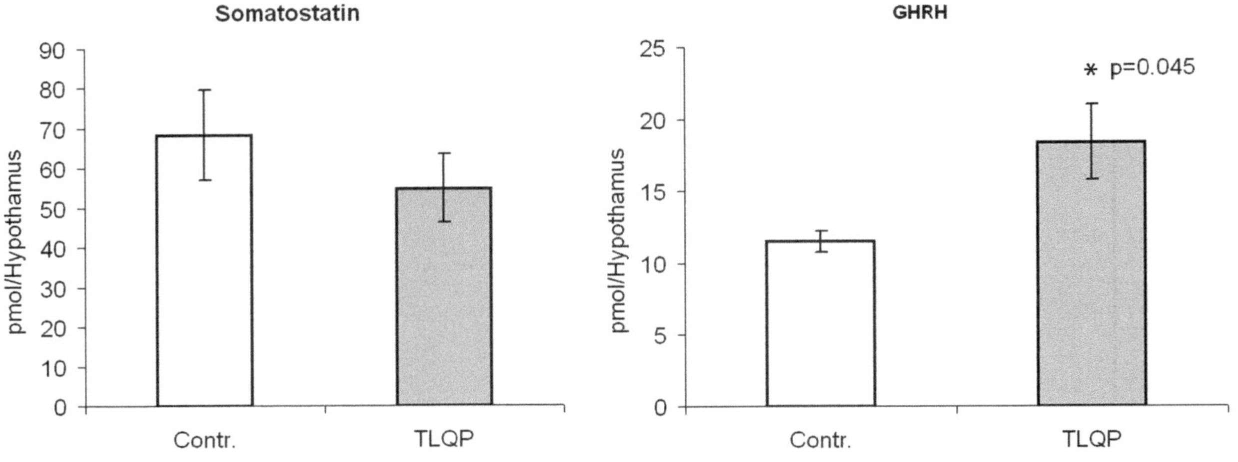

Figure 7. TLQP-21 in *in vitro* experiments. TLQP-21 included in the medium of hypothalamic samples up-regulates the secretion of growth-hormone-releasing hormone (GHRH). Contr.: control medium analysed by ELISA without the addition of TLQP-21 *versus* the medium including the peptide (TLQP column).

neither extracted, nor treated before assays. While examples of the binding of VGF peptides to other components are provided above, the possibility that at least some of the VGF-immunoreactive large MW forms found in plasma may represent actual VGF precursor cannot be excluded.

On this context, the selective differential MW profiles of the VGF peptides were found in parallel with a striking modulation in their tissue levels across the estrous cycle.

With respect to the TLQP peptides, as mentioned, they were found within median eminence somatostatin neurones, gonadotropic and ovary cells with high tissue levels especially in ovary and plasma. In the blood, their low levels in ovariectomised rats showed the ovary as a major source of circulating TLQP peptides. During the cycle, we showed an increase in pituitary TLQP levels on metestrus–diestrus. This is according to the increase in LH secretion obtained after TLQP-21 *icv* administration in adult female rats on the same diestrous phase [25]. Moreover, we reported here that, on proestrus, the TLQP ovary levels were augmented, but during the following phases (including the diestrus), the same ovary reduced its TLQP peptide content that concurrently augmented in blood. The possible involvement of TLQP peptides in endocrine mechanisms related to reproduction is suggested also by the reported increase in LH secretion after system *ip* administration of TLQP-21 on prepubertal rats [25]. Hence, from our results, one may hypothesize that during the diestrus-metestrus, circulating TLQP peptides secreted from the ovary, may stimulate the pituitary secretion of LH, perhaps through an augment of the same TLQP content in the pituitary. The involvement of TLQP peptides on female reproductive mechanisms has so far been reported to be related to the LH production at the pituitary [25] but not at the gonad level. As to the potential TLQP receptors, the same C3a/C3AR1 molecules that have been found to modulate the pituitary hormonal activity [43] have been reported to be the targets of the TLQP-21 in the hamster ovary cell lines [44]. Hence, the same ovary that secretes TLQP peptides into the blood could be regulated by its own derived peptides, or alternatively the circulating TLQP peptides reacting to the ovary receptors could originate, at least in part, from the hypophysis. This is suggested by our finding in estrous phase, where a marked reduction in TLQP pituitary levels (according to a minor number of immnolabeled cells) was found in parallel with a TLQP plasmatic increase.

Moreover, we cannot exclude the possibility that TLQP peptides could also act through a paracrine and/or autocrine way, in view of their presence in the same organs (pituitary and ovary) that contain their potential receptors. This autocrine/paracrine role could involve the regulation of LH secretion, according to the mentioned augment in TLQP pituitary levels on the same phase in which the LH secretion was found to increase [25]. Indeed, an autocrine role have been already demonstrated for other VGF peptides as NERPs that being present within the vasopressin cells, regulated the same vasopressin production [16,34]. On the other end, our results showed also that TLQP peptides in the pituitary and hypothalamus could be up-regulated by the oestradiol/progesterone.

These hormones regulate also somatostatin [45], and being TLQP peptides present in such neurones, it is possible that steroid hormones could modulate both TLQP and somatostatin by the same mechanisms. Regarding the role of TLQP peptides in the median eminence, in view of their close relation to somatostatin seen also in pancreas [46] and stomach [30], we tried to elucidate a possible bioactivity of TLQP-21 on somatostatin and on its GHRH neurone targets. We found that TLQP-21 up-regulated the GHRH production suggesting that such peptide could act promoting the growth at the hypothalamic level. When adult male mice were chronically treated (by *icv* injection) with TLQP-21, physiological, molecular and behavioral parameters related to the GH axis were investigated, however, TLQP-21 did not modulate the GH axis [47]. One could hypothesize that TLQP-21 may regulate GHRH through somatostatin neurones selectively at the median eminence level, instead when the same peptide is injected, only a little part could reach the median eminence. Further experiments are needed to ascertain the precise role of TLQP-21 on the growth mechanisms and the possible connections with the cycle. Regarding the other VGF peptides, also C-and N-terminus peptides changed in the hypothalamus, pituitary and plasma. However, for these peptides is more difficult to hypothesize mechanisms of action in view of the rare information regarding their involvement on reproduction. It could be only suggested that these peptides could have a neuroendocrine and/or endocrine activity on the estrous cycle, and their presence into kisspeptin neurones is intriguing because of the importance of this hormone in reproductive mechanisms [48,49]. Furthermore, also the presence of PGH peptides in gonadotrophs, GnRH neurones, plasma and especially within the oocyte, needs more investigation. In conclusion, various VGF peptides may regulate the hypothalamus-pituitary complex *via* specific neuroendocrine mechanisms. In particular, for TLQP peptides we may hypothesize different possible interacting ways of action on the reproduction including endocrine pathways largely involving the ovary as well as paracrine/autocrine mechanisms at both the pituitary and ovary levels.

In addition, we also found evidence for an involvement of TLQP-21 on neuroendocrine mechanisms acting on promoting growth at the median eminence level.

Supporting Information

Data S1 TLQP and C-terminus assay results. For each assay, data referring to picomoles per gram or milliliter revealed by ELISA for each single animal case in each tissue tested through the 4 cycle phases.

Data S2 N-terminus and PGH assay results. For each assay, data referring to picomoles per gram or milliliter revealed by ELISA for each single animal case in each tissue tested through the 4 cycle phases.

Data S3 TLQP, C-terminus, N-terminus and PGH assay results. For each assay, data referring to picomoles per gram and milliliter revealed by ELISA for each single animal case in each tissue tested using ovariectomised rats without any hormonal tratment (OVX) and treated with estrogen-progesterone (OVX + EP).

Data S4 Somatostatin and GHRH assay results. For each assay, data referring to picomoles per well, grams per well, total grams of hypothalamus, as well as picomoles per hypothalamus and milliliter obtained using each single hypothalamic sample with (TLQP: B1 to B8) and without (contr: controls, A1 to A6) the addition of the TLQP-21 peptide to the culture medium.

Acknowledgments

We thank C. Mostallino at the National Research Council, Institute of Neuroscience, Cagliari, for rat stabulation. Dr. Peter Berger, National Institute of Diabetes and Digestive and Kidney Diseases and Dr. A.F. Parlow for providing antibodies.

Author Contributions

GLF raised antisera. Conceived and designed the experiments: BN CC. Performed the experiments: BN FD CB. Analyzed the data: BN CC CB. Contributed reagents/materials/analysis tools: GLF. Contributed to the writing of the manuscript: CC GLF.

References

1. Hahm S, Mizuno TM, Wu TJ, Wisor JP, Priest CA, et al. (1999) Targeted deletion of the vgf gene indicates that the encoded secretory peptide precursor plays a novel role in the regulation of energy balance. Neuron 23: 537–548.
2. Levi A, Eldridge JD, Paterson BM (1985) Molecular cloning of a gene sequence regulated by nerve growth factor. Science 229: 393–5.
3. Salton SR, Fischberg DJ, Dong KW (1991) Structure of the gene encoding VGF, a nervous system-specific mRNA that is rapidly and selectively induced by nerve growth factor in PC12 cells. Mol Cell Biol 11(5): 2335–2349.
4. Snyder SE, Pintar JE, Salton SR (1998) Developmental expression of VGF mRNA in the prenatal and postnatal rat. J Comp Neurol 394: 64–90.
5. Snyder SE, Salton SR (1998) Expression of VGF mRNA in the adult rat central nervous system. J Comp Neurol 394(1): 91–105.
6. Van den Pol AN, Decavel C, Levi A, Paterson B (1989) Hypothalamic expression of a novel gene product, VGF: immunocytochemical analysis. J Neurosci 9: 4122–4137.
7. Van den Pol AN, Bina K, Decavel C, Ghosh P (1994) VGF expression in the brain. J Comp Neurol 347: 455–469.
8. Levi A, Ferri GL, Watson E, Possenti R, Salton SR (2004) Processing, distribution, and function of VGF, a neuronal and endocrine peptide precursor. Cell Mol Neurobiol: 24 517–33.
9. Salton SR, Ferri GL, Hahm S, Snyder SE, Wilson AJ, et al. (2000) VGF: a novel role for this neuronal and neuroendocrine polypeptide in the regulation of energy balance. Front Neuroendocrinol 21: 199–219.
10. Possenti R, Rinaldi AM, Ferri GL, Borboni P, Trani E, et al. (1999) Expression, processing, and secretion of the neuroendocrine VGF peptides by INS-1 cells. Endocrinology 140: 3727–3735.
11. Trani E, Ciotti T, Rinaldi AM, Canu N, Ferri GL, et al. (1995) Tissue-specific processing of the neuroendocrine protein VGF. J Neurochem 65: 2441–2449.
12. Trani E, Giorgi A, Canu N, Amadoro G, Rinaldi AM, et al. (2002) Isolation and characterization of VGF peptides in rat brain. Role of PC1/3 and PC2 in the maturation of VGF precursor. J Neurochem 81: 565–574.
13. Canu N, Possenti R, Rinaldi AM, Trani E, Levi A (1997) Molecular cloning and characterization of the human VGF promoter region. J Neurochem 68: 1390–1399.
14. Bartolomucci A, La Corte G, Possenti R, Locatelli V, Rigamonti AE, et al. (2006) TLQP-21, a VGF-derived peptide, increases energy expenditure and prevents the early phase of diet-induced obesity. Proc Natl Acad Sci U S A 103(39): 14584–14589.
15. Bozdagi O, Rich E, Tronel S, Sadahiro M, Patterson K, et al. (2008) The neurotrophin-inducible gene vgf regulates hippocampal function and behavior through a brain-derived neurotrophic factor-dependent mechanism. J Neurosci 28: 9857–69.
16. Yamaguchi H, Sasaki K, Satomi Y, Shimbara T, Kageyama H, et al. (2007) Peptidomic identification and biological validation of neuroendocrine regulatory peptide-1 and -2. J Biol Chem 282: 26354–26360.
17. Rizzi R, Bartolomucci A, Moles A, D'Amato F, Sacerdote P, et al. (2008) The VGF-derived peptide TLQP-21: a new modulatory peptide for inflammatory pain. Neurosci Lett 441: 129–133.
18. Chen YC, Pristerá A, Ayub M, Swanwick RS, Karu K, et al. (2013) Identification of a receptor for neuropeptide VGF and its role in neuropathic pain. J Biol Chem: 288 34638–34646.
19. Razzoli M, Bo E, Pascucci T, Pavone F, D'Amato FR, et al. (2012) Implication of the VGF-derived peptide TLQP-21 in mouse acute and chronic stress responses. Behav Brain Res 229(2): 333–339.
20. Severini C, La Corte G, Improta G, Broccardo M, Agostini S, et al. (2009) In vitro and in vivo pharmacological role of TLQP-21, a VGF-derived peptide, in the regulation of rat gastric motor functions. Br J Pharmacol. 157(6): 984–93.
21. Ferri GL, Gaudio RM, Cossu M, Rinaldi AM, Polak JM, et al. (1995) The VGF protein in rat adenohypophysis: sex differences and changes during the estrous cycle and after gonadectomy. Endocrinology 136: 2244–2251.
22. Brancia C, Nicolussi P, Cappai P, La Corte G, Possenti R, et al. (2005) Differential expression and seasonal modulation of VGF peptides in sheep pituitary. J Endocrinol 186: 97–107.
23. Babbitt CC, Tung J, Wray GA, Alberts SC (2012) Changes in gene associated with reproductive maturation in wild female baboons. Genome Biol Evol 4(2): 102–109.
24. Pinilla L, Pineda R, Gaytán F, Romero M, García-Galiano D, et al. (2011) Characterization of the reproductive effects of the anorexigenic VGF-derived peptide TLQP-21: in vivo and in vitro studies in male rats. Am J Physiol Endocrinol Metab 300(5): E837–847.
25. Aguilar E, Pineda R, Gaytán F, Sánchez-Garrido MA, Romero M, et al. (2013) Characterization of the reproductive effects of the VGF-derived peptide, TLQP-21, in female rats: in vivo and in vitro studies. Neuroendocrinology 98(1): 38–50.
26. Cocco C, Melis GV, Ferri GL (2003) Embedding media for cryomicrotomy: an applicative reappraisal. Appl Immunohistochem Mol Morphol 11(3): 274–80.
27. Ferri GL, Cocco C, Melis GV, Aste L (2002) Equipment testing and tuning: the cold-knife cryomicrotome microm HM-560. Appl Immunohistochem Mol Morphol 10(4): 381–386.
28. D'Amato F, Noli B, Brancia C, Cocco C, Flore G, et al. (2008) Differential distribution of VGF-derived peptides in the adrenal medulla and evidence for their selective modulation. J Endocrinol 197: 359–369.
29. Cocco C, D'Amato F, Noli B, Ledda A, Brancia C, et al. (2010) Distribution of VGF peptides in the human cortex and their selective changes in Parkinson's and Alzheimer's diseases. J Anat 217: 683–93.
30. Brancia C, Cocco C, D'Amato F, Noli B, Sanna F, et al. (2010) Selective expression of TLQP-21 and other VGF peptides in gastric neuroendocrine cells and modulation by feeding. J Endocrinol 207: 329–341.
31. Bernay B, Gaillard M-C, Guryca V, Emadali A, Kuhn L, et al. (2009) Discovering New Bioactive Neuropeptides in the Striatum Secretome Using in Vivo Microdialysis and Versatile Proteomics. Mol Cell Proteomics 8(5): 946–58.
32. Sasaki K, Takahashi N, Satoh M, Yamasaki M, Minamino N (2010) A Peptidomics Strategy for Discovering Endogenous Bioactive Peptides. Journal of Proteome Research 9: 5047–5052.
33. Rozek W, Kwasnik M, Debski J, Zmudzinski JF (2013) Mass spectrometry identification of granins and other proteins secreted by neuroblastoma cells. Tumor Biol 34: 1773–1781.
34. Fujihara H, Sasaki K, Mishiro-Sato E, Ohbuchi T, Dayanithi G, et al. (2012) Molecular Characterization and Biological Function of Neuroendocrine Regulatory Peptide-3 in the Rat. Endocrinology 153(3): 1377–86.
35. Sasaki K, Osaki T, Minamino N (2012) Large-scale identification of endogenous secretory peptides using electron transfer dissociation mass spectrometry. Mol Cell Proteomics 12(3): 700–9.
36. Yuan X, Desiderio DM (2005) Human cerebrospinal fluid peptidomics. J Mass Spectr 40: 176–181.
37. Carrette O, Demalte I, Scherl A, Yalkinoglu O, Corthals G, et al. (2003) A panel of cerebrospinal fluid potential biomarkers for the diagnosis of Alzheimer's disease. Proteomics 3: 1486–1494.
38. Ruetschi U, Zetterberg H, Podust VN, Gottfries J, Li S, et al. (2005) Identification of CSF biomarkers for frontotemporal dementia using SELDI-TOF. Experimental Neurology 196: 273–281.
39. Busse S, Bernstein HG, Busse M, Bielau H, Brisch R, et al. (2012) Reduced density of hypothalamic VGF-immunoreactive neurons in schizophrenia: a potential link to impaired growth factor signaling and energy homeostasis. Eur Arch Psychiatry Clin Neurosc 262(5): 365–74.
40. Asano T, Koizumi S, Takagi A, Hatori T, Kuwabara K, et al. (2011) Identification of a novel biomarker candidate, a 4.8-kDa peptide fragment from a neurosecretory protein VGF precursor, by proteomic analysis of cerebrospinal fluid from children with acute encephalopathy using SELDI-TOF-MS. Neurology 11: 101.
41. Bai Y, Markham K, Chen F, Weerasekera R, Watts J, et al. (2005) The in vivo brain interactome of the amyloid precursor protein. Mol Cell Proteomics (1): 15–34.
42. Wijte D, McDonnell LA, Balog CI, Bossers K, Deelder AM, et al. (2012) A novel peptidomics approach to detect markers of Alzheimer's disease in cerebrospinal fluid. Methods 56(4): 500–7.
43. Francis K, Lewis BM, Akatsu H, Monk PN, Cain SA (2003) Complement C3a receptors in the pituitary gland: a novel pathway by which an innate immune molecule releases hormones involved in the control of inflammation. FASEB J 17(15): 2266–8.
44. Hannedouche S, Beck V, Leighton-Davies J, Beibel M, Roma G, et al. (2013) Identification of the C3a receptor (C3AR1) as the target of the VGF-derived peptide TLQP-21 in rodent cells. J Biol Chem 288(38): 27434–27443.
45. Van Vugt HH, Van de Heijning BJ, Van der Beek EM (2008) Somatostatin in the rat periventricular nucleus: sex differences and effect of gonadal steroids. Exp Brain Res 188(4): 483–491.
46. Cocco C, Brancia C, Pirisi I, D'Amato F, Noli B, et al. (2007) VGF metabolic-related gene: distribution of its derived peptides in mammalian pancreatic islets. J Histochem Cytochem 55: 619–628.

47. Bartolomucci A, Rigamonti AE, Bulgarelli I, Torsello A, Locatelli V, et al. (2007) Chronic intracerebroventricular TLQP-21 delivery does not modulate the GH/IGF-1-axis and muscle strength in mice. Growth Horm IGF Res 17(4): 342–5.
48. Navarro VM, Castellano JM, Fernández-Fernández R, Tovar S, Roa J, et al. (2005) Effects of KiSS-1 peptide, the natural ligand of GPR54, on follicle-stimulating hormone secretion in the rat. Endocrinology 146(4): 1689–1697.
49. Adachi S, Yamada S, Takatsu Y, Matsui H, Kinoshita M, et al. (2007) Involvement of anteroventral periventricular metastin/kisspeptin neurons in estrogen positive feedback action on luteinizing hormone release in female rats. J Reprod Dev 53(2): 367–78.

Short and Long Term Effects of Left and Bilateral Repetitive Transcranial Magnetic Stimulation in Schizophrenia Patients with Auditory Verbal Hallucinations: A Randomized Controlled Trial

Leonie Bais[1,2*], Ans Vercammen[3], Roy Stewart[4], Frank van Es[5,7], Bert Visser[5], André Aleman[1,6], Henderikus Knegtering[1,2,7]

1 University of Groningen, University Medical Center Groningen, Department of Neuroscience and BCN NeuroImaging Center, Groningen, The Netherlands, **2** Lentis Psychiatric Institute, Groningen, The Netherlands, **3** Australian Catholic University, Strathfield, Australia, **4** University of Groningen, University Medical Center Groningen, Department of Health Sciences, Community and Occupational Medicine, Groningen, The Netherlands, **5** University of Groningen, University Medical Center Groningen, Department of Psychiatry, Groningen, The Netherlands, **6** University of Groningen, Department of Psychology, Groningen, The Netherlands, **7** University of Groningen, University Medical Center Groningen, Rob Giel Research Center, Groningen, The Netherlands

Abstract

Background: Repetitive transcranial magnetic stimulation of the left temporo-parietal junction area has been studied as a treatment option for auditory verbal hallucinations. Although the right temporo-parietal junction area has also shown involvement in the genesis of auditory verbal hallucinations, no studies have used bilateral stimulation. Moreover, little is known about durability effects. We studied the short and long term effects of 1 Hz treatment of the left temporo-parietal junction area in schizophrenia patients with persistent auditory verbal hallucinations, compared to sham stimulation, and added an extra treatment arm of bilateral TPJ area stimulation.

Methods: In this randomized controlled trial, 51 patients diagnosed with schizophrenia and persistent auditory verbal hallucinations were randomly allocated to treatment of the left or bilateral temporo-parietal junction area or sham treatment. Patients were treated for six days, twice daily for 20 minutes. Short term efficacy was measured with the Positive and Negative Syndrome Scale (PANSS), the Auditory Hallucinations Rating Scale (AHRS), and the Positive and Negative Affect Scale (PANAS). We included follow-up measures with the AHRS and PANAS at four weeks and three months.

Results: The interaction between time and treatment for Hallucination item P3 of the PANSS showed a trend for significance, caused by a small reduction of scores in the left group. Although self-reported hallucination scores, as measured with the AHRS and PANAS, decreased significantly during the trial period, there were no differences between the three treatment groups.

Conclusion: We did not find convincing evidence for the efficacy of left-sided rTMS, compared to sham rTMS. Moreover, bilateral rTMS was not superior over left rTMS or sham in improving AVH. Optimizing treatment parameters may result in stronger evidence for the efficacy of rTMS treatment of AVH. Moreover, future research should consider investigating factors predicting individual response.

Trial Registration: Dutch Trial Register NTR1813

Editor: Ryouhei Ishii, Osaka University Graduate School of Medicine, Japan

Funding: This project was supported by the University of Groningen (www.rug.nl). The University of Groningen had no role in study design, data collection and analysis, decision to publish, or preparation of the manuscript.

* Email: l.bais@umcg.nl

Introduction

About 50–70% of the patients fulfilling the criteria for schizophrenia experience auditory verbal hallucinations (AVH) on a frequent basis [1]. Antipsychotic medication is often chosen as the first treatment for this disabling symptom of schizophrenia. However, in 25% of the patients, hallucinations appear to be refractory to adequate treatment trials with antipsychotic medication [2]. The high level of burden accompanied with AVH urges for the development of more efficient treatments.

Understanding the underlying neural basis of AVH may be helpful in the development of better treatment options. AVH have been related to both structural and functional anomalies in frontal, temporal and parietal regions [3,4]. Furthermore, cingular, subcortical and cerebellar areas have shown involvement as well (for an overview, see: [5]). Several theories about the genesis of AVH have been suggested, but the most popular theory argues that AVH are a result of misattributions of inner speech to an external source [6]. Allen et al. [5] postulated a neurocognitive model in which they state that over-activation of primary and secondary auditory cortices may be associated with bottom-up over-perceptualization. Meanwhile, aberrant activation in Broca's area (speech production), and reduced connectivity between Broca's area and the anterior cingulate (monitoring) and Wernicke's area (speech reception), may lead to reduced top-down control, ultimately resulting in the experience of auditory verbal hallucinations.

Given the hyperactivation within speech perception areas during the experience of AVH, it seems plausible that modulation of the neuronal activity could reduce AVH. The left temporo-parietal junction area (TPJ) is strongly connected with primary and secondary auditory cortices, and has therefore been proposed as a target region for treatment with low frequency repetitive Transcranial Magnetic Stimulation (rTMS). rTMS constitutes the administration of brief magnetic pulses with an electro-magnetic coil on the scalp. Low frequency rTMS can reduce cortical excitability within the underlying cortical tissue and connected deeper brain tissues in healthy volunteers [7–9]. Although the exact mechanism of action is not yet understood, the effect of low frequency rTMS is being explained in terms of long-term depression (LTD)-like changes in synaptic efficacy [10]. In rats, it has been shown that the inhibiting effect on cortical excitability endures after multiple rTMS sessions [11]. Researchers have therefore begun to apply this technique in the treatment of neurological and psychiatric disorders [12] associated with aberrant cortical activity. Hoffman et al. [13,14] pioneered this intervention in schizophrenia patients experiencing AVH. Since the early 2000's a number of rTMS trials have been initiated, aiming to treat AVH, with the majority targeting the left TPJ area [15–31]. Recent basic cognitive rTMS studies have shown the relevance of the TPJ area in the language and AVH network [32–36].

Meta-analytical reviews of the treatment studies have shown moderate to large effect sizes [37–39]. However, the majority of these effect sizes are based on the severity of symptoms immediately after treatment. Little is known about the duration effects of rTMS for AVH. Only a few studies have been published on the effects after more than four weeks [16,19,20,28]. From a clinical perspective, insight into long-term effects of this type of treatment would be highly advantageous.

Despite neuroimaging findings on the involvement of both the left and right temporal cortex in the genesis of AVH [3,4], most treatments have restricted stimulation of low frequency rTMS to the left TPJ area. This treatment has been found to influence characteristics like frequency and attentional salience of AVH [15,16]. The right hemisphere is considered to be dominant for the processing of emotions [40], especially negative emotions [41]. As AVH are often negative in emotional content [42,43], it is conceivable that low frequency rTMS treatment over the right hemisphere down-regulates this negative content.

As an extension of the trial reported by Vercammen et al. [44], we report on a randomized controlled trial in schizophrenia patients with 1 Hz rTMS over the left TPJ area, compared to sham stimulation over the left TPJ area. To investigate whether stimulation over the right TPJ area would have an additional effect, we added an extra treatment arm of bilateral TPJ area stimulation. We included follow-up measures at four weeks and three months after treatment. We hypothesized that 1 Hz rTMS over the left TPJ area would result in improvement of AVH, compared to sham stimulation, and that reduction of AVH would be further enhanced after bilateral stimulation, compared to both left TPJ stimulation and sham.

Materials and Methods

The protocol for this trial and supporting CONSORT checklist are available as supporting information; see Checklist S1 and Protocol S1.

Participants

From July 2006 to March 2012, patients were recruited at University Medical Center Groningen (UMCG), and collaborating regional mental health foundations: Lentis, GGz Friesland, GGz Drenthe and Mediant. All patients met DSM-IV criteria for schizophrenia; diagnoses were confirmed using Schedules for Clinical Assessment in Neuropsychiatry [45]. Only patients reporting frequent (at least daily) medication resistant AVH were included. Medication resistance was defined as daily occurring AVH despite at least two adequate trials of antipsychotic medication for at least four weeks prior to study inclusion. Medication dose remained unchanged for the duration of the study. To minimize the risk of inducing seizures by rTMS, patients with a personal or family history of epileptic seizures were excluded. Other exclusion criteria were: a history of severe head trauma or neurological disorder, the presence of intra-cerebral or pacemaker implants, inner ear prosthesis or other metal prosthetics/implants, severe behavioral disorder, current substance abuse, and pregnancy.

This study was approved by the licensed local medical ethical committee of the University Medical Center Groningen (number 2006/052) and conducted in accordance with the latest version of the Declaration of Helsinki (Protocol S1). As it was not yet customary in The Netherlands to register non-pharmaceutical trials when our trial started in 2006, we registered the trial in 2009 in the Dutch trial register when it was advised to do so (www.trialregister.nl, number: NTR1813). The authors confirm that all ongoing and related trials for this intervention are registered. Only patients who were competent to give informed consent were included. Prior to the study, all subjects gave oral and written informed consent after the procedure had been fully explained. All obtained subject data was handled anonymously.

This study was a double-blind randomized controlled trial. Treatments were given in the University Center of Psychiatry of the UMCG. Before the start of the trial, envelopes were numbered sequentially with participant ID numbers. An independent colleague drew tokens for one of the three treatment conditions, which were subsequently put into the envelopes. The envelopes were sealed, and prior to the start of each participant's treatment period, the researcher (AV or LB) opened the envelope with the number that corresponded to the participant's allocated ID number. Participant ID numbers were allocated consecutively based on date of participant intake, which was not controlled by the TMS administrator. Only the persons who administered the TMS (either the researchers or a trained nurse) were aware of the treatment condition. All other people involved – participants, clinical raters and clinicians – were kept blind. To check for blinding success, the participants completed a questionnaire. Participants were informed about the received treatment when the last follow-up measurement at three months was completed.

During the trial, patients were either admitted to an inpatient care unit, a day-hospital, or visited the hospital twice a day. Demographic and clinical characteristics at baseline are provided in Table 1.

rTMS procedure

We used a Magstim Rapid System (Magstim Company Ltd, Whitland, Wales) with a 70 mm figure-of-eight coil. Sham stimulation was administered using a coil that produced the same clicking sound, without delivering a measurable magnetic field. Before the first treatment session, resting motor threshold was only determined in patients enrolled in an active treatment condition. The resting motor threshold is defined as the minimum intensity to induce a noticeable movement of the dominant hand in five out of ten pulses administered on the contralateral primary motor cortex [46]. We did not determine the motor threshold in the patients that were to receive sham treatment, to reduce the risk of unblinding the participant to the treatment condition, as our sham procedure produces no physical sensation, but the motor threshold determination does.

The localization of the TPJ area was based on the 10–20 International System of EEG electrode positions. Both active and sham stimulation of the left TPJ area were administered halfway between T3 and P3 electrode positions. In the bilateral condition the left TPJ area was stimulated for the first 10 minutes of the session, after which the coil position was switched to the right TPJ area, halfway between T4 and P4 electrode positions. The 10–20 system has been commonly used in previous rTMS trials for AVH [16,19–24,26,27,47], because it is a patient-friendly compromise between time efficiency and individual variability, as it takes individual head size into account [48].

Treatment was conducted for six consecutive days (except during the weekends), twice daily, for 20 minutes at 1 Hz on 90% of resting motor threshold. Patients thus received a total of 14400 pulses during the treatment. There was always a minimum period of five hours between two treatment sessions.

Power calculation

Previous research using a similar design and rTMS parameters [22] found significant effects of the treatment on behavioral variables (Auditory Hallucination Rating Scale). An effect size of 1.22 was observed [22,37]. With the inclusion of 16 subjects in each treatment arm, and an alpha of <.05, a power of.90 would be acquired.

Outcome parameters

All participants were interviewed with the semi-structured Positive and Negative Syndrome Scale (PANSS) [49] before and immediately after treatment by two trained raters. For the analyses we used the scores on hallucination item P3, as well as scores on the subscales for Positive symptoms, Negative symptoms and

Table 1. Demographic data and baseline characteristics of the sample.

		Left TMS (n = 16)	Bilateral TMS (n = 15)	Sham TMS (n = 16)	p
Age (years)	Mean (+/− SD)	37.2 (14.9)	33.9 (9.2)	37.3 (11.6)	0.688
Sex (m/f)	N	9/7	8/7	10/6	0.869
Education (years)	Mean (+/− SD)	13.7 (2.0)	13.4 (1.2)	13.7 (2.1)	0.870
Age of onset (years)	Mean (+/− SD)	26.4 (10.2)	23.1 (4.2)	21.8 (6.9)	0.230
Duration of illness (months)	Mean (+/− SD)	150.4 (123.2)	135.8 (123.4)	186.7 (149.4)	0.559
Type of medication					
Clozapine		6	7	6	
Olanzapine		4	2	4	
Risperidone		3	3	3	
Aripiprazole		3	1	3	
Quetiapine		2	3	1	
Sulpiride		–	–	1	
Haloperidol		–	–	3	
Other first generation		1	3	4	
None		1	–	1	
Motor threshold	Mean (+/− SD)	60.2 (7.4)	56.7 (9.5)	–	0.366
AHRS frequency item	Mean (+/− SD)	6.9 (2.8)	5.9 (2.7)	5.9 (3.0)	0.521
AHRS total	Mean (+/− SD)	28.3 (5.7)	25.6 (6.7)	24.8 (6.0)	0.241
PANSS P3 (Hallucinations)	Mean (+/− SD)	5.2 (0.7)	4.6 (0.6)	4.7 (0.7)	0.036
PANSS Positive	Mean (+/− SD)	16.3 (4.8)	15.8 (3.9)	16.7 (4.6)	0.856
PANSS Negative	Mean (+/− SD)	15.1 (4.7)	13.7 (4.7)	16.6 (5.6)	0.269
PANSS General					
Psychopathology	Mean (+/− SD)	30.1 (8.9)	27.7 (6.2)	32.4 (9.5)	0.300

M = male; F = female; AHRS = Auditory Hallucinations Rating Scale [20]; PANSS = Positive and Negative Syndrome Scale [24]; PANAS = Positive and Negative Affect Scale [50]. Groups were compared using analysis of variance (ANOVA), followed by Bonferroni's post-hoc tests in case of significant effects. The chi square test was applied to test group differences on the nominal variable sex.

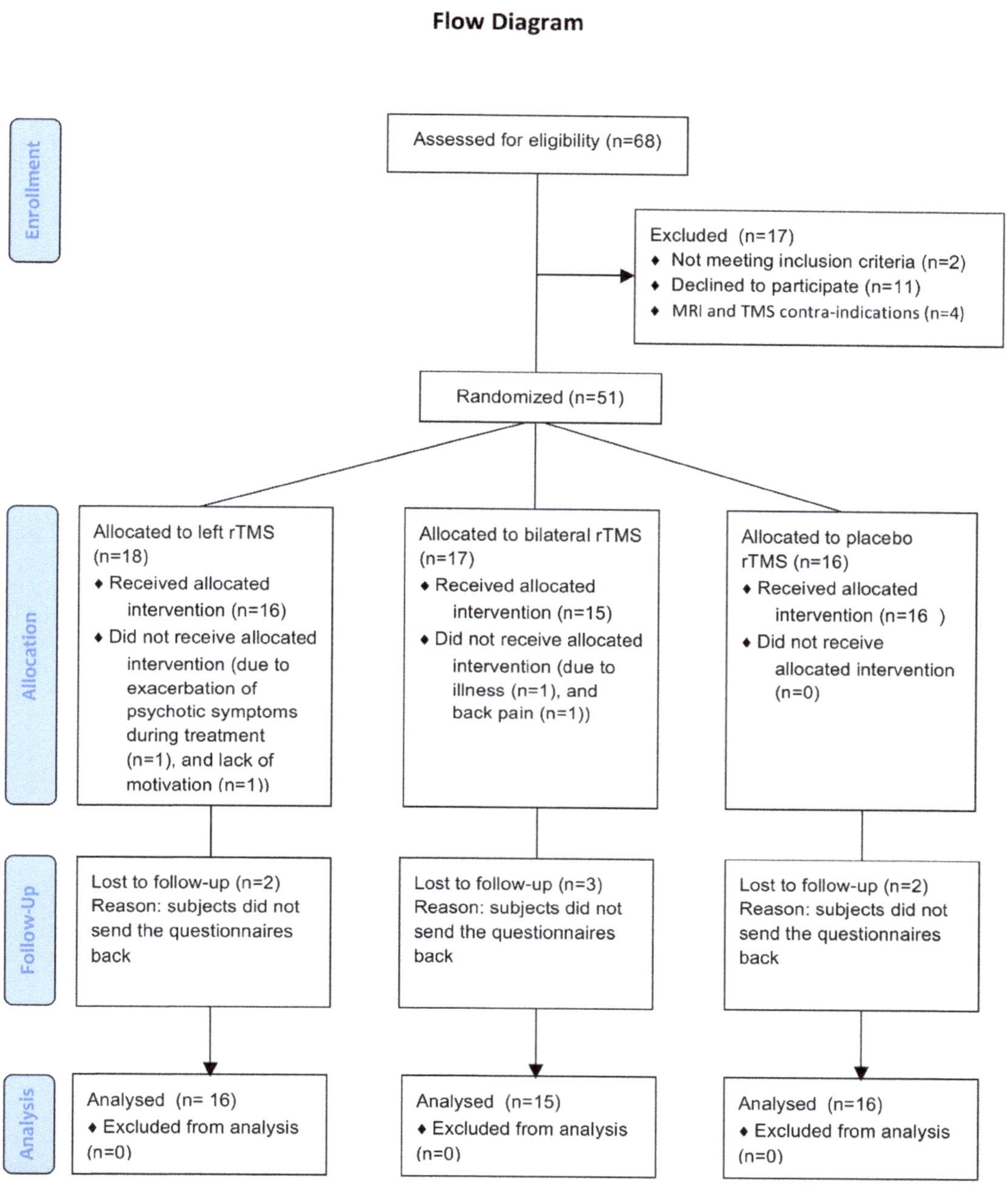

Figure 1. Flow diagram demonstrating the progress of the trial.

General Psychopathology. Characteristics of the AVH were measured with the Auditory Hallucinations Rating Scale (AHRS), which is a self-report questionnaire [15]. It comprises seven items (frequency, reality, loudness, number of voices, length, attentional salience, distress level). AHRS frequency scores and total AHRS scores were used for the analysis. Positive and negative emotional affective states were measured with the Positive and Negative Affect Scale (PANAS) [50] adapted for hallucinations (note that this is a different scale than the PANSS). Participants were instructed to indicate to what extent they experienced ten positive and ten negative affective states during AVH. Items had to be rated on a five-point scale, ranging from 1 = very slightly to 5 = extremely. Sum scores of all positive and all negative items were calculated and used for analysis. Both the AHRS and PANAS were administered before and immediately after treatment. For the measurements at four weeks and three months follow-up we sent the questionnaires by mail to the participants.

fMRI procedure

In 36 participants, fMRI scans were made before and after rTMS treatment, the results of the fMRI analyses are discussed elsewhere [51].

Statistics

Differences in demographic characteristics and baseline data between the three treatment groups were tested with analysis of variance (ANOVA), followed by Bonferroni's post-hoc tests in case of significant effects. Chi-square tests were applied to the nominal variables.

The influence of patients, time, and treatment on the outcome measures of the PANSS (Hallucination item P3, Positive symptoms, Negative symptoms and General Psychopathology), AHRS (Frequency and Total) and PANAS (Positive and Negative) were analyzed using multilevel modeling, because this technique handles missing data better than single level designs. It does not require balanced designs (e.g. same sample sizes in each level of the design) and is more flexible.

A two-level random intercept model was fitted to the data. Repeated measurements in Time (for the PANSS: baseline and end of treatment; for the AHRS and PANAS: baseline, end of treatment, four weeks follow-up and three months follow-up) were nested within patients. Group (left rTMS, bilateral rTMS and sham rTMS) was added as a covariate. The main effects of Time and Group are given, as well as their interactions. In case of significant main or interaction effects, estimates of fixed effects are presented, to clarify which differences caused the effects. P-values of $<.05$ were considered statistically significant. We used the IBM software package SPSS version 21 to fit the multilevel model to the data.

Results

Participants

The flow diagram (Figure 1) demonstrates the progress of the trial. 68 patients were assessed for eligibility, and eventually 51 patients were included in the trial. A total of four patients withdrew from the study, for various reasons, which are described in the safety and tolerability section. So, 47 participants completed the study, with 16 patients in the left group, 15 patients in the bilateral group, and 16 patients in the sham group. Demographic characteristics did not differ significantly between the three treatment groups (Table 1). There were no baseline differences between groups in hallucination severity as reflected by the AHRS. Baseline scores on hallucination item P3 of the PANSS were not equal between the three groups; however post-hoc testing revealed no significant differences between the groups (Table 1).

Short term-efficacy measured with the PANSS P3 item and subscales

Mean scores on the PANSS are displayed in Table 2. There was no significant main effect of group on the PANSS Hallucination item P3 ($F(2,44.0) = 1.034$, $p = 0.364$). However, the main effect of time (pre- vs. post-treatment) was significant ($F(1,44.0) = 5.942$, $p = 0.019$). The interaction between time and treatment group showed a trend for significance ($F(2,44.0) = 2.545$, $p = 0.090$), which was caused by a small decrease of hallucination severity in the left treatment group. Figure 2 illustrates the individual courses in hallucination scores. Each line represents how many subjects showed a specific change in hallucination score, separate for the three treatment groups.

Treatment group or time did not have significant effects on the total positive symptoms, negative symptoms and general psychopathology subscales.

Short term and long term efficacy, as measured with the AHRS

Mean scores on the AHRS are displayed in Figure 3 and Table 2. Analysis revealed a significant main effect of the factor time for the AHRS Frequency scores ($F(3,41.6) = 4.92$, $p = 0.005$). Table 3 summarizes the results of pairwise comparisons and shows that the means on all post treatment measurements decreased significantly compared to baseline. So AHRS frequency scores were significantly lower at the end of treatment, when compared to the measurement at baseline and remained on a lower level for at least three months (Table 3). The reduction of AHRS frequency scores over time was independent of the treatment condition, as there was no main effect of treatment, or interaction between time and treatment.

Total AHRS scores also decreased over time ($F(3,40.9) = 2.89$, $p = 0.047$). However, pairwise comparisons only showed trends for significance between the mean at baseline and the means at four weeks follow-up and three months follow-up (Table 3). Again, main effects of treatment and the interaction between treatment and time were not significant.

Short term and long term efficacy, as measured with the PANAS

Mean scores on the PANAS are displayed in Table 2. Both negative and positive affect scores as measured with the PANAS showed significant decreases in time ($F(3,38.0) = 5.69$, $p = 0.003$; $F(3,40.5) = 6.29$, $p<0.001$, respectively). In case of the PANAS negative scores, this effect was caused by significant decreases after four weeks follow-up compared to baseline, and remained decreased until three months follow-up. The PANAS positive scores decreased during the treatment and stayed on a constant level for three months (Table 3). There were no main effects for treatment or interaction effects on either PANAS positive or negative scores.

Responder analysis

Eight patients in the left group improved one point or more on the PANSS Hallucination item P3, against five patients in the bilateral group and four in the sham group. In five patients from the sham group, the scores increased one point, against one patient in the bilateral group and none in the left group.

When considering a reduction of three points or more on the AHRS frequency item as a response, five patients in the left group were responders, and one patient in the bilateral group, against three in the sham group.

Blinding

Not all data on blinding success were available. Out of the sixteen participants surveyed in the left group, ten thought they received real treatment (62.5%), in the bilateral group nine out of twelve surveyed thought they received real treatment (75%), against ten out of sixteen patients surveyed in the sham group that believed they received sham rTMS (62.5%).

TMS safety and tolerability

Four patients withdrew from the study, for the following reasons: increase of psychotic symptoms; severe back pain that the patient attributed to the rTMS treatment; and inability to visit the hospital due to illness.

In the patients that completed the treatment, rTMS was well tolerated and no serious adverse events occurred. Side-effects reported in the active rTMS groups were: twitching facial muscles (ten patients), light-headedness (one patient), earache (one patient), tingling sensation in the arm on the contralateral side of rTMS stimulation, and minor pain in the left arm (one patient). These side-effects were confined to the actual stimulation session, and disappeared immediately after stimulation. One patient that received active rTMS experienced restless legs during stimulation, but she already had these complaints before participating in the trial. Nine participants in the active groups and two in the sham

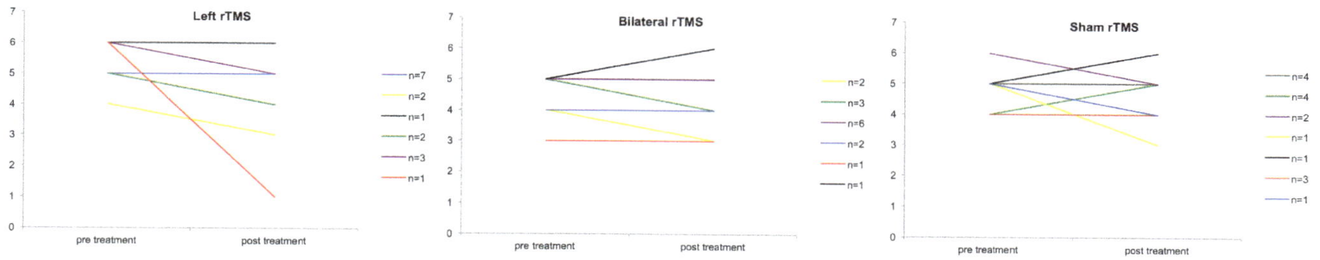

Figure 2. Changes in PANSS hallucination scores. This figure illustrates the individual courses in hallucinations score. Each line represents how many subjects showed a specific change in hallucination score, separate for the three treatment groups.

group reported mild transient headache following (at least one) stimulation session. Other side-effects reported in the sham group were a tingling sensation near the ear (one patient) and blunted affect (one patient) during the stimulation session. One patient in the sham group reported concentration problems during the treatment period.

Discussion

In this trial we randomized 51 schizophrenia patients with treatment resistant auditory verbal hallucinations to receive 1 Hz rTMS treatment of the left or bilateral TPJ area, or sham rTMS. The present study was conducted as an extension of the RCT reported by Vercammen et al. [44] on 36 patients. This is the first study on hallucinations that included an extra treatment arm of bilateral stimulation to allow for the comparison of different treatment configurations. We hypothesized that stimulation of the left TPJ area would result in decreased frequency, loudness or attentional salience of AVH through diminution of left-hemispheric hyperactivation, and that bilateral stimulation would additionally reduce affect-based aspects of AVH thought to originate in the right hemisphere. This would theoretically result in a more complete management of AVH. We observed a significant decrease in mean hallucination score that remained stable for three months. Although left-sided rTMS showed a trend to significance on the PANSS, neither left nor bilateral rTMS treatment was superior over sham treatment in reducing hallucination severity as measured with the AHRS and PANAS.

As the durability of rTMS effects is of specific interest to clinicians, we included two follow-up measurements with the AHRS and PANAS, at four weeks and three months. At each time point a reduction of AVH was found, but it was irrespective of treatment condition. This corroborates findings of other studies that included long-term follow-up assessments [20,24,28]. It is remarkable that hallucination severity tends to decrease over time in a relatively stable and chronically ill sample, both after active and sham treatment. It is conceivable that participating in an rTMS trial to reduce auditory verbal hallucinations, promotes awareness and a realization that AVH are a product of 'abnormal' neural processes, residing in the brain, rather than originating from some external source. From this point of view, it may become easier for patients to cope with their hallucinations and/or they may even find a way to influence them.

By stimulating bilaterally, we applied an unconventional approach in the study of rTMS for AVH. Three previous studies compared the effects of right-sided rTMS with left-sided rTMS and sham stimulation, but did not observe superior effects of right-sided stimulation [21,25,26]. Contrary to our study, the rationale for adding a third treatment arm of right-sided rTMS in these former studies was not specifically based on the hypothesis that the right hemisphere might influence the emotional states accompanied with the AVH. We assessed positive and negative emotional states associated with the experience of hallucinations, observing an overall decrease in the scores of both positive and negative emotional states during the study period in all three treatment groups. Thus, our hypothesis that low-frequency bilateral stimulation specifically would result in more complete management of AVH could not be confirmed. The possibility should be considered that the lack of beneficial effects of bilateral stimulation is due to a neurophysiological process referred to as transcallosal inhibition. Thiel et al. [52] have shown that low frequency rTMS of the left inferior frontal gyrus resulted in increased activity in the right inferior frontal gyrus. In our design, inhibition of the left TPJ area might have caused disinhibition of its corresponding contralateral area, and vice versa, which may have produced a null-effect. Theoretically, low frequency rTMS of the left TPJ area, combined with high frequency rTMS of the right TPJ area, may induce a stronger effect. As various bilateral approaches are possible, further exploratory work will be necessary to clarify which configuration would be most advantageous in the treatment of hallucinations. Another explanation for the lack of improvement in the bilateral condition may be that each hemisphere received 50% fewer rTMS pulses than in the left rTMS condition, such that the total amount of pulses applied to participants was equal in every treatment condition. Perhaps 20 minutes of 1 Hz rTMS on each side, might have achieved a significant treatment effect.

Nevertheless, as we did not observe improvement in either of the active rTMS conditions, it may be more plausible that the overall lack of substantial, clinically relevant improvements can be ascribed to methodological variables. Increasing stimulation intensity, varying frequency, and extending duration of treatment may positively influence efficacy. For instance, a two-day high-frequency treatment has demonstrated remarkable efficacy in two studies [47,53]. Moreover, it is still debatable whether the left TPJ area – which is assumed to be hyperactive – should be stimulated in isolation. Recent imaging findings revealed reduced connectivity and information flow between left frontal and temporal areas in schizophrenia patients with AVH [54–56]. Additionally, hypofrontality has been reported in schizophrenia patients [57,58]. Taking this into account, high-frequency rTMS over the left frontal area combined with low-frequency rTMS over the left TPJ area, may strengthen fronto-temporal pathways, potentially resulting in a more efficacious reduction of hallucination severity. To our knowledge, this type of stimulation has not been performed yet with rTMS. However, Brunelin et al. [59] obtained interesting results using transcranial Direct Current Stimulation (tDCS). With tDCS, cathodal and anodal electrodes are applied, which respectively result in decreased or increased membrane potentials of neurons underlying the respective stimulation sites. Cathodal

Table 2. PANSS, AHRS and PANAS scores at all four measurement moments.

		Baseline			End of treatment			4 weeks follow-up			3 months follow-up		
	Group	**mean**	**SD**	**n**	**mean**	**SD**	**n**	**mean**	**SD**	**n**	**mean**	**SD**	**n**
PANSS	Left	5.19	0.66	16	4.44	1.21	16	–			–		
Item P3	Bilateral	4.60	0.63	15	4.33	0.90	15	–			–		
	Sham	4.69	0.70	16	4.69	0.70	16	–			–		
PANSS	Left	16.31	4.76	16	15.06	5.64	16	–			–		
Positive	Bilateral	15.80	3.88	15	15.21	4.14	15	–			–		
	Sham	16.69	4.60	16	16.56	3.88	16	–			–		
PANSS	Left	15.12	4.70	16	14.50	4.40	16	–			–		
Negative	Bilateral	13.67	4.67	15	14.00	4.95	15	–			–		
	Sham	16.63	5.57	16	16.81	5.04	16	–			–		
PANSS	Left	30.12	8.85	16	28.38	9.04	16	–			–		
General	Bilateral	27.67	6.20	15	26.71	5.81	15	–			–		
	Sham	32.50	9.41	16	31.56	7.50	16	–			–		
AHRS Frequency	Left	6.88	2.83	16	5.50	3.06	16	5.07	3.13	14	5.14	3.18	14
Frequency item	Bilateral	5.87	2.70	15	5.13	3.07	15	5.83	3.19	12	5.42	3.23	12
	Sham	5.88	2.96	16	4.75	3.00	16	4.14	2.91	14	4.14	2.83	14
AHRS	Left	28.31	5.67	16	26.13	5.55	16	24.79	8.76	14	24.29	9.43	12
Total	Bilateral	25.60	6.73	15	23.27	7.09	15	22.50	8.10	12	23.92	7.10	14
	Sham	24.75	5.97	16	21.63	9.95	16	20.00	10.41	14	21.79	9.41	14
PANAS	Left	28.79	10.60	14	24.47	9.67	15	24.33	10.34	15	24.19	10.1	16
Positive	Bilateral	25.67	10.10	15	19.93	8.08	15	21.53	7.92	15	22.13	7.99	15
	Sham	21.08	6.97	14	19.14	7.16	14	17.69	6.86	13	17.62	6.20	13
PANAS	Left	21.50	7.98	14	20.13	8.40	15	18.27	6.72	15	18.94	8.44	16
Negative	Bilateral	23.40	10.53	15	21.80	11.20	15	19.40	9.42	15	19.53	9.14	15
	Sham	29.43	10.30	13	25.43	10.60	14	24.92	11.93	13	26.46	13.0	13

Means, standardg deviations and the number of participants in each measurement are presented for the three treatment groups. AHRS = Auditory Hallucinations Rating Scale [20]; PANSS = Positive and Negative Syndrome Scale [24]; PANAS = Positive and Negative Affect Scale [50].

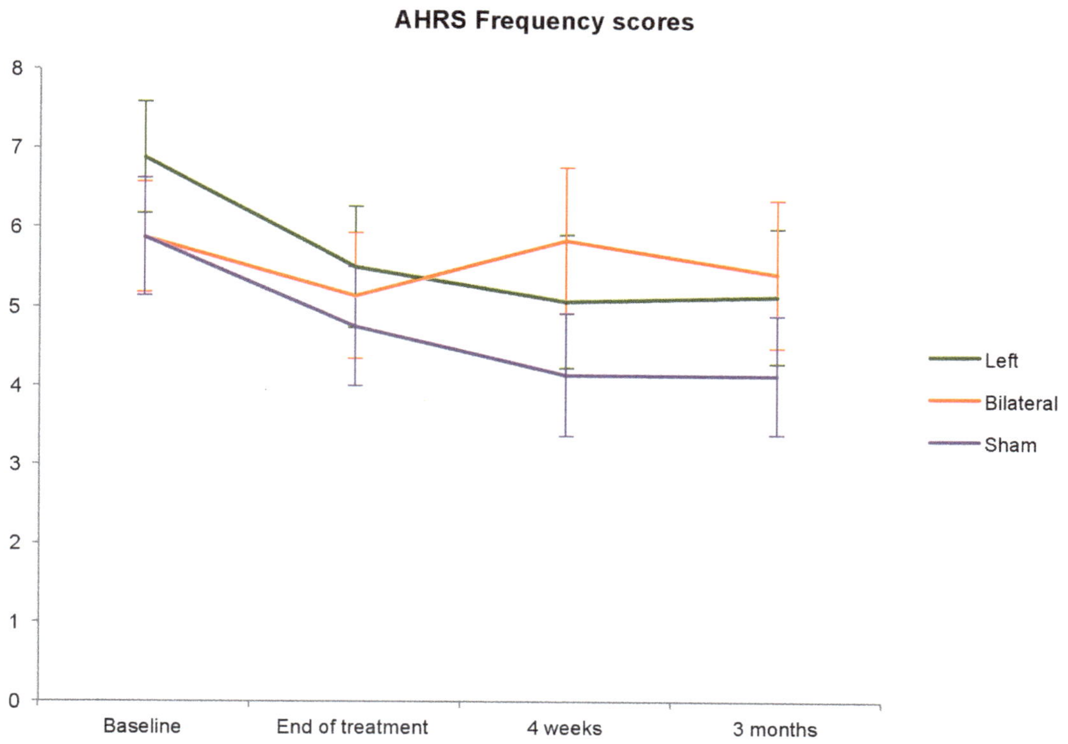

Figure 3. Changes in AHRS Frequency scores. The three lines represent the mean AHRS Frequency scores for each treatment group during the four measurements at baseline, end of treatment, and at four weeks and three months follow-up.

left TPJ area stimulation to decrease underlying tissue activity and anodal left dorsolateral prefrontal stimulation to elicit an increase in activity resulted in a substantial decrease in AVH after 5 days. In addition, this improvement sustained for at least three months in the treatment group, whereas the sham group did not show significant improvement. It goes without saying that replication studies are required to substantiate this initial finding [60].

Aside from variability in stimulation parameters, variability between subjects in response to rTMS treatment should also be taken into account. Although not clinically significant, responder analysis demonstrated that in the left rTMS group, twice as many patients improved at least one point on the PANSS hallucination item compared to the sham group. This finding might suggest that left-sided rTMS does have some effect on AVH. It is conceivable that the stimulation parameters were not optimally matched to the individuals to elicit statistically and clinically relevant reductions of AVH. This is in accordance with the increasing support for the approach of personalized medicine in the treatment of schizophrenia. Examining individual differences could expose factors contributing to response. Accordingly, variability in brain structure, such as size, lateralization and gyrification might lead to unreliable estimations of the localization of the TPJ area. Although the International 10–20 EEG system we used for localization does take variability in head size into account, it is difficult to account for differences in brain morphology. Frameless stereotactic neuronavigation using anatomical MRI scans may allow for more accurate individual targeting. Few rTMS trials for the treatment of AVH applied this method of localization, with mixed results [25,30,31].

Not only brain structure, but also patterns of associated brain activation during AVH may differ between patients [61,62]. One study that used fMRI-guided rTMS, based on individually defined areas of maximal activation during AVH, did not reveal additional benefits [28]. Homan et al. [63] on the other hand, assessed resting state perfusion in patients prior to treatment with rTMS. Those patients who eventually responded to rTMS treatment were

Table 3. Pairwise comparisons between post-treatment measurements and baseline.

	AHRS Frequency	AHRS Total	PANAS Positive	PANAS Negative
	Mean difference	Mean difference	Mean difference	Mean difference
End of Treatment - Baseline	1.08**	2.55	4.57**	1.85
4 weeks follow-up - Baseline	1.26**	3.35*	4.77**	3.63**
3 months follow-up - Baseline	1.31**	3.03*	4.04**	3.61**

**significant at p≤0.05. *trend for significance: 0.01<p<0.05. AHRS = Auditory Hallucinations Rating Scale [20]; PANSS = Positive and Negative Syndrome Scale [24]; PANAS = Positive and Negative Affect Scale [50].

characterized by increased cerebral blood flow in the left STG, suggesting that resting-state activity of STG could serve as a biomarker of treatment response in schizophrenia patients with AVH. In a PET study by Klírová et al. [29], resting regional brain metabolism has been used for stereotactic neuronavigation to determine the optimum area for stimulation, and found this method to be superior over the traditional method and sham stimulation. Albeit it requires further clarification, assessment of functional brain activity before treatment may be valuable in the prediction of treatment success.

Functional neuroimaging studies can also provide information about the effect of rTMS on the underlying neural basis of AVH. However, only few studies have assessed brain activation before and after treatment. In a subgroup of present study sample, resting state connectivity was investigated. Reduction in hallucinations in the active rTMS group was correlated with an increased connectivity between the left TPJ area and the right insula [51]. Kindler et al. [36] assessed patients with AVH before and after treatment. The active treatment group showed both clinical improvement and decreased blood flow in the primary auditory cortex, left Broca's area and the cingulate gyrus, whereas no changes in activity occurred in the sham group. So indeed, the left TPJ area appears an accurate target for influencing brain activity within the AVH network. One study that investigated the effect of rTMS on Broca's area did not observe changes on a clinical or neural level [64]. This supports the idea that the speech perception areas in the temporal cortex, rather than speech production areas in the frontal cortex are important for the experience of AVH [65].

Since many of the rTMS studies in patients with AVH are characterized by small sample sizes, we recommend the initiation of large multi-center trials, and the validation of practical and reliable clinical measures in order to enhance power and draw stronger conclusions about the utility of rTMS in reducing AVH. To improve blinding, studies should employ sham coils that mimic the scalp sensation produced by real rTMS.

To summarize, although we observed a trend for AVH reduction in the left rTMS group as measured by clinicians, this improvement was not confirmed with self-reported hallucination scores. We thus conclude that we did not find evidence for the efficacy of left-sided rTMS, compared to sham stimulation. Moreover, bilateral rTMS was not superior over left-sided rTMS or sham in improving AVH. Mean self-reported hallucination scores, and negative and positive emotional content as measured with AHRS and PANAS were reduced during rTMS treatment and over the course of a three-month follow-up period, but its overall effect did not seem to be specific to either rTMS of the left or bilateral TPJ area, or sham treatment. Optimizing treatment parameters may yield more convincing evidence for efficacy of rTMS treatment of AVH. Moreover, for future studies it is recommended to incorporate evaluation of treatment effects with neuroimaging. And in order to develop individually tailored treatments, studies should focus on individual differences that may influence treatment response.

Supporting Information

Checklist S1 CONSORT checklist 2010.

Protocol S1 The approved protocol of the study.

Data S1 All data of the participants.

Acknowledgments

The authors would like to thank all the participants; the mental health care workers of the University Center of Psychiatry Groningen UMCG, Lentis, GGz Drenthe, GGz Friesland and Mediant for referring their patients to our study; the colleagues of the BCN NeuroImaging Center UMCG for conducting patient interviews and the staff of the University Center of Psychiatry for their assistance during the study and inpatient care.

Author Contributions

Conceived and designed the experiments: AV AA HK. Performed the experiments: LB AV BV. Analyzed the data: LB RS. Contributed reagents/materials/analysis tools: FE BV RS AA. Contributed to the writing of the manuscript: LB AV RS FE BV AA HK. Coordination of patient recruitment and data collection: LB AV. Literature search and drafted the first version of the manuscript: LB. Responsible for the selection assessments and recruitment of study participants: FE HK. Supervising the manuscript preparation: AA HK.

References

1. Andreasen NC, Flaum M (1991) Schizophrenia: The Characteristic Symptoms. Schizophrenia Bulletin 1: 27–49.
2. Shergill SS, Murray RM, McGuire PK (1998) Auditory hallucinations: a review of psychological treatments. Schizophr. Res. 3: 137–150.
3. Shergill SS, Brammer MJ, Williams SC, Murray RM, McGuire PK (2000) Mapping auditory hallucinations in schizophrenia using functional magnetic resonance imaging. Arch. Gen. Psychiatry 11: 1033–1038.
4. Lennox BR, Park SB, Medley I, Morris PG, Jones PB (2000) The functional anatomy of auditory hallucinations in schizophrenia. Psychiatry Res. 1: 13–20.
5. Allen P, Laroi F, McGuire PK, Aleman A (2008) The hallucinating brain: a review of structural and functional neuroimaging studies of hallucinations. Neurosci. Biobehav. Rev. 1: 175–191.
6. Waters F, Allen P, Aleman A, Fernyhough C, Woodward TS, et al. (2012) Auditory hallucinations in schizophrenia and nonschizophrenia populations: a review and integrated model of cognitive mechanisms. Schizophr. Bull. 4: 683–693.
7. Fitzgerald PB, Fountain S, Daskalakis ZJ (2006) A comprehensive review of the effects of rTMS on motor cortical excitability and inhibition. Clin. Neurophysiol. 12: 2584–2596.
8. Di Lazzaro V, Oliviero A, Mazzone P, Pilato F, Saturno E, et al. (2002) Short-term reduction of intracortical inhibition in the human motor cortex induced by repetitive transcranial magnetic stimulation. Exp. Brain Res. 1: 108–113.
9. Pascual-Leone A, Davey N, Rothwell J, Wassermann EM, Puri BK (2002) Handbook of transcranial magnetic stimulation. 1st ed. London: Arnold; 2002.
10. Post RM, Kimbrell TA, Frye M, George M, McCann U, et al. (1997) Implications of kindling and quenching for the possible frequency dependence of rTMS. CNS Spectrums 54–60.
11. Froc DJ, Chapman CA, Trepel C, Racine RJ (2000) Long-term depression and depotentiation in the sensorimotor cortex of the freely moving rat. J. Neurosci. 1: 438–445.
12. Hoffman RE, Cavus I (2002) Slow transcranial magnetic stimulation, long-term depotentiation, and brain hyperexcitability disorders. Am. J. Psychiatry 7: 1093–1102.
13. Hoffman RE, Boutros NN, Berman RM, Roessler E, Belger A, et al. (1999) Transcranial magnetic stimulation of left temporoparietal cortex in three patients reporting hallucinated "voices". Biol. Psychiatry 1: 130–132.
14. Hoffman RE, Boutros NN, Hu S, Berman RM, Krystal JH, et al. (2000) Transcranial magnetic stimulation and auditory hallucinations in schizophrenia. Lancet 9209: 1073–1075.
15. Hoffman RE, Hawkins KA, Gueorguieva R, Boutros NN, Rachid F, et al. (2003) Transcranial magnetic stimulation of left temporoparietal cortex and medication-resistant auditory hallucinations. Arch. Gen. Psychiatry 1: 49–56.
16. Hoffman RE, Gueorguieva R, Hawkins KA, Varanko M, Boutros NN, et al. (2005) Temporoparietal transcranial magnetic stimulation for auditory hallucinations: safety, efficacy and moderators in a fifty patient sample. Biol. Psychiatry 2: 97–104.
17. McIntosh AM, Semple D, Tasker K, Harrison LK, Owens DG, et al. (2004) Transcranial magnetic stimulation for auditory hallucinations in schizophrenia. Psychiatry Res. 1–2: 9–17.
18. Fitzgerald PB, Benitez J, Daskalakis JZ, Brown TL, Marston NA, et al. (2005) A double-blind sham-controlled trial of repetitive transcranial magnetic stimulation in the treatment of refractory auditory hallucinations. J. Clin. Psychopharmacol. 4: 358–362.

19. Poulet E, Brunelin J, Bediou B, Bation R, Forgeard L, et al. (2005) Slow transcranial magnetic stimulation can rapidly reduce resistant auditory hallucinations in schizophrenia. Biol. Psychiatry 2: 188–191.
20. Chibbaro G, Daniele M, Alagona G, Di Pasquale C, Cannavo M, et al. (2005) Repetitive transcranial magnetic stimulation in schizophrenic patients reporting auditory hallucinations. Neurosci. Lett. 1–2: 54–57.
21. Lee SH, Kim W, Chung YC, Jung KH, Bahk WM, et al. (2005) A double blind study showing that two weeks of daily repetitive TMS over the left or right temporoparietal cortex reduces symptoms in patients with schizophrenia who are having treatment-refractory auditory hallucinations. Neurosci. Lett. 3: 177–181.
22. Brunelin J, Poulet E, Bediou B, Kallel L, Dalery J, et al. (2006) Low frequency repetitive transcranial magnetic stimulation improves source monitoring deficit in hallucinating patients with schizophrenia. Schizophr. Res. 1: 41–45.
23. Saba G, Verdon CM, Kalalou K, Rocamora JF, Dumortier G, et al. (2006) Transcranial magnetic stimulation in the treatment of schizophrenic symptoms: a double blind sham controlled study. J. Psychiatr. Res. 2: 147–152.
24. Rosa MO, Gattaz WF, Rosa MA, Rumi DO, Tavares H, et al. (2007) Effects of repetitive transcranial magnetic stimulation on auditory hallucinations refractory to clozapine. J. Clin. Psychiatry 10: 1528–1532.
25. Loo CK, Sainsbury K, Mitchell P, Hadzi-Pavlovic D, Sachdev PS (2010) A sham-controlled trial of left and right temporal rTMS for the treatment of auditory hallucinations. Psychol. Med. 4: 541–546.
26. Jandl M, Steyer J, Weber M, Linden DE, Rothmeier J, et al. (2006) Treating auditory hallucinations by transcranial magnetic stimulation: a randomized controlled cross-over trial. Neuropsychobiology 2: 63–69.
27. de Jesus DR, Gil A, Barbosa L, Lobato MI, Magalhaes PV, et al. (2011) A pilot double-blind sham-controlled trial of repetitive transcranial magnetic stimulation for patients with refractory schizophrenia treated with clozapine. Psychiatry Res. 2: 203–207.
28. Slotema CW, Blom JD, de Weijer AD, Diederen KM, Goekoop R, et al. (2011) Can low-frequency repetitive transcranial magnetic stimulation really relieve medication-resistant auditory verbal hallucinations? Negative results from a large randomized controlled trial. Biol. Psychiatry 5: 450–456.
29. Klirova M, Horacek J, Novak T, Cermak J, Spaniel F, et al. (2013) Individualized rTMS neuronavigated according to regional brain metabolism ((18)FGD PET) has better treatment effects on auditory hallucinations than standard positioning of rTMS: a double-blind, sham-controlled study. Eur. Arc h. Psychiatry Clin. Neurosci. 6: 475–484.
30. Hoffman RE, Wu K, Pittman B, Cahill JD, Hawkins KA, et al. (2013) Transcranial magnetic stimulation of Wernicke's and Right homologous sites to curtail "voices": a randomized trial. Biol. Psychiatry 10: 1008–1014.
31. Blumberger DM, Christensen BK, Zipursky RB, Moller B, Chen R, et al. (2012) MRI-targeted repetitive transcranial magnetic stimulation of Heschl's gyrus for refractory auditory hallucinations. Brain Stimul 4: 577–585.
32. Fitzgerald PB, Sritharan A, Benitez J, Daskalakis ZJ, Jackson G, et al. (2007) A preliminary fMRI study of the effects on cortical activation of the treatment of refractory auditory hallucinations with rTMS. Psychiatry Res. 1: 83–88.
33. Costanzo F, Menghini D, Caltagirone C, Oliveri M, Vicari S (2012) High frequency rTMS over the left parietal lobule increases non-word reading accuracy. Neuropsychologia 11: 2645–2651.
34. Maiza O, Herve PY, Etard O, Razafimandimby A, Montagne-Larmurier A, et al. (2013) Impact of Repetitive Transcranial Magnetic Stimulation (rTMS) on Brain Functional Marker of Auditory Hallucinations in Schizophrenia Patients. Brain Sci. 2: 728–743.
35. Homan P, Kindler J, Hauf M, Walther S, Hubl D, et al. (2013) Repeated measurements of cerebral blood flow in the left superior temporal gyrus reveal tonic hyperactivity in patients with auditory verbal hallucinations: a possible trait marker. Front. Hum. Neurosci. 304.
36. Kindler J, Homan P, Jann K, Federspiel A, Flury R, et al. (2013) Reduced Neuronal Activity in Language-Related Regions After Transcranial Magnetic Stimulation Therapy for Auditory Verbal Hallucinations. Biol Psychiatry 73: 518–524.
37. Aleman A, Sommer IE, Kahn RS (2007) Efficacy of slow repetitive transcranial magnetic stimulation in the treatment of resistant auditory hallucinations in schizophrenia: a meta-analysis. J. Clin. Psychiatry 3: 416–421.
38. Slotema CW, Aleman A, Daskalakis ZJ, Sommer IE (2012) Meta-analysis of repetitive transcranial magnetic stimulation in the treatment of auditory verbal hallucinations: Update and effects after one month. Schizophr. Res. 1–3: 40–45.
39. Slotema CW, Blom JD, van Lutterveld R, Hoek HW, Sommer IE (2014) Review of the Efficacy of Transcranial Magnetic Stimulation for Auditory Verbal Hallucinations. Biol. Psychiatry 2: 101–110.
40. Heller W, Nitschke JB, Miller GA (1998) Lateralization in Emotion and Emotional Disorders. Current Directions in Psychological Science 1, Evolving Perspectives on Lateralization of Function: 26–32.
41. Silberman EK, Weingartner H (1986) Hemispheric lateralization of functions related to emotion. Brain Cogn. 3: 322–353.
42. Honig A, Romme MA, Ensink BJ, Escher SD, Pennings MH, et al. (1998) Auditory hallucinations: a comparison between patients and nonpatients. J. Nerv. Ment. Dis. 10: 646–651.
43. Daalman K, Boks MP, Diederen KM, de Weijer AD, Blom JD, et al. (2011) The same or different? A phenomenological comparison of auditory verbal hallucinations in healthy and psychotic individuals. J. Clin. Psychiatry 3: 320–325.
44. Vercammen A, Knegtering H, Bruggeman R, Westenbroek HM, Jenner JA, et al. (2009) Effects of bilateral repetitive transcranial magnetic stimulation on treatment resistant auditory-verbal hallucinations in schizophrenia: a randomized controlled trial. Schizophr. Res. 1–3: 172–179.
45. Giel R, Nienhuis FJ (1996) SCAN-2.1: Schedules for Clinical Assessment in Neuropsychiatry (in Dutch). Geneva/Groningen: WHO; 1996.
46. Schutter DJ, van Honk J (2006) A standardized motor threshold estimation procedure for transcranial magnetic stimulation research. J. ECT 3: 176–178.
47. Dollfus S, Larmurier-Montagne A, Razafimandimby A, Allio G, Membrey JM, et al. (2008) Treatment of auditory hallucinations by combining high-frequency repetitive transcranial magnetic stimulation and functional magnetic resonance imaging. Schizophr. Res. 1–3: 348–351.
48. Herwig U, Satrapi P, Schonfeldt-Lecuona C (2003) Using the international 10–20 EEG system for positioning of transcranial magnetic stimulation. Brain Topogr. 2: 95–99.
49. Kay SR, Fiszbein A, Opler LA (1987) The positive and negative syndrome scale (PANSS) for schizophrenia. Schizophr. Bull. 2: 261–276.
50. Watson D, Clark LA, Tellegen A (1988) Development and validation of brief measures of positive and negative affect: the PANAS scales. J. Pers. Soc. Psychol. 6: 1063–1070.
51. Vercammen A, Knegtering H, Liemburg EJ, den Boer JA, Aleman A (2010) Functional connectivity of the temporo-parietal region in schizophrenia: effects of rTMS treatment of auditory hallucinations. J. Psychiatr. Res. 11: 725–731.
52. Thiel A, Habedank B, Herholz K, Kessler J, Winhuisen L, et al. (2006) From the left to the right: How the brain compensates progressive loss of language function. Brain Lang. 1: 57–65.
53. Montagne-Larmurier A, Etard O, Razafimandimby A, Morello R, Dollfus S (2009) Two-day treatment of auditory hallucinations by high frequency rTMS guided by cerebral imaging: a 6 month follow-up pilot study. Schizophr. Res. 1: 77–83.
54. Spalletta G, Tomaiuolo F, Marino V, Bonaviri G, Trequattrini A, et al. (2003) Chronic schizophrenia as a brain misconnection syndrome: a white matter voxel-based morphometry study. Schizophr. Res. 1: 15–23.
55. Seok JH, Park HJ, Chun JW, Lee SK, Cho HS, et al. (2007) White matter abnormalities associated with auditory hallucinations in schizophrenia: a combined study of voxel-based analyses of diffusion tensor imaging and structural magnetic resonance imaging. Psychiatry Res. 2: 93–104.
56. Curcic-Blake B, Liemburg E, Vercammen A, Swart M, Knegtering H, et al. (2012) When Broca Goes Uninformed: Reduced Information Flow to Broca's Area in Schizophrenia Patients With Auditory Hallucinations. Schizophr. Bull.
57. Weinberger DR, Berman KF, Illowsky BP (1988) Physiological dysfunction of dorsolateral prefrontal cortex in schizophrenia. III. A new cohort and evidence for a monoaminergic mechanism. Arch. Gen. Psychiatry 7: 609–615.
58. Wang CS, Yang YK, Chen M, Chiu NT, Yeh TL, et al. (2003) Negative symptoms and regional cerebral blood flow in patients with schizophrenia: a single photon emission computed tomography study. Kaohsiung J. Med. Sci. 9: 464–469.
59. Brunelin J, Mondino M, Gassab L, Haesebaert F, Gaha L, et al. (2012) Examining transcranial direct-current stimulation (tDCS) as a treatment for hallucinations in schizophrenia. Am. J. Psychiatry 7: 719–724.
60. Sommer IE, Aleman A, Slotema CM, Schutter DJ (2012) Transcranial stimulation for psychosis: the relationship between effect size and published findings. Am. J. Psychiatry 11: 1211.
61. Sommer IE, de Weijer AD, Daalman K, Neggers SF, Somers M, et al. (2007) Can fMRI-guidance improve the efficacy of rTMS treatment for auditory verbal hallucinations? Schizophr. Res. 1–3: 406–408.
62. Sommer IE, Diederen KM, Blom JD, Willems A, Kushan L, et al. (2008) Auditory verbal hallucinations predominantly activate the right inferior frontal area. Brain Pt 12: 3169–3177.
63. Homan P, Kindler J, Hauf M, Hubl D, Dierks T (2012) Cerebral blood flow identifies responders to transcranial magnetic stimulation in auditory verbal hallucinations. Transl. Psychiatry. e189.
64. Hoffman RE, Hampson M, Wu K, Anderson AW, Gore JC, et al. (2007) Probing the pathophysiology of auditory/verbal hallucinations by combining functional magnetic resonance imaging and transcranial magnetic stimulation. Cereb. Cortex 11: 2733–2743.
65. Moseley P, Fernyhough C, Ellison A (2013) Auditory verbal hallucinations as atypical inner speech monitoring, and the potential of neurostimulation as a treatment option. Neurosci. Biobehav. Rev. 10 Pt 2: 2794–2805.

Permissions

All chapters in this book were first published in PLOS ONE, by The Public Library of Science; hereby published with permission under the Creative Commons Attribution License or equivalent. Every chapter published in this book has been scrutinized by our experts. Their significance has been extensively debated. The topics covered herein carry significant findings which will fuel the growth of the discipline. They may even be implemented as practical applications or may be referred to as a beginning point for another development.

The contributors of this book come from diverse backgrounds, making this book a truly international effort. This book will bring forth new frontiers with its revolutionizing research information and detailed analysis of the nascent developments around the world.

We would like to thank all the contributing authors for lending their expertise to make the book truly unique. They have played a crucial role in the development of this book. Without their invaluable contributions this book wouldn't have been possible. They have made vital efforts to compile up to date information on the varied aspects of this subject to make this book a valuable addition to the collection of many professionals and students.

This book was conceptualized with the vision of imparting up-to-date information and advanced data in this field. To ensure the same, a matchless editorial board was set up. Every individual on the board went through rigorous rounds of assessment to prove their worth. After which they invested a large part of their time researching and compiling the most relevant data for our readers.

The editorial board has been involved in producing this book since its inception. They have spent rigorous hours researching and exploring the diverse topics which have resulted in the successful publishing of this book. They have passed on their knowledge of decades through this book. To expedite this challenging task, the publisher supported the team at every step. A small team of assistant editors was also appointed to further simplify the editing procedure and attain best results for the readers.

Apart from the editorial board, the designing team has also invested a significant amount of their time in understanding the subject and creating the most relevant covers. They scrutinized every image to scout for the most suitable representation of the subject and create an appropriate cover for the book.

The publishing team has been an ardent support to the editorial, designing and production team. Their endless efforts to recruit the best for this project, has resulted in the accomplishment of this book. They are a veteran in the field of academics and their pool of knowledge is as vast as their experience in printing. Their expertise and guidance has proved useful at every step. Their uncompromising quality standards have made this book an exceptional effort. Their encouragement from time to time has been an inspiration for everyone.

The publisher and the editorial board hope that this book will prove to be a valuable piece of knowledge for researchers, students, practitioners and scholars across the globe.

List of Contributors

Miklós Sárvári
Laboratory of Endocrine Neurobiology, Institute of Experimental Medicine, Hungarian Academy of Sciences, Budapest, Hungary

Pál Kocsis, Levente Deli, Dávid Gajári, Szabolcs Dávid, Zsófia Pozsgay, Nikolett Hegedűs and Károly Tihanyi
Preclinical Imaging Center, Gedeon Richter Ltd., Budapest, Hungary

Zsolt Liposits
Laboratory of Endocrine Neurobiology, Institute of Experimental Medicine, Hungarian Academy of Sciences, Budapest, Hungary
Faculty of Information Technology, Pázmány Péter Catholic University, Budapest, Hungary

Shinichi Harada, Yui Yamazaki and Shogo Tokuyama
Department of Clinical Pharmacy, School of Pharmaceutical Sciences, Kobe Gakuin University, Kobe, Japan

Shuichi Koda
Asubio Pharma Co., Ltd., Kobe, Japan

Alberto Gallace, Giovanna Soravia and Zaira Cattaneo
Department of Psychology, University of Milano-Bicocca, Milan, Italy

G. Lorimer Moseley
The Sansom Institute for Health Research, University of South Australia, Adelaide, Australia
Neuroscience Research Australia, Sydney, Australia

Giuseppe Vallar
Department of Psychology, University of Milano-Bicocca, Milan, Italy
IRCCS Istituto Auxologico Italiano, Milano, Italy

Naoki Tajiri, Yuji Kaneko and Cesar V. Borlongan
Center of Excellence for Aging & Brain Repair, Department of Neurosurgery and Brain Repair, University of South Florida College of Medicine, Tampa, Florida, United States of America

David M. Quach, Stephanie Wu, David Lee, Tina Lam, Ken L. Hayama, Thomas G. Hazel and Karl Johe
Neuralstem, Inc., Rockville, Maryland, United States of America

Michael C. Wu
Neurodigitech, LLC., San Diego, California, United States of America

Richard L. Hoffman
Ohio Musculoskeletal & Neurological Institute (OMNI), Ohio University, Athens, Ohio, United States of America

Petra S. Williams
Ohio Musculoskeletal & Neurological Institute (OMNI), Ohio University, Athens, Ohio, United States of America
Department of Physical Therapy and Athletic Training, Northern Arizona University, Flagstaff, Arizona, United States of America

Brian C. Clark
Ohio Musculoskeletal & Neurological Institute (OMNI), Ohio University, Athens, Ohio, United States of America
Department of Biomedical Sciences, Ohio University, Athens, Ohio, United States of America
Department of Geriatric Medicine and Gerontology, Ohio University, Athens, Ohio, United States of America

Zhen-Yu Zhang, Jian Xu, Ying Mao, Liang-Fu Zhou, Ping Zhong and Yu Yao
Department of Neurosurgery, Huashan Hospital, Fudan University, Shanghai, China

Yong Ren
Department of Pathology, Wuhan General Hospital of Guangzhou Command, People's Liberation Army, Wuhan, China

Kay Ka-Wai Li and Ho-Keung Ng
Department of Anatomical and Cellular Pathology, Prince of Wales Hospital, The Chinese University of Hong Kong, Hong Kong, China

Scott E. Cooper and Andre M. Machado
Cleveland Clinic, Center for Neurological Restoration, Cleveland, Ohio, United States of America

Klaus G. Driesslein and Christopher R. Butson
Medical College of Wisconsin, Departments of Neurology & Neurosurgery, Biotechnology and Bioengineering Center, Milwaukee, Wisconsin, United States of America

Angela M. Noecker and Cameron C. McIntyre
Case Western Reserve University, Department of Biomedical Engineering, Cleveland, Ohio, United States of America

Tonya M. Moloney and Alice G. Witney
Department of Physiology, Trinity College Institute of Neuroscience and Trinity Centre for BioEngineering, Trinity College, Dublin, Ireland
Junle Qu and Wenda Peng
College of Optoelectronics Engineering, Shenzhen University, Shenzhen, China

Shuhua Mu and Jian Zhang
College of Optoelectronics Engineering, Shenzhen University, Shenzhen, China
School of Medicine, Shenzhen University, Shenzhen, China

Jiachuan Wang, Guangqian Zhou, Zhendan He, Zhenfu Zhao and CuiPing Mo
School of Medicine, Shenzhen University, Shenzhen, China
Paul A. Muller and Sameer C. Dhamne
Department of Neurology, Boston Children's Hospital, Harvard Medical School, Boston, Massachusetts, United States of America

Andrew M. Vahabzadeh-Hagh and Alexander Rotenberg
Department of Neurology, Boston Children's Hospital, Harvard Medical School, Boston, Massachusetts, United States of America
Berenson-Allen Center for Noninvasive Brain Stimulation, Beth Israel Deaconess Medical Center, Harvard Medical School, Boston, Massachusetts, United States of America

Alvaro Pascual-Leone
Berenson-Allen Center for Noninvasive Brain Stimulation, Beth Israel Deaconess Medical Center, Harvard Medical School, Boston, Massachusetts, United States of America
Institut Universitari de Neurorehabilitació Guttmann, Universidad Autónoma de Barcelona, Badalona, Spain

Frances E. Jensen
Department of Neurology, Perelman School of Medicine, University of Pennsylvania Health System, Philadelphia, Pennsylvania, United States of America

Erik W. Schluter, Andrew R. Mitz and Bruno B. Averbeck
Laboratory of Neuropsychology, Division of Intramural Research, National Institute of Mental Health, National Institutes of Health, Bethesda, Maryland, United States of America

Joseph F. Cheer
Department of Anatomy and Neurobiology, University of Maryland School of Medicine, Baltimore, Maryland, United States of America

Toru Fukuhara, Mizuho Aoi and Yoichiro Namba
Department of Neurological Surgery, National Hospital Organization Okayama Medical Center, Okayama, Japan

Katherine E. Davis, Sarah Fox and John Gigg
Faculty of Life Sciences, University of Manchester, Manchester, United Kingdom

Graham K. Sheridan
Department of Physiology, Development and Neuroscience, University of Cambridge, Cambridge, United Kingdom

Emad Moeendarbary
Hughes Hall, University of Cambridge, Cambridge, United Kingdom

Mark Pickering
School of Medicine and Medical Science, Health Sciences Centre, University College Dublin, Dublin, Ireland

John J. O'Connor
UCD School of Biomolecular and Biomedical Science, Conway Institute, University College Dublin, Dublin, Ireland

Keith J. Murphy
Neurotherapeutics Research Group, UCD School of Biomolecular and Biomedical Science, Conway Institute, University College Dublin, Dublin, Ireland

James R. Houston, Christopher Buzzelli, Xuan Li and A. Katherine Harrington
Department of Psychology, University of Akron, Akron, Ohio, United States of America

Philip A. Allen and Joshua W. Pollock
Department of Psychology, University of Akron, Akron, Ohio, United States of America
Conquer Chiari Research Center, University of Akron, Akron, Ohio, United States of America

Bryn A. Martin and Francis Loth
Conquer Chiari Research Center, University of Akron, Akron, Ohio, United States of America
Department of Mechanical Engineering, University of Akron, Akron, Ohio, United States of America

Mei-Ching Lien
School of Psychological Science, Oregon State University, Corvallis, Oregon, United States of America

Jahangir Maleki
Neurological Center for Pain, Cleveland Clinic Foundation, Cleveland, Ohio, United States of America

Mark G. Luciano
Department of Neurological Surgery, Cleveland Clinic Foundation, Cleveland, Ohio, United States of America

Clinton B. McCracken and Zelma H. T. Kiss
Department of Clinical Neurosciences and Hotchkiss Brain Institute, University of Calgary, Calgary, Alberta, Canada

Elisabeth Cannon
Neuropsychiatric Institute, Prince of Wales Hospital, Randwick, NSW, Australia

Perminder S. Sachdev and Adith Mohan
Neuropsychiatric Institute, Prince of Wales Hospital, Randwick, NSW, Australia
Centre for Healthy Brain Ageing, School of Psychiatry, The University of New South Wales, Sydney, Australia

John D. Crawford
Centre for Healthy Brain Ageing, School of Psychiatry, The University of New South Wales, Sydney, Australia

Paul Silberstein and Raymond Cook
North Shore Private Hospital, St. Leonards, Sydney, NSW, Australia

Terrence Coyne and Peter A. Silburn
Centre for Clinical Research, University of Queensland, Herston, QLD, Australia
St. Andrew's War Memorial Hospital, Spring Hill, QLD, Australia

Stéphane Vinit and Emilie Keomani
Université de Versailles Saint-Quentin-en-Yvelines, Unité End:icap, UFR des Sciences de la Santé-Simone Veil, Montigny-le-Bretonneux, France

Thérèse B. Deramaudt
Université de Versailles Saint-Quentin-en-Yvelines, Unité End:icap, UFR des Sciences de la Santé-Simone Veil, Montigny-le-Bretonneux, France
LIA-BAHN (Laboratoire International Associé-Biologie Appliquée Handicap Neuromusculaire), CSM (Centre Scientifique de Monaco), Monaco, Monaco

Victoria M. Spruance, Tatiana Bezdudnaya and Michael A. Lane
Drexel University College of Medicine, Department of Neurobiology and Anatomy, Philadelphia, Pennsylvania, United States of America

Marcel Bonay
Université de Versailles Saint-Quentin-en-Yvelines, Unité End:icap, UFR des Sciences de la Santé-Simone Veil, Montigny-le-Bretonneux, France
LIA-BAHN (Laboratoire International Associé-Biologie Appliquée Handicap Neuromusculaire), CSM (Centre Scientifique de Monaco), Monaco, Monaco
Service de Physiologie-Explorations Fonctionnelles, Hôpital Ambroise Paré, Assistance Publique-Hôpitaux de Paris (AP-HP), Groupe Hospitalier Paris Ile-de-France Ouest, Boulogne-Billancourt, France

Michel Petitjean
Université de Versailles Saint-Quentin-en-Yvelines, Unité End:icap, UFR des Sciences de la Santé-Simone Veil, Montigny-le-Bretonneux, France
Service de Physiologie-Explorations Fonctionnelles, Hôpital Ambroise Paré, Assistance Publique-Hôpitaux de Paris (AP-HP), Groupe Hospitalier Paris Ile-de-France Ouest, Boulogne-Billancourt, France

Barbara Noli, Carla Brancia, Filomena D'Amato, Gian-Luca Ferri and Cristina Cocco
Department of Biomedical Sciences, University of Cagliari, Monserrato (Cagliari), Italy

Leonie Bais
University of Groningen, University Medical Center Groningen, Department of Neuroscience and BCN NeuroImaging Center, Groningen, The Netherlands
Lentis Psychiatric Institute, Groningen, The Netherlands

Ans Vercammen
Australian Catholic University, Strathfield, Australia

Roy Stewart
University of Groningen, University Medical Center Groningen, Department of Health Sciences, Community and Occupational Medicine, Groningen, The Netherlands

Frank van Es
University of Groningen, University Medical Center Groningen, Department of Psychiatry, Groningen, The Netherlands
University of Groningen, University Medical Center Groningen, Rob Giel Research Center, Groningen, The Netherlands

Bert Visser
University of Groningen, University Medical Center Groningen, Department of Psychiatry, Groningen, The Netherlands

André Aleman
University of Groningen, University Medical Center Groningen, Department of Neuroscience and BCN NeuroImaging Center, Groningen, The Netherlands
University of Groningen, Department of Psychology, Groningen, The Netherlands

Henderikus Knegtering
University of Groningen, University Medical Center Groningen, Department of Neuroscience and BCN NeuroImaging Center, Groningen, The Netherlands
Lentis Psychiatric Institute, Groningen, The Netherlands
University of Groningen, University Medical Center Groningen, Rob Giel Research Center, Groningen, The Netherlands

Index

A

Alzheimer's Disease, 128, 137, 141-142, 210

Anesthesia, 31, 97-99, 101-104, 106, 177, 180, 190-191, 194

Anova, 3, 5, 7, 12, 23, 33, 45, 52, 82-83, 89, 99-100, 130, 132, 134, 146, 161, 170, 191, 203, 214-215

Auditory Verbal Hallucinations, 212, 217, 221

B

Bovine Serum Albumin, 12, 146

Bradykinesia, 68-69, 71-72, 76, 177, 179

Brain Damage, 21, 166

C

Cervicomedullary, 38-44, 46, 48, 50, 57, 59, 195-196

Chemotherapy, 60, 62-64, 66-67

Chiari Malformation, 157-158, 163-164, 166-167

Chronic Pain, 24, 78-79, 85, 157-158, 163-165

Comatose Patients, 120-121, 124-125, 127

Corpus Callosum, 29, 33, 35-36

Cortical Excitability, 39-40, 56-57, 78-80, 82-85, 97-98, 103-104, 199, 213, 220

Craniospinal Irradiation, 60

D

Deep Brain Stimulation, 68, 76-77, 106, 118-119, 168, 178-181, 186-188, 195

E

Elbow Flexor, 41, 47, 56, 58

Elbow Flexors, 38-43, 52-54

Electromyography, 80, 97-98

Endocannabinoid, 1-2, 5, 7, 9

Endocannabinoid Signaling, 1-2, 5, 7, 9

Energy Balance, 1-3, 5, 7-9, 200, 210

Entopeduncular Nucleus, 168-170, 175, 178-179

Episodic Memory, 128, 137, 141, 157-159, 163-165

F

Fast-scan Cyclic Voltammetry, 105, 118-119

Fatiguing Contractions, 38-39, 43-44, 49-52, 57-59

Fibromyalgia, 78, 85

First Dorsal Interosseous, 80

Functional Recovery, 10, 30, 35-37, 87, 90, 94-95, 190

G

Gene Transcription, 20, 143, 153

Globus Pallidus Interna, 179, 181, 186-187

Growth Hormone, 1, 8-9, 200, 202

H

Hedonic Brain, 1

Huntington's Disease, 87-88, 94-96

I

In-hospital Mortality, 120-123, 125

Induced Pluripotent Stem Cells, 87, 95

Intracerebral Hemorrhage, 120, 127

Intracerebral Transplantation, 29, 35

Ischemic Stroke, 19-20, 29-30, 35-37, 127

L

Limbic System, 1, 165

Long-term Depression, 97, 99, 104, 155, 213, 220

M

Magnetic Resonance Imaging, 1, 76, 188, 221

Mechanical Ventilation, 120, 125

Mechanical Ventilator, 121

Medulloblastoma, 60-64, 66-67

Micromanipulator, 98, 105

Middle Cerebral Artery, 10-11, 29, 31

Motor Cortex, 23, 38-41, 43-44, 46, 53, 56-59, 73, 77-80, 82-86, 97, 101, 103-104, 112, 119, 168-170, 173, 175, 177-179, 189, 193-197, 199, 214, 220

Motor Cortical Excitability, 78, 82, 97, 103-104, 199, 220

Motor Evoked Potential, 39, 42, 48, 50, 97, 193, 199

Motor Evoked Potentials, 78, 80, 104, 189, 199

Multisensory Brain, 21, 27

Muscle Fatigue, 38-39, 47, 53-54, 57-58

N

Nervous System, 1, 9-10, 19-20, 39-40, 57, 60-61, 66, 85, 88, 104, 118-119, 190, 196, 210

Nervous System Tumors, 60

Neural Stem Cells, 29, 36-37, 94

Neurological Function, 31

Neuronal Hormone, 1

Neurotransmitter, 76, 103, 147, 180

Nmdar Antagonists, 97-98, 102-103
Non-invasive Cortical Stimulation, 78-79
Nucleus Accumbens, 1, 3-9, 117, 178-179, 188

P
Post-tetanic Oscillations, 153
Posterior Parietal Cortex, 21, 25-28
Pressure Pain Thresholds, 78-80, 82-83, 85
Primary Motor Cortex, 78, 82, 85-86, 103, 112, 168, 170, 173, 175, 179, 189, 194, 196, 214
Primary Somatosensory Cortex, 21, 25-26

Q
Quantitative Sensory Testing, 78-79, 81-82

R
Radiation Therapy, 60-63, 66
Real-time Dopamine, 105
Repetitive Transcranial Magnetic Stimulation, 21, 28, 78, 85-86, 97, 99, 103-104, 199, 212, 220-221

S
Somatosensory Cortex, 21-22, 25-28, 84
Spatial Learning, 143-144, 146, 152-154
Spinal Cord Resistance, 38, 57
Spinal Mechanisms, 38, 40, 57-58
Stem Cell Therapy, 29-30, 36-37, 88, 94-95
Stem Cells, 29, 33, 36-37, 87, 94-96
Stereotaxic Space, 75
Stroke, 10, 19-22, 27-31, 33, 35-37, 88, 94-96, 124, 127
Subthalamic Nucleus, 68, 76-77, 117, 119, 177-180, 185, 188
Suprachiasmatic Nucleus, 1, 3-5
Synaptic Plasticity, 8, 82, 97, 103-104, 132, 139, 142-144, 149, 153-155, 199
Synaptic Transmission, 129, 132, 140, 142-144, 153-156, 178

T
Task Failure, 38-42, 45-47, 49-50, 54-59
Thermoregulatory Control, 21-22, 24-27
Theta-burst Stimulation, 143-145, 149, 151-154
Tourette Syndrome, 178, 181, 186-187
Transcranial Direct Current Stimulation, 57-58, 78, 85, 217
Transcranial Magnetic
Stimulation, 21, 27-28, 38-39, 43, 58-59, 78, 85-86, 97, 99, 103-104, 189-190, 199, 212-213, 220-221
Transplant Surgery, 30

V
Ventral Striatum, 105-106, 112-113, 115-117, 188
Ventral Tegmental Area, 3, 5-6, 8-9, 105, 118-119
Ventromedial Nucleus, 1, 3-6
Voltage-dependent Calcium Channels, 144, 155

Z
Zona Incerta, 68, 72-73, 76-77, 193